PRAISE FOR *YOGA FOR WELLNESS*

"Gary Kraftsow is one of America's leading sources on Yoga therapy. He represents the best of the generation of people who went to India in the seventies to learn Yoga. Because of his mature understanding and experience, *Yoga for Wellness* is a treasure. It should be included on every Yoga practitioner's bookshelf."

—Swami Chetanananda, Abbott, Nityananda Institute,
and author of *Choose to Be Happy*

"Gary has done a great service to the Yoga world by putting his understanding of Viniyoga on paper. There is so much valuable information within these pages. Read it and learn!"

—Erich Schiffmann,
author of *Yoga: The Spirit and Practice of Moving into Stillness*

"A profound and detailed guide to yoga therapy and yoga for healing. It contains one of the most sophisticated presentations of asanas in print, showing how to adapt the Yoga poses to special individual health and energy requirements."

—David Frawley,
author of *Yoga and Ayurveda* and *Ayurveda and the Mind*

ABOUT THE AUTHOR

Gary Kraftsow's interest in the spiritual dimension of life was awakened at a very young age. His connection to Yoga and the spiritual traditions of India was strengthened through his studies at Colgate University, where he graduated with honors. At the age of nineteen, he traveled to Madras to meet T.K.V. Desikachar and T. Krishnamacharya, initiating a link to the Viniyoga tradition that was to become his lifelong dedication.

Gary has taught Yoga and has practiced Yoga therapy since 1976. In 1983 he completed a Master's program in psychology and religion at the University of California, Santa Barbara, focusing his study on health as a paradigm for spiritual transformation. Gary is an internationally known educator in the Viniyoga lineage, conducting retreats, trainings, and seminars throughout the United States and Europe. He currently offers in-depth training programs for both teachers and therapists and has received the Viniyoga Special Diploma, recognizing his ability to train teachers and therapists in this lineage. Gary continues his studies with T.K.V. Desikachar. He lives on the island of Maui with his family.

PENGUIN COMPASS

Yoga for Wellness

Healing with the Timeless Teachings of Viniyoga

GARY KRAFTSOW

FOREWORD BY SCOTT GERSON, M.D.

MEDICAL ILLUSTRATIONS BY SUSAN GILBERT

PENGUIN COMPASS

COMPASS
Published by the Penguin Group
Penguin Putnam Inc., 375 Hudson Street,
New York, New York 10014, U.S.A.
Penguin Books Ltd, 27 Wrights Lane, London W8 5TZ, England
Penguin Books Australia Ltd, Ringwood, Victoria, Australia
Penguin Books Canada Ltd, 10 Alcorn Avenue,
Toronto, Ontario, Canada M4V 3B2
Penguin Books (N.Z.) Ltd, 182–190 Wairau Road,
Auckland 10, New Zealand

Penguin Books Ltd, Registered Offices:
Harmondsworth, Middlesex, England

First published in Arkana 1999

15 16 17 18 19 20

A NOTE TO THE READER

The information in this book is not intended as a substitute for the advice of physicians or other qualified health professionals. It is not intended to be prescriptive with reference to any specific ailment or condition or to the general health of the reader, but, rather, descriptive of one approach to fostering health and wellness. The reader is advised to consult with his or her physician before undertaking any of the practices contained in this book. The reader should also continue to consult regularly with his or her physician in matters relating to his or her health, particularly in respect to any symptoms that may require diagnosis or medical treatment. Neither the author nor the publisher shall be liable or responsible for any loss, injury, or damage allegedly arising from the use of any information contained in this book.

ISBN 0 14 01.9569 6
(CIP data available)

Printed in the United States of America
Set in Hiroshige
Designed by Kathryn Parise

For Matteo and future generations

Foreword

It has been more than twenty years since I first arrived in south India to begin my study of Āyurveda, the traditional system of Indian medicine. Naturally, I have an avid interest in the origins and influences of this healing system and have taken every opportunity to delve into the original ancient texts for evidence of its philosophical and intellectual underpinnings. We know, for example, from archeological remains that Āyurveda can be traced to the ancient cities of Mohenjo-Daro and Harappa in the region known as the Indus Valley. At that time a system of healing prevailed, amongst a people known as the Aryans, in which sophisticated medicines of vegetable, animal, and mineral origin were used. The Ṛgveda, the oldest known document from the Aryan civilization, contains abundant references to plants and herbal medicines. The concepts of *agni* and *soma*, the seed concepts for later medical theories of digestion and reproduction, are likewise discussed in detail in this ancient metrical scripture. The Ṛgveda and the other two early Vedas (Yajurveda and Samaveda) are distinctly ritualistic and magical, full of references to sacrifice and deities. The deities were often personifications of natural forces, such as sun, wind, and earth. The later text of the Vedic period, the Arthavaveda, provides a much more specific and detailed view of medicine as it existed in ancient India. The detailed description of the human body is evidence of a highly developed knowledge of anatomy. In addition, we find a great many disease conditions delineated including hṛdyota (heart disease), kustha (leprosy), rajayaksma (consumption), asmari (kidney stones), and unmada (insanity), to mention only a few. There is also mention in the Arthavaveda of a great many plants used in the treatment of specific diseases. Certainly, Āyurveda can be said to have its roots in this Arthavavedic era.

Gradually, with the dawning of scientific thought, these early Vedic concepts of anatomy, physiology, pathology, and pharmacology were greatly expanded and developed. Finally, during the first and second centuries A.D., these ideas were organized and recorded as the famous encyclopedic compendiums of Charaka and Sushruta. Even today these books are regarded as the main textbooks of Indian medicine.

It was during this period that the Āyurvedic vavidyās began to incorporate ideas from other schools of thought apart from the Sāṃkhya doctrine that was its main affiliation. One of these schools was the Yoga School, the most celebrated and earliest text of which is ascribed to Patañjali, a sage who lived at the end of the second century A.D. This school set forth the concept of psychophysiological constitutions of human beings, a system of controlling the mind and body through physical and behavioral disciplines, and methods of attaining one-pointed concentration. This latter goal could lead the aspirant to knowledge of the spirit untainted by matter.

One of the features that sets Gary Kraftsow's book apart from hundreds of others on the subject is its inclusion of an enlightening discussion of negative emotions and conditioning, which are obstacles to our evolution into conscious beings. Gary draws on modern neurophysiology to help us understand ancient concepts of ahamkāric self-limiting misconceptions of ourselves and our world. The prāṇāyāma-āsana-meditation triad of interventions which are beautifully elucidated with clinical cases is practical and inspiring. In this section generous references are also made to concentrative and visualization techniques as therapeutic tools. Although it is commonly assumed that Patañjali was the founder of the Yoga system, his own compendium, Yoga Sūtra, states he was only the compiler and editor. The origin of the Yoga system is more accurately ascribed to more ancient priest-physicians of the Vedic era. The system of Yoga, although popularized in the West as a system of physical āsanas, was originally considerably medical in its purpose. The Yoga system speaks of understanding disease, its etiology and course, and the methods by which to best eliminate it. This is in close agreement with the Āyurvedic approach to disease. It is clear that Charaka was greatly influenced by the Yoga School. Among the health-promoting measures common to Yoga and Āyurveda are the use of mantras, dietary measures, fasting, controlled breathing practices, fomentation, relaxation, adherence to natural urges, and abstinence from excess and immoral behavior. Perhaps the most important link, however, is their common grounding in the tenets of the Sāṃkhya philosophy.

For example, there is a discussion in the Charaka Samhita of the relation between Yoga and *moksha* (CS, 2:137–156). Moksha, the summum bonum of human life, is defined by Charaka as the "complete annihilation of all material attachments," *moksho nivṛttirnihśesha* (CS, ibid., 137). Chakrapani, another noted Āyurvedic commentator, defines moksha as "absolute annihilation of the body" (*atyantika sariradyucchedeh*). Both of these physicians identify Yoga as the means of attaining this ultimate state of human liberation. Patañjali takes this idea further and provides the practical means beginning with his second sūtra: *yogaś citta vṛtti nirodhaḥ* ("Yoga is the control of fluxes in the mind").

Today, there is a great need to clearly elucidate the therapeutic applications of Yoga and its āsanas. Although much is known, not much is written on the uses of āsanas in the treatment of specific diseases. Among informed Āyurvedic physicians interested in well-founded Yoga research, the general consensus today is that three Indian institutions are conducting well-designed Yoga research. Of the three, the most respected is the Krishnamacharya Yoga Mandiram in Madras, where ground-breaking research is currently addressing the role of Yoga in mentally retarded children. Other renowned institutions include the Kaivalyadhama Samiti Yogic Health Center in Lonavia and the Vivekananda Kendra in Bangalore. However, these two latter schools, in my opinion, share the limitation of their research having a notable lack of correlation with modern medical understanding of disease. Another limitation is that often the recommended asanas are beyond the ability of the individual in need. The message of Yoga according to Patañjali is *prayatna śaithilyānanta samāpattibhyām* (YS, 2:47), which means that the force and effort expended in doing āsanas should be the minimum. The postures are intended to be comfortable and steady (*sthira sukham āsanam*, YS, 2:46). A third limitation of many Yoga instructions is the emphasis on the achievement of a fixed, rigid form of each āsana; this negates the individual constitutional differences of each practitioner and can even be injurious. Finally, the importance of the breath as the key to one's Yoga practice is often not emphasized enough.

The present volume adeptly addresses all of these issues and brilliantly fulfills the needs of the beginner and the initiate. Gary Kraftsow is one of the most highly respected contemporary teachers of Viniyoga, a tradition that invites, even demands, self-awareness and attunement to one's physical, emotional, and mental reality.

Its ultimate goal is to bring about nothing less than a complete transformation of its sincere students. One of the distinguishing features of this Yoga system to which the reader is directed is the concept of *release valves*. These unconscious compensatory movements that dilute the value of an āsana are extremely relevant for all of us who practice any form of therapeutic movement. Throughout the book the author makes us aware of these patterns and offers methods of adaptation. Viniyoga, practiced regularly, can no doubt transform the physically and mentally limited individual into a harmonious and balanced being. We witness the fulfillment of this tradition to a large extent in the author, who has pursued the path of Yoga full-time for more than twenty years. He is a teacher and guide to many individuals, among whom are many knowledgeable and experienced health-care providers.

What makes this volume unique and fresh is not only that it has arisen from years of personal discovery, but also that Gary has in addition years of experience in clearly expounding these techniques to students of all levels of practice. I am gratified and astonished how well the grace and wisdom of this man translates into words. This is certainly not a book to be read cursorily and then put down. Herein lies a gold mine of practical knowledge for enlivening all aspects of the physiology. It is a book worthy of study, which no doubt will enlighten the reader in unexpected ways each time it is opened. I therefore urge you to read this book and take the time to digest the words; practice the postures and breathing techniques as you proceed. This book will guide you with patience and refreshing insight, born out of years of teaching experience, through the often daunting challenge of self-discovery. With some perseverance and much letting-go, you will be amply rewarded. And may the next step on your journey bring surprise and delight.

SCOTT GERSON, M.D.
The National Institute of Ayurvedic Medicine
Brewster, New York

Acknowledgments

I learned the most about the meaning of Yoga, the practice of Yoga, and the methods of Yoga therapy from my teacher, Sri T.K.V. Desikachar of Madras, India. I began my study with him in Madras in 1974. I am continually grateful for his perceptive and patient instruction. I bow to the greatness of Sri T. Krishnamacharya, my teacher's teacher, who brought forth this teaching from the depths of his practice and devotion.

I learned the most about teaching Yoga and practicing Yoga therapy from my students and clients. I am continually grateful for their trust and inspiration. I also want to acknowledge them for their patience with me as I mature over the years.

I am deeply grateful to Mirka, my wife, and her sister Mara. Writing such an exhaustive book has taken time and concentration. I wrote this book as our son Matteo lived through his second and third years! It was only through their loving support that I was able to complete this project.

I want to thank my friend (who wishes to remain anonymous) for his photography and his tireless efforts in the darkroom; Susan Gilbert for her medical illustrations; Nur Gibson for her rendition of Ananta; Barry Kaplan for the cover photo; and Dr. Scott Gerson for his interest in my work and for writing the foreword to this book.

I also want to thank all of the models, who are actually students at our school, for their participation: Phyllis Addison, Keith Bailey, Melanie Bohn-Bailey, Julie Gayer, Sara Grigsby, Brian Griswold, Justin Groode, Ronald Kawahara, Matteo Kraftsow, Vance Koenig, Mirka Scalco-Kraftsow, Jenn Fredricksen, Mika Nakamura, Natalie Maisel, Barbara Plunkett, Robert Ward, and Gary Weber.

I am grateful to my literary agent, Ling Lucas, for believing in my work; to Mary Lou Mellinger, who has given countless hours to help me disseminate my work, including organizing the massive number of photographs for this book; to Margo Morris, who offered her assistance at the outset of this project and gave generously of her time throughout the years to see it to completion; to Mrs. Latha Satish, Ph.D., of Madras for her technical assistance; to Pat Sheldon for her editorial assistance; and to Dr. Ken Wolkoff for generously sharing his medical knowledge.

I want to thank Jariya Wanapun and Leda Scheintaub of Penguin Putnam for making my dream of the ideal relationship between an author and a publisher come true. Thank you both for your clarity, kindness, and good work. And thank you to the rest of the Penguin team: Dawn Drzal, Janet Goldstein, Kathie Parise for your elegant text design, Dolores Reilly, Nelly Bly, and Nancy Seitz.

Finally, I relied on Frederic Martini's *Fundamentals of Anatomy and Physiology*, published by Prentice-Hall in 1992, as a reference for the scientific information found in the "Common Aches and Pains" and "Chronic Disease" sections of the book.

Contents

Introduction

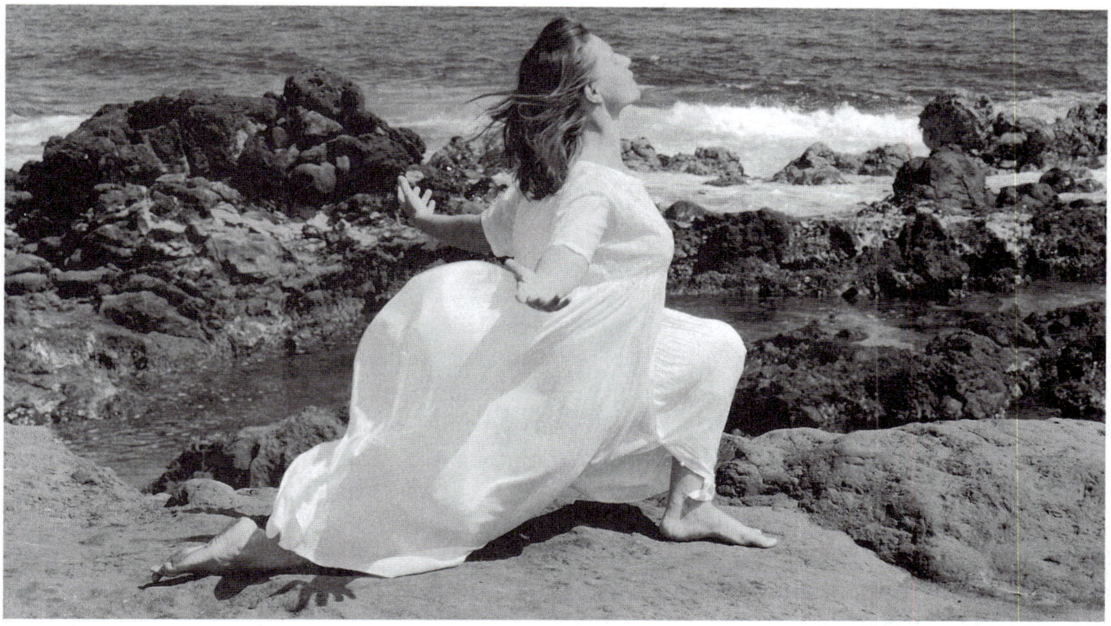

The Yoga star is rising: this child of the East is becoming a citizen of the world. At the end of the twentieth century, the teachings of Yoga are transcending racial, cultural, and religious barriers as never before—and Yoga's deep and lasting value as a comprehensive system for self-development is being discovered by people from every culture, in every part of the globe.

Yoga is for everyone and always has been. Since ancient times, Yoga has been continuously adapted to suit the needs of individuals from different times, cultures, and traditions. The young have come to explore and develop their potential. The sick and aged have come for healing and a fresh perspective. Spiritual seekers have come to find freedom from the burdens of the material world or to find peace at the feet of God. All who come are welcome.

In the hands of the wise teacher, Yoga meets the individual as he is and where he is, addressing each person's unique interests and concerns. Unfortunately, however, in transcending those barriers that once separated it from the West, the Yoga tradition has too often been turned into a mixture of fact and fantasy, filled with misunderstanding and misinterpretation.

Today, more and more people in the Western world are becoming health conscious. This renewed attention to health may reflect our sense of imbalance with accelerated technological growth: while we witness our incredible potential to transform the outer world, at the same time we experience a growing thirst for inner transformation. We want to live healthy, productive, and meaningful lives with a sense of inner contentment.

Following the current trend toward improving the quality of life, the health industry has blossomed. New prepackaged, generalized, get-healthy-quick programs continually appear—and Yoga, too, has been brought into the market. Yoga schools can already be found in almost every city of the Western world; they are now starting to spread throughout eastern Europe, South America, and East Asia.

This is a great and beneficial development. It is important, though, that in the midst of this expansion the deeper, more truly practical relevance of Yoga not be lost; that, with an eye to the marketplace, we not lose sight of the essential principles underlying this profound tradition.

As human beings, we are a complex of interrelated systems (including the various components of our anatomy, physiology, and psychology) existing within a larger complex of interrelated systems, including our interpersonal relationships and our environment. There is a reciprocal relation between these various structural components and the metabolic functioning of the body as a whole. The body possesses an intrinsic, organic wholeness, and the key to health lies in the balanced interaction of all these systems.

We have all noticed that there are some people who always seem healthy, while others have chronic problems—and we may tend to think of these differences as being largely ingrained, especially today, as we learn more and more about the role of genetic inheritance in individual health. Yet, while it is true that we are each born with certain genetically predetermined characteristics that influence our health, who we are and how we feel is strongly influenced by our day-to-day activity. This means that we have an opportunity, through changing our actions, to effect great changes in our degree of wellness. If we understand who we are, we can refine and improve how we feel, no matter what our genetic predisposition.

The process of achieving wellness, however, is complicated by the fact that our day-to-day activity is influenced by our *conditioning:* what is known in the Yoga tradition as saṃskāra. For each of us, this conditioning has been forming since early childhood. It is the result of our particular relation to our interpersonal and social environments; the result, in fact, of all our past actions.

At birth most of our movements are instinctive: we experience hunger or fear, and we respond by crying. As we grow, our movements gradually become more and more active, more intentional, and as the mind develops, it begins in turn to program the functioning brain and body. Learning how to walk, to talk, to play, to relate with other people—acquiring these skills—we impose onto our neuromuscular structure an order that becomes programmed, through repetition, into our pre-motor cortex in the form of increasingly conditioned reflexes. Where we once had to focus all our attention on a movement as seemingly simple as walking, we are gradually patterned to move reflexively, unconsciously. This learning process is the beginning of our conditioning, and it is why we tend, even if we don't like to admit it, to walk, talk, and behave like our parents or the people who raised us.

As we continue to grow, even beyond childhood, the development of our body and mind continues to be conditioned by these twin processes of neuromuscular organization and socialization. Meanwhile, those particular patterns we each acquire and develop are always imperfect in some way, in relation to wellness: even though they allow us to function—in fact, *because* they allow us to function and are therefore reinforced—they inhibit our optimal development. The consequence of this conditioning is imbalance at various levels of our system, accumulation of stress, and, ultimately, dis-ease.

The good news is that things are always changing! If we can become *reflectively self-conscious* of our conditioned behavior, we can break the cycle by introducing new patterns of behavior that will, over time, replace the old ones and help us regain control of the direction of change in our lives. This liberation from the effects of conditioning, on all levels, is the purpose of Yoga.

In normal behavior our attention is primarily focused outward, into the world. As a result, we are generally unaware of the mechanical and repetitive nature of our actions, both physical and mental. Thus, the starting point in breaking these cycles and changing the quality of our lives must be *interiorizing our attention.* This is the key to the Yoga process and the meaning of what I call *personal practice.*

This process begins with the discipline of body, breath, and mind, known in the Yoga tradition as āsana practice. At the most basic level, this practice involves consciously moving the body into specific postures—āsanas—remaining in these postures for some time, and organizing them together in particular sequences. Āsana practice was developed as a means of purifying and restructuring the body, bringing to it the qualities of stability, strength, flexibility, stillness, and a sense of clarity and well-being. It does this by introducing some nonmechanical elements into our daily life, through which we free ourselves from conditioning and effect positive change.

Since ancient times, the āsanas have been defined in terms of relatively precise forms; by mastering these forms, an individual demonstrated his or her mastery of certain basic principles of movement. Yet it was also generally understood that the practical application of these principles must be based on *each individual's actual condition*. An individual's way of doing each posture was therefore worked out between teacher and student. In this sense, the transformational value of a posture was always seen in relation to its *function,* not to its form.

Unfortunately, chief among the popular misconceptions about Yoga (including among many practitioners and even teachers of Yoga) is the idea that the value of each posture lies in achieving its precise, fixed form. Thus, emphasis has too often been placed on superficial details of positioning and the development of the body in the direction of preconceived, external standards of perfection—and the forms have been crystallized into rigid, static postures in which the living quality of the āsana is lost.

But if we strive in this way to meet external standards, without first recognizing our actual condition and developing our practice accordingly, we may actually *re-enforce* dysfunctional patterns and completely miss the deeper value of āsana practice. In such a case, Yoga practicioners generally attempt to achieve a form (based on ideas of how it *should* be) through a willful effort of muscular contraction; but the achievement of a form through static contraction creates rigidity and, ultimately, other problems, such as compression at the joints and restriction of blood flow. The body creates resistance, stress is absorbed in vulnerable areas, and problems almost inevitably develop, either immediately or after some time. Our efforts to achieve the precise form of an āsana then become an actually harmful imposition on the body, of an order that has no relation to the *actual needs of the body.*

If we analyze the classical āsanas in terms of their *function and interrelation,* however, we can see them as a systematic record of the structural potential of the human body. According to this view, the benefits to be achieved from these postures derive not at the level of form but at the level of function. We should therefore consider the practice of āsanas as a study in *movement potential,* not in the attainment of perfect form.

For each of us, actualizing the potential represented in the āsanas involves understanding the effects of movement and adapting our own movement in relation to our individual structural needs and capabilities. This is the functional orientation—the Viniyoga orientation—to āsana practice, and it is the one taught in this book.

Among Yoga traditions, the Viniyoga tradition uniquely offers an articulated science from which a *personal practice,* the foundation for health, can grow. From the Viniyoga perspective, āsana practice is not simply another mechanical system of exercise. The study of āsanas in Viniyoga always begins from an understanding of the individual body's unique condition, both theoretically and actually: in order to get anywhere, we must begin from where we are. This study then continues according to certain principles of adaptation: thus, as we come to understand ourselves more deeply, we are able to continually adjust our practice to meet our individual needs.

The Viniyoga tradition also teaches us that we must be clear about the *goals* of Yoga practice. In general, the whole movement of āsana practice should be one toward understanding more deeply *the mechanisms that are responsible for our present condition*. Achieving this understanding is more important than achieving proficiency in any particular āsana, or even all the āsanas. From this point of view, āsana practice is a means of *deepening our self-awareness*—and self-awareness is the key to any process of self-transformation.

With this understanding as its basis, āsana practice becomes a means of improving the function of each of the body's systems and of those systems' interaction with each other. We learn, through the process of conscious movement, to use our bodies more efficiently. In turn, harmonious and efficient movement prevents wear and tear on the system and dissipates less energy. Ultimately, with proper application, we can change habitual patterns at a neuromuscular level, develop new patterns that decrease physical stress and promote skeletal alignment, mechanical freedom, and organic unity, and lead ourselves toward optimum wellness.

To achieve all this, your āsana practice must be adapted to your individual skeletal structure and muscular and organic functions. You must *evolve*, on an individual basis, a method of working with the āsanas that increases your own, unique movement potential.

This evolution must begin with a basic understanding of the principles of Yoga. In Part I, "Yoga: A Developmental Approach," I set forth these general principles as they are articulated in the Viniyoga tradition, in order to develop a context for your understanding of the specific practices to follow. In Chapter 1, "Principles of Practice," we explore the fundamental principles of practice, including āsana, breath, adaptation, and sequencing.

In Chapter 2, "Biomechanics of Movement," I present a comprehensive series of sequences that work the entire body and can be used to develop and maintain a high level of health and well-being. Each of these seven sequences is organized around a fundamental movement of the spine. Although each sequence emphasizes certain areas, all of them are well balanced; however, although each sequence stands on its own, the program will be most effective if you practice all of them on a rotating basis. Taken together, the sequences offer a comprehensive program for bringing your system to an optimal level of functioning.

For the most part, Yoga has grown in popularity as a balanced system of health and fitness. In over two decades of work in this field, however, I have been most strongly touched by the healing potential of Yoga therapy. Time and again I have watched individuals be transformed from conditions of illness and dependency to wellness and self-sufficiency. Thus, in Part II, "Yoga: A Therapeutic Approach," I introduce the tradition of Yoga therapy. This section is divided into three chapters: "Common Aches and Pains," "Chronic Disease," and "Emotional Health." In each section, there is a basic description of a particular bodily system, as well as a discussion of some of the common problematic conditions that can affect it. Each section closes with actual case studies followed by practice sequences developed for each case.

Of course, the practices offered represent only a sample of the work that can be done, using Yoga therapy methods, to help the healing process. They are obviously not prescriptive but rather descriptive of a methodology for working with particular conditions.

It is my hope that you will be inspired to work toward developing a personal practice, according to principles of adaptation you'll have learned by reading this book. As your lifestyle evolves, your condition will change—and your key to wellness will be your continuing ability to adapt to changing circumstances. Through understanding the principles outlined throughout this book—through developing a personal practice—you will become well equipped to face the challenges of life and to work to further your own evolution.

With most learned skills, the test is in the performance. This involves going through a learning phase to develop a skill that gradually, with proper training, becomes refined and finally mastered. In tennis competition, for example, the movements must come spontaneously, reflexively: if you have to think yourself through the movements, you won't be able to win.

In Yoga practice, the performance doesn't consist of striving to achieve perfection in executing the āsanas; in a sense, it doesn't ultimately have to do with āsana practice itself. No, in Yoga the performance is *life itself*. Āsana practice is, as it were, the learning phase of a generalized *skill in movement and action:* it gives you the necessary reflexes for proper and efficient action in the game of life.

Developing skill in movement and action isn't quite the same thing as mastering one's backhand. As you evolve your own Yoga practice, therefore, don't be discouraged by any difficulties you encounter with particular postures or sequences. It is the process and your understanding of how the process is working in you that matter.

So observe, learn . . . and remember: according to the Viniyoga perspective, there is *no doubt* that you can achieve proficiency, regardless of your individual physical liabilities, regardless of your individual ability to achieve "perfection." Develop the potentials for movement inherent in *your* body, without damaging or disrupting that body's natural order and integrity, and your body *will* be transformed, moving toward greater balance, strength, and flexibility. Keep an attitude open to investigation, experimentation, and discovery, and your practice will stay alive and fresh—and, in a gradual, progressive way, become an endlessly fruitful ground for experience, learning, and growth.

Part I

YOGA: A Developmental Approach

Chapter 1

Principles of Practice

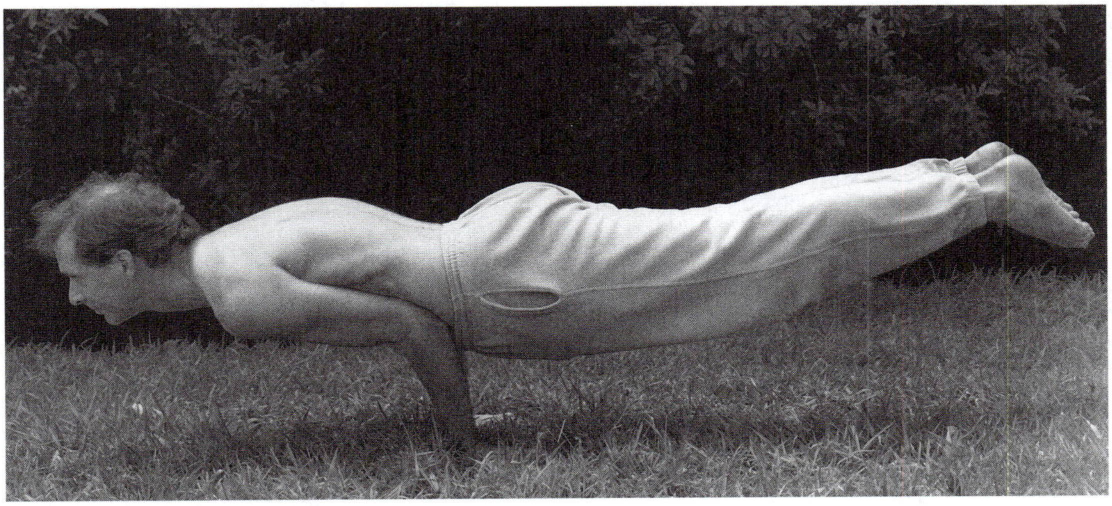

Introduction to Āsana

The Sanskrit word *āsana* derives from the verbal root *as,* meaning "to sit" or "to be present," and, in the context of the Yoga tradition, means "to be established in a particular posture." Historically the term refers to a wide range of bodily postures that have been transmitted by teachers in India for thousands of years. Because the forms of many of these postures have been more or less precisely defined in the classic texts of the Haṭha Yoga tradition, each āsana is characterized by certain objective criteria; and, in fact, one traditional definition of āsana is "the arrangement of the different components of the body in a specific way." However, the history of āsana is *not* a record of the possibilities of bodily contortion, nor simply a record of an ancient form of physical culture; rather, āsana evolved as an integral part of a comprehensive spiritual practice oriented toward purification, accomplishment, and realization.

Whether or not we are on the path to achieving our highest spiritual potential, āsana practice, in and of itself, promotes structural stability, physiological immunity, and emotional health. If we have the good fortune to begin āsana practice when we are young, it will help our bodies develop in a balanced way; or if we come to it as adults, it will help us restore and maintain balance as we grow older. Structurally, proper practice will promote stability, strength, flexibility, skeletal alignment, and mechanical freedom.

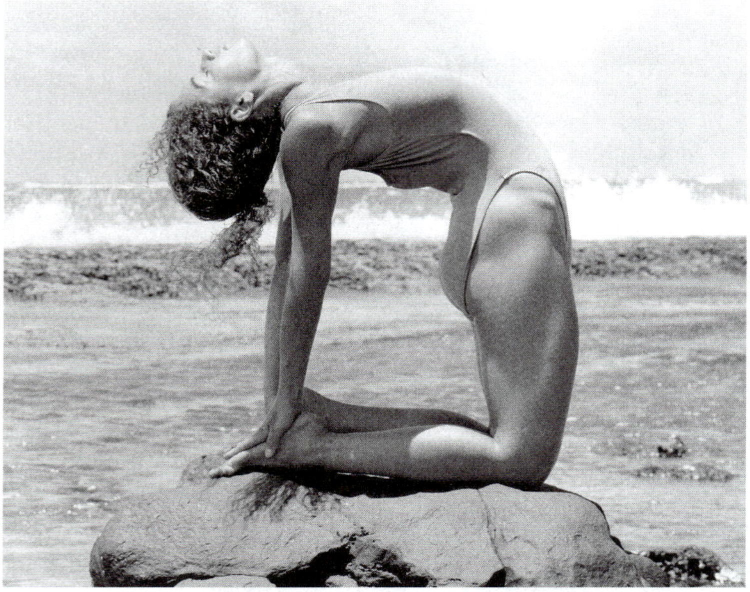

Physiologically, proper practice will balance neurological and hormonal activity, strengthen cardiovascular and respiratory functioning, improve absorption of nutrients and elimination of wastes, and strengthen the body's ability to resist and even overcome chronic disease. Emotionally, proper practice will increase our self-confidence, our tolerance for those different than us, our compassion for the suffering of ourselves and others, our capacity to withstand change, and our appreciation for the gift of life.

The essential qualities of āsana practice are given to us by Patañjali, the ancient authority on Yoga, in his Yoga Sūtras. These qualities are the following:

Sthira:	to be conscious, alert, present, firm, stable
Sukha:	to be relaxed, comfortable, at ease, without pain or agitation

Sthira and *Sukha* are symbolized by the ancient Hindu story of Ananta, the Ādi Śeṣa, king of the Nāgas, who carries the world on his head and the Lord on his lap; and it is these qualities along with certain organizational principles and objective criteria that give us the guidelines to develop a safe and effective practice. According to this authoritative text, our ability to be present and aware in an āsana is through the breath. It is *through the breath that we can truly link the mind to the body,* not at an imaginary level but as an actual and tangible experience.

On a practical level, Ananta symbolizes the goal of our practice: the ability to take full responsibility for being a healthy human being in the context of our personal, social, and physical environment while at the same time being relaxed and at peace in our body, mind, and heart. Our āsana practice should be as if we are becoming Ananta: doing our work with full attention while at the same time providing a comfortable resting place for God in our hearts.

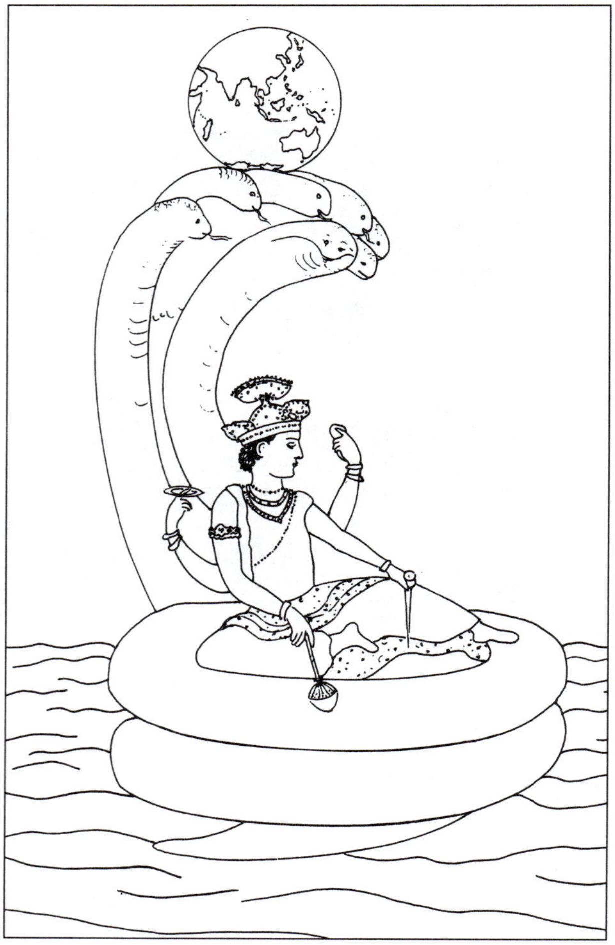

Ananta

Though we all have the same basic structural and organic parts, we are nonetheless unique in our structural, physiological, and emotional functioning; and though we all have certain deep constitutional tendencies that remain constant, our own condition changes from day to day. Thus the key to the art of personal practice lies in learning how to accurately assess our present condition, how to set appropriate goals, and how to develop an appropriate practice.

Learning to accurately assess our present condition involves looking at what is really happening in our body as we practice. For example, we may accomplish the form of a posture beautifully and still actually miss the potential benefits or even neglect to see the potential harm of that posture! This may happen for two reasons: We may fail to recognize our own *release valves;* and/or we may be so focused on the form of a posture that we fail to consider its function, i.e., we fail to ask what we are really trying to accomplish by using it.

Release valves are compensatory mechanisms that occur when we are unable to stabilize a part of the body because of excessive mobility or restriction, habitual movement patterns, or lack of understanding and/or attention. There are many possible release valves in any posture; and because our ability to observe, identify, and block our own release valves is so fundamental to achieving the benefits of āsana practice, a full presentation of them appears in the chapters ahead.

The form-function problem, on the other hand, concerns the relationship between the classical form of a posture and its *actual functional value.* While it is true that the forms of the classical postures reveal a systematic record of the structural potential of the human body, achieving one of these forms does not necessarily indicate that we have achieved its function. The true value of these postures lies in their functional benefit to our own body, not in the objective character of their classical forms. Therefore, rather than focusing on the achievement of objective standards, we should focus on what is actually happening in our body as we practice. The classical postures should be used initially as mirrors to help us discover something about that actual condition. Then the information gained from this observation should be used to help us determine the direction of our practice.

Setting appropriate goals for our practice involves the ability to recognize change. Because our condition is always changing, we must continually redefine and renew our practice. With this in mind, we will explore throughout this book a broad spectrum of possible goals, including relieving chronic aches and pains, balancing conditions of excess or deficiency, promoting emotional health, and developing the body through challenging postures.

Because the spine is the structural core of the body, developing an appropriate āsana practice necessarily involves studying the structural relations between the various parts of the spine, analyzing the specific movements of āsana practice in relation to their effect on the spine, and developing movement patterns that bring all of the parts into proper relationship. In the chapters immediately ahead, we will explore the principles for planning an appropriate practice, including the role of the breath, the principles of adaptation, the science of sequencing, and the principles of movement.

Repetition versus Stay

When the information gained in the process of self-observation—using the classical postures as mirrors to discover our actual condition—is combined with the principles mentioned above, we can adapt an āsana practice that truly respects our changing condition and our changing goals. Such a practice will include both the repetitive movements of the body into and out of particular postures, and the holding of particular postures for extended periods of time. Through alternate stretching and contracting, repetition increases circulation to the larger superficial skeletal muscles, making them stronger and more flexible. Thus repetition prepares us for holding postures for extended periods of time with minimal resistance. Through conscious movement with attention to our release valves, repetition helps us to identify habitual movement patterns and to develop new ones that are adapted to the structural and functional needs of our body. Thus repetition transforms the way we use our body in normal daily activity. In fact, according to the Viniyoga tradition, the most significant musculoskeletal and neuromuscular transformation occurs through this repetitive movement.

On the other hand, the most significant inner purification and physiological transformation occurs through holding postures for an extended period of time. Through the application of specific deep breathing techniques while holding a relatively fixed posture, subtle but powerful internal movements are created that activate the deepest layers of the

Repetition

Stay in position

spinal musculature. These movements act as "prāṇa pumps," which increase circulation to specific areas of the body, providing great benefit to the spine, organs, and glands.

Unless the body is sufficiently prepared, however, holding certain postures will be either impossible or useless. For example, tight joints, a big belly, or a muscle-bound body may inhibit one's ability to even get into certain postures or, once in them, create too much tension for one to realize the postures' benefits. On the other hand, while hypermobility of the joints may make it easy to get into certain postures, they may still be without benefit. In the first case, the use of repetition is called for to help the body develop in the direction of the particular postures. In the second case, the use of adaptation is called for to help block the release valves so that the benefits of the postures may be achieved.

Considering this, a question emerges: How do we use āsanas in such a way that the movements promote new and more useful possibilities for our body, rather than increasing stress and tension or simply re-enforcing existing conditions? The answer: By bringing our full attention to the integrated relationship between the breath, movement, and the spine. By *linking our awareness to the spine through our breath,* instead of focusing on the external form of a posture, we are able to feel from the inside how our body is responding to the movement. Once this awareness has been established, then we can proceed to find the most effective combination of repetition and hold, of adaption of form and use of breath, and of sequencing, without losing touch with the essential purpose of Yoga practice.

In this way, āsana practice becomes an experimental ground in which we experience, learn, and grow. With this kind of an open attitude of investigation and discovery, our practice will stay alive and fresh. In a gradual and progressive way our body will be transformed toward greater balance, strength, and flexibility; and the result will be a deep and effective āsana practice, regardless of the mechanical possibilities of our body.

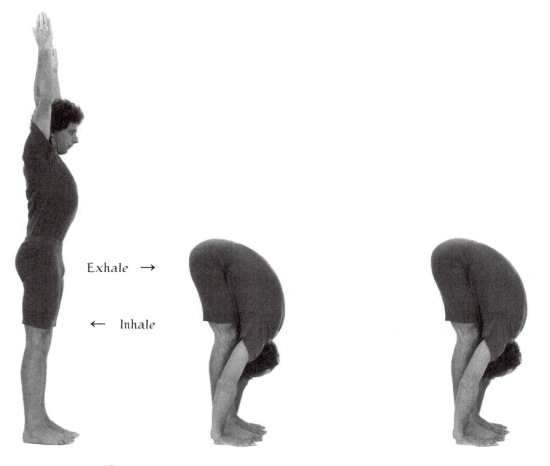

Introduction to Breath

The six vital functions—the life breath, the faculty of speech, the eye, the ear, the mind, and the semen—were disputing among themselves about which was most excellent. They brought their dispute to Brahma, who told them, "One of you is most excellent after whose departure the body is thought to be worse off."

The organ of speech departed and, having remained absent for a year, came back and said, "How have you been able to live without me?" They said, "As the dumb, not speaking with speech but breathing with the breath, seeing with the eye, hearing with the ear, knowing with the mind, procreating with the semen. Thus we have lived."

The eye departed and, having remained absent for a year, came back and said, "How have you been able to live without me?" They said, "As the blind, not seeing with the eye, but breathing with the breath, speaking with the speech, hearing with the ear, knowing with the mind, procreating with the semen. Thus we have lived."

The ear departed and, having remained absent for a year, came back and said, "How have you been able to live without me?" They said, "As the deaf, not hearing with the ear, but breathing with the breath, speaking with the speech, seeing with the eye, knowing with the mind, procreating with the semen. Thus we have lived."

The mind departed and, having remained absent for a year, came back and said, "How have you been able to live without me?" They said, "As the stupid, not knowing with the mind, but breathing with the breath, speaking with the speech, seeing with the eye, hearing with the ear, procreating with the semen. Thus we have lived."

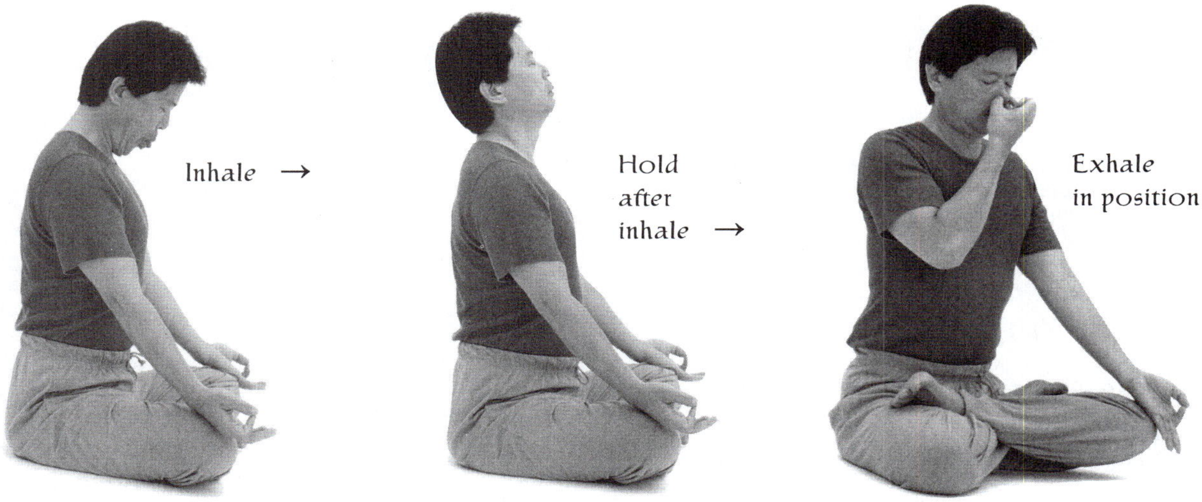

Then semen departed and, having remained absent for a year, came back and said, "How have you been able to live without me?" They said, "As the impotent, not procreating with the semen, but breathing with the breath, speaking with the speech, seeing with the eye, hearing with the ear, knowing with the mind. Thus we have lived."

Then as the life breath was about to depart, even as a large and spirited horse might pull up the pegs to which his feet are tied, even so did it pull up those other vital functions together. They gathered around him and said, "Venerable Sir, do not depart, verily, we shall not be able to live without you. You are the most excellent among us."

BṚHAD-ĀRANYAKA UPANIṢAD VI, 1–13.
CHĀNDOGYA UPANIṢAD VI, 6–12.*

* Translation by S. Radhakrishnan, *The Principal Upaniṣads* (George Allen Unwin/London: Humanities Press, 1953).

From ancient times, the breath has been recognized as the key to our life. In fact, in the root languages of modern cultures, the word for breath is also the word for spirit, life force, even God.

While normal unconscious breathing is controlled by the autonomic nervous system, the breath is readily accessible to conscious control and can therefore provide a link between our conscious mind and our anatomy, physiology, deeper emotional states, and our deepest spiritual potential. And it is this unique quality of the breath that qualifies it as the primary concern of the science of self-development that we find in the Yoga tradition. For the moment, we will specifically focus on the structural aspects of the breath as they relate to āsana practice, leaving the deeper aspects for a later consideration. The particular techniques of breathing used in āsana practice are designed to maximize certain structural effects of inhale and exhale; and the postures themselves can be considered as a way to deepen or extend these structural effects of the breath. Moreover, all movement in āsana is initiated through the action of the breath and is guided by the breath. In other words: Breath is always initiated prior to movement; it evokes a natural movement of the spine, and the action of an āsana is coordinated with this movement. An analogy can be made to swimming in a river, the current of the river being the breath; and, while there are exceptions, the general rule of āsana practice is to first feel the current, and then swim with it.

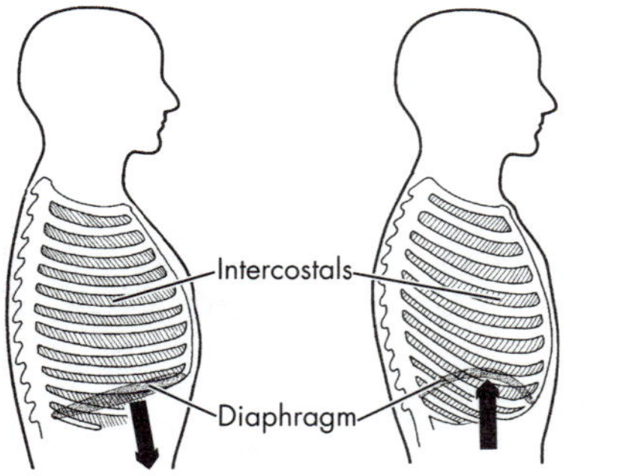

Inspiration: External intercostal muscles and diaphragm contract during inspiration.

Expiration: External intercostal muscles and diaphragm relax during expiration.

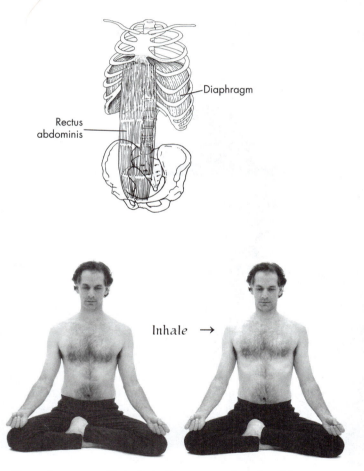

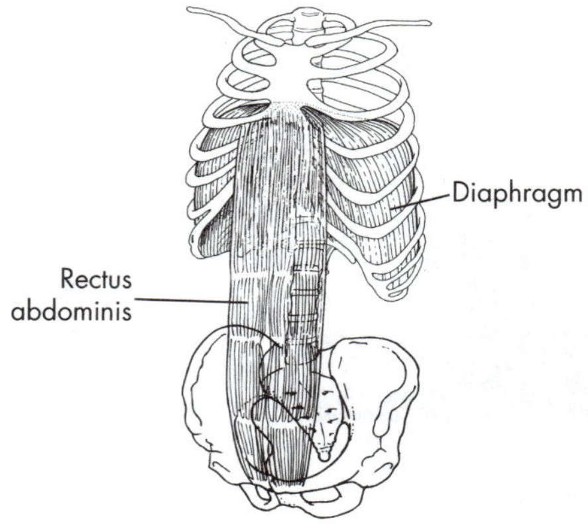

Inhalation

Like all movement in the body, the mechanics of breathing are related to muscular contraction; and inhalation is specifically initiated as a result of the contraction of the intercostal muscles (the muscles between the ribs) and the diaphragm. This process is as follows: The intercostals contract; the rib cage elevates; the diaphragm contracts downward; the elevation of the rib cage, combined with the downward movement of the diaphragm, creates a negative density in the thoracic cavity, allowing air to be sucked into the lungs; and the result is an expansion of the thoracic cavity. Other muscles involved in the process include the erector spinae, the semispinalis, the multifidus, the serratus posterior group, and the interspinalis—all of which contribute to the elevation of the rib cage, expansion of the chest, flattening of the thoracic curve, and vertical extension of the spine.

Conscious use of inhale in āsana practice should enhance this natural process, and all of the following movements, when linked to inhale, are designed for this purpose: raising the arms, expanding the chest, arching the back, moving into backward bends and extension postures, and straightening of the spine from a forward bend, a twist, or a lateral position.

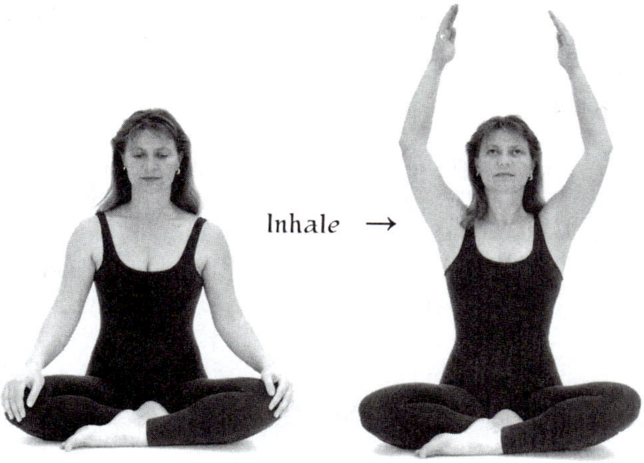
Inhale →

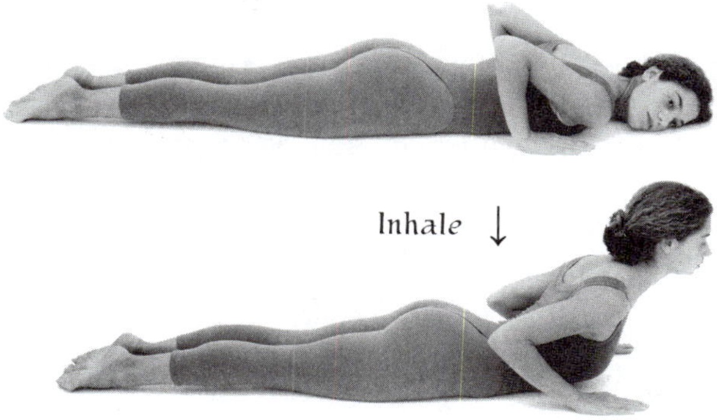
Inhale ↓

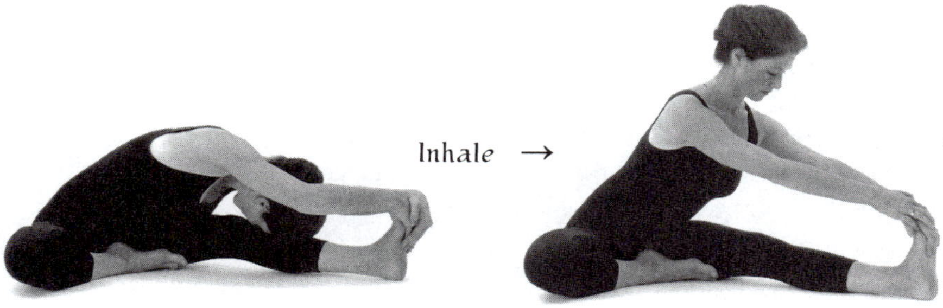
Inhale →

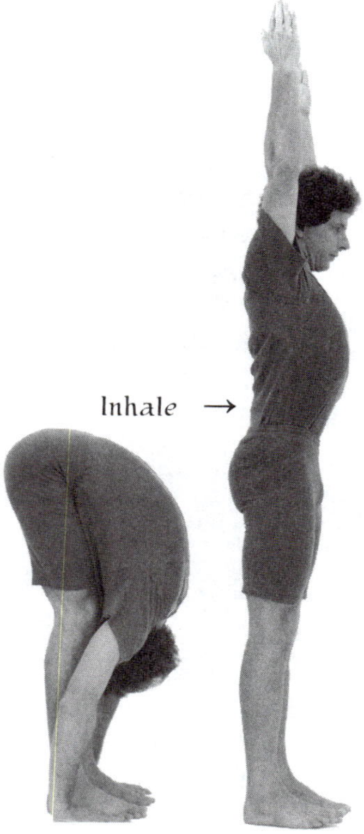
Inhale →

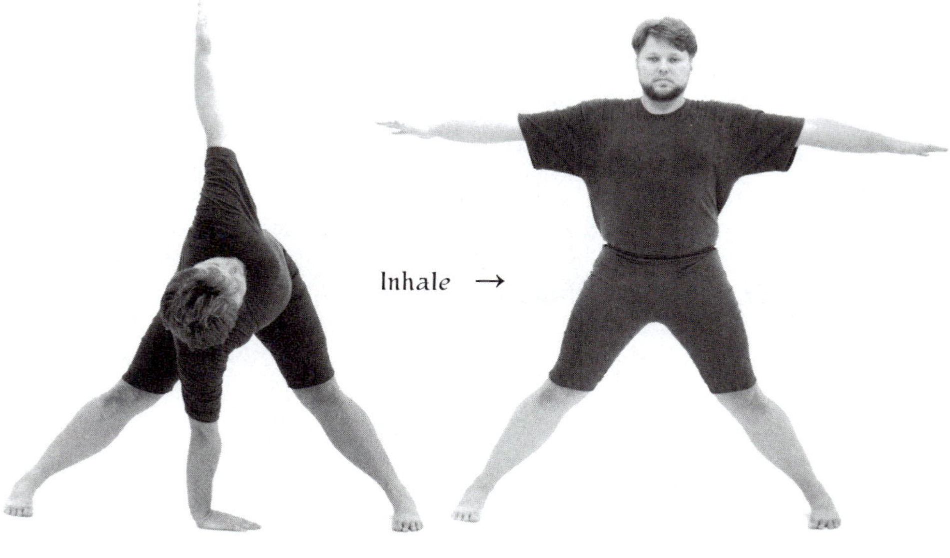
Inhale →

The technique of inhalation is one of the most commonly confused issues in āsana practice because, although its basic mechanics are as described above, a number of variations can be introduced for the purpose of producing special effects; and these variations somewhat modify the effects of the breath itself. Such variations include emphasizing the expansion of the upper, middle, or lower rib cage; emphasizing the expansion of the abdomen; or emphasizing some combination of these events. However, according to the Viniyoga tradition, the general rule is to begin the inhale with the expansion of the upper chest. As the inhalation progresses, move the expansion down into the middle and, finally, into the lower portion of the rib cage. In the last part of the inhale, the abdominal contraction initiated on exhalation (see below) can be released, beginning from the top and then releasing progressively downward.

Exhalation

Where inhalation is a function of muscular contraction, the normal unconscious exhalation is the result of the relaxation of the muscles responsible for inhalation. This process is as follows: As the intercostal muscles relax, the rib cage returns from its elevated position; as the diaphragm relaxes, it raises up; and the result is the expulsion of air from the lungs.

Unlike inhalation, conscious use of exhalation in āsana practice does not follow this natural process. Instead, rather than simply relaxing the muscles contracted to create the inhalation, we intentionally contract the abdominal muscles progressively from the pubic bone to the navel. This contraction is initiated at the rectus abdominis, and then engages both the obliques and transverse abdominis. In certain circumstances, we may also intentionally contract the superficial and deep musculature of the perineal floor, including the anal sphincter, the urethral sphincter, the levator ani muscles, and the deep transverse perineus. This action stabilizes the pelvic-lumbar relationship, creates more structural stability, helps in the flattening of the lumbar lordosis, and, when there is contraction of all the muscles mentioned above, it also supports the organs of the pelvis and lower abdomen.

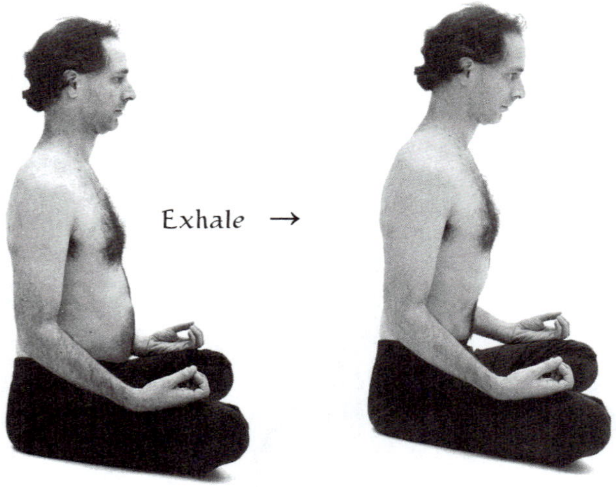

Movements linked to exhale are designed to increase this intentional effect, and they include lowering the arms; compression of the abdomen, which happens when moving into forward bends, twists, and lateral bends; and moving out of backward bends.

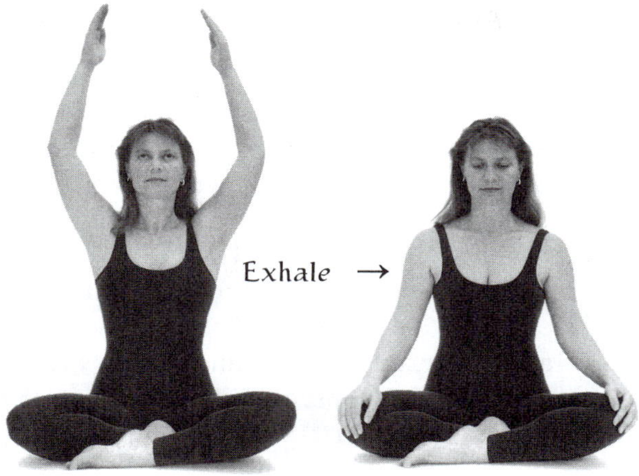

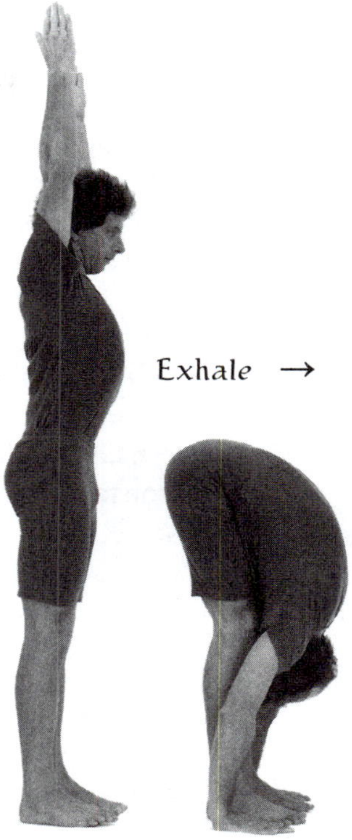

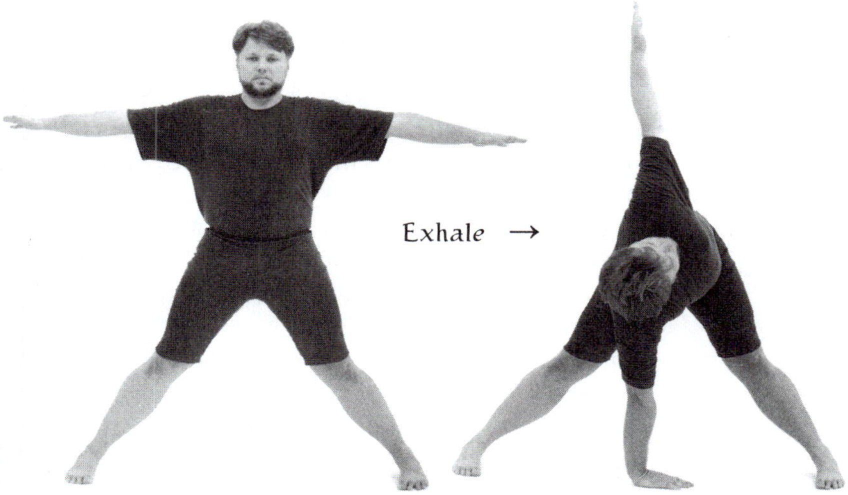

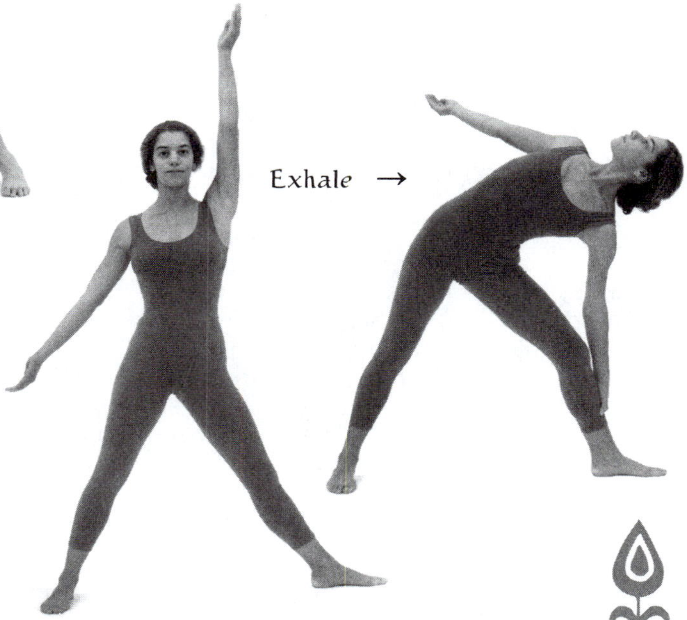

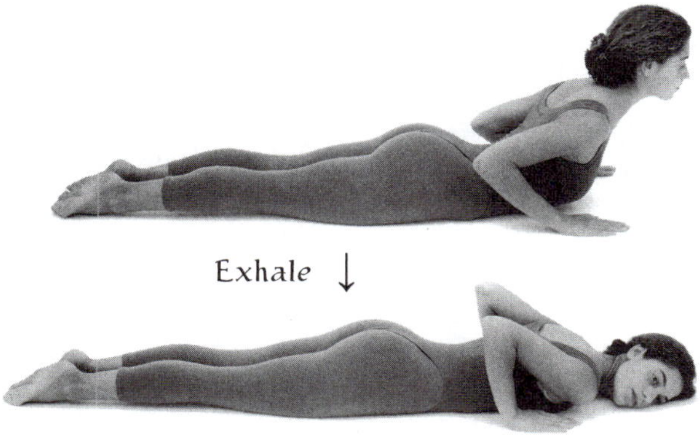

There is a paradox in the fact that as the structure moves upward on inhale, the attention should move downward, following the breath; and as the structure moves downward on exhale, the attention should move upward, following the breath. In other words: On inhale, the ribs are elevated and the spine extends upward, but the diaphragm and the attention move downward with the breath as it flows down into the lungs; and on exhale, the ribs drop downward, but the diaphragm and the attention moves upward with the breath as it flows up and out of the body.

In āsana practice, the main focus of attention should be on the movement of the spine through the breath. This is important because the mechanics of breathing help us to mobilize the spine in particular ways, and, at the same time, the conscious control of the breath enables us to link our attention directly to the movement of the spine. Because the spine is the core of all movement, linking our awareness to the spine brings a deeper level of awareness to all our movements. In short: instead of moving mechanically, we begin to move consciously.

In fact, throughout āsana practice, the mind should control the breath, staying aware of how the spine is moving through the breath and how we are allowing the breath to guide our movements. In this way our postures are developed from the inside out; and instead of focusing on the external form of the posture, we begin to feel from the inside how the body is responding to the movement that is taking place. In this way, instead of using the will to impose form onto our structure, as we follow the lead of the breath, we begin to discover how to adapt the form of a posture to fulfill its function.

Principles of Adaptation

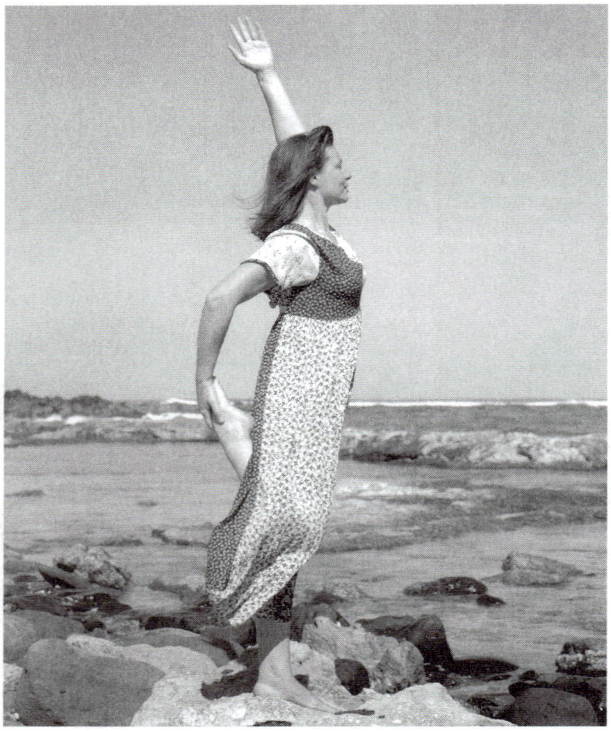

Why We Adapt

Perhaps one of the most important reasons to adapt our practice is to keep it from becoming mechanical. Our bodies become habituated by any kind of repetitive activity to move in particular patterns, until we can successfully perform these patterns with little or no conscious attention. We are much more likely to give our full attention to something that is new. Therefore, changing the practice helps keep it alive, awakens new interest, keeps familiarity from leading to inattention, and helps us stay present throughout the process.

Another reason to adapt our practice is that our physical and mental condition is always changing: one morning we may wake up with a stiff neck and another with a pain in our lower back; one afternoon we may have low energy but want to go out for the evening; or after a celebration, we come home with an upset stomach. Therefore, by adapting the practice, we are able to work on specific conditions as they arise.

In addition to managing day-to-day changes, adaptation is essential when working with any long-term problematic condition. Accordingly, these principles of adaptation are the basis for Yoga therapy, and examples of their application for common aches and pains, chronic diseases, and emotional health can be found in the chapters ahead.

Beyond this therapeutic application, adaptation is the way to develop our potential and achieve something new through our practice. For example, if our hips are very tight, elevating our buttocks in a seated forward bend will facilitate the forward rotation of our pelvis and thus help us stretch our low back.

On the other hand, if our hips are very loose, elevating our heels in a seated forward bend will inhibit the forward rotation of our pelvis and thus help us stretch our low back.

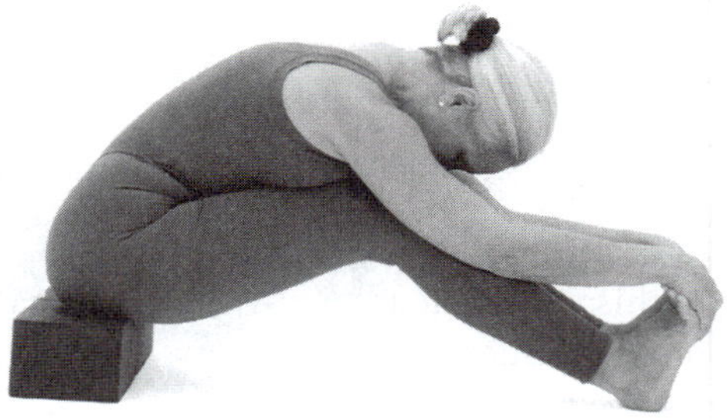

Paścimatānāsana

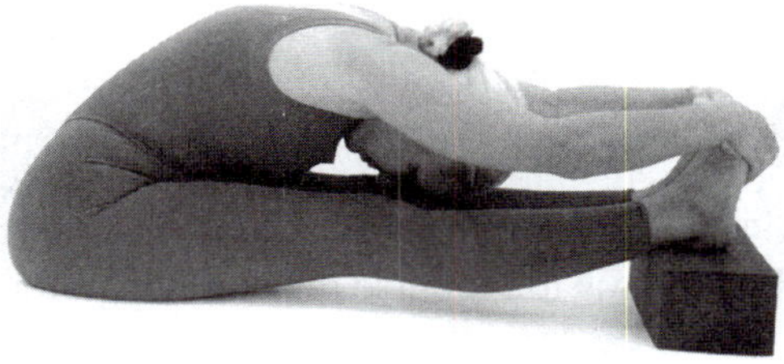

Paścimatānāsana

We can also use adaptation to emphasize different aspects of the same posture. For example, in the case of Vīrabhadrāsana this symmetric adaptation emphasizes flattening the thoracic curve, while this asymmetric adaptation emphasizes stretching the psoas muscles.

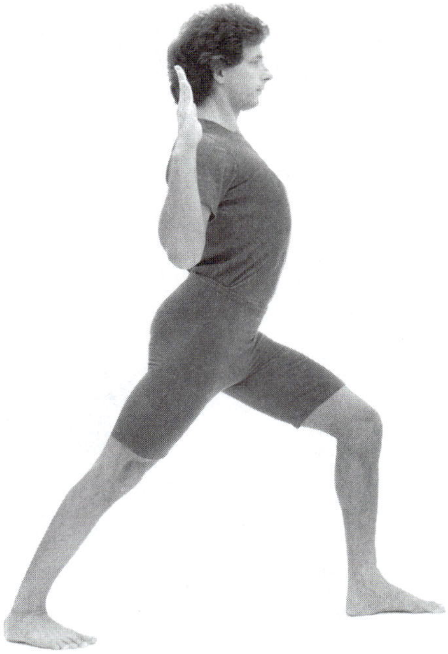

Vīrabhadrāsana

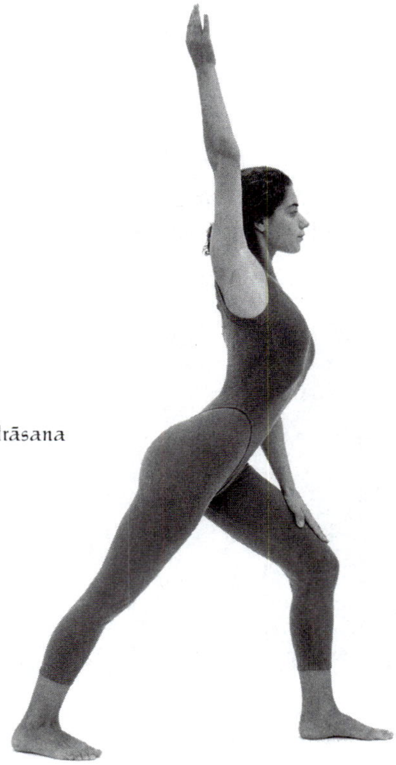

Vīrabhadrāsana

In Parivṛtti Trikoṇāsana we can shift the location of spinal rotation by changing the placement of the hand on the floor. When the hand is midway between the feet, the primary rotation is in the mid-back; as the hand moves closer to the opposite foot, the primary rotation moves down the spine.

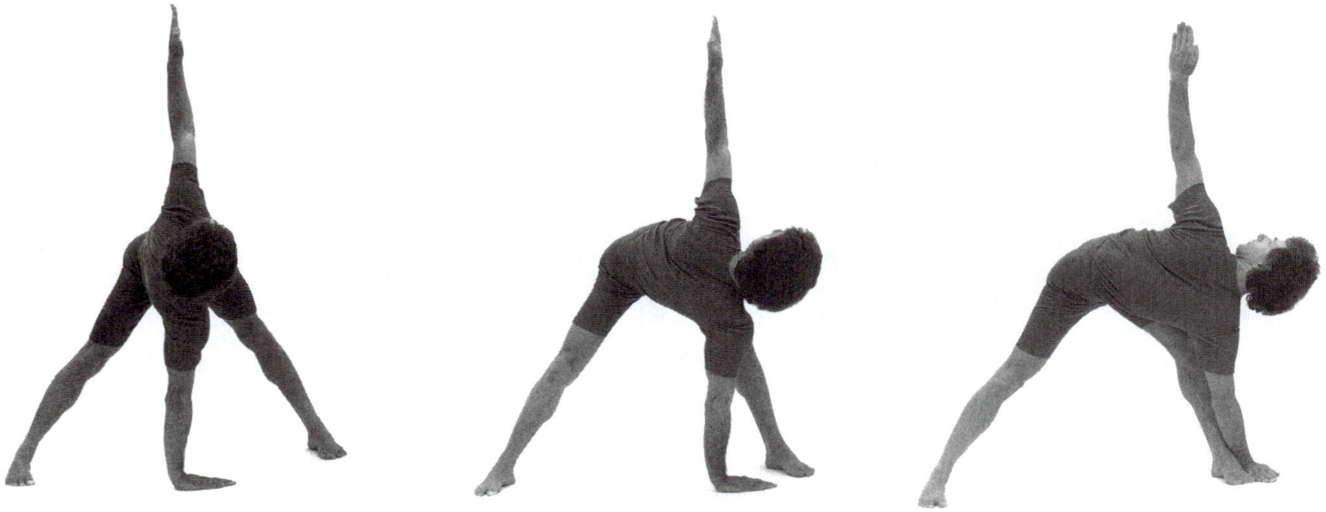

Parivṛtti Trikoṇāsana

Vary arm position

It is important to have a clear intention and orientation at the beginning of each practice. If we are clear, our practice will be efficient, effective, and safe; but if our intention is confused, we may actually end up doing harm to ourselves. For example, there is a tradition of sitting in the full lotus posture for prāṇāyāma (breathing) practices, and some schools suggest not practicing prāṇāyāma until this is possible for you. This is an unfortunate misrepresentation of the tradition, for although a well-conceived and adapted practice can help prepare the body for this posture, many people will never be able to sit in full lotus safely, and yet they would benefit greatly from prāṇāyāma. In fact, it is surprising how many Yoga teachers have had knee surgery because of inappropriate use of this posture. Therefore, the intention and orientation of our practice should be based on a realistic assessment of our needs, limitations, and potentials.

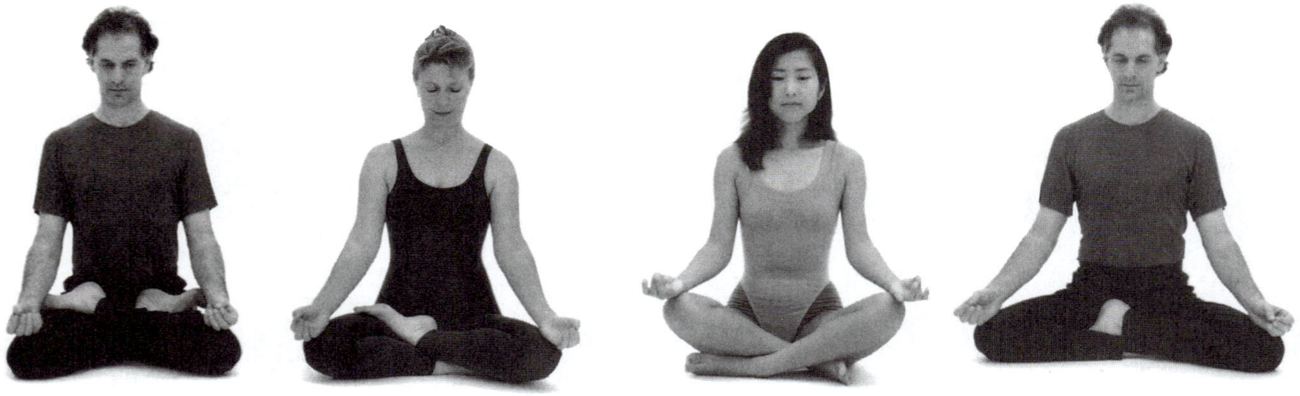

Padmāsana Brahmāsana Sukhāsana Siddhāsana

Alternative prāṇāyāma positions

Adapting the Form of a Posture

Using Arm Variations

In most postures, use of the arms can be adapted to make the postures more or less challenging, and can even be used to shift the postures' effects altogether. Look, for example, at these different possibilities:

- **Using one rather than both arms**

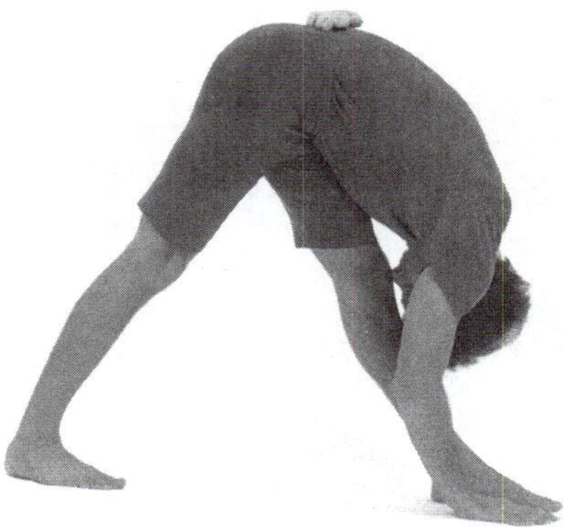

Pārśvottānāsana

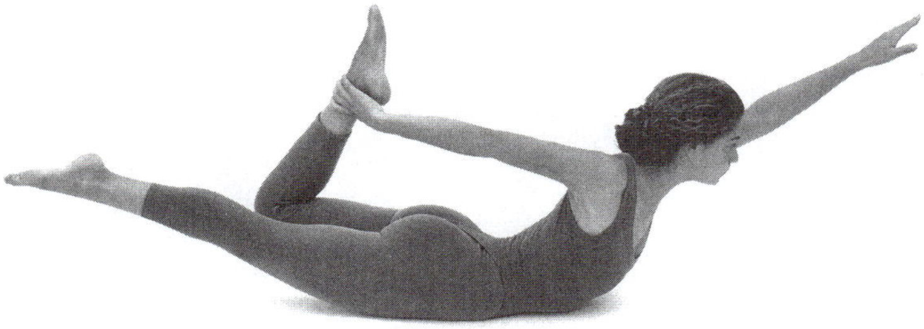

Ardha Dhanurāsana

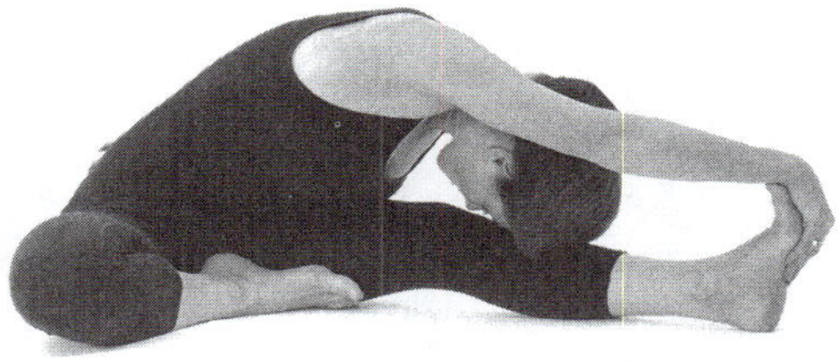

Jānu Śirṣāsana

- **Using sweeping arm movements, with one or both arms**

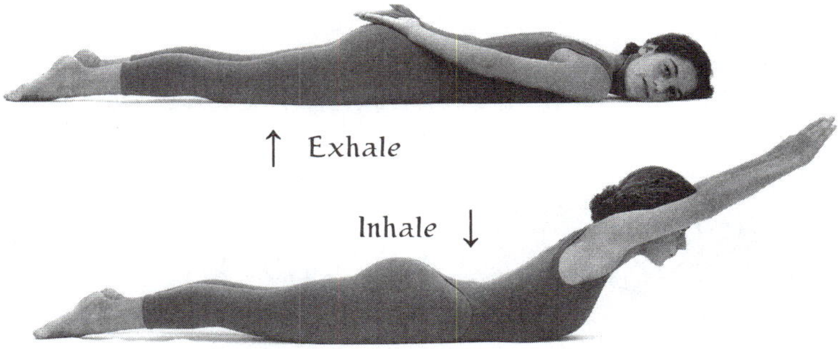

Bhujaṅgāsana

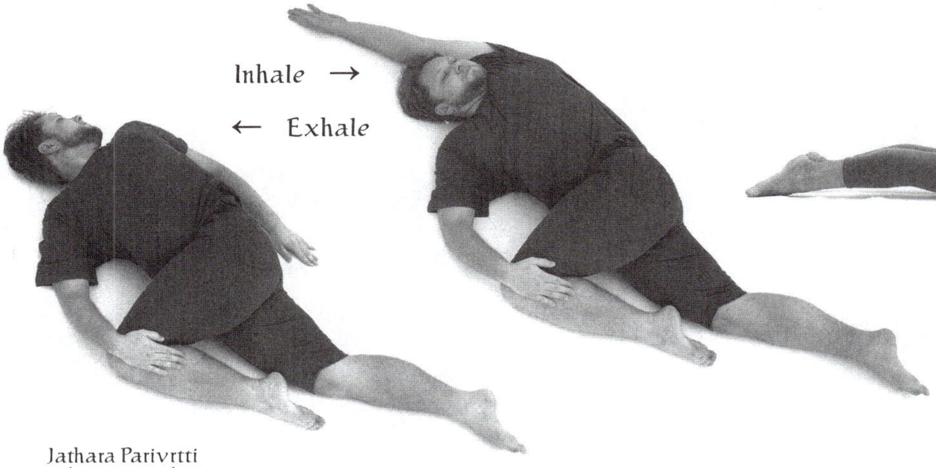

Jaṭhara Parivṛtti

♦ **Using arm/head movement combinations**

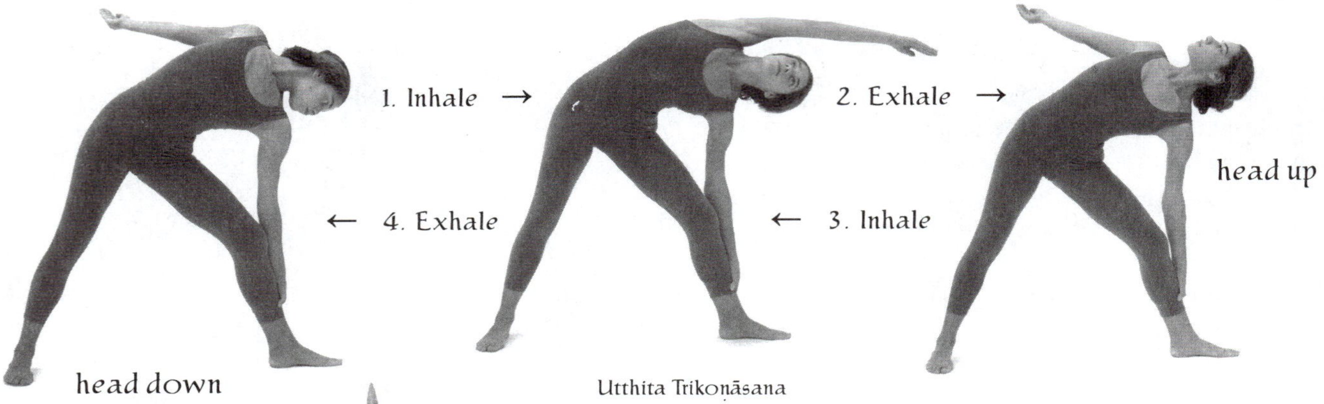
1. Inhale →
2. Exhale →
head up
← 4. Exhale
← 3. Inhale
head down

Utthita Trikoṇāsana

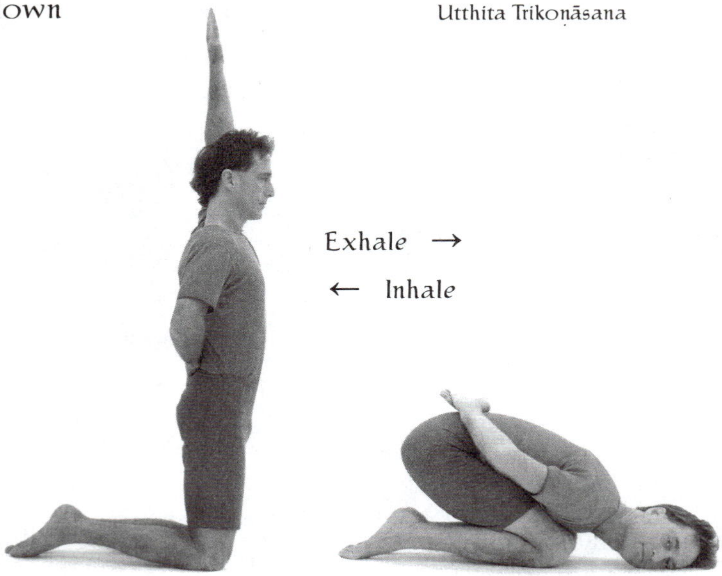
Exhale →
← Inhale

Vajrāsana

♦ **Bending the arms, or alternately bending and straightening one or both arms**

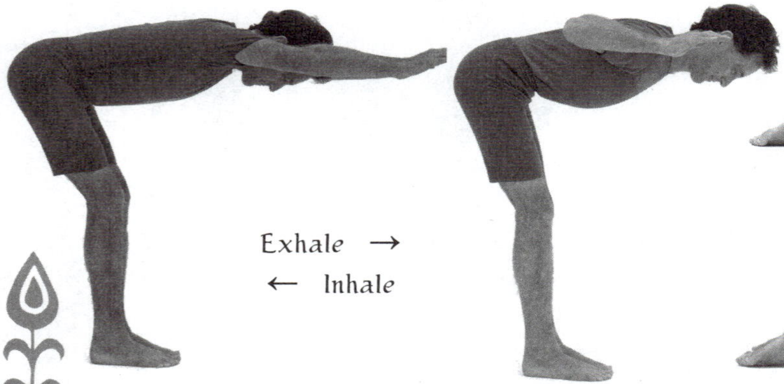
Exhale →
← Inhale

Ardha Uttānāsana

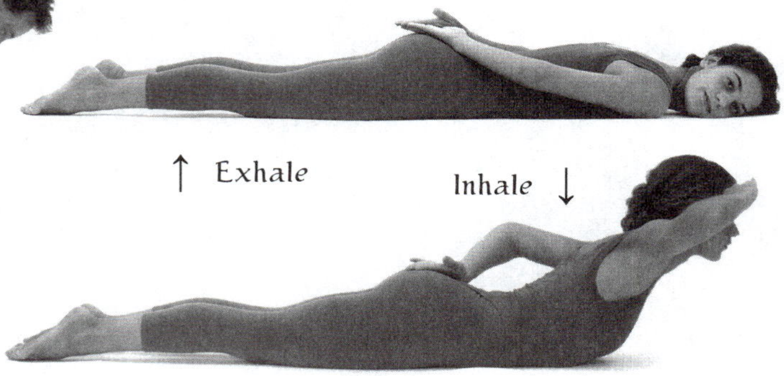
↑ Exhale
Inhale ↓

Bhujaṅgāsana

♦ **Using the arms as levers**

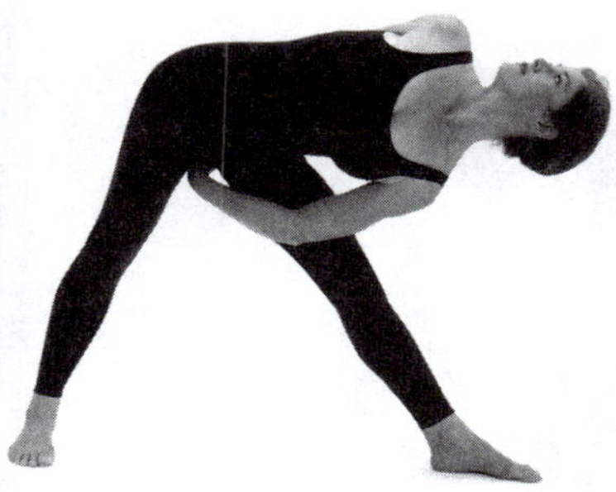

Utthita Trikoṇāsana

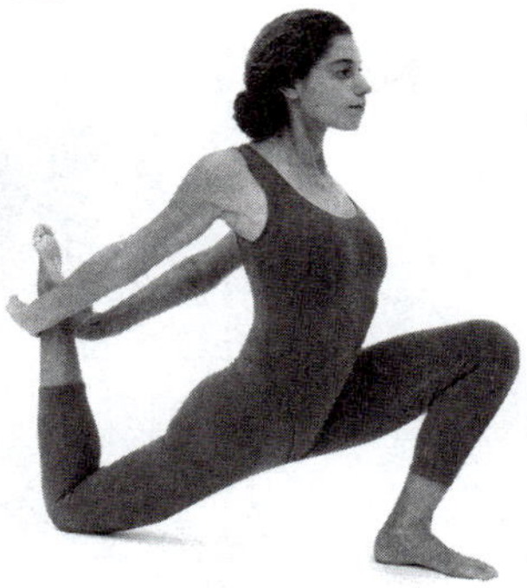

Ekapāda Uṣṭrāsana

One-arm variations lessen the work load, reduce stress in the neck and shoulders, and emphasize each side independently. Sweeping arm movements also lessen the workload and reduce stress in the neck and shoulders, and when used in combination with head movements, they also help to stretch and strengthen the neck and shoulders. Bending the arms reduces stress in the neck and shoulders, and bending and straightening the arms helps bring awareness to the thoracic curve and facilitates flattening it. Using the arms as levers increases the potential to work deeper into the posture, although there is also an increased risk to the joints. Also, as can be seen from these examples, the same type of arm adaptation can be applied in different types of movements. For example, when one-arm sweeping movements are used in combination with turning the head in a forward bend, a twist, or a backward bend, the benefit of this adaptation to the neck and shoulders is increased.

Using Leg Variations

In most postures, the position of the legs can be adapted to make the postures more or less challenging, and can even be used to shift their effects altogether. Look, for example, at these different possibilities:

♦ **Bending the knees**

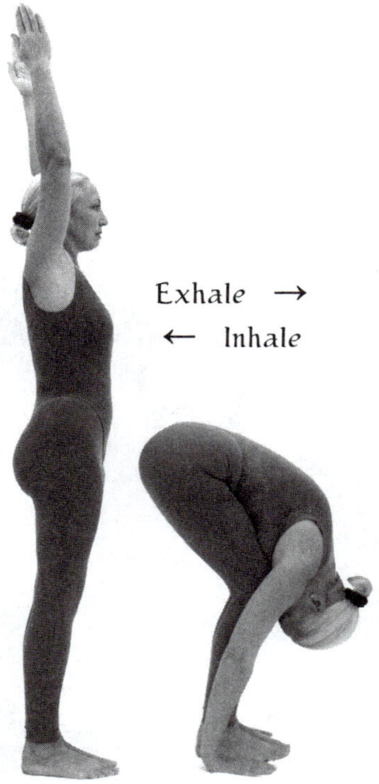

Uttānāsana

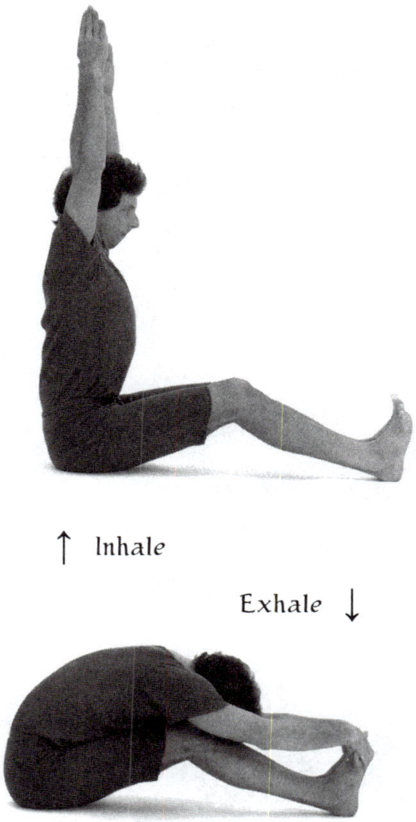

Paścimatānāsana

♦ **Changing the distance between the legs and feet**

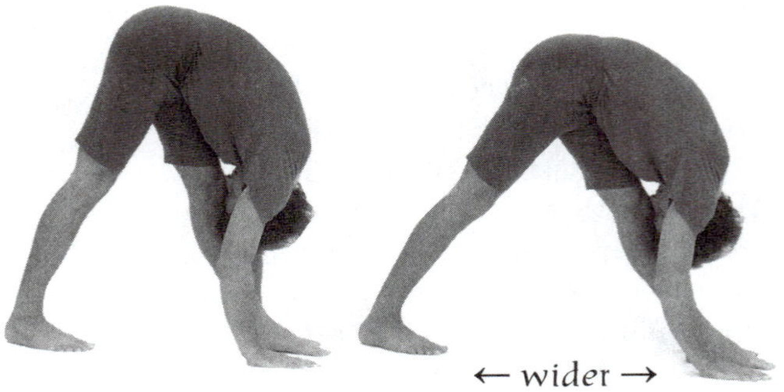

← wider →

to increase stretching: Pārśvottānāsana

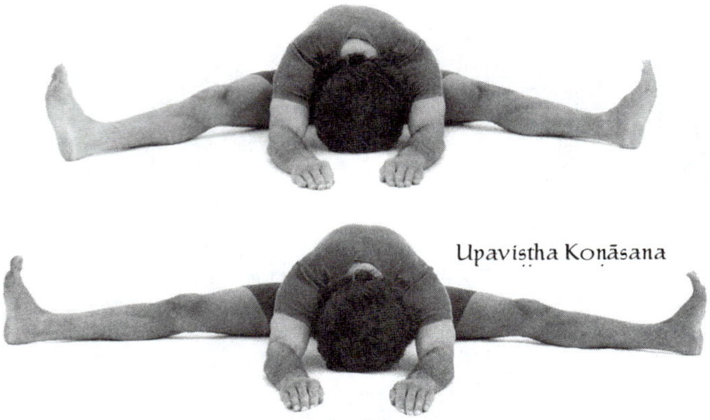

Upaviṣṭha Koṇāsana

← wider →

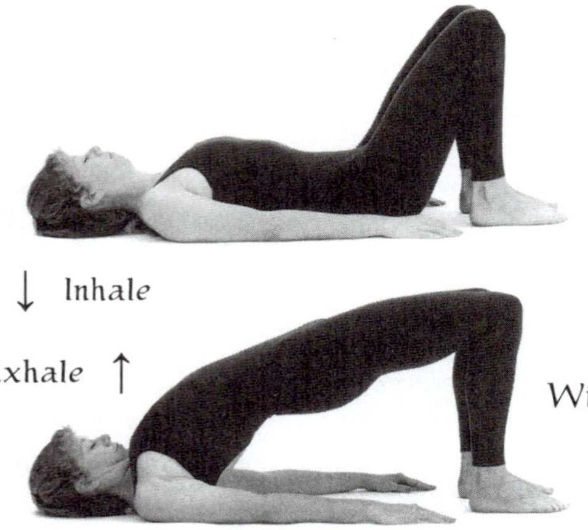

↓ Inhale

Exhale ↑

Widen feet

to increase strength: Dvipāda Pīṭham

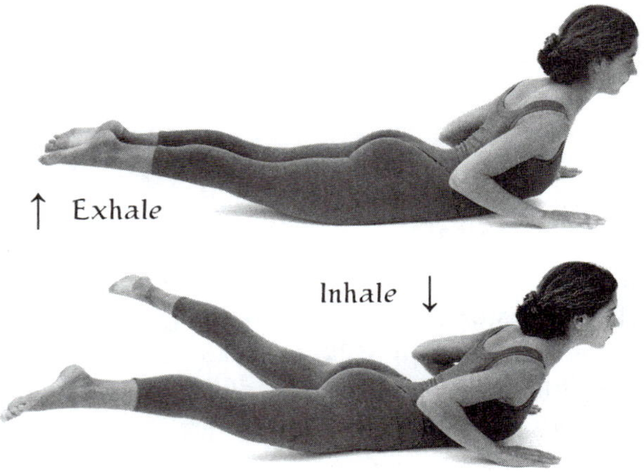

↑ Exhale

Inhale ↓

Vimanāsana

♦ **Displacing one knee backward**

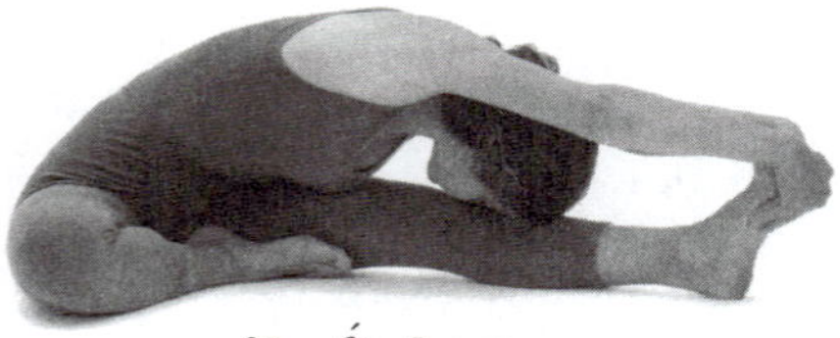

Jānu Śirṣāsana

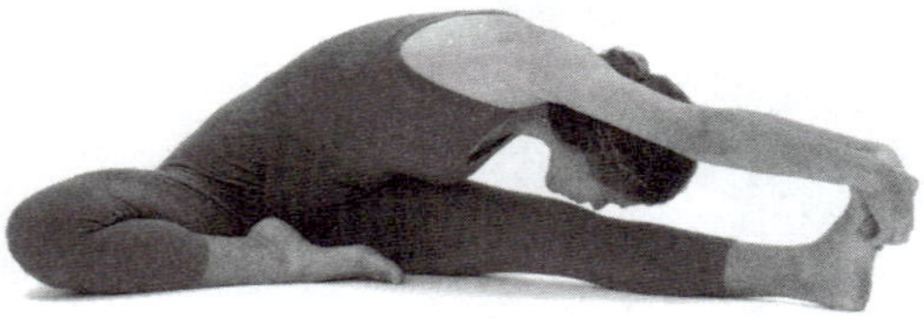

← wider →

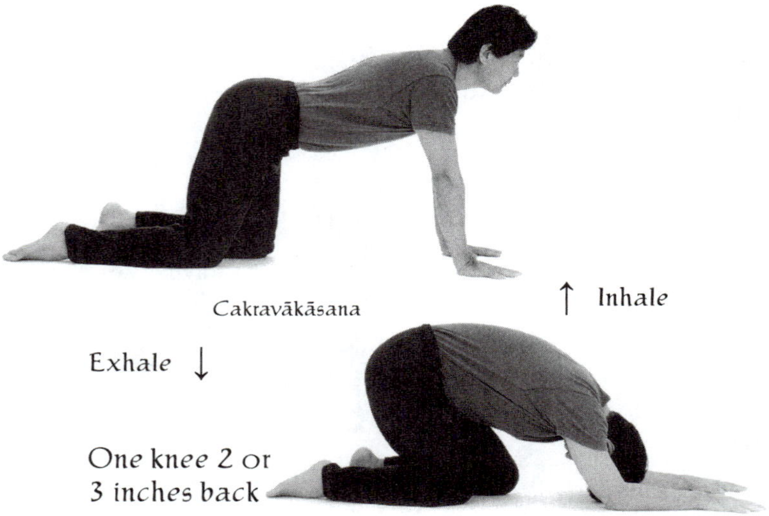

Cakravākāsana

↑ Inhale

Exhale ↓

One knee 2 or 3 inches back

♦ Rotating the leg externally

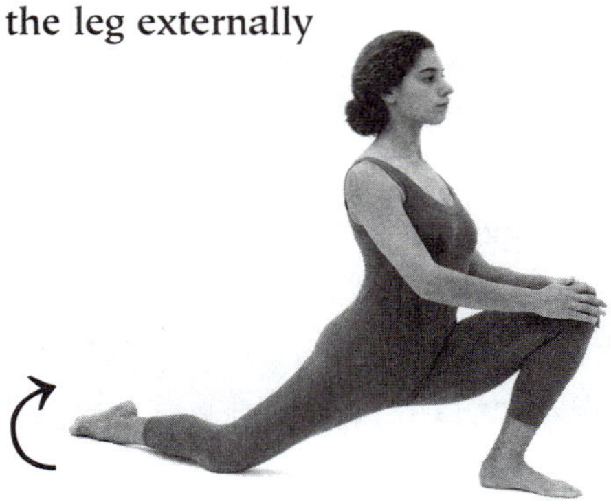

Ekapāda Uṣṭrāsana

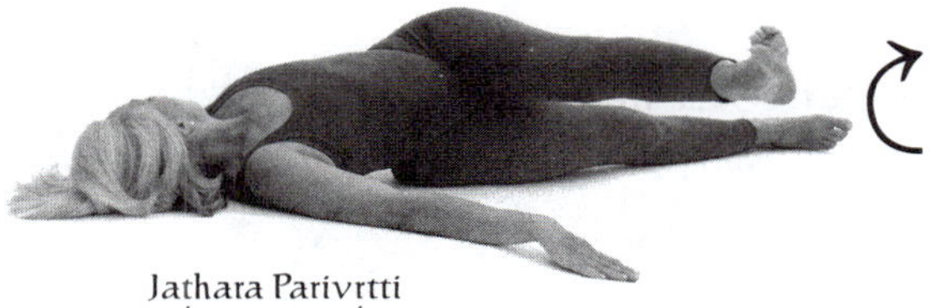

Jaṭhara Parivṛtti

Bending the knees in standing postures lowers the center of gravity and facilitates the stretching of the low back. Bending the knees in seated postures can be used to either facilitate or inhibit the forward rotation of the pelvis, and often reduces stress in the low back. Increasing the distance between the feet in standing or seated postures increases and modifies the stretching of the legs. Widening the feet in the prone and supine postures above increases the contraction of the musculature of the hips. Displacing one knee backward increases the stretching of that side of the back. Rotating the knee externally, in the kneeling posture, increases the stretching of the inner thigh; and, in the supine twist, it increases the contraction of the musculature of the hip.

Adapting the Movement into and out of a Posture

Origin of Movement

The place of origin determines the effect of a movement. For example: in a standing forward bend, originating the movement in the abdomen inhibits the forward rotation of the pelvis, while originating the movement in the hips facilitates it.

Direction of Movement

Moving into a posture in different ways also changes the effect of the posture. For example: coming up into Ardha Uttānāsana encourages the flattening of the upper back, and is most appropriate if you have a normal to excessive thoracic curve; while moving down into Ardha Uttānāsana encourages the rounding of the upper back, and is most appropriate if you have a normal to flattened thoracic curve.

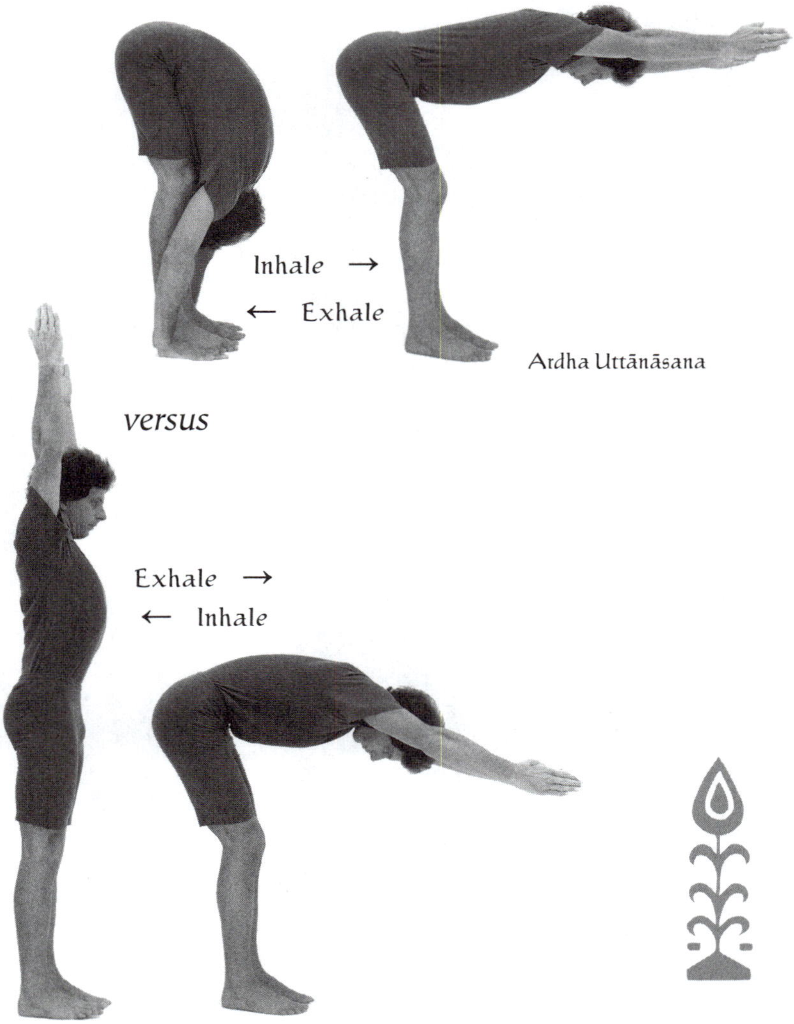

Ardha Uttānāsana

Another example is how to apply the force of the arms when coming up into Bhujangāsana: pushing down on the hands and lifting the chest deepens the arching effect in the lower back; while pulling back on the hands and pushing the chest forward deepens the arching effect in the upper back.

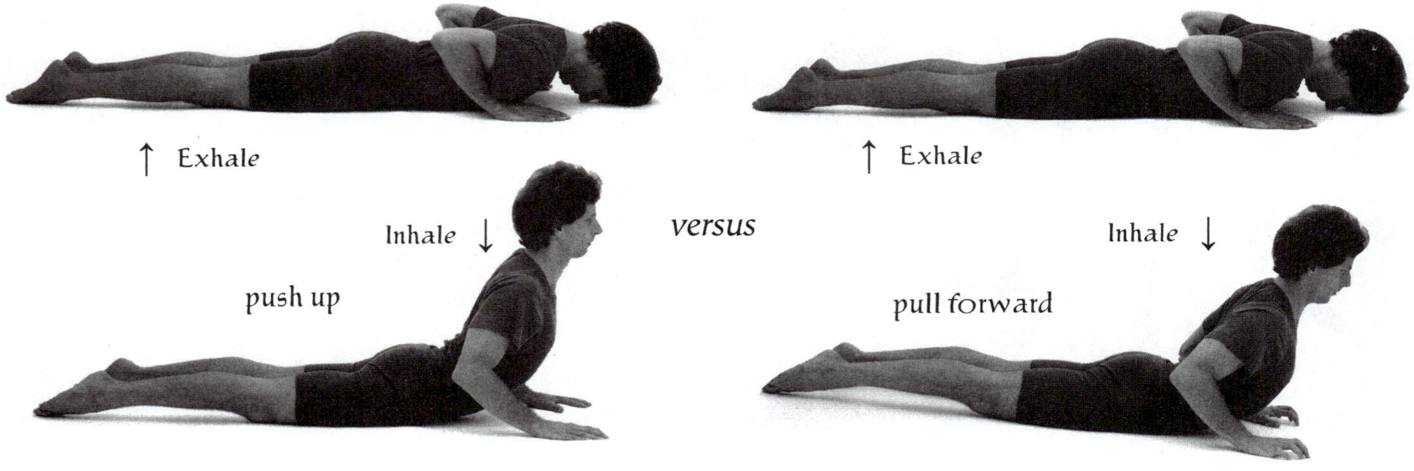

Bhujaṅgāsana

Range of Motion

It is not correct to assume that the goal in any āsana is to move as far into the posture as possible; and sometimes the ability to move fully into a particular posture may even interfere with the ability to truly benefit from it. If you are one of those people who can easily drop into a posture like Upaviṣṭha Koṇāsana without any resistance, try bending one or both knees and keeping your sit bones on the floor as you bend forward. You will not go as far into the posture but will much more effectively stretch your low back.

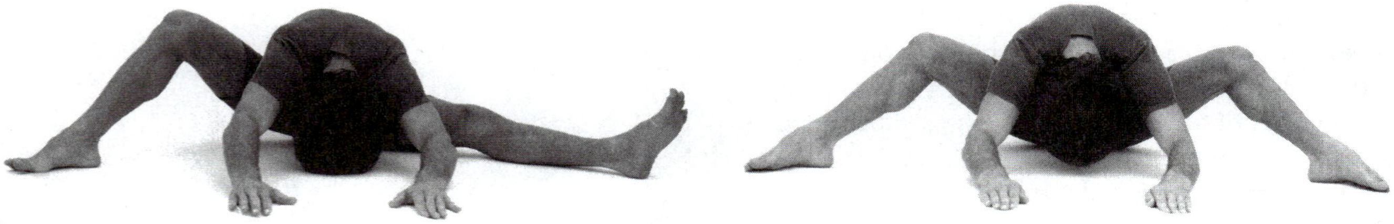

Upaviṣṭha Koṇāsana

Moving in Stages

Breaking a movement into stages can deepen its effect.

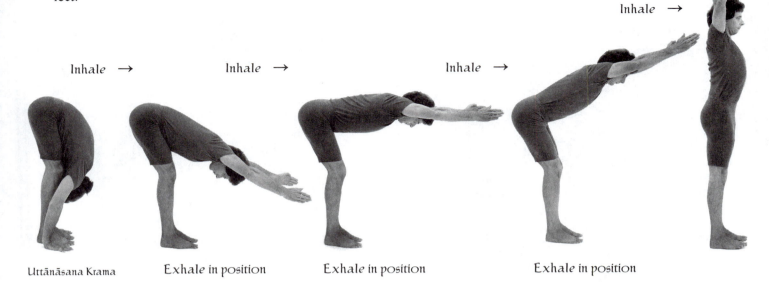

Inhale →
Inhale →
Inhale →
Inhale →
Exhale in position
Exhale in position
Exhale in position

Uttānāsana Krama

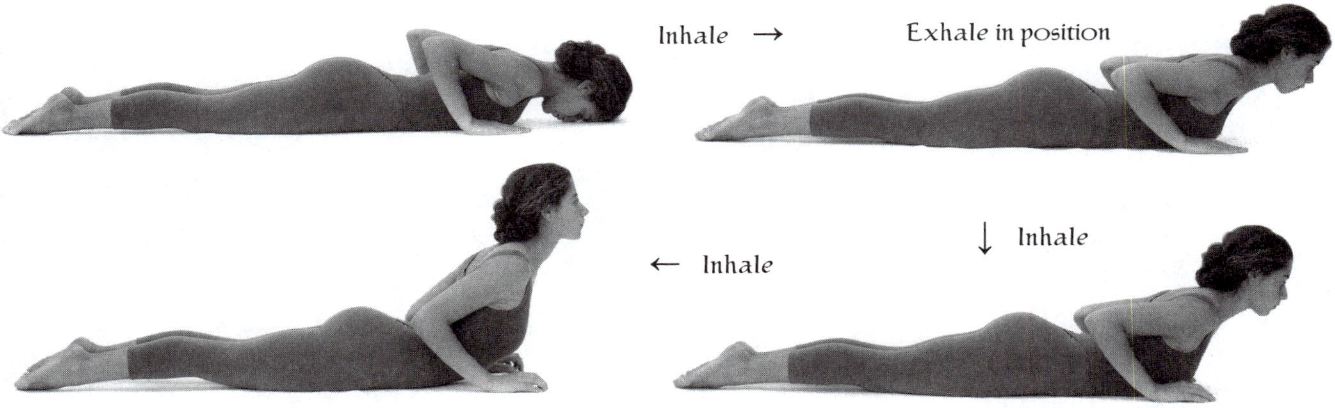
Inhale →
Exhale in position
↓ Inhale
← Inhale
Exhale in position

Bhujaṅgāsana Krama

Speed of Movement

Speed of movement should always be coordinated with the length of a full breath. Speed influences the effect of movement: in general, faster movements being more energizing and slower movements more calming. However, if the movement is too quick it is easy to slip into unconscious movement patterns or to avoid sustained muscular work.

Combining Movement with Staying in a Posture

In general, we use the repetitive movement into and out of a posture as a preparation for staying in it. We can create various combinations of moving and staying to modify the effects of the positions.

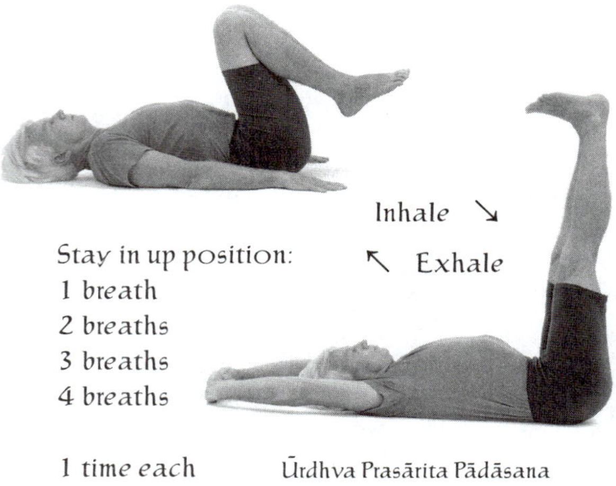
Inhale ↘
↖ Exhale
Stay in up position:
1 breath
2 breaths
3 breaths
4 breaths
1 time each

Ūrdhva Prasārita Pādāsana

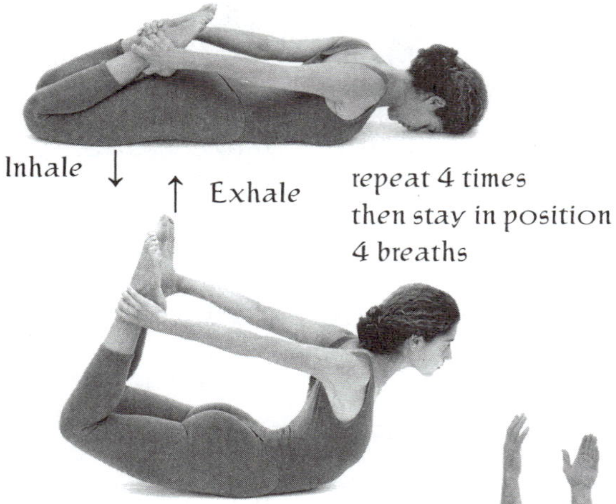
Inhale ↓
↑ Exhale
repeat 4 times
then stay in position
4 breaths

Dhanurāsana

Combining Two or More Postures Together

This is done with postures that can be linked together easily to create a flowing sequence.

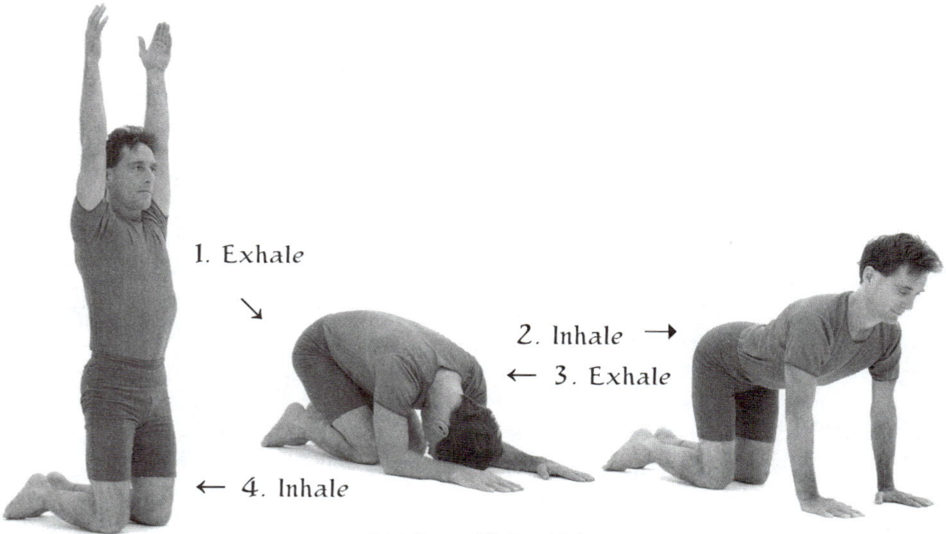
1. Exhale ↘
2. Inhale →
← 3. Exhale
← 4. Inhale

Vajrāsana/Cakravākāsana

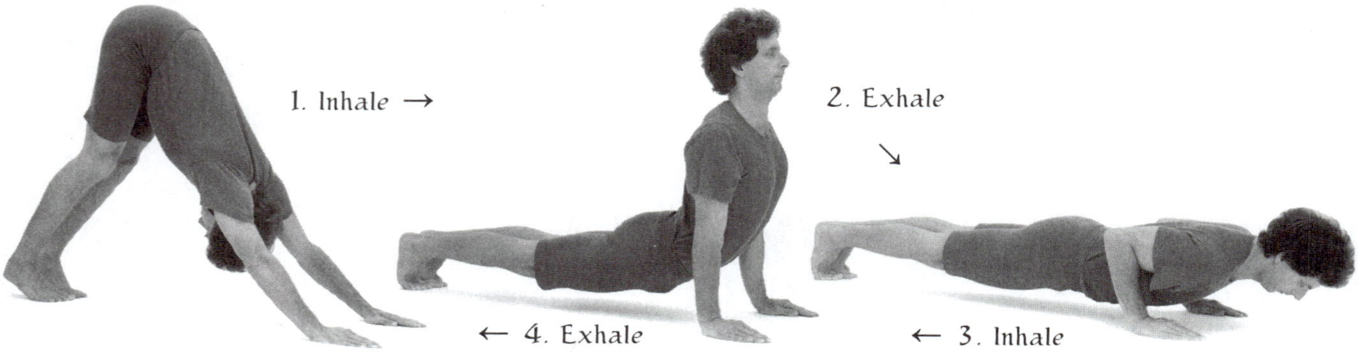
1. Inhale →
2. Exhale ↘
← 3. Inhale
← 4. Exhale

Adho / Ūrdhva Mukha Śvānāsana / Caturaṅga Daṇḍāsana

Shifting the Attention

Generally, we suggest keeping attention on the breath and the parts of the body where the most action is occurring. However, shifting the focus of attention can also change the effect of a posture in surprising ways. For example, try moving into and out of Pārśvottānāsana four times on each side. On the first repetition, keep the attention on the back heel; on the second, keep the attention on the abdomen; on the third, keep the attention on the hands; and on the fourth, try to keep your attention on all three points at the same time. Notice how, each time, the effects of the movement shift.

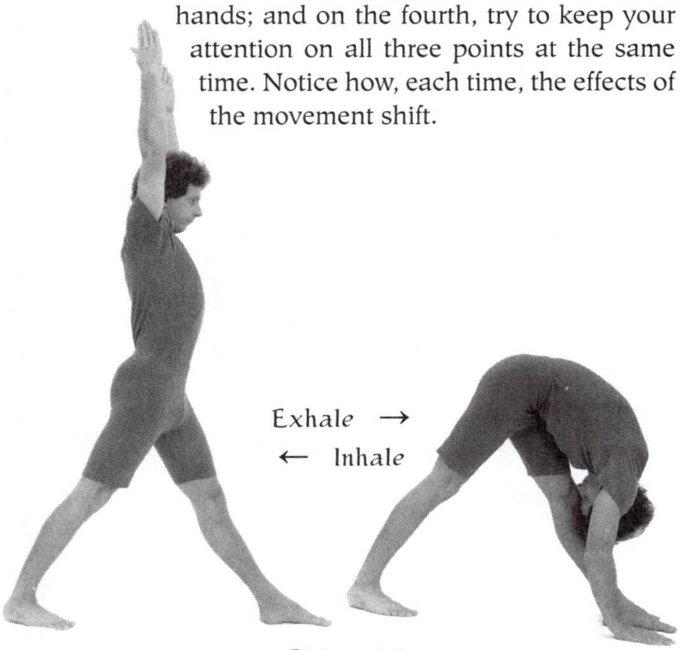

Pārśvottānāsana

At a different level, try placing your attention on a quality, such as kindness, and hold that in your thoughts. With this focus, you may notice that your practice softens and deepens.

Or, allow yourself to sincerely connect to the mysterious source of life itself, and hold that in your heart. With this focus, you may notice that your practice becomes a kind of prayer.

Adapting the Breath

The breath can be adapted in a variety of ways to deepen the practice and produce different effects. Look, for example, at these different possibilities:

1. Creating a deep flowing inhale and exhale, without a fixed length or proportional ratio between them.
2. Establishing a fixed length to inhale and/or exhale. For example, fix the inhale and exhale at six seconds, or fix the exhale at six seconds and leave the inhale free.
3. Establishing a proportional relationship between inhale and exhale. For example: make the inhale six seconds and the exhale ten seconds. (Only rarely should inhale be greater than exhale, and commonly exhale is longer than inhale.)
4. Changing the length of the breath without changing the proportional relationship. For example: start with inhale and exhale equal at six seconds each; increase after several breaths to eight seconds each; and then to ten seconds each. The capacity to lengthen inhale and exhale in challenging positions is a measure of structural integrity, stamina, and inner strength.
5. Progressively lengthening either inhale or exhale and leaving the other free or fixed. For example: in certain postures, inhalation may be fixed at six seconds but exhalation progressively lengthened from six to twelve seconds.
6. Changing the breathing patterns by making the breath very silent and subtle, or more audible and intense, significantly alters the effects of the movements.
7. Introducing holding of the breath after inhale and/or exhale significantly intensifies the effects of the postures.

   Holding after inhale generally extends the effects of the inhalation and is therefore usually applied in positions that emphasize inhalation. Holding after exhale generally extends the effects of exhalation and is therefore usually applied in positions that emphasize exhalation.

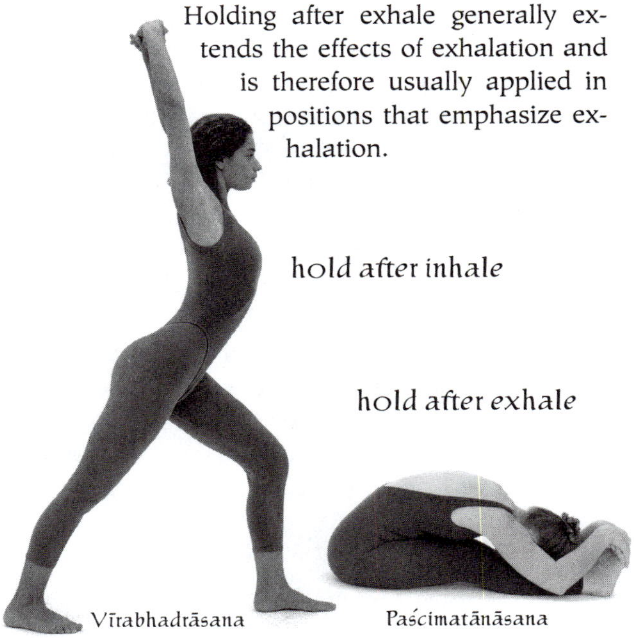

Vīrabhadrāsana Paścimatānāsana

8. Modifying the technique by which the breath is taken. For example: focusing the inhale in the solar plexus may be useful if the upper back and neck are stiff and inhale in the chest is creating tension.
9. Changing the normal breathing pattern. For example: doing a movement on exhale that is normally done on inhale.

   Or doing a movement while holding after exhale that is normally done on exhale.
10. Breathing in segments—known as *krama* breathing. For example: inhale one-third of the comfortable capacity at a time, pausing between each segment of the inhale.

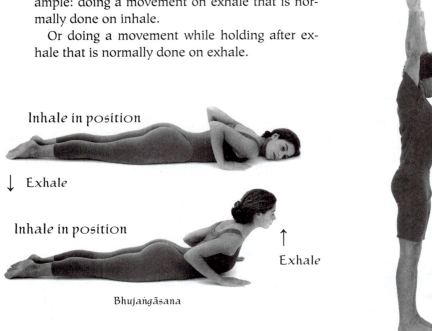

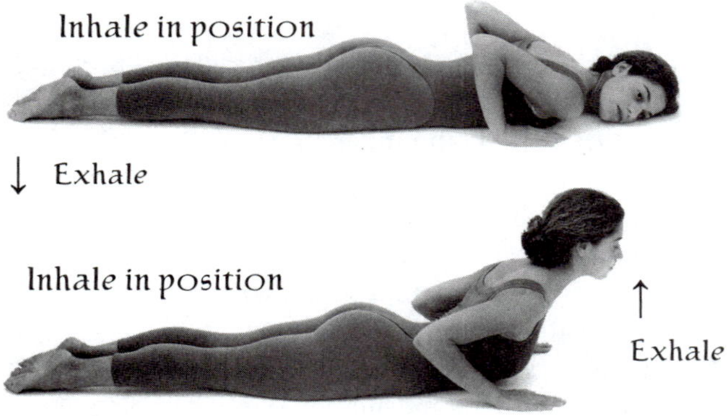
Inhale in position
↓ Exhale
Inhale in position
↑
Exhale

Bhujaṅgāsana

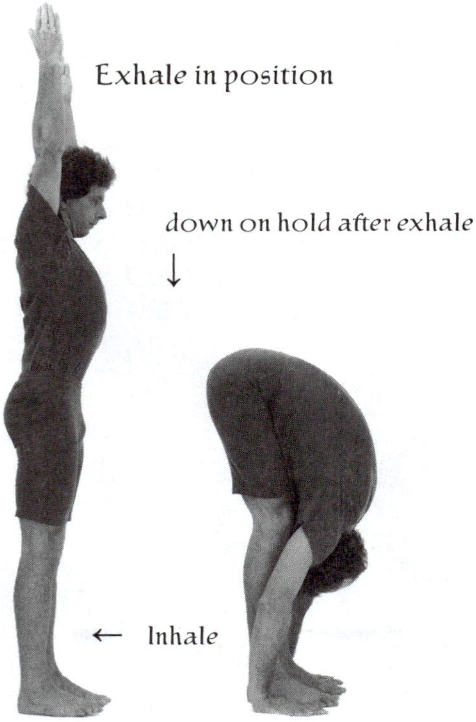
Exhale in position
down on hold after exhale
↓
← Inhale

Uttānāsana

Using Sound

Using vocal sound techniques in combination with postures effectively intensifies practice, focuses attention, deepens exhalation, increases circulation to the organs, and balances the emotions. Sound creates internal vibrations that increase circulation to different parts of the body.

The main factors that determine the effects of the sounds that are used are their particular vowels and consonants (*varna*), their pitch (*svara*), and their volume (*bala*). Though different traditions give different explanations about the use of the different vowel and consonant sounds, we can explore for ourselves how these various sounds resonate in our own bodies. There seems to be universal agreement that higher pitched sounds tend to resonate higher in the body and energize the system, while lower pitched sounds tend to resonate lower in the body and calm the system; and that louder sounds tend to awaken the energy and externalize the attention, while softer sounds tend to pacify the energy and internalize the attention.

Vocal sound techniques include humming, chanting simple syllables, chanting simple phrases that have certain meanings, and chanting more complete songs or prayers. Examples of the therapeutic uses of sound for common aches and pains, chronic diseases, and emotional health can be found in the chapters ahead.

Using Props

Props are useful when the capacity for movement is restricted due to structural limitations. They can be particularly useful in therapeutic application. They can also be useful to intensify work in a particular area. Props can include a wall, a table, a chair, blocks, cushions to support the body, straps for help with achieving closed-frame postures, and weights to intensify the effects of open-frame postures.

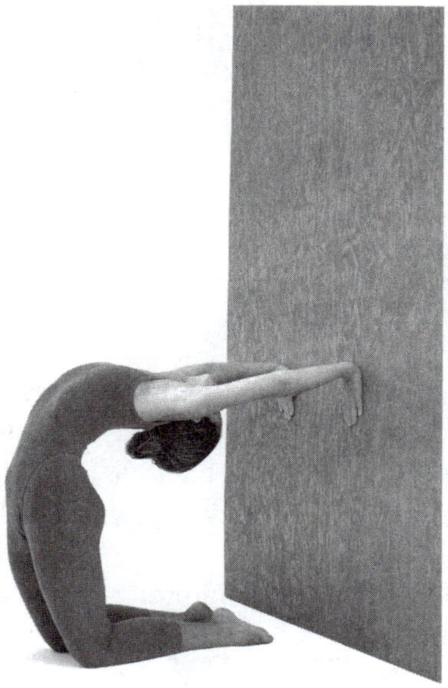

Vajrāsana against a wall

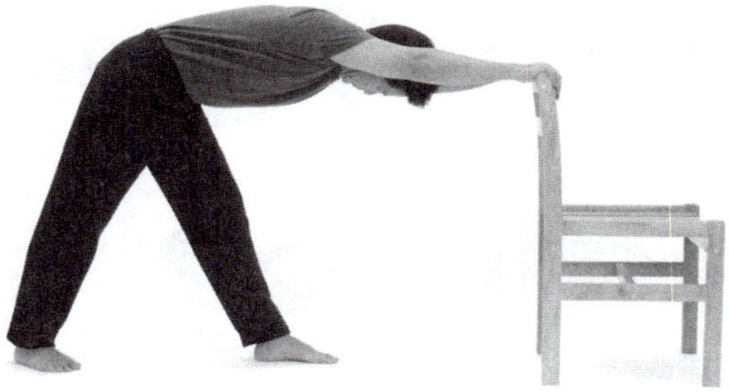

Pārśvottānāsana to a chair

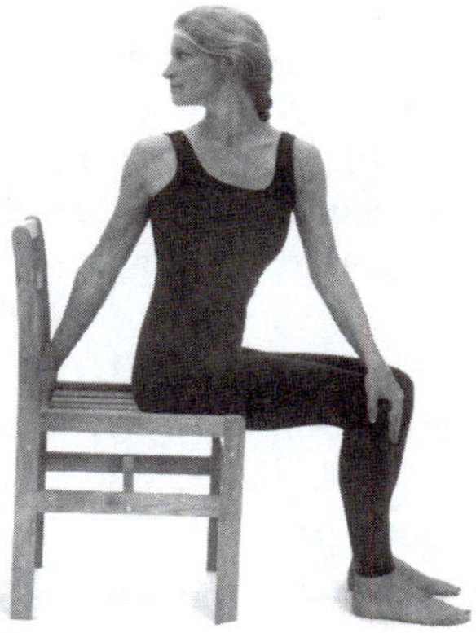

Ardha Matsyendrāsana on a chair

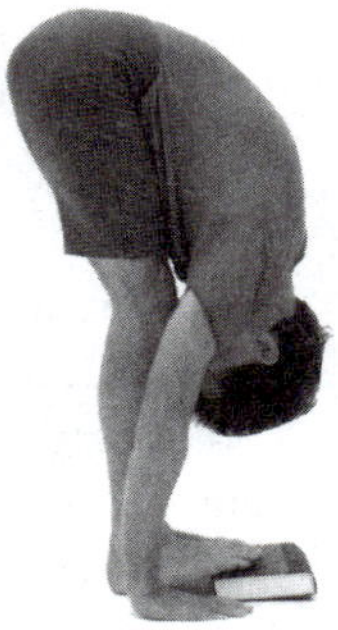

Uttānāsana with a book

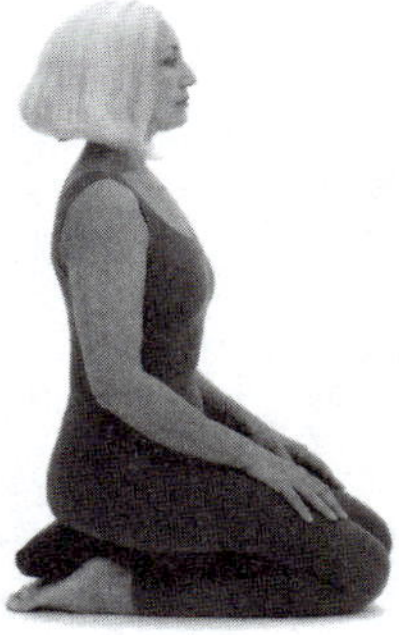

Vajrāsana on a cushion

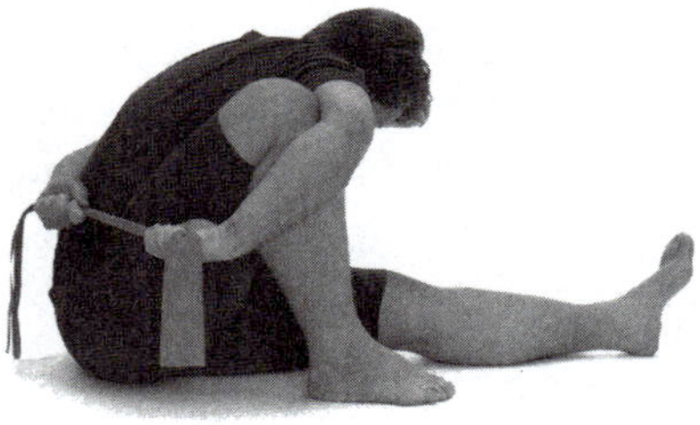

Marīcyāsana with a strap

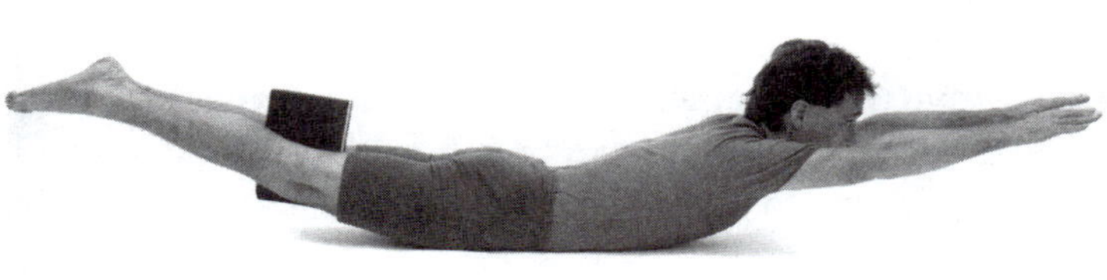

Śalabhāsana with a book

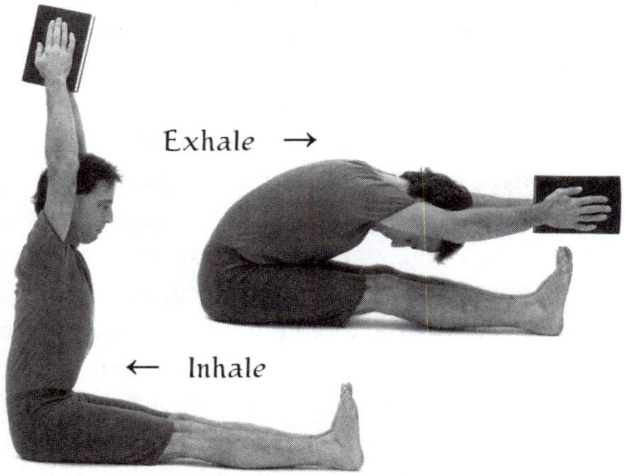

Paścimatānāsana with a book

The Art and Science of Sequencing

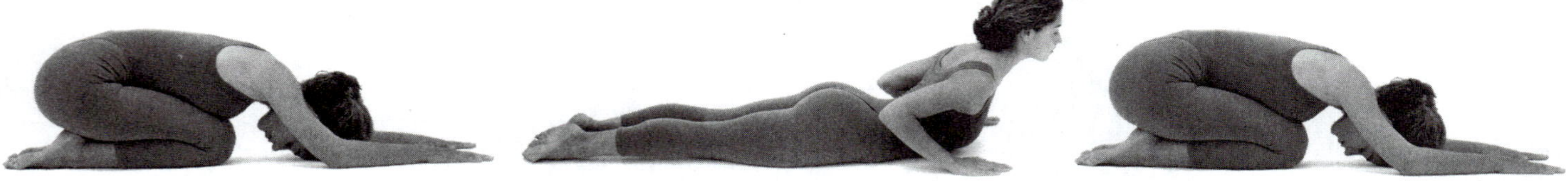

A well-conceived sequence is the key to an effective practice. Such a sequence has the qualities of order, harmony, and efficiency throughout, each posture and adaptation being selected and placed purposefully to create an integrated whole. Building effective sequences is at once an art and a science based on definite principles. So if you study and apply the principles detailed in this chapter, you will find your practices becoming progressively more elegant, refined, and relevant to your changing needs and interests, and in time, you will master the fine art of sequencing.

The many sequences appearing in this book are presented as models for approaching different specific conditions through practice. However, because no individual can be characterized by one specific condition alone, the sequences are necessarily descriptive rather than prescriptive, and each must be further adapted to respect your total situation, including your age, physical and emotional condition, profession, and personal interests. Therefore, the information in this chapter is also intended to help you in this process of adaptation.

Your Yoga practice should help to enhance the flow of your day; it should not be a predetermined and fixed affair that you fit in whenever you can. This means that the character of the sequences you use should change, depending upon the time of day, the activities that proceed practice, and the activities that follow it. For example, in the morning, you may want to do a more general warming up and energizing practice to prepare you for the day ahead. In the evening, on the other hand, you may want to do a more specific and relaxing practice to unwind from the stresses of the day. How you spend your day will also influence your practice. For example, if your work is physically demanding, you may want to use your practice to compensate for the physical stresses of your work and to help return balance to your body. If, on the other hand, your work is physically sedentary, you may want to use your practice to work out your body, to help release mental stress, and to achieve a clear mind.

The components of your practice are variable and can include any combination of the following elements: āsana, prāṇāyāma, chanting, meditation, prayer, and ritual. The keys to the science of combining these elements and arranging them in a particular order are the principles of *Viṅyāsa* and *Pratikriyā*, which apply to all of the above-mentioned elements of a Yoga practice and to most activities in daily life as well.

Viṅyāsa

Viṅyāsa, literally "arranging" or "placing," refers to the preparatory steps required to move the mind, breath, and/or body in a particular direction. The general idea of viṅyāsa is to move progressively from the gross to the subtle, from the external to the internal, from the simple to the complex, and from the easy to the difficult. For example, āsana is more external than prāṇāyāma, and prāṇāyāma is more external than meditation. Therefore, you can use āsana to prepare the body and breath for prāṇāyāma, and prāṇāyāma to prepare the breath and mind for meditation.

In āsana practice, viṅyāsa refers to the steps that must be taken in order to achieve a particular goal.

Such goals might include achieving proficiency in a particular āsana, as demonstrated in the sequences in the chapters on āsana practice; working on a particular area of the structure, as demonstrated in the sequences in the chapters on common aches and pains; or producing an overall effect in the body, as demonstrated in the sequences in the chapters on chronic disease.

In preparing for a particular posture, it is helpful to progressively warm up the body by using simpler postures that move the body in the same direction. For example, simple forward bends can be used to prepare for deeper forward bends, simple back bends can be used to prepare for deeper back bends, et cetera. In making specific choices along these lines, characteristics of the main posture as well as specific body needs should also be considered. The sequences appearing on the following page are good examples for illustrating these principles. Both sequence A and sequence B are preparations for Krauñcāsana, using asymmetrical forward bends, in some cases with both hands holding the foot of the extended leg as in Krauñcāsana itself. **Sequence A shows increased back bend preparation.** If there is an exaggerated thoracic curve, this preparation will help in keeping the chest lifted while stretching the extended leg. **Sequence B shows increased twisting preparation.** If there is tightness in the low back and hips, this preparation will help in keeping the hips rotated forward while one leg is inwardly rotated and folded back.

Sequence A

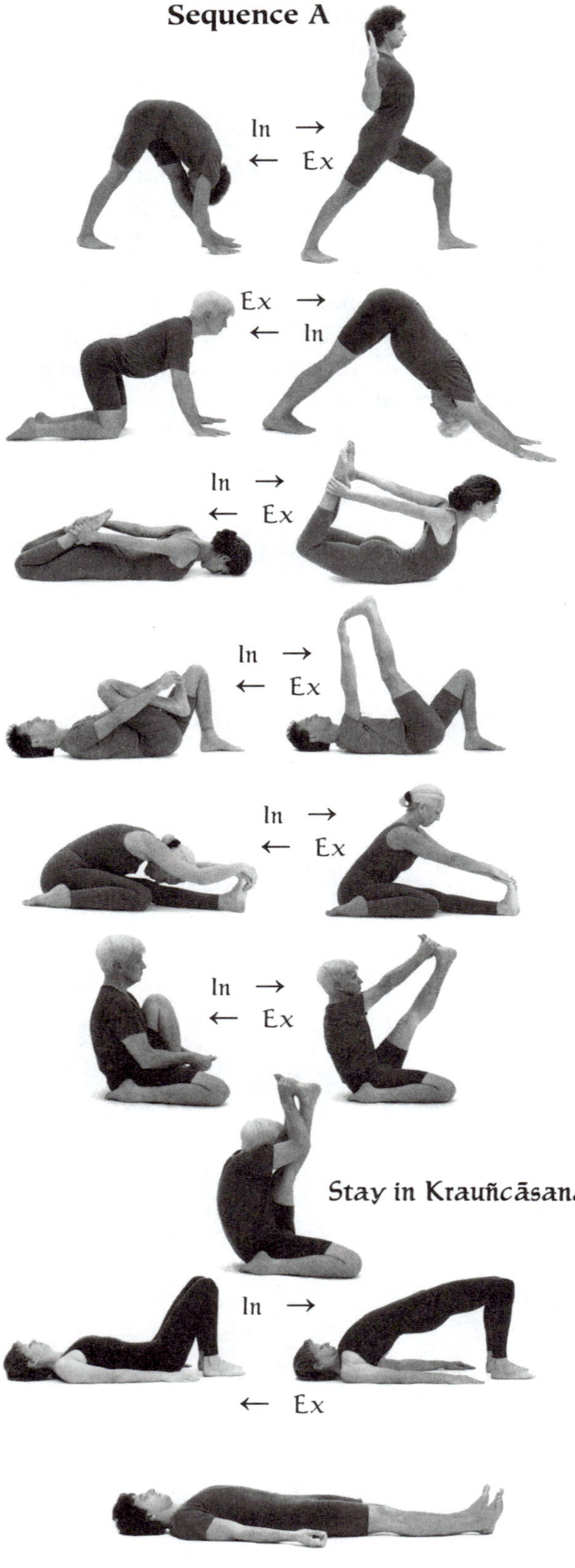

Sequence B

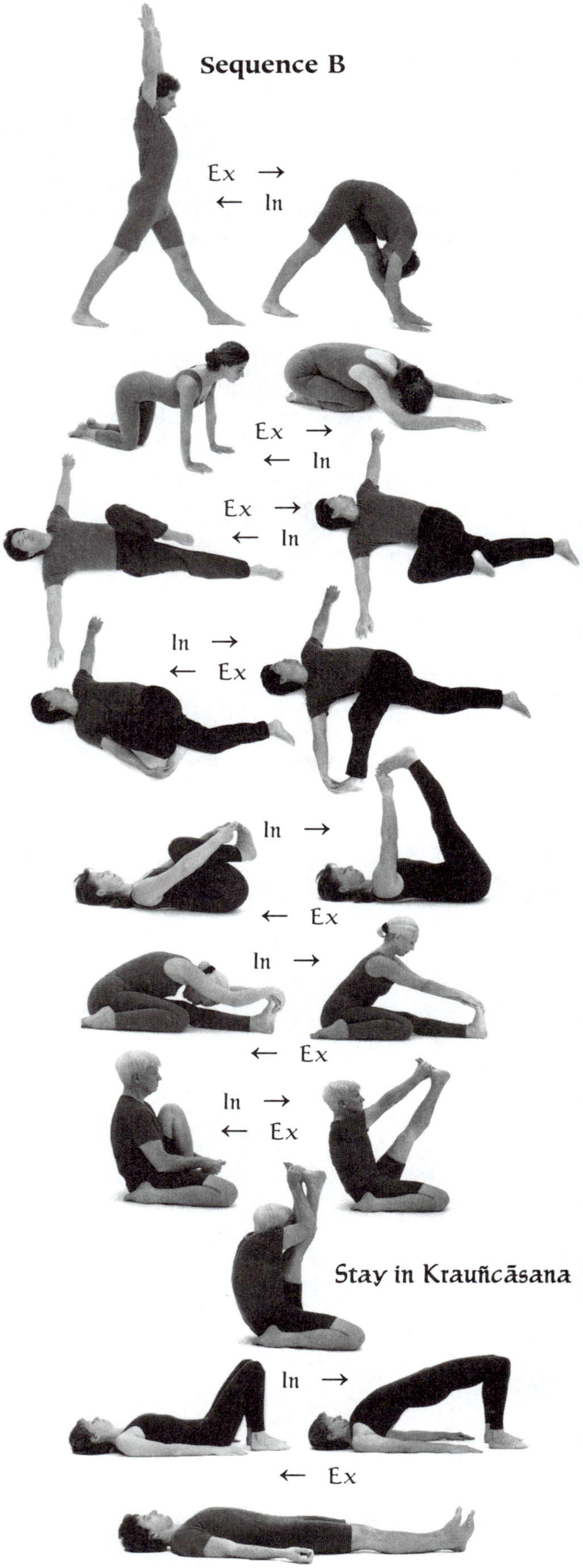

The effectiveness of any posture is influenced by the other postures it is combined with. If you look at the two sequences that appear below, you will notice examples of this interrelationship. **Sequence A shows a general forward bending preparation for Paścimatānāsana.** If there is tightness in the hips and/or low back, this preparation will help you to move further into the posture by progressively working to release the hips and stretch the low back. **Sequence B, on the other hand, shows an unusual back bending preparation for Paścimatānāsana.** If there is excessive looseness in the hips and/or loose low back, this preparation will help you experience the effects of the posture by progressively working to stabilize the hips and tighten the low back.

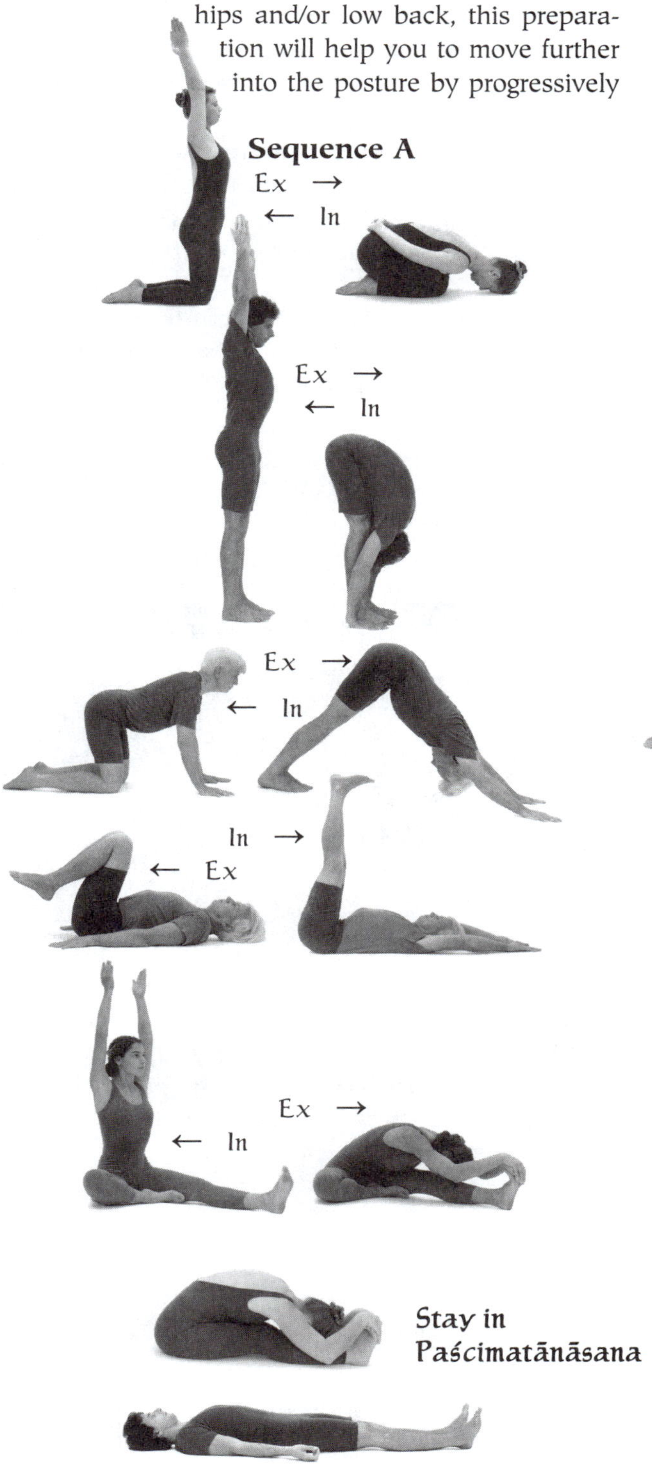
Sequence A
Ex →
← In
Ex →
← In
Ex →
← In
In →
← Ex
Ex →
← In
Stay in Paścimatānāsana

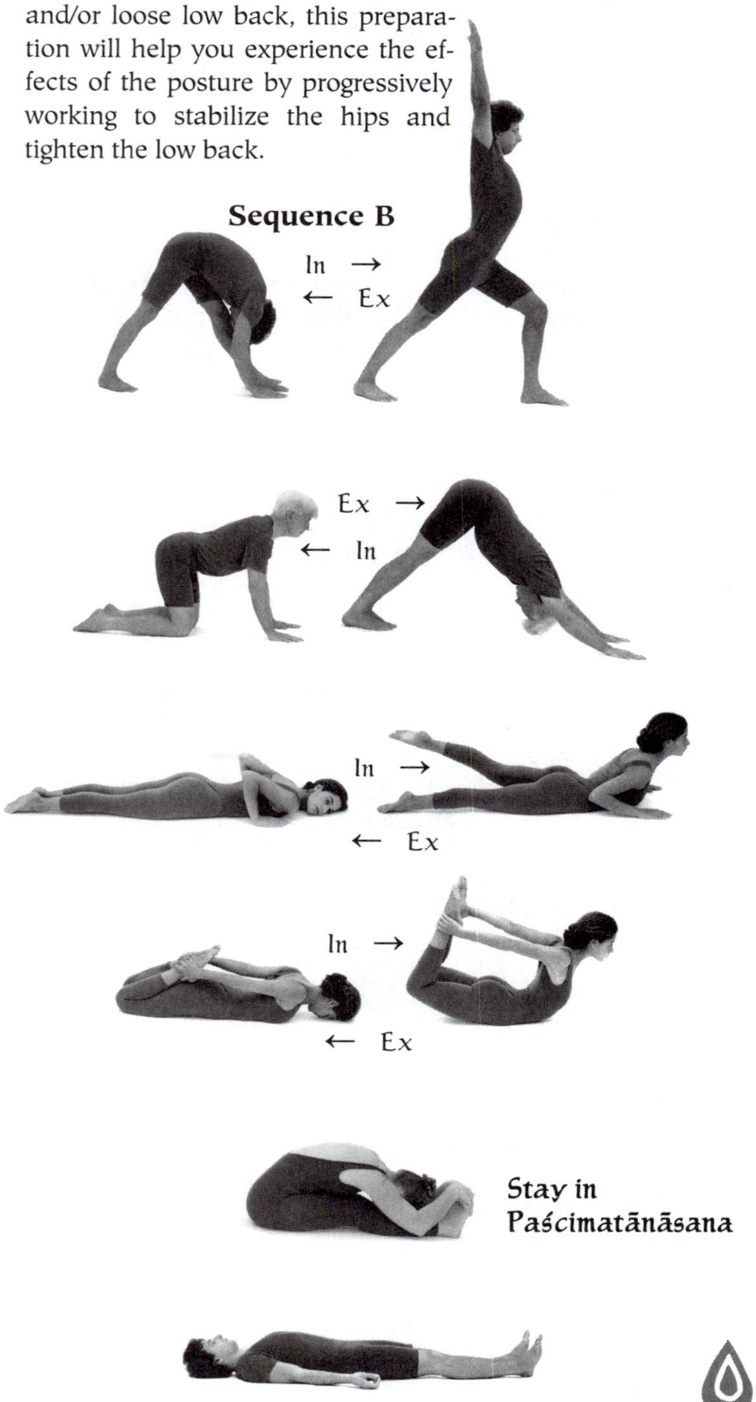
Sequence B
In →
← Ex
Ex →
← In
In →
← Ex
In →
← Ex
Stay in Paścimatānāsana

Pratikriyā

Pratikriyā, literally "counteracting," refers to the compensatory steps required to return the mind, breath, and/or body to a neutral condition. The general idea of pratikriyā is that balance can be progressively restored by moving from the internal to the external, from the complex to the simple, and from the difficult to the easy. For example, simple prāṇāyāma can be used to reintegrate the body and the breath after a complex āsana practice; simple meditation can be used to reintegrate the breath and the mind after a deep prāṇāyāma practice; and simple āsana can be used to reintegrate the mind and the body after a long meditation.

In relation to āsana practice, pratikriyā specifically refers to the steps that can be taken to maintain or restore balance to the body. For example, such steps may be concerned with avoiding stress to a particular part of the body in the midst of a practice, or returning the body to a balanced and neutral condition at the end of a practice. Such appropriate compensation usually involves a simple posture or group of postures that will neutralize the stress accumulated from the preceding ones, and, accordingly, they relate to the specific areas of accumulated stress. For example, on different days you may need different counterposes to the same posture, depending on how your body is responding at the particular moment.

In sequence A below, the counterpose is for the neck and upper back. In sequence B the counterpose is for the lower back.

Sequence A

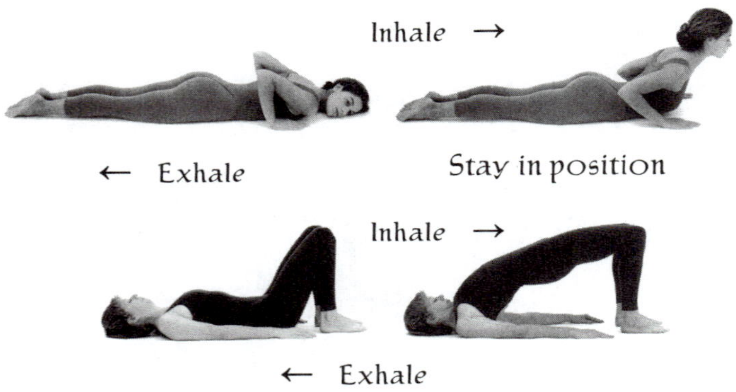

Sequence B

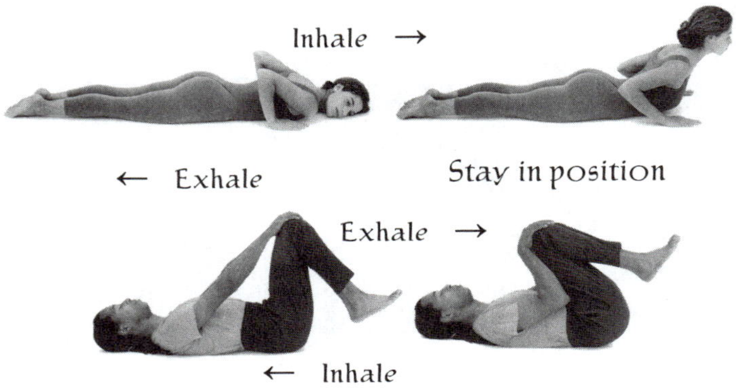

Often several postures will be required to return the body to a balanced and neutral condition. For example, after a deep back bend, you will need to balance the low back, hips, upper back, neck, and shoulders, and the order of these counterposes will depend on the needs of your own body. In sequence **A on the next page, the priority is to the low back and hips. In sequence B, the priority is to the upper back, neck, and shoulders.**

Sequence A

Sequence B

If your aim is to develop your body, challenging postures will be the major focus of your practice. You can begin with simpler movements, build progressively to more challenging postures, neutralize with simpler postures again, and end with a simple prāṇāyāma practice and rest.

If your aim is to develop your breath, prāṇāyāma will be the major focus of your practice. In this case, you can begin with some simple āsana practice to prepare the body and breath, then start the prāṇāyāma simply and move progressively into deeper and/or more complex techniques, neutralize with simpler breathing again, and end with a simple meditation and rest.

If your aim is to develop your mind, meditation will be the major focus of your practice. With this focus, you can begin with simple āsana, prāṇāyāma, and chanting to prepare the body, breath, and mind for the practice; then move into the meditation practice, and end with some simple āsana, to relieve any structural stress from extended sitting; and rest.

If your aim is to open your mind and heart to the sacred dimension of life, prayer and ritual will be the major focus of your practice. However, āsana, prāṇāyāma, chanting, and meditation can also be an integral part of your practice, helping to prepare for the pinnacle of the practice as well as to reintegrate to normal awareness after it is finished.

And if your aim is to do a therapeutic practice, any combination of the above elements may be appropriate, depending upon your condition.

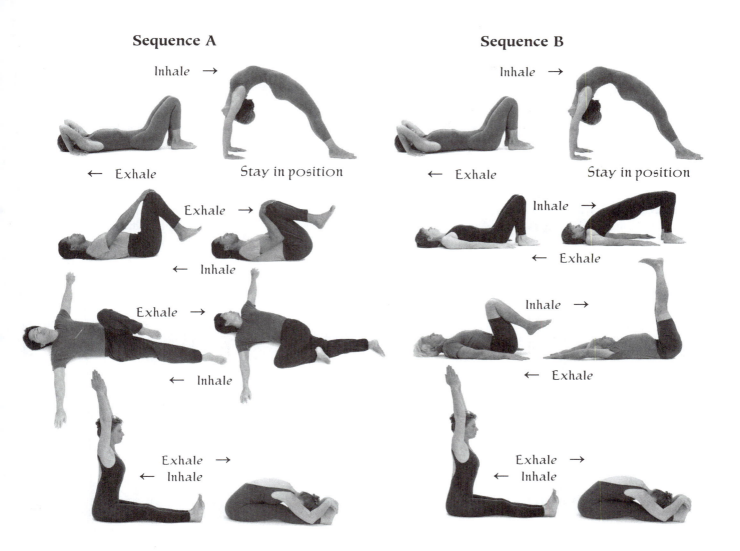

General Principles for Designing an Āsana Sequence

1. ***Intention:*** Set an intention or goal for your practice. For example, your intention may be to achieve certain postures, to work a certain area or condition in your body, or to prepare for a prāṇāyāma and/or meditation practice.

2. ***Efficiency:*** Limit the number of postures and adaptations. Link your choices purposefully to the intention of your practice. A focused course can be more powerful, useful, and specific than a general one. In fact, too many postures can dilute the effect of the practice, just as eating too many foods at one meal can limit (overload) the body's ability to absorb the nutrients.

3. ***Breath:*** Use the breath to link your attention to the spine and to move the spine. Maintain a deep and even breathing pattern throughout the practice. Use retention of the breath purposefully, and link it to the overall intention of the practice.

4. ***Transition:*** Take time to make the transition from other activities into your practice. Also within the practice, make transitions smooth. For example, use kneeling postures to transition from standing postures to postures on your back or stomach.

5. ***Cumulative stress:*** Use appropriate compensation for stresses that accumulate in the neck, shoulders, hips, and knees. For example, use arm movements to release stress accumulated in the shoulders from postures where the arms are fixed.

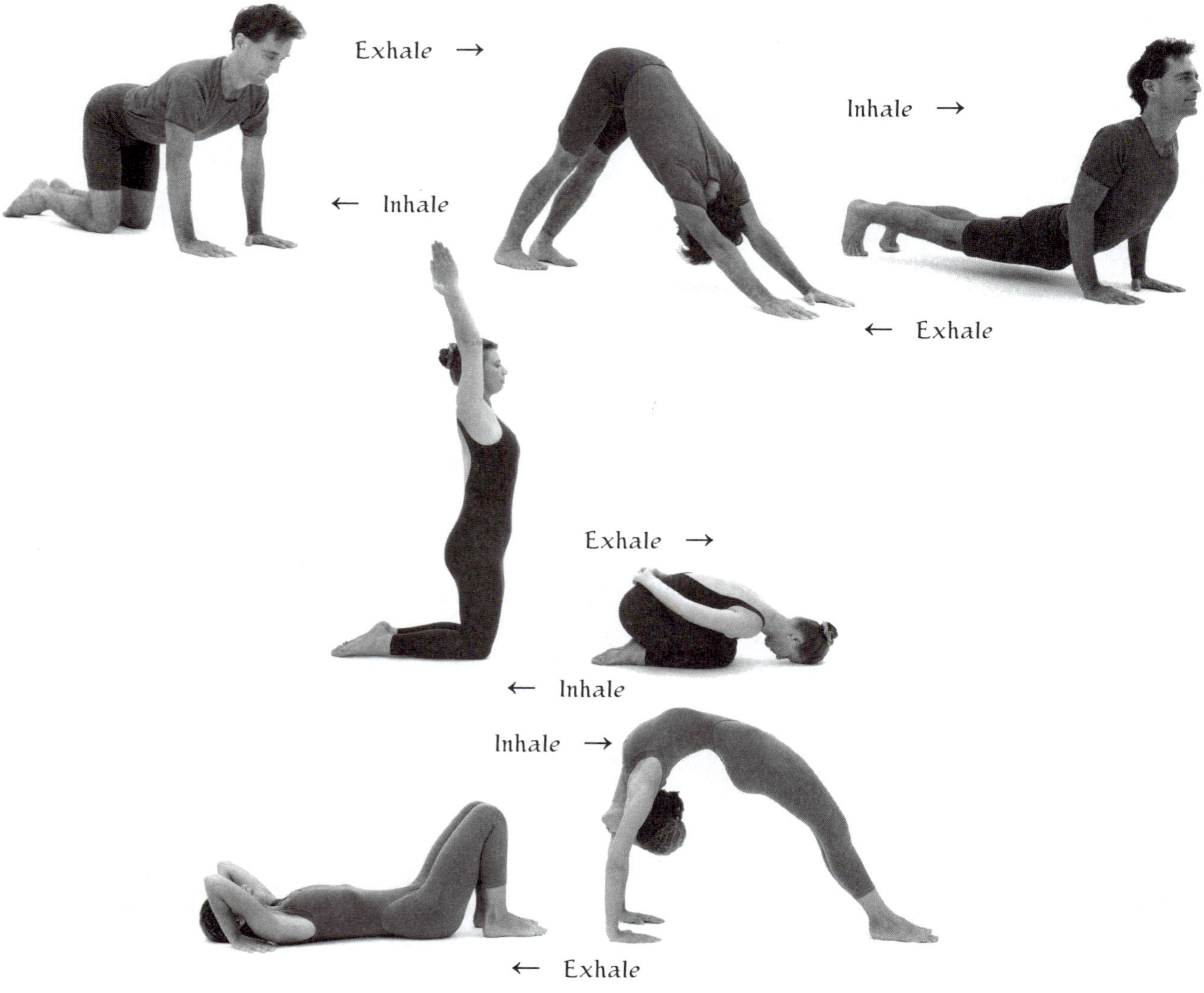

6. ***Risk:*** Postures that are risky for the joints should follow sufficient preparation. Usually, riskier postures are placed toward the end of the practice, followed by simple counterposes to leave the body in a neutral condition.

7. ***Rest:*** Use rest appropriately. For example, rest when the breath becomes unsteady, after difficult postures, or when transitioning from one direction to another. The position in which you rest should be one in which you feel relaxed and supported without residual stress. A longer rest at the end of the practice is important in order to both absorb more fully the deeper effects of the practice and to make a transition to the next activity.

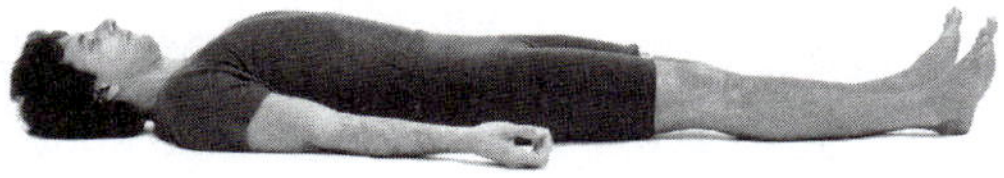

or

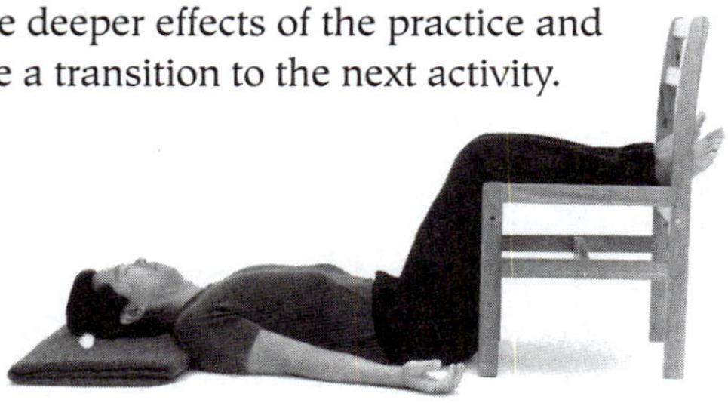

Specific Principles for Posture Combination

In relation to āsana practice, forward bending is considered the hub of the wheel, and back bending, twisting, and lateral bending are considered the spokes. Forward bending is used to transition into and out of other movements. For example, forward bends are used to transition from a back bend to a twist, from a lateral bend to a back bend, and even from a twist to a lateral bend. The following examples can be used as a general guideline for beginning to work with combining postures, respecting their general biomechanical requirements.

Sequence A

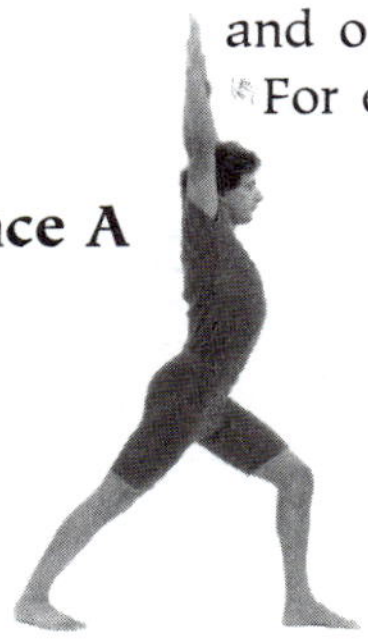

Standing back bend

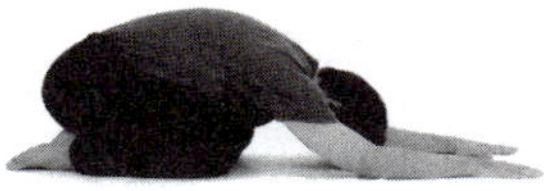

Kneeling forward bend

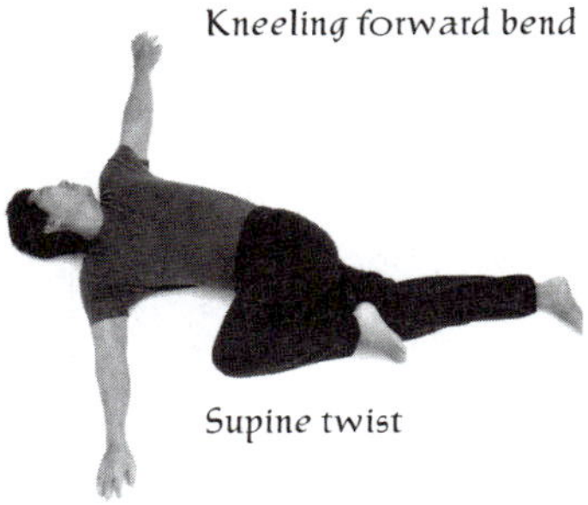

Supine twist

Sequence B

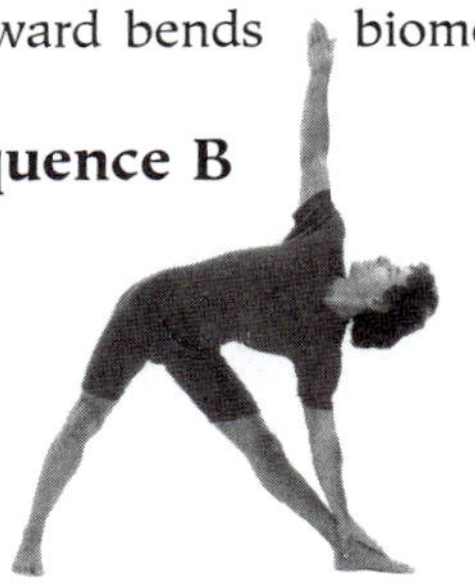

Standing lateral bend

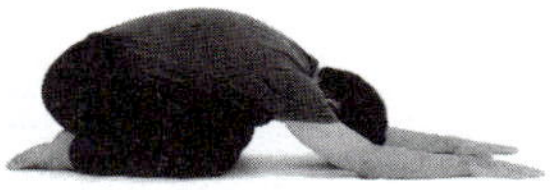

Kneeling forward bend

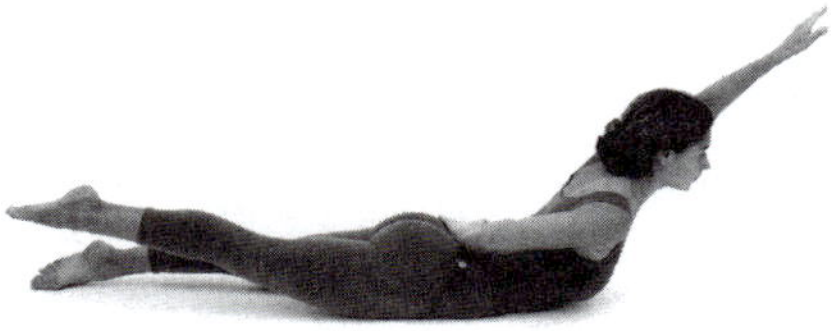

Prone back bend

Sequence C

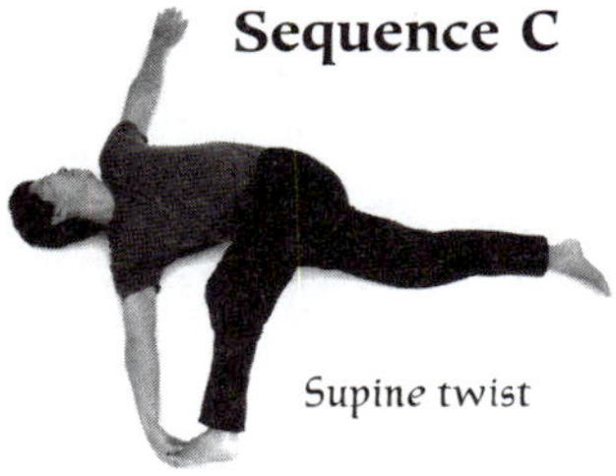

Supine twist

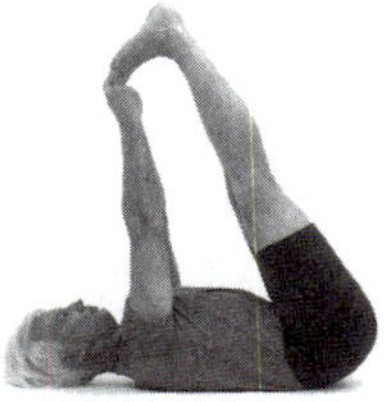

Supine forward bend

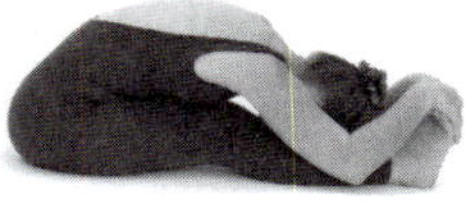

Seated forward bend

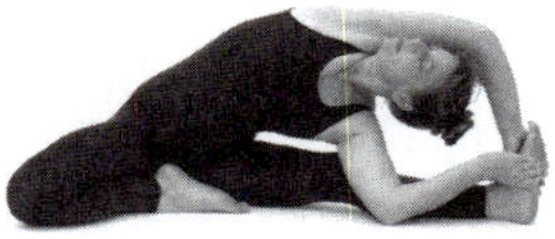

Seated lateral bend

Postures can be done standing, kneeling, on the back, inverted, on the stomach, and seated. Standing and kneeling postures are generally useful for warming up the body. Standing postures are stronger, and kneeling postures more stable. Kneeling postures are good for transitioning from standing to lying on the back or stomach. Postures on the back are generally relaxing, although they can be adapted to create deep stretching of the legs, hips, and low back as well as the neck and shoulders. They can also be good preparation for inverted postures. Both headstand and shoulder stand require good preparation and compensation and are therefore usually placed between half and two-thirds of the way through the practice. In the Viniyoga tradition, the shoulderstand is considered the classic counterpose to headstand. Postures on the stomach can be good compensation for the shoulderstand; generally stronger than other postures, they are useful for strengthening and stabilizing the back, and they are also good preparation for deeper back bends. Seated postures generally place more stress on the low back; they can be good compensation for deeper back bends; they are also good preparation for the extended sitting required in prāṇāyāma and/or meditation; and they are usually placed at the end of the practice.

Respecting these principles, different strategies can be used for combining postures. For example, if you are tired in the morning and want to warm up slowly and then go off to work, you may begin lying on your back, transition through your knees to standing, and end resting on a chair. If, on the other hand, you come home form work in the evening feeling hyperactive, and want to relax before going to sleep, you may begin standing and transition through your knees to lying on your back.

Chapter 2

Biomechanics of Movement

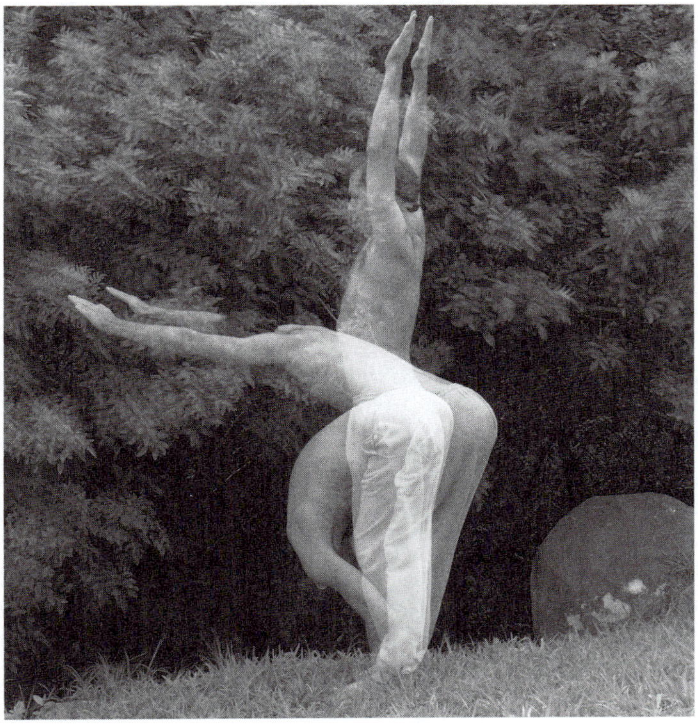

Stretching the West: An Introduction to Forward Bends

Primary and Secondary Intentions

Facing the rising sun as they practiced, the ancient yogis called forward bending "stretching the west." Forward bends stretch and strengthen the back portion of the spine, shoulder and pelvic girdles, and legs. They stretch and strengthen the entire length of the erector spinae muscles, which extend all the way from the sacrum to the cervical spine; the deep spinal extensor muscles and intervertebral ligaments, which interconnect and stabilize each vertebrae; the posterior muscles, which bind the shoulder girdle to the spine; and the posterior muscles of the pelvis and legs. In addition they strengthen the abdominal muscles, which contract as we bend forward; gently compress the abdominal organs (particularly the intestines), providing a visceral massage; and stretch the kidney/adrenal area, stimulating the function of these organs.

From a biomechanical perspective, according to

the Viniyoga tradition, the *primary intention* of forward bending is to stretch the structures of the lumbo-sacral spine.

Above the lumbar spine, the *secondary intention* of forward bending is to stretch the posterior structures of the upper back, shoulder girdle, and neck.

Below the lumbar spine, the secondary intention of forward bending is to stretch the posterior musculature of the pelvic girdle and legs, particularly the hamstrings.

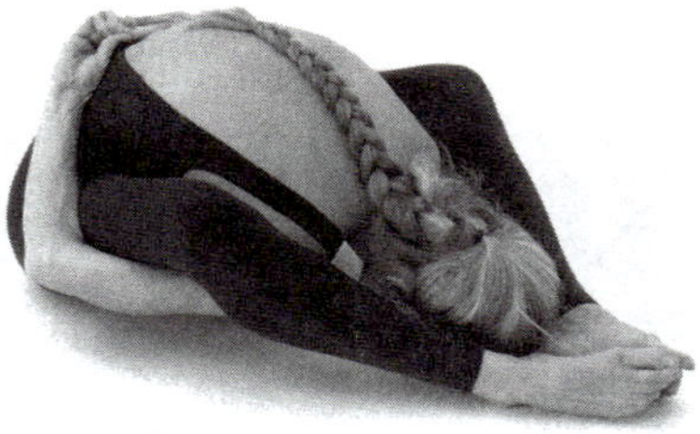
Kūrmāsana

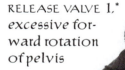

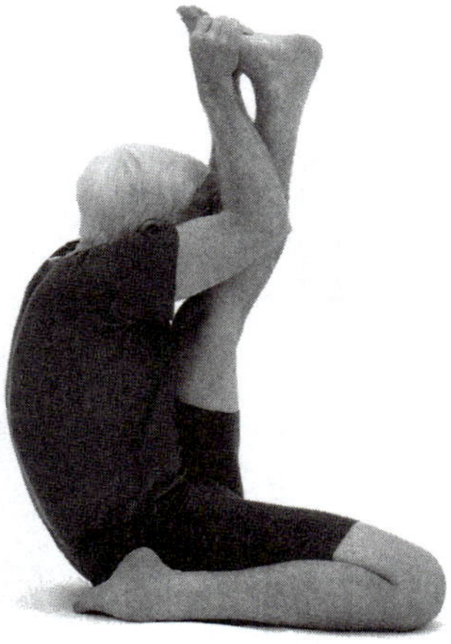
Krauñcāsana

Technique

The key to forward bends is the ability to control the proportional relation between the progressive flattening and potential reversal of our lumbar curvature and the forward rotation of our pelvis at the hip joints.

The proportional relation between these two actions is known as *lumbar-pelvic rhythm.* In normal activity, we are usually unaware of this rhythm and, therefore, one aspect is often overemphasized.

Forward rotation of the pelvis may be excessive because of actual structural conditions, such as loose hip ligaments and tight low back muscles, or the result of training: for example, due to habitually bending from the hips with a "straight" back in standing forward bends. Bending in this way, in fact, increases the contraction of the low back muscles, inhibiting effective stretching, and places tremendous stress on the musculature, ligaments, and tendons of the hip joints. The possible long-term result of this practice is instability in the hip joints, chronic contraction of the lumbar muscles, and posterior intervertebral disc compression.

Reversal of the lumbar curve may be excessive because of actual structural conditions, such as tight hip ligaments and leg muscles (hamstrings), which restrict pelvic rotation, or the result of training: for example habitually insisting on straight legs in seated forward bends.

RELEASE VALVE 1,* excessive forward rotation of pelvis

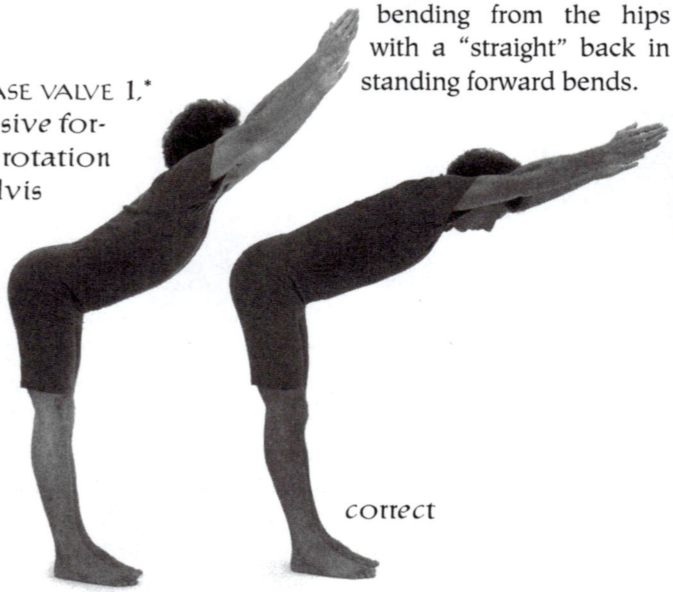

correct

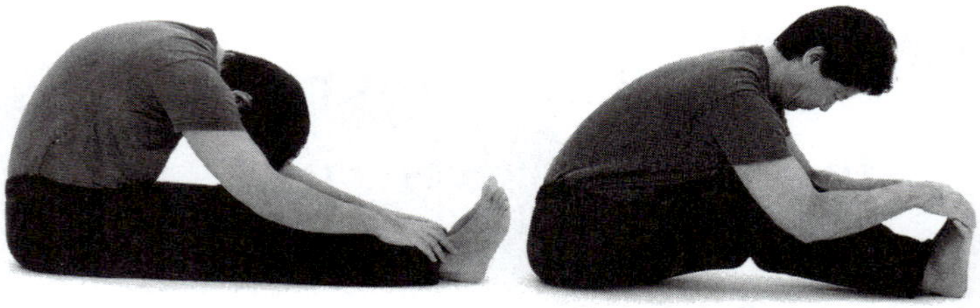

RELEASE VALVE 2, chest collapsed over belly

correct

* For a list of common release valves for forward bends, see page 44.

Bending in this way may, in fact, lead to a backward rotation of the pelvis and to a collapsing of the chest over the belly at the thoracic-lumbar junction. The possible long-term result of this practice is anterior intervertebral disc compression.

Low back pain is often the direct result of a poor mechanical relationship between the lumbar spine and pelvis. In fact, many chronic low back conditions originate in forward bended positions. And yet, it is also through the forward bend that we can improve our lumbar-pelvic rhythm and thereby strengthen and stabilize our body.

The key to the lumbar-pelvic rhythm, and therefore all forward bends, is the technique of abdominal contraction on exhale. At the initiation of exhalation, contract the abdominal muscles at their insertion into the pubic bone, thereby checking excessive forward rotation of the pelvis, promoting progressive reversal of the lumbar spine, and maximizing the stretching of the low back.

If you have either a deep lumbar curve and/or very loose hips, lift the pubic bone slightly upward at the beginning of the forward bend and focus on the stretching of the low back.

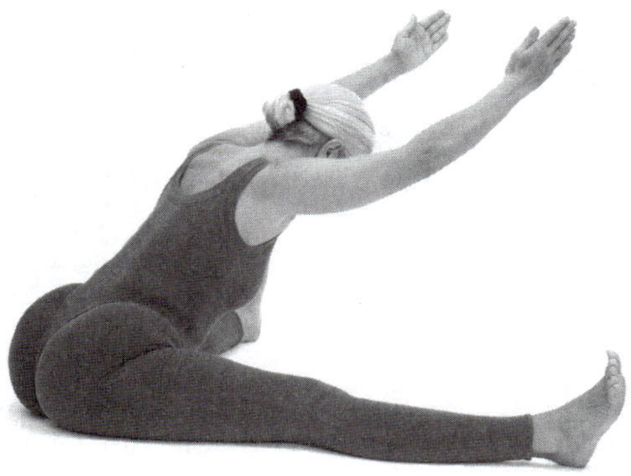

for deep lumbar curve
and loose hips (RELEASE VALVE 1),

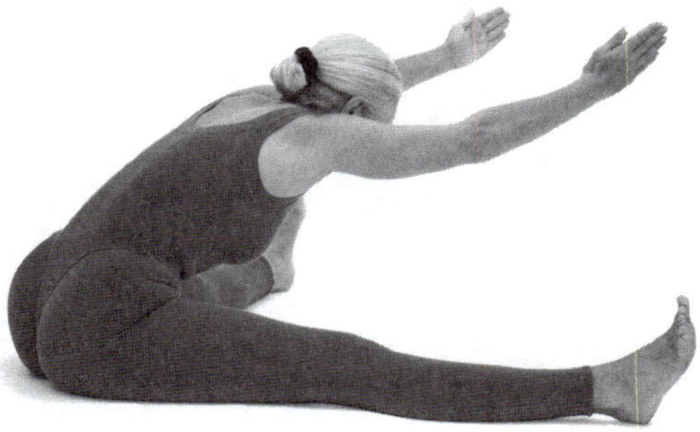

lift pubic bone

If you have tight hips, encourage the pelvis to rotate forward and focus on the stretching of the low back. In either case, be careful to avoid anterior compression of your lumbar spine.

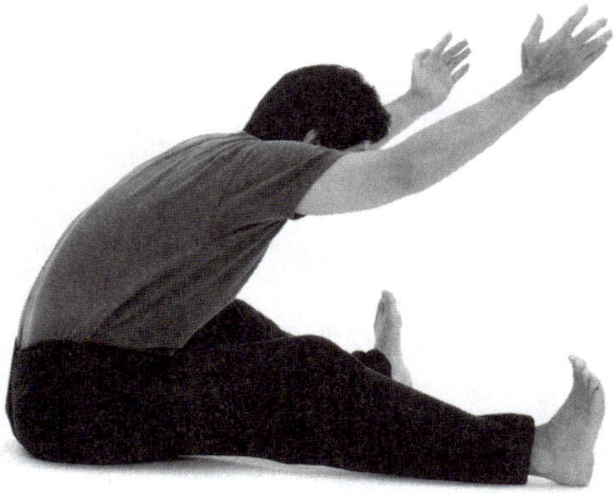

for tight hips,

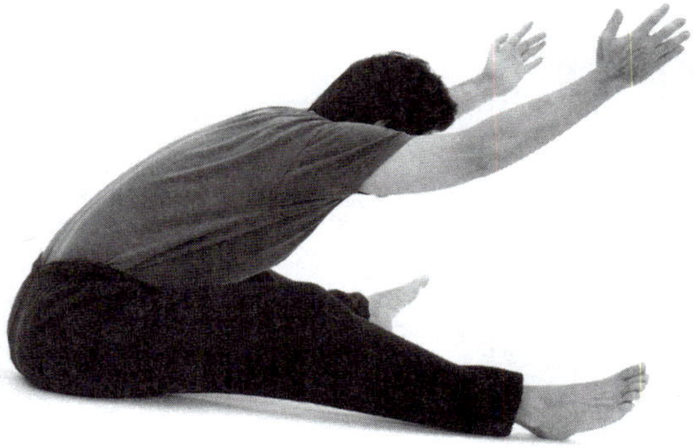

rotate pelvis forward

As the forward bend proceeds, contract your abdominal muscles from the pubic bone to the navel. Bend your knees progressively throughout the movement, as much as necessary to feel the maximum stretching of your low back without strain.

The natural curve of the thoracic spine may create a tendency to collapse the rib cage over the belly as you bend forward. This can be avoided by lengthening between the chest and belly on inhale and maintaining that length throughout the forward bend. This is especially important if your thoracic curve is naturally excessive. If, on the other hand, your thoracic curve is slightly flattened, then you can allow it to round slightly as you bend.

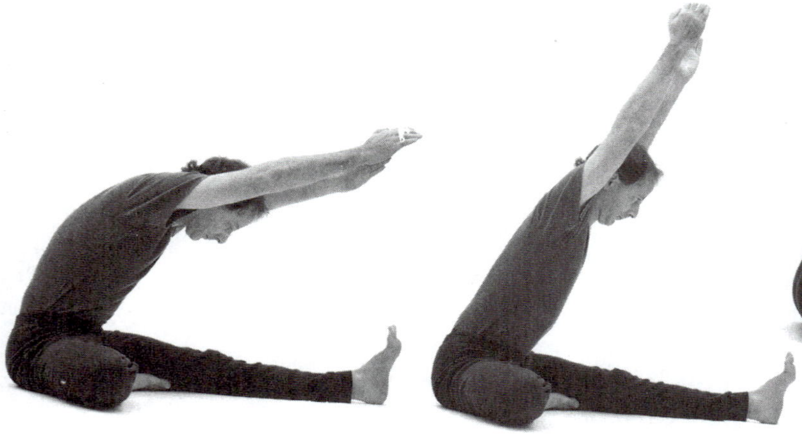

for excessive thoracic curve, lift chest away from belly

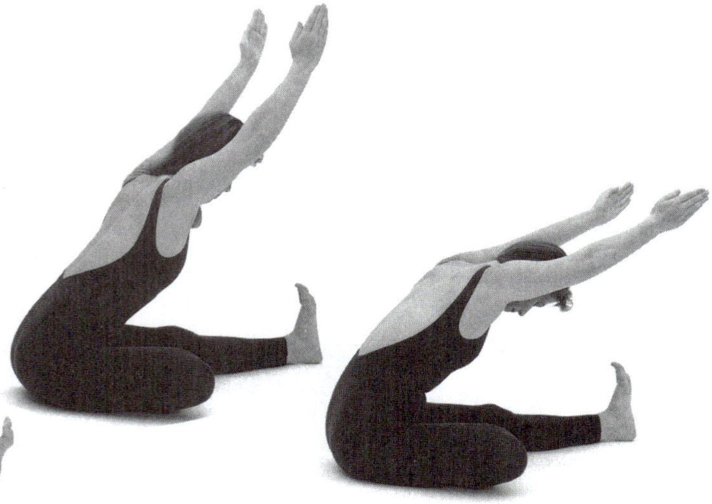

for flattened thoracic curve, allow upper back to round

In coming up from a forward bend, lead with your chest from the initiation of inhale, pulling the entire thoracic cavity away from the abdomen and stretching in the solar plexus area. Maintain a partial abdominal contraction on the way up, preventing your pelvis from rotating excessively forward, in order to protect your low back from strain (particularly in standing postures).

RELEASE VALVE 3,
excessive forward rotation

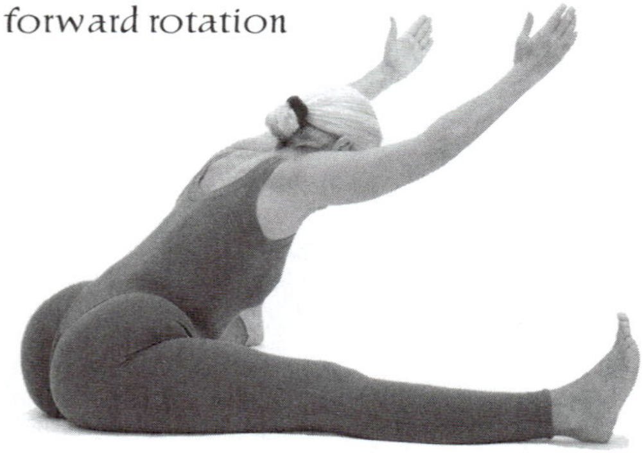

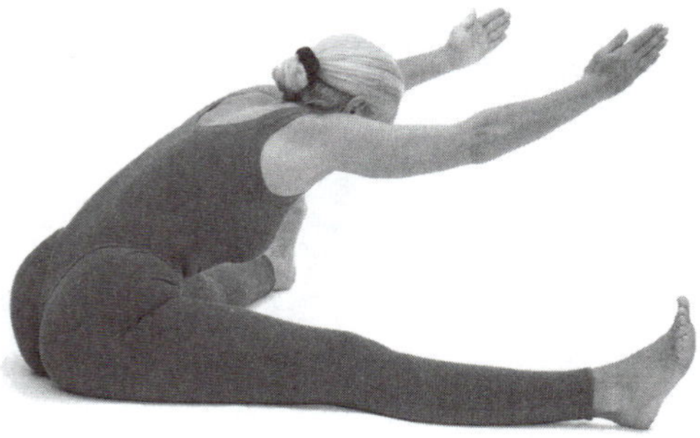

correct

This will also facilitate elevating the rib cage and reversing any exaggeration of the thoracic curve.

Though the cervical spine can flex easily, many people tend to arch their necks in the process of bending forward, either because of actual structural conditions, such as tightness in the muscles of the upper back and neck, or because of training: for example, habitually lifting the chin while bending forward.

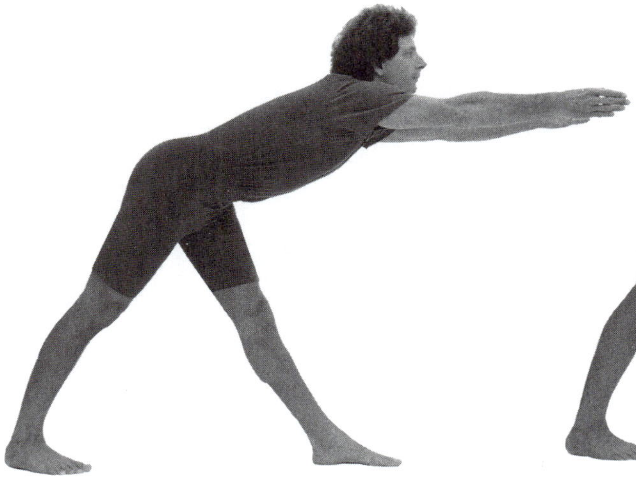

RELEASE VALVE 4, increased cervical arch

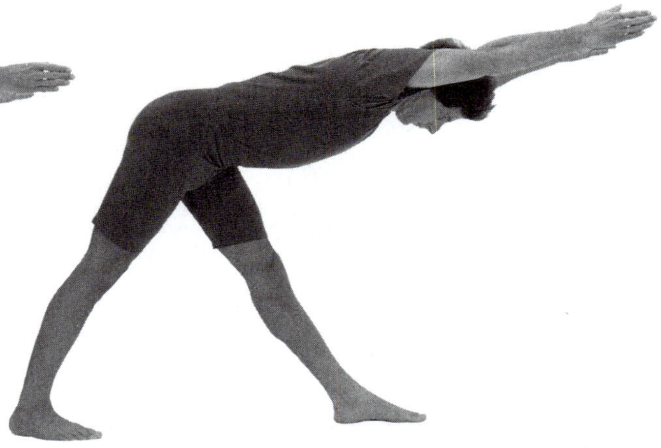

correct

This practice, over time, creates tension in the neck and shoulders, may lead to headaches, and also limits the effectiveness of the forward bend itself. Instead, we suggest that you tuck the chin in gently toward the throat while displacing the head slightly backward, until the ears are aligned above the shoulders. This technique straightens the cervical curve, helps straighten the thoracic curve, and increases the stretching of the muscles of the upper back and neck.

Raising the arms overhead, in coordination with the movement of the thoracic cavity on inhale, aids the extension of the spinal curves. Classically, the arms, chest, and head are held in alignment while moving into and out of forward bends. However, as this technique may create tension in the neck and shoulders, the arm position can be adapted to minimize stress and/or emphasize a particular effect.

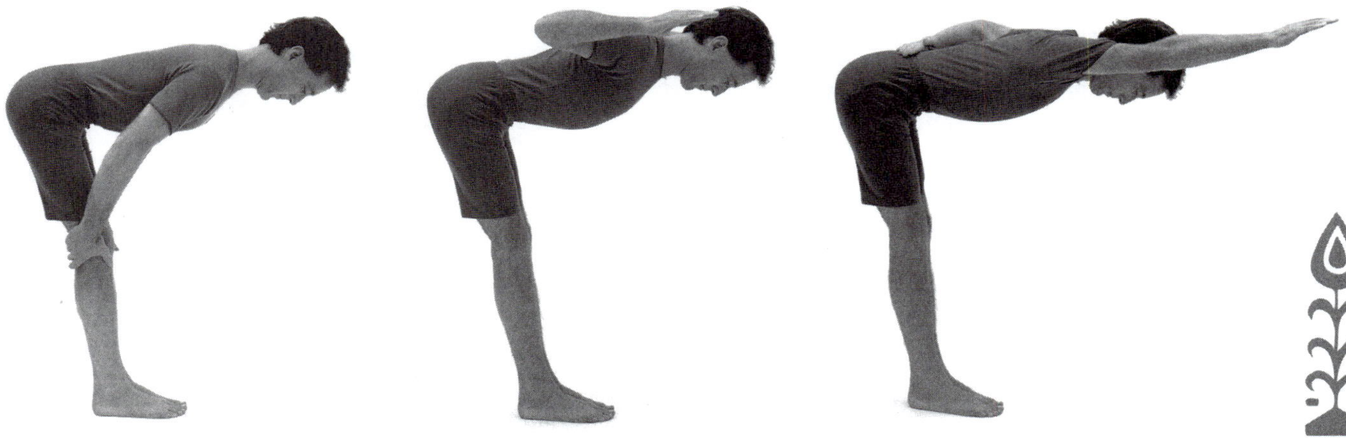

Further examples of arm variations can be seen in the therapy section later in the book. **In general, to avoid tension, it is important to allow the arms and/or head to follow the lead of the spine, rather than to themselves lead.**

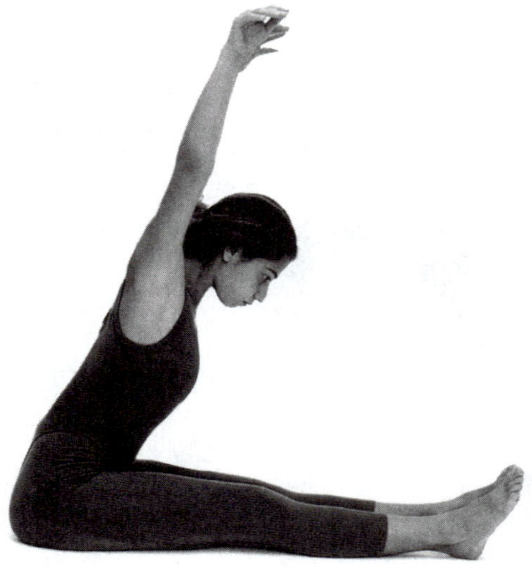

shoulder tension

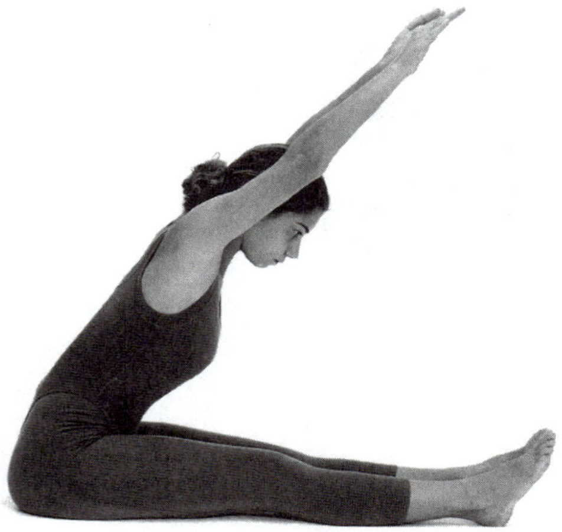

correct

Forward bends can be done supine (on the back), kneeling, standing, and seated. Supine and kneeling postures are generally simple, stable, and safe. Standing postures allow the greatest range of unrestricted motion and, therefore, are usually safe and effective for warming up and working the large musculature of the spine, pelvis, and legs. Seated postures are the most restricted, and while they provide the deepest stretching, they also incur the greatest risk to the musculature and ligaments of the spine, shoulders, pelvis, and legs.

Types of Forward Bends

♦ GROUP 1

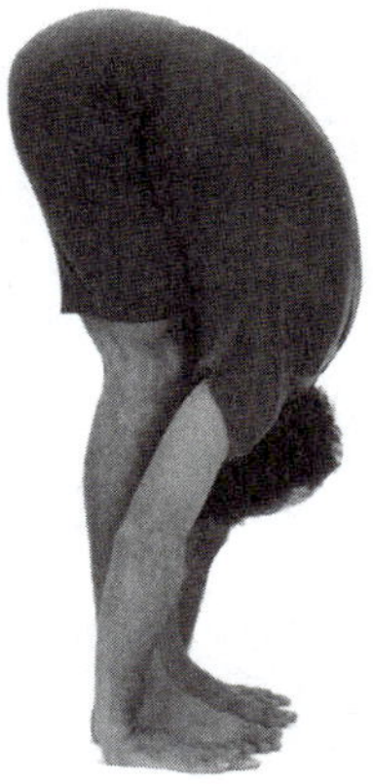

Uttānāsana

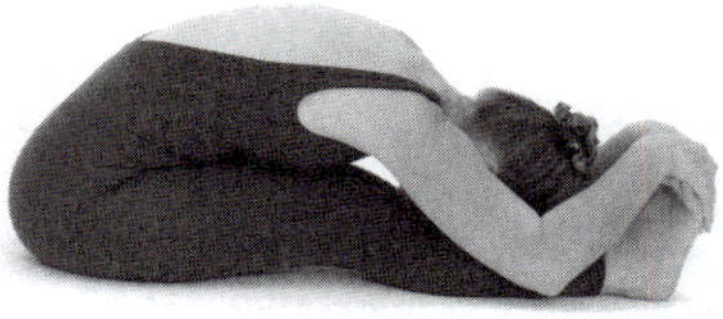

Paścimatānāsana

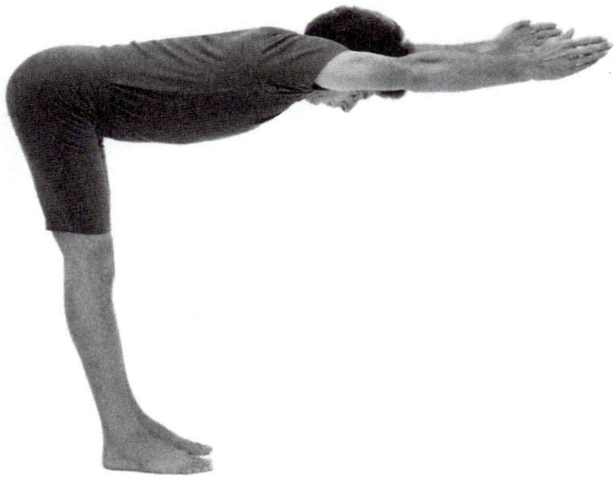

Ardha Uttānāsana

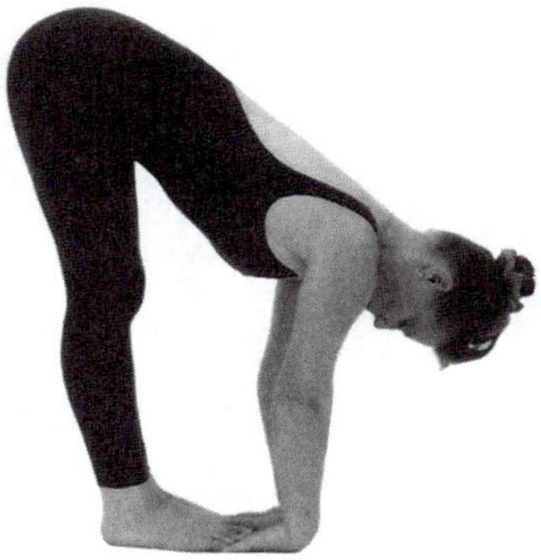

Pādahastāsana

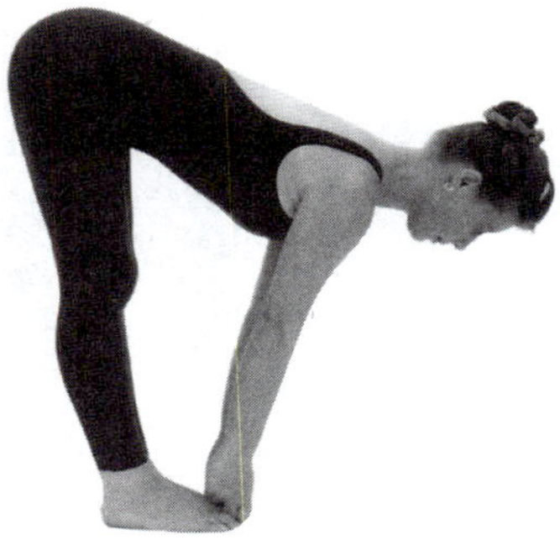

Pādāṅguṣṭhāsana

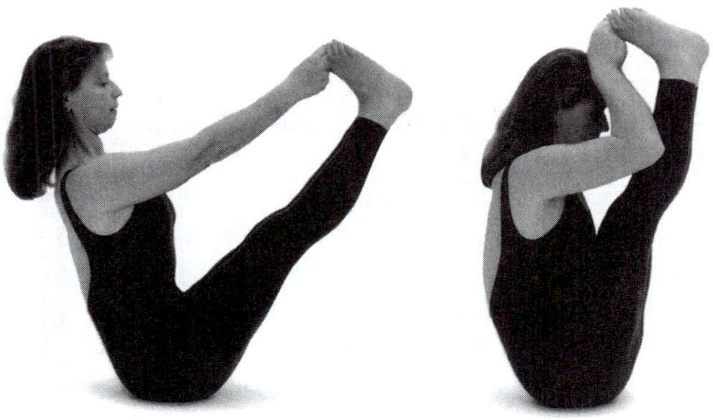

Ubhaya Pādāṅguṣṭhāsana

The first group of postures includes open- and fixed-frame symmetric standing and seated forward bends, with the legs extended and feet close together. Although classically the feet are together, we suggest that they remain slightly apart, vertically below the thigh bone's (femur) junction (acetabulum) with the pelvis.

Ardha Uttānāsana builds strength in the posterior spinal musculature.

Pādahastāsana, Pādāṅguṣṭhāsana, and Ubhaya Pādāṅguṣṭhāsana are fixed-frame postures. The leverage created when the hands hold the feet deepens the forward bend. Paścimatānāsana can also be adapted as a fixed-frame posture.

♦ GROUP 2

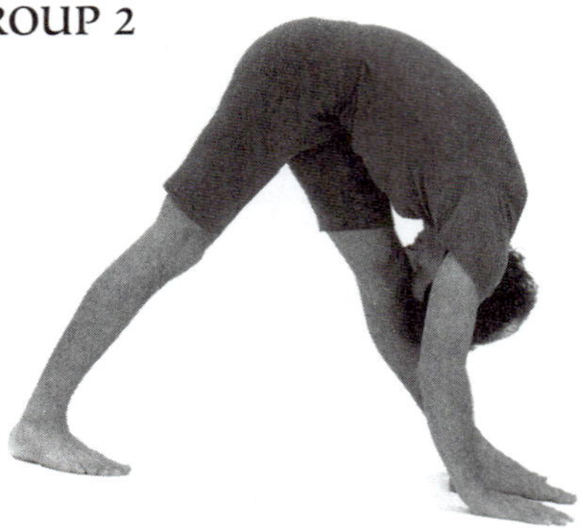

Pārśvottānāsana

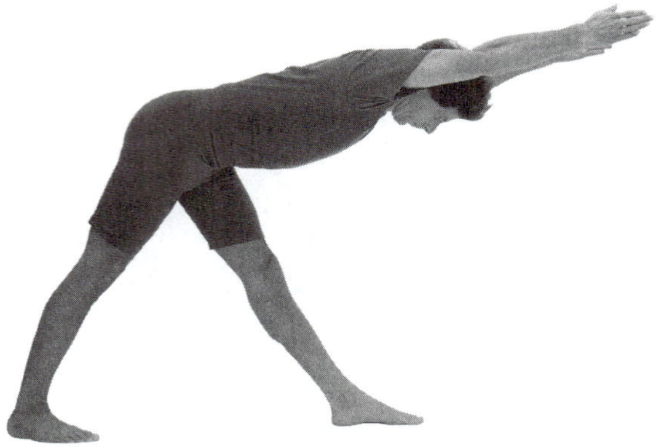

Ardha Pārśvottānāsana

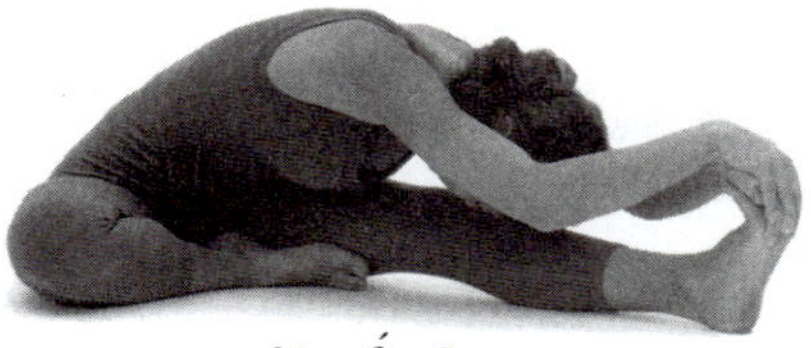

Jānu Śirṣāsana

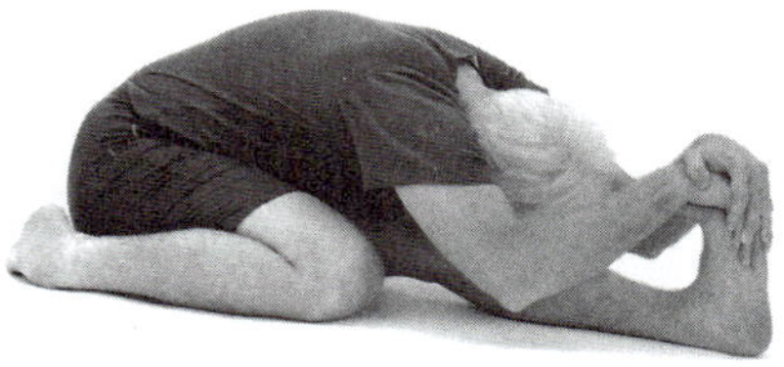

Tiryaṅgmukha Ekapāda Paścimatānāsana

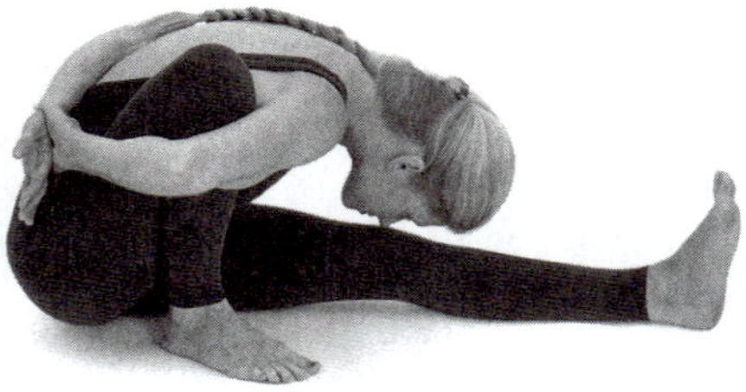

Marīcyāsana

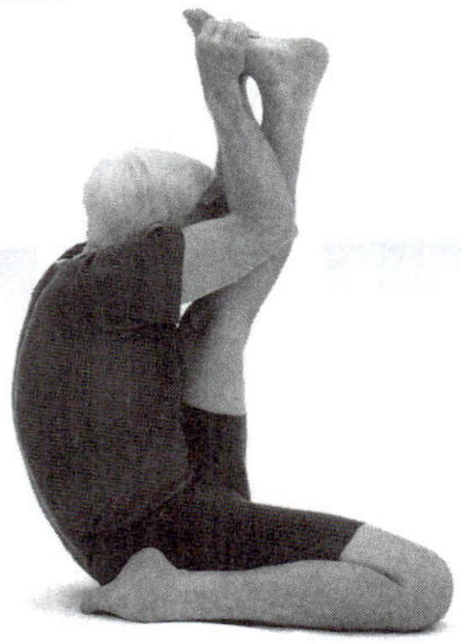

Krauñcāsana

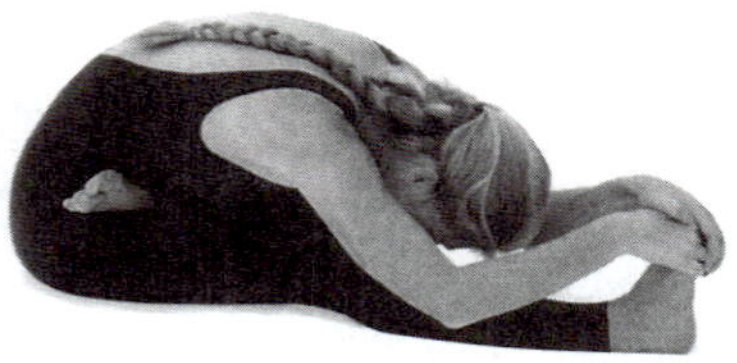

Ardha Padma Paścimatānāsana

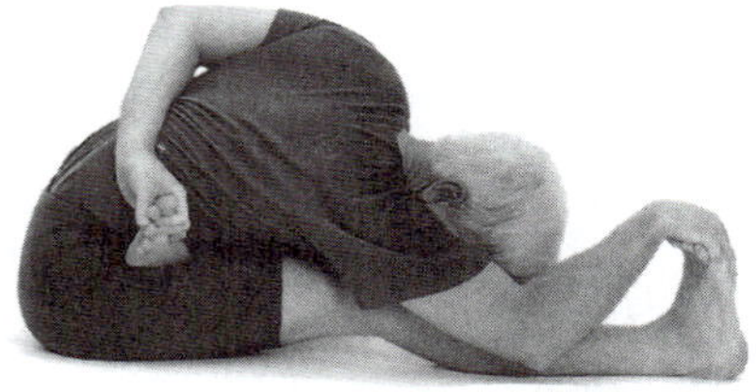

Ardha Baddha Padma Paścimatānāsana

This group of postures includes open- and fixed-frame asymmetric standing and seated forward bends. In the seated forward bends, one leg is extended and the other folded and rotated either externally or internally. The position of the leg significantly influences the effect of the forward bends. Generally, asymmetric positions isolate and intensify the stretching effects on one side of the back and in one leg. Ardha Pārśvottānāsana builds strength in the muscles of the back.

Marīcyāsana, Krauñcāsana, Ardha Padma Paścimatānāsana, and Ardha Baddha Padma Paścimatānāsana are fixed-frame postures, using the arms and legs as levers in different ways to modify and deepen the effects of the postures. Marīcyāsana stretches the deep and superficial posterior muscles that bind the shoulder and arm to the spine. Krauñcāsana strongly stretches the back of the extended leg. Ardha Baddha Padma Paścimatānāsana strongly stretches the hip rotators of the folded leg.

♦ GROUP 3

This group of postures includes open- and fixed-frame symmetric forward bends, in which the knees are near the chest and the buttocks near the heels. This position offers a safe and effective stretching of the lower back. Apānāsana is the simplest of all forward bends. Utkaṭāsana strongly develops the big muscles of the thighs.

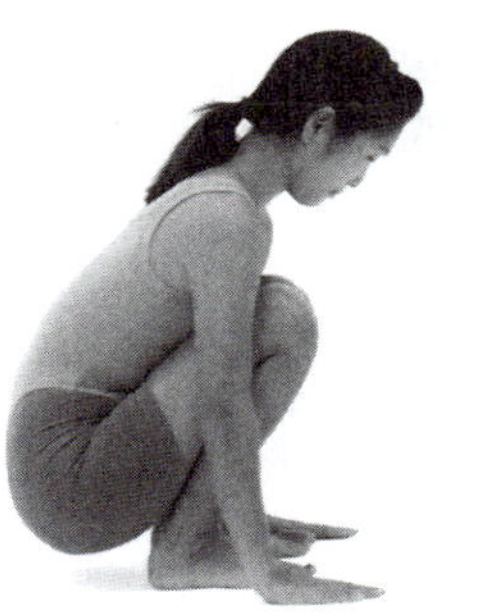

Utkaṭāsana

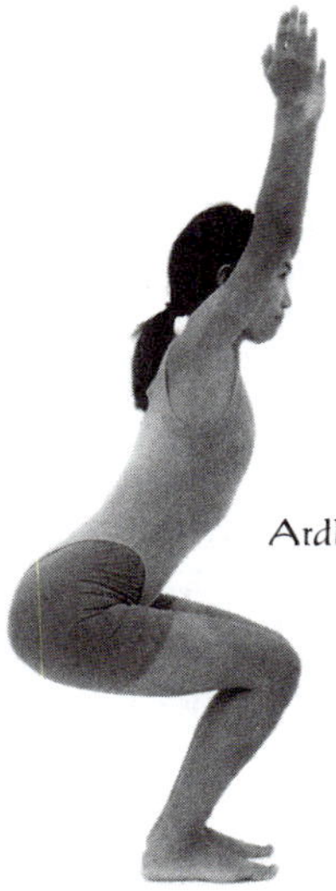

Ardha Utkaṭāsana

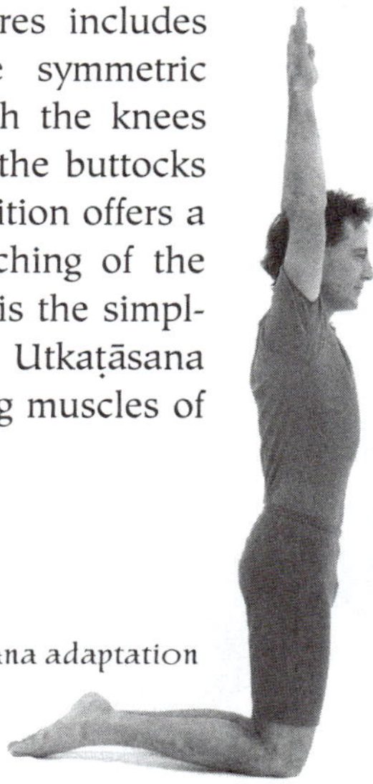

Vajrāsana adaptation

Exhale →
← Inhale

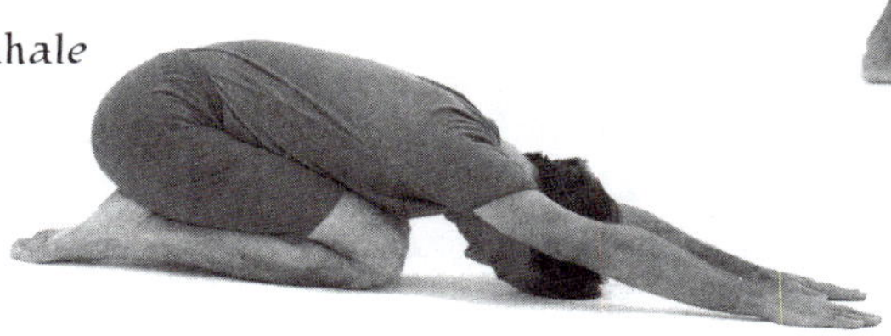

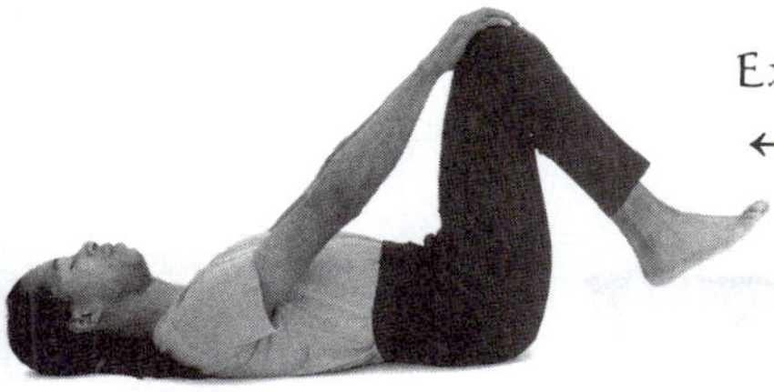

Exhale →
← Inhale

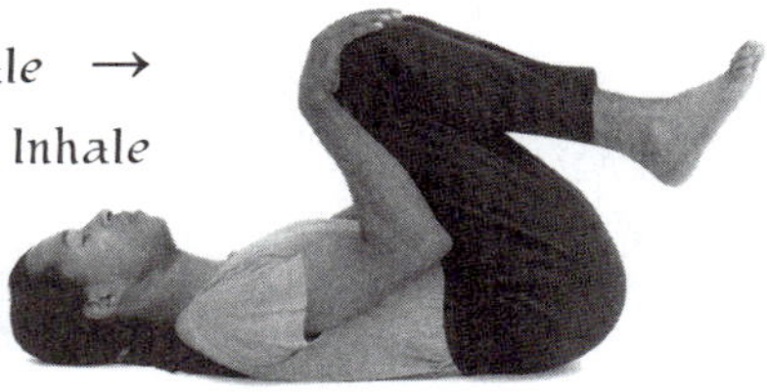

Apānāsana

♦ GROUP 4

This group of postures includes open- and fixed-frame symmetric standing and seated forward bends with spread legs. This position of the legs facilitates the forward rotation of the pelvis and increases the stretching of the inner thighs.

In Kūrmāsana, the arms wrap under the legs and the hands are grasped behind the back. The leverage generated by the arms and legs makes this one of the deepest forward bends. If you can master this posture, you will experience the truly calming and internalizing potential of forward bends.

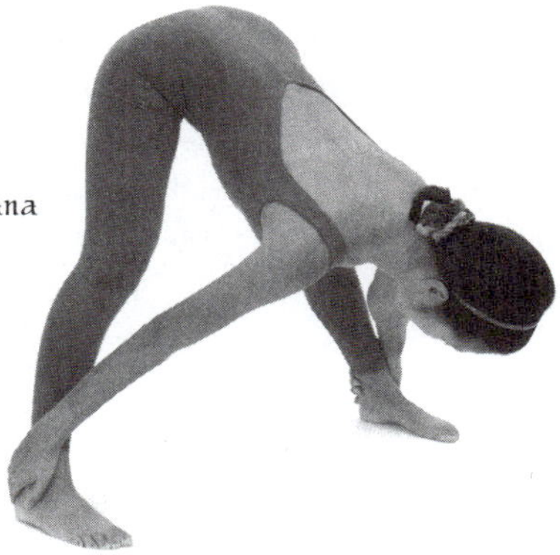

Prasarīta Pādottānāsana

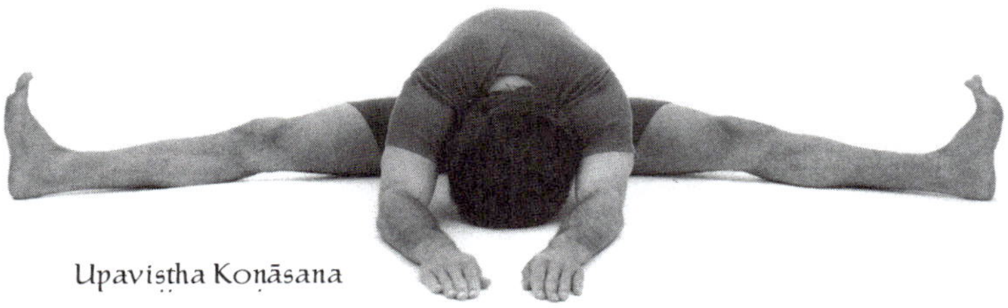

Upaviṣṭha Koṇāsana

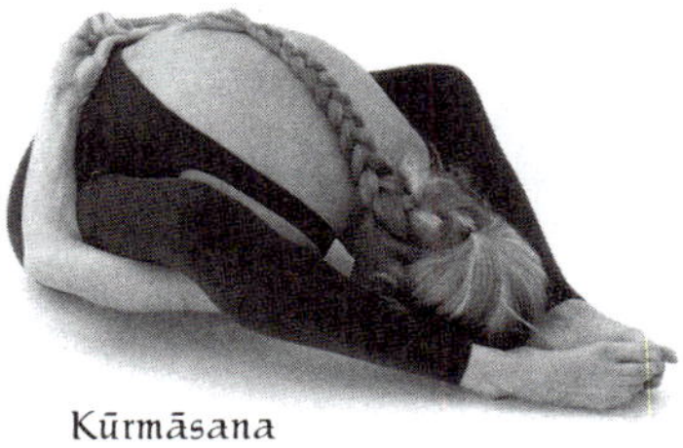

Kūrmāsana

Common Release Valves for Forward Bends

1. Rotating the pelvis excessively forward allows the lumbar curve to remain intact during a forward bend, preventing an effective stretch of the low back.
2. Collapsing the chest over the belly limits the ability to achieve extension of the spine, increases the risk of anterior compression, and inhibits the stretching of the low back, the upper back, and the neck.
3. Pivoting from the lumbar spine when coming out of forward bends, rather than lifting from the upper back, limits the benefits in the chest and upper back, while increaing the risks of compression in the low back.
4. Jutting the chin forward, increasing the cervical arch, when going into or coming out of forward bends, creates tension in the neck and prevents the full stretching of the upper back.
5. Rotating the hips, knees, or feet excessively inward or outward limits the full stretching of the muscles of the low back, pelvis, and legs.

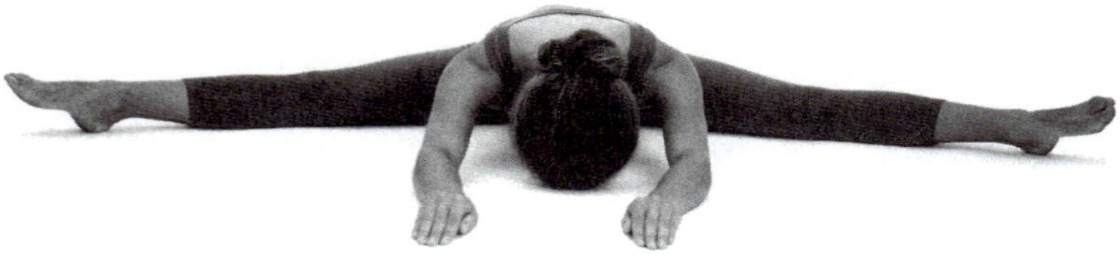

RELEASE VALVE 5, internal rotation

♦ GROUP 5

Nāvāsana is the sole member of this group. This open-frame posture is unique in its function as a forward bend. Unlike other forward bends, the primary intention is strengthening and stabilizing the lumbar-pelvic relationship rather than stretching the lumbosacral spine.

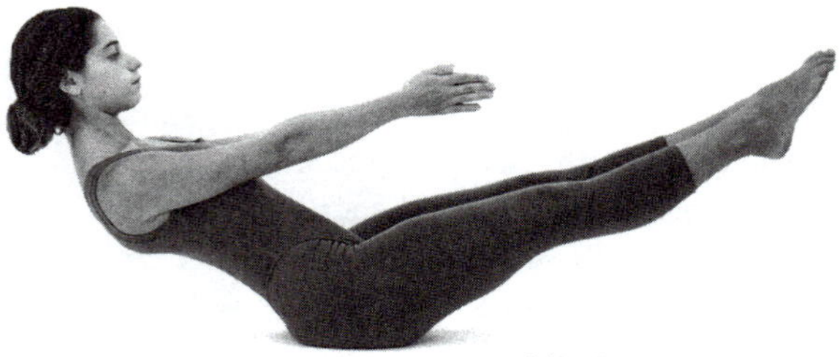

Nāvāsana

Common Risks

The greatest risk in forward bends is to the lumbosacral spine. If, in standing-forward bends, the lumbar curve is maintained too long when going down, or regained too soon when coming up, there can be low back strain and excessive posterior disc compression. If, in seated-forward bends, the hips cannot rotate forward, there can be excessive anterior disc compression. In either case, if the sacroiliac joint is weak, there can be strain to the ligaments.

There is also risk in forward bends to the musculature and ligaments of the hip joints. Excessive forward rotation of the pelvis, over time, may create instability in the hip joints and a susceptibility to injury. Developing the proper pelvic-lumbar rhythm will minimize risks to both the low back, sacrum, and hips.

There is some risk of strain in the area of the upper back, shoulder girdle, and neck in coming up from a forward bend. Adapting the position of the arms and avoiding pulling the spine with the head will usually alleviate this stress.

Forward Bending Practice (for Kūrmāsana)

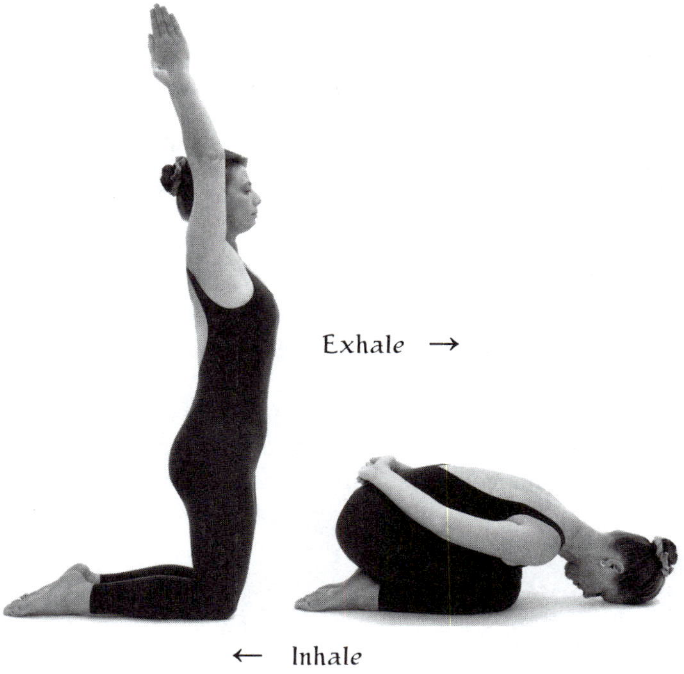

1.
POSTURE: Vajrāsana.
EMPHASIS: To warm up body. To stretch low back.
TECHNIQUE: Stand on knees with arms over head.

On exhale: Bend forward, sweeping arms behind back, and bringing hands to sacrum, keeping palms up.

On inhale: Return to starting position.

NUMBER: 8 times.
DETAILS: *On exhale:* Bring chest to thighs before bringing buttocks to heels. Rotate arms so palms are up and hands are resting on sacrum. *On inhale:* Expand chest and lift it up off of knees as arms sweep wide.

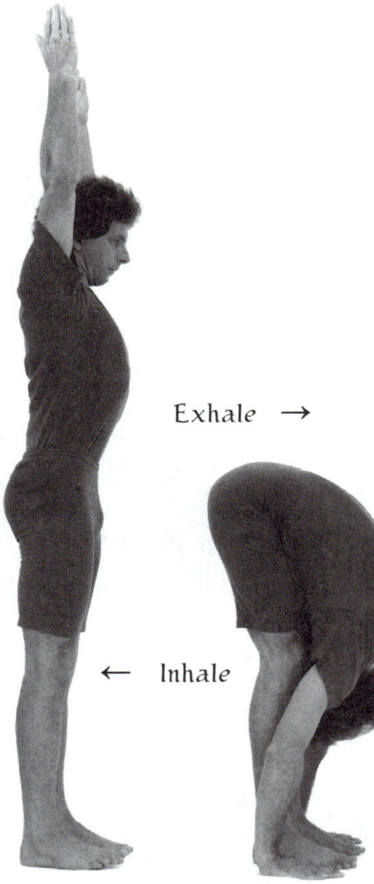

2.
POSTURE: Uttānāsana.
EMPHASIS: To warm up back and legs.
TECHNIQUE: Stand with arms over head.

On exhale: Forward bend, bringing belly and chest toward thighs and bringing hands to feet.

On inhale: return to starting position.

NUMBER: 6 times.
DETAILS: *On exhale:* Bend knees to facilitate stretching of low back. Move chin down toward throat. *On inhale:* Lift chest up and away from thighs, flattening upper back. Keep knees bent until end of movement.

3.

POSTURE: Parivṛtti Trikoṇāsana.
EMPHASIS: To stretch legs, back, and shoulders.
TECHNIQUE: Stand with feet spread wider than shoulders, with arms out to sides and parallel to floor.

On exhale: Bend forward and twist, bringing left hand to floor, pointing right arm upward, and twisting shoulders right. Turn head down toward left hand.

On inhale: Maintaining rotation, and with right shoulder vertically above left, bring right arm up over shoulder and forward, turning head to center and looking at right hand.

On exhale: Return to previous position with right arm pointing upward. Turn head up, looking toward right hand.

On inhale: Return to starting position.

Repeat on other side.

NUMBER: 6 times each side, alternately.
DETAILS: Keep down arm vertically below its respective shoulder, and keep weight of torso off arm. Knees can bend while moving into twist.

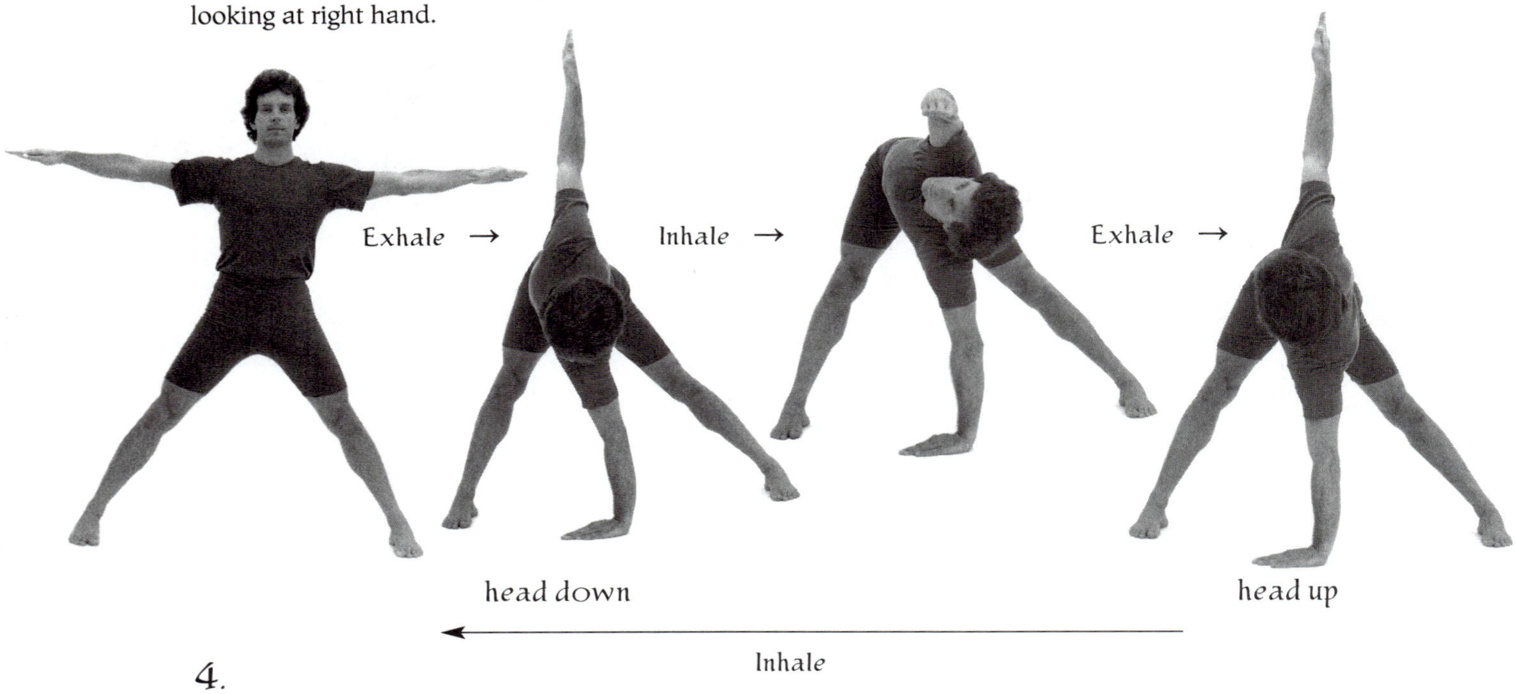

Exhale →
Inhale →
Exhale →
head down
head up
Inhale

4.

POSTURE: Cakravākāsana.
EMPHASIS: To make transition from standing to supine position. To stretch rib cage on inhale and low back on exhale.
TECHNIQUE: Get down on hands and knees, with shoulders vertically above wrists and with hips above knees.

On inhale: Lift chest up and away from belly.

On exhale: Gently contract belly, round low back, and bring chest toward thighs.

NUMBER: 8 times.
DETAILS: *On inhale:* Lead with chest, keeping chin slightly down. Avoid compressing low back; rather, feel chest expanding. *On exhale:* Round low back without collapsing chest over belly. Avoid increasing curvature of upper back. Let chest lower toward thighs sooner than hips toward heels.

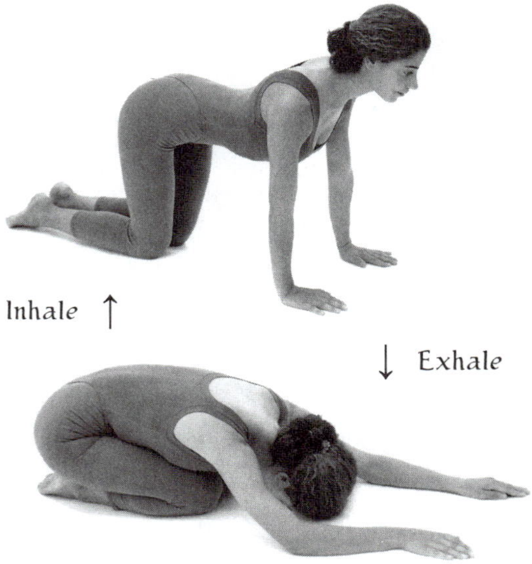

Inhale ↑
↓ Exhale

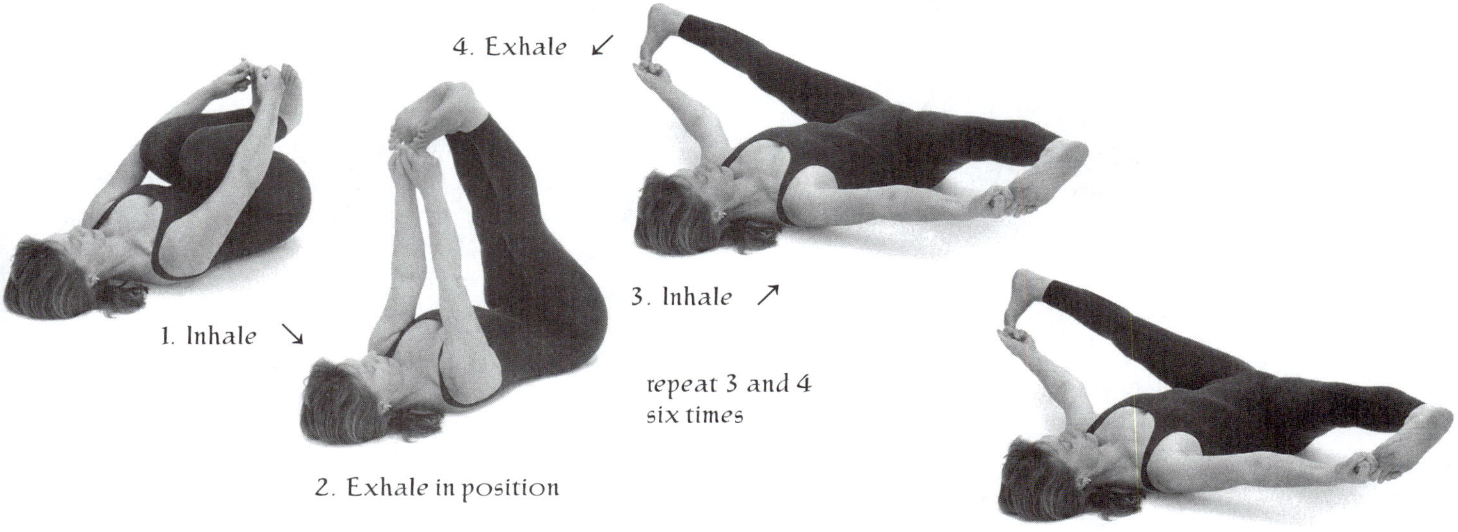
4. Exhale ↙
1. Inhale ↘
3. Inhale ↗
repeat 3 and 4
six times
2. Exhale in position
5. Stay in position six breaths

5.

POSTURE: Supta Prasārita Pādāṅguṣṭhāsana.
EMPHASIS: To stretch musculature of lower back, backs of legs, and inner thighs in preparation for seated forward bends.
TECHNIQUE: Lie on back with knees lifted toward chest and with hands holding respective toes.

On inhale: With hands holding toes, lift heels upward, straightening legs.

On exhale: Stay in position.

On inhale: Open legs wide, pulling legs apart gently with arms.

On exhale: close legs.

Repeat 6 times; then stay open 6 breaths.

DETAILS: Keep sacrum, chin, and shoulders down throughout movement. If legs are loose, hold balls of feet while staying in final position.

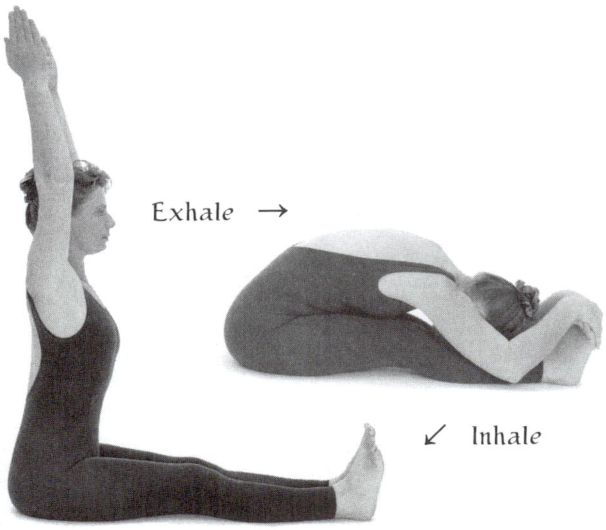
Exhale →
↙ Inhale

6.

POSTURE: Paścimatānāsana.
EMPHASIS: To stretch back and legs in preparation for Kūrmāsana.
TECHNIQUE: Sit with legs forward, back straight, and arms raised over head.

On exhale: Bending knees slightly, bend forward, bringing chest to thighs and palms to balls of feet.

On inhale: Return to starting position.

NUMBER: 6 times.
DETAILS: *On exhale:* Bend knees to facilitate stretching low back and bring belly and chest to thighs. Move chin down toward throat. *On inhale:* Lift chest up and away from thighs, flattening upper back.

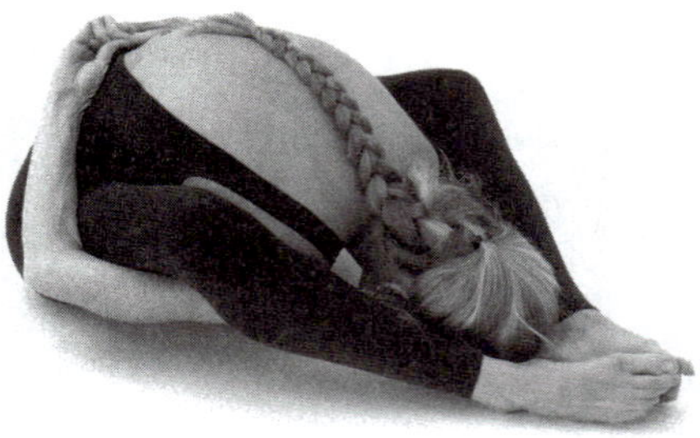

7.

Posture: Kūrmāsana.
Emphasis: To stretch musculature of back, shoulders, and legs. To experience one of the deepest forward bends.
Technique: Sit with legs straight forward and apart wider than shoulders. Bend forward, with bent knees, and slide arms under knees, wrapping them around torso, clasping hands behind back. Stay in position 8 breaths. Extend legs progressively straighter.

8.

Posture: Dvipāda Pīṭham.
Emphasis: To relax back and stretch belly.
Technique: Lie on back with arms down at sides, knees bent, and feet on floor, slightly apart and comfortably close to buttocks.

On inhale: Pressing down on feet and keeping chin down, raise pelvis up toward ceiling, until neck is gently flattened on floor.

On exhale: Return to starting position.

Number: 6 times.
Details: *On inhale:* Lift spine, vertebra by vertebra, from bottom up. *On exhale:* Unwind spine, coming down vertebra by vertebra.

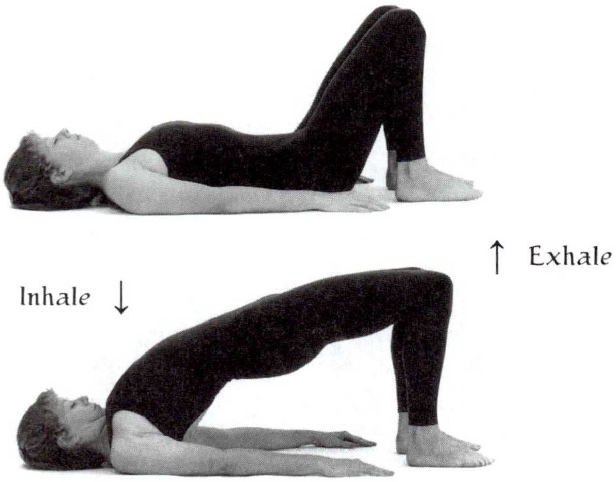

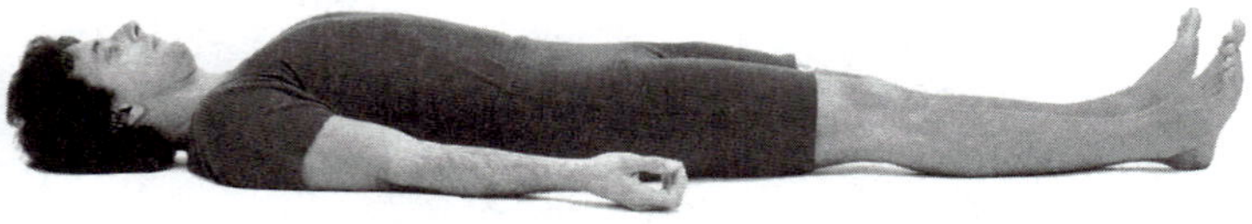

9.

Posture: Śavāsana.
Emphasis: To rest.
Technique: Lie flat on back, with arms at sides, palms up, and legs slightly apart. Close eyes. Relax body fully, keeping mind relaxed and alert to sensations in body.
Duration: Minimum 3 to 5 minutes.

Stretching the East: An Introduction to Backward Bends

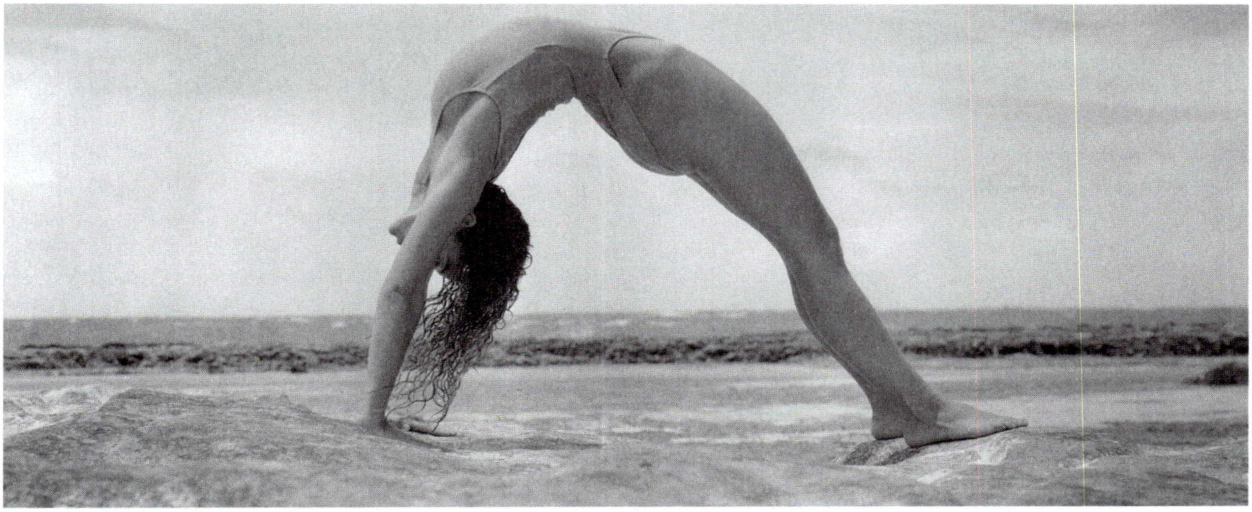

Primary and Secondary Intentions

As part of their sunrise practice, the ancient yogis called backward bending "stretching the east." Backward bends stretch and strengthen the front portion of the torso, the shoulder and pelvic girdles, and the legs. They stretch and strengthen the iliopsoas muscles, which lay deep under the anterior musculature of the abdomen and pelvis and bind the legs to the spine; the diaphragm and intercostals, which are the primary musculature of respiration; the anterior muscles, which bind the shoulder girdle to the spine; and the anterior muscles of the legs. In addition, they strengthen the superficial and deep muscles of the back, which contract as we bend backward; strengthen the posterior muscles of the shoulder girdle; stretch the abdominal organs, relieving visceral compression; gently compress the kidney/adrenal area, stimulating its function; and stretch the anterior muscles of the neck and throat, including the area of the thyroid and thymus glands.

From a biomechanical perspective, according to the Viniyoga tradition, the *primary intention* of backward bending is to expand and stretch the anterior structures of the chest and shoulder girdle, and to stretch the anterior musculature of the solar plexus, abdomen, hips, and thighs. The primary focus in different back bends can be the chest and shoulders, the solar plexus and abdomen, the hips and thighs, or equally distributed among them all.

The *secondary intention* of backward bending is to strengthen the musculature of the back. In certain backward bends, this strengthening is actually more important than the anterior stretching.

Technique

The key to backward bends is the ability to control the proportional relation between lengthening and flattening the thoracic curve and deepening the lumbar curve.

The proportional relation between these two actions is known as the thoraco-lumbar rhythm. Though the thoracic spine has a limited capacity for arching backward, due to the structure of the spinous processes and the rib cage, the lumbar spine can arch deeply. The tendency to excessively arch the lumbar spine in backward bending may be increased by individual structural conditions, such as an increased lumbar curve, or as the result of training: for example, habitually rotating the pelvis forward to create the back bend.

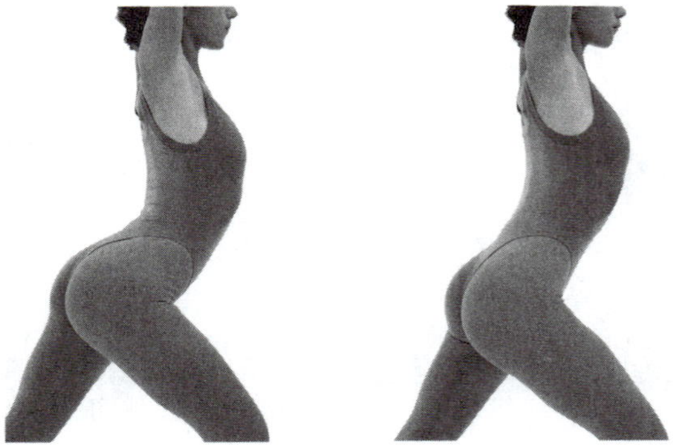

RELEASE VALVE 1,*
excessive lumbar arch *correct*

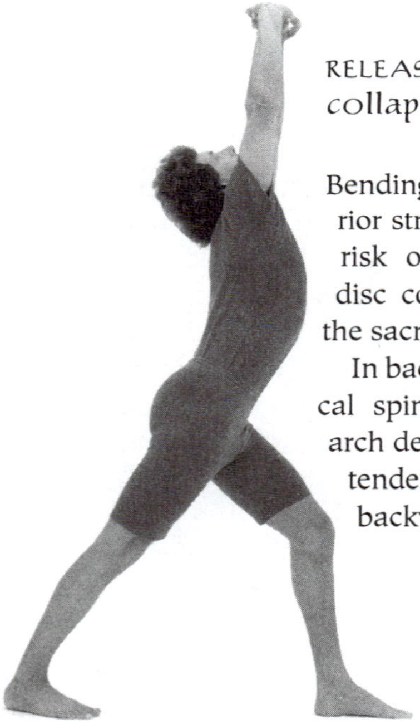

RELEASE VALVE 2,
collapsed neck

Bending in this way limits anterior stretching and increases the risk of posterior intervertebral disc compression and strain to the sacroiliac ligaments.

In backward bending, the cervical spine, like the lumbar, can arch deeply backward, creating a tendency to collapse the head backward.

This again may be the result of individual structural conditions, such as weakness in the neck, or the result of training: for example, habitually initiating the backbend by pulling the spine with the head. This practice increases the risk of posterior strain and compression to the neck and, by giving the illusion of an intense backward bend, may also actually limit our efforts to work more deeply.

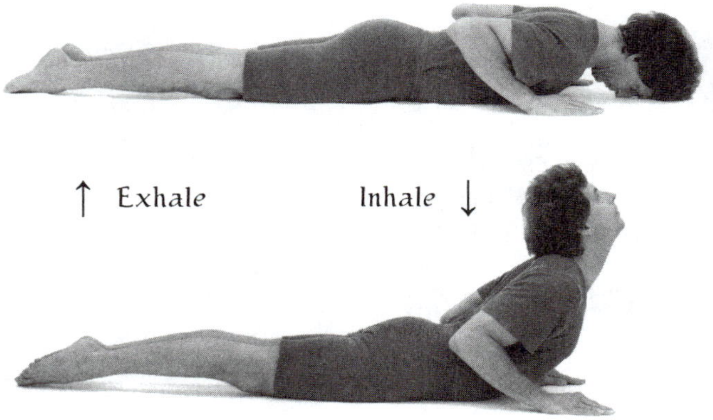

RELEASE VALVE 3, *leading with head*

versus

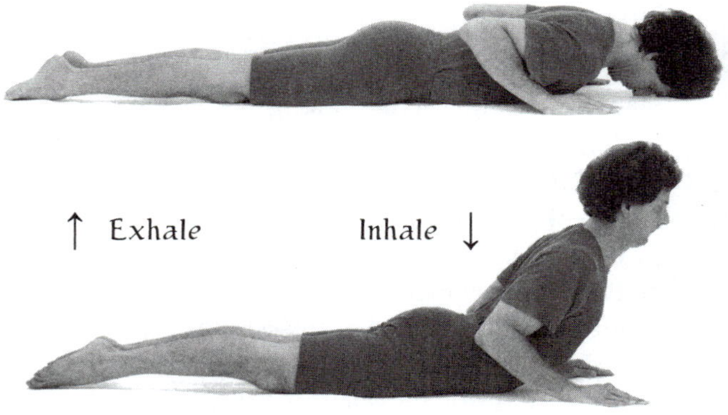

head follows spine

* For a list of common release valves for backward bends, see page 55.

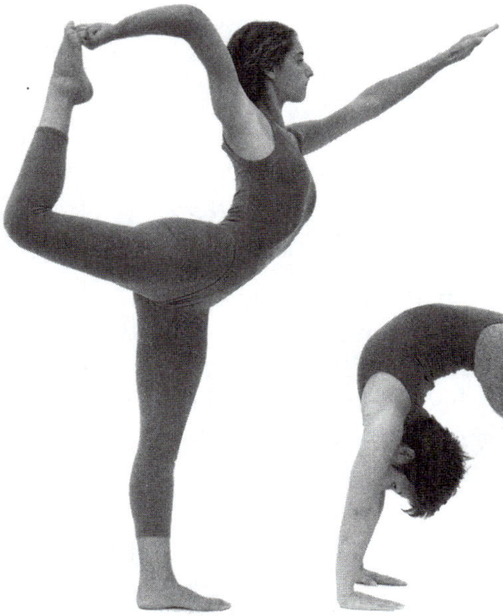

correct

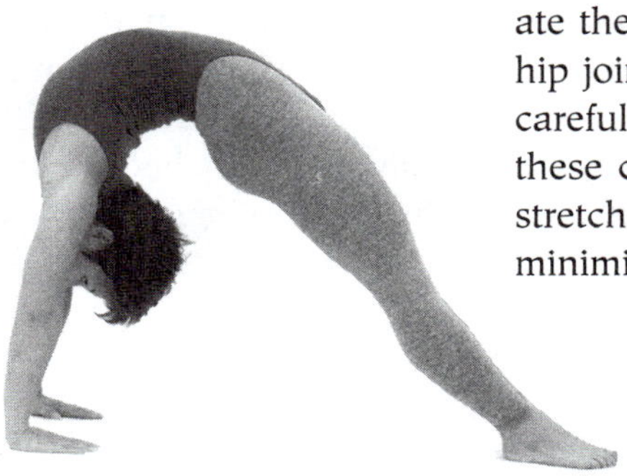

correct

In the shoulders as well as the hips, the range of backward extension depends on many factors, including, with respect to the shoulders, the condition of the cervical and thoracic spine and their supporting muscles; and, with respect to the hips, the condition of the lumbar-pelvic structures and their supporting muscles.

When the arms and legs are used as levers to create the back arch, there is risk to the shoulder and hip joints. So, in order to avoid injury, we must be careful not to apply excessive muscular force in these cases. As we are able to open the chest and stretch the front of the abdomen and pelvis, we will minimize the risks to the shoulders and hips.

The key to the thoraco-lumbar rhythm, and therefore all backward bends, is the technique of expanding the chest on inhale while *maintaining the abdominal contraction* initiated on exhale. At the initiation of the inhale expand the chest and lift the ribs, thereby lengthening the thoracic spine and stretching the front of the torso, and, as the chest expands, open the shoulders and pull them down and back. As the volume of air is reduced in the lungs on exhale, if you have a normal to excessive thoracic curve, in order to flatten it, contract the muscles of the upper back, pull the shoulders back, and push the mid-thoracic forward; or, if your thoracic curve is already flattened, focus on the vertical extension of the spine and avoid pushing the mid-thoracic forward. Then, on all successive *inhales,* maintain a slight abdominal contraction, in order to prevent excessive forward rotation of the pelvis and posterior lumbar intervertebral compression. And on the next and all successive *exhales,* use the increased abdominal contraction to stabilize the pelvic-lumbar relationship; focus the arching in the upper back; allow the head to rise away from the shoulders, creating as much space as possible between the cervical vertebrae; and keep the chin level, or even slightly tucked in, to enhance the lengthening of the cervical spine, lifting it only toward the end of the inhale in order to stretch the front of the neck and throat.

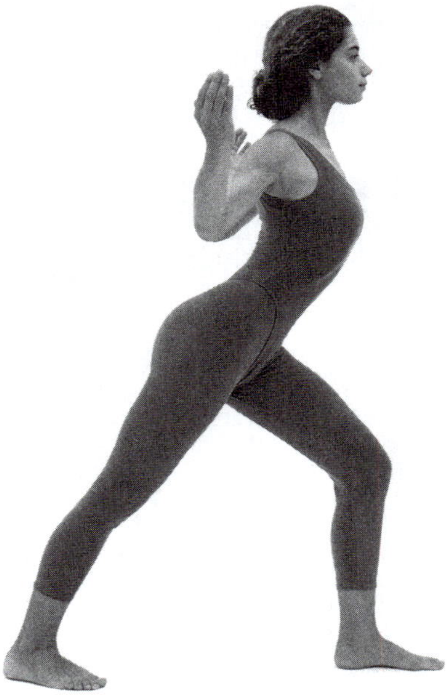

for excessive thoracic curve

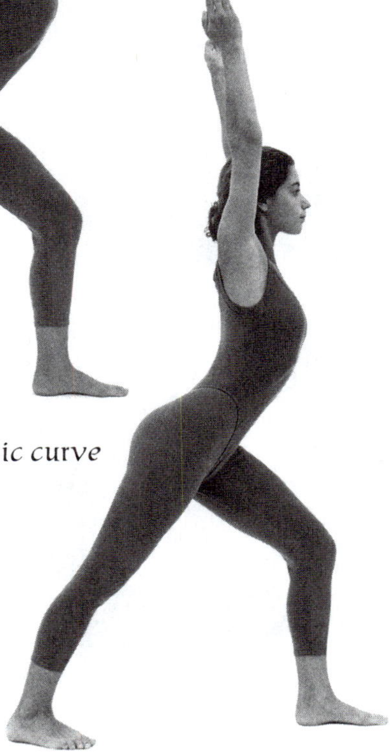

for flattened thoracic curve

Types of Backward Bends

♦ GROUP 1

The first group of postures includes open-frame back bends initiated from the prone position, which utilize primarily the contraction of the posterior muscles of the back (spinal extensor) and hips (hip extensors) to generate the back bend, aided in some cases by the backward extension of the arms. In these postures, the primary intention is the development of strength and resiliency in these muscles. Vimanāsana uniquely isolates and strengthens the muscles that support the sacroiliac joints.

The Viniyoga tradition gives special importance to these postures, which are relatively safe and universally beneficial, because they significantly strengthen the posterior musculature of the spine.

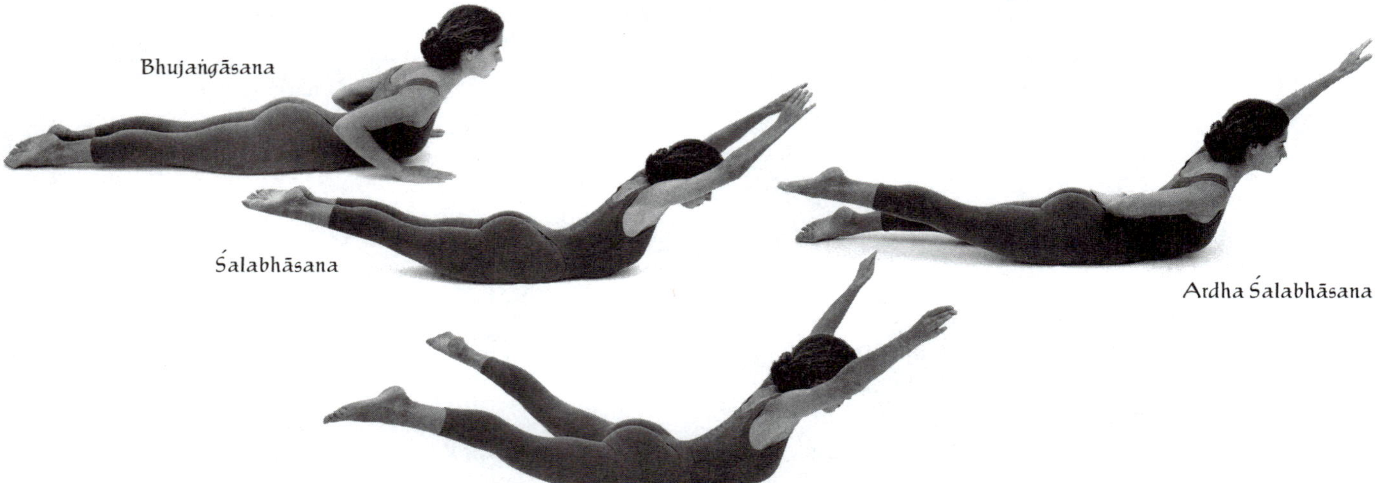

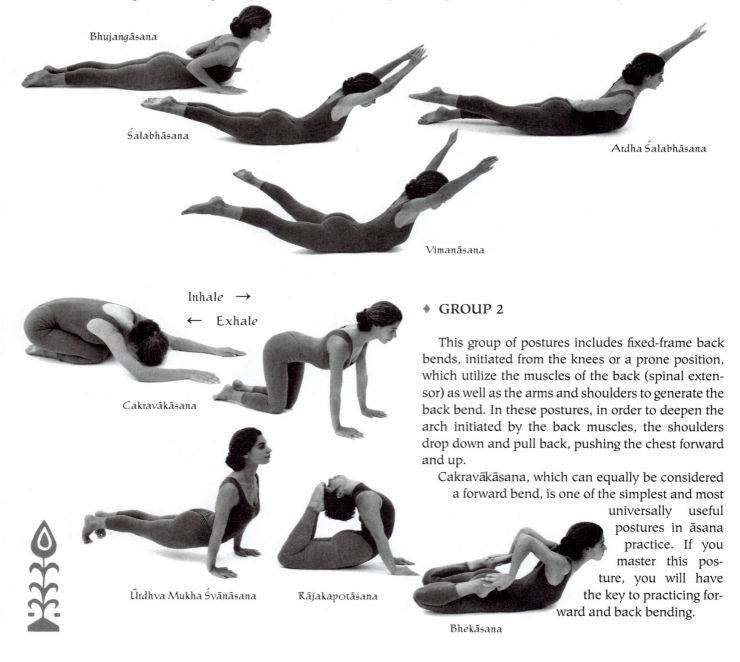

Bhujaṅgāsana

Śalabhāsana

Ardha Śalabhāsana

Vimanāsana

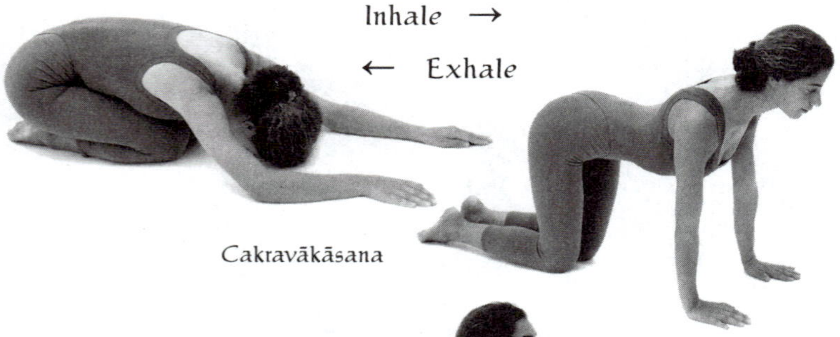

Cakravākāsana

♦ GROUP 2

This group of postures includes fixed-frame back bends, initiated from the knees or a prone position, which utilize the muscles of the back (spinal extensor) as well as the arms and shoulders to generate the back bend. In these postures, in order to deepen the arch initiated by the back muscles, the shoulders drop down and pull back, pushing the chest forward and up.

Cakravākāsana, which can equally be considered a forward bend, is one of the simplest and most universally useful postures in āsana practice. If you master this posture, you will have the key to practicing forward and back bending.

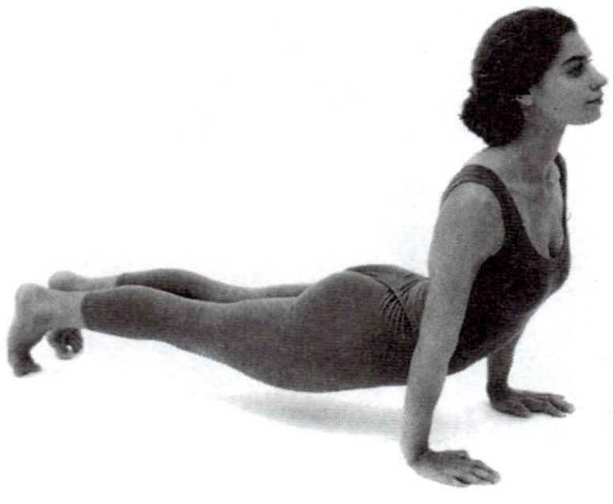

Ūrdhva Mukha Śvānāsana

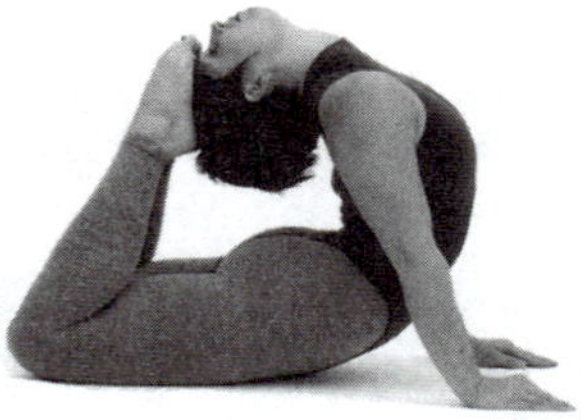

Rājakapotāsana

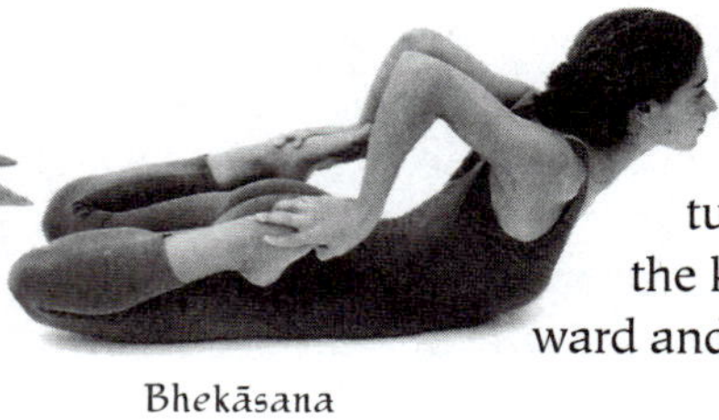

Bhekāsana

♦ GROUP 3

This group of postures includes standing and kneeling back bends that can be practiced as open- or close-frame postures. In addition to providing anterior stretching of the chest and abdominal areas, the asymmetric quality of these postures facilitates a deep stretching of the iliopsoas muscles. These muscles are often chronically contracted and can cause excessive anterior compression of the lumbar discs and low back pain. Asymmetric postures enable us to isolate and intensify the stretching of these important muscles, increasing their strength and flexibility.

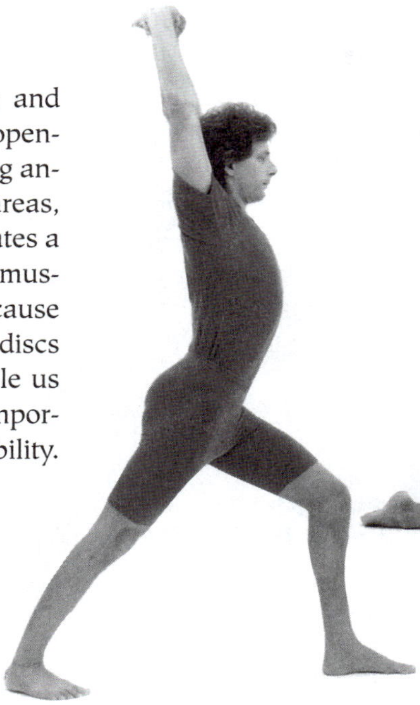
Vīrabhadrāsana

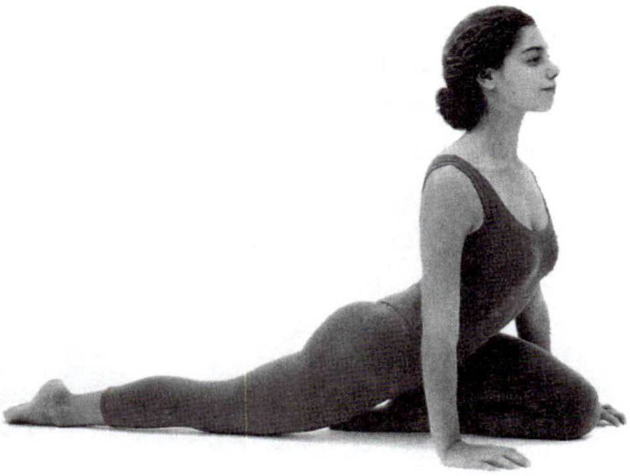
Godhāpīṭham

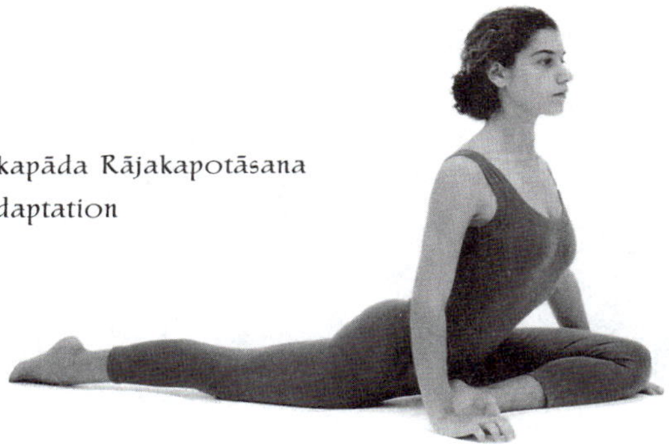
Ekapāda Rājakapotāsana adaptation

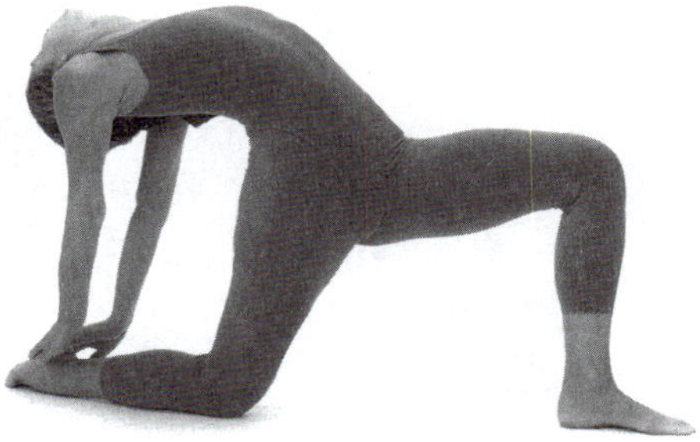
Ekapāda Uṣṭrāsana classic posture

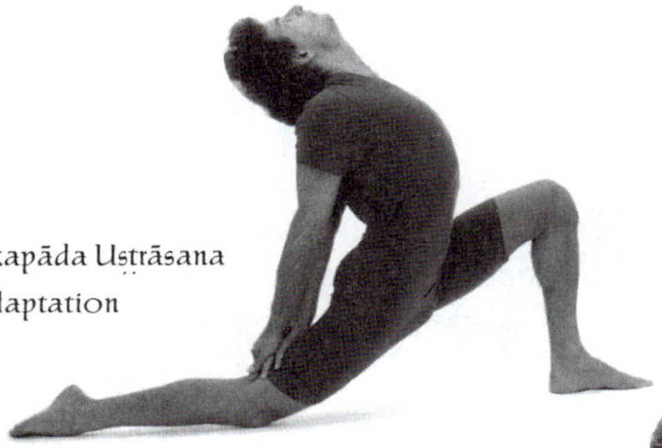
Ekapāda Uṣṭrāsana adaptation

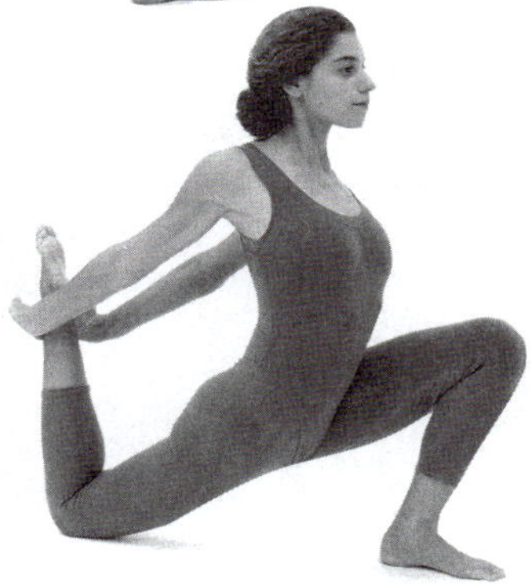
Ekapāda Uṣṭrāsana adaptation

Though Vīrabhadrāsana can be adapted to emphasize the iliopsoas muscles (see page 13), it is particularly useful for expanding the chest, stretching the intercostals and diaphragm, flattening the thoracic curve, and strengthening the hips and legs.

In the classical version of Ekapāda Uṣṭrāsana, it is difficult to avoid excessive posterior lumbar compression. This adaptation reduces the risk to the lumbar while increasing the beneficial stretching of the iliopsoas and thighs.

♦ GROUP 4

This group of postures includes fixed-frame back bends initiated from the supine (on the back), kneeling, or prone (on the stomach) positions, which utilize primarily the muscles of the arms, shoulders, legs, and hips to generate the arch. In all of these postures, because of the leverage generated by the arms and legs, deeper back bending is possible. This both increases the anterior stretching and the risk to posterior strain and compression.

In most of these postures, the shoulders are dropped down, the shoulder blades are pulled back, the arms are at the sides, and the hands push against the floor or either pull the legs or are pulled by them. This action expands the chest, flattens the thoracic spine, and deepens the back arch. In Ūrdhva Dhanurāsana, however, the arms are raised over the head and extended behind the spine. If you can master this posture, you will experience the truly energizing and expanding quality of back bending.

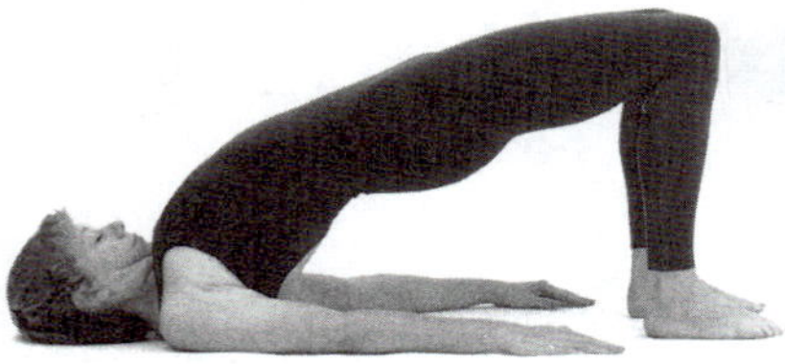
Dvipāda Pīṭham

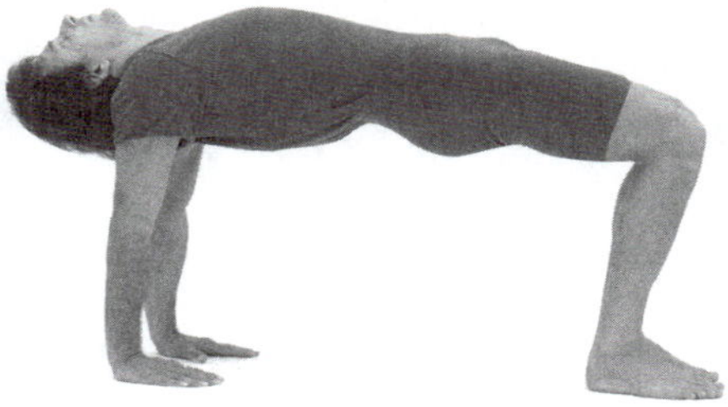
Catuṣpādapīṭham

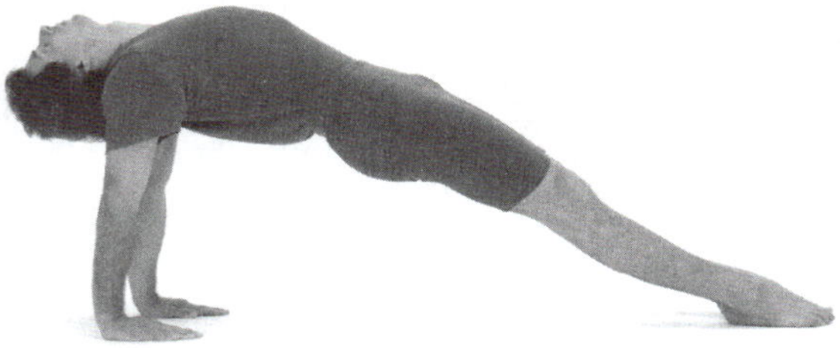
Pūrvatānāsana

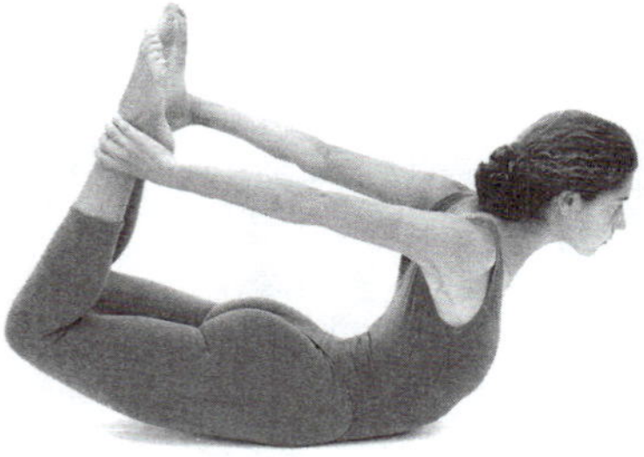
Dhanurāsana

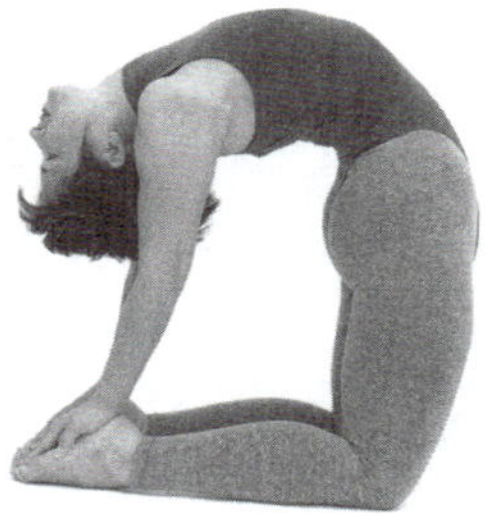
Uṣṭrāsana

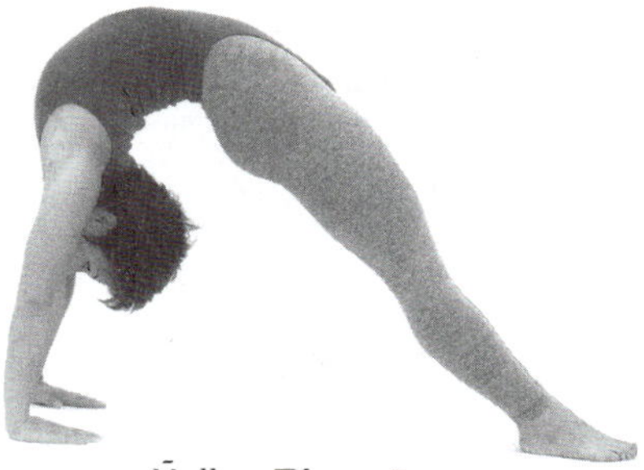
Ūrdhva Dhanurāsana

♦ GROUP 5

These are fixed-frame back bends in which the weight of the upper torso is supported by the top of the head. They are similar in form and function with respect to the upper torso and neck. Their primary intention is stretching the chest, the front of the neck, and throat, and strengthening the muscles of the upper back and back of the neck. In practicing these postures, press your head firmly down, engaging the muscles in the back of the neck and upper back to help expand the chest, and avoid collapsing your head backward.

Uttāna Pādāsana uniquely strengthens the iliopsoas muscles and stabilizes the pelvic-lumbar relationship.

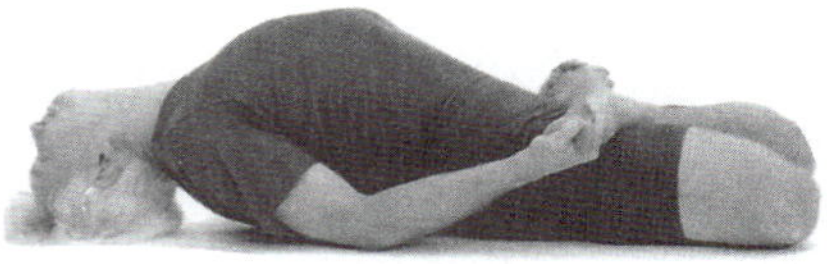
Matsyāsana

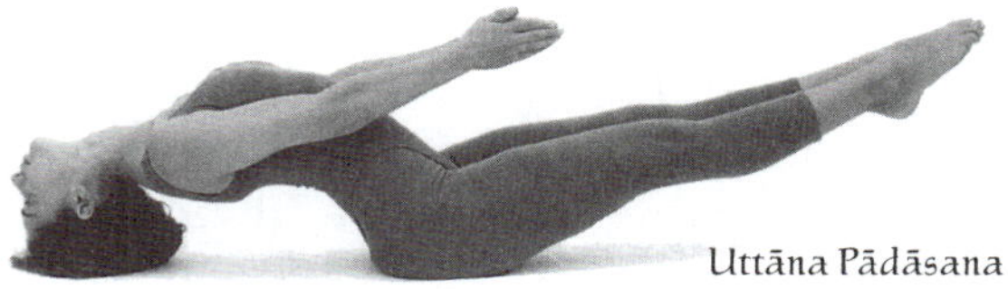
Uttāna Pādāsana

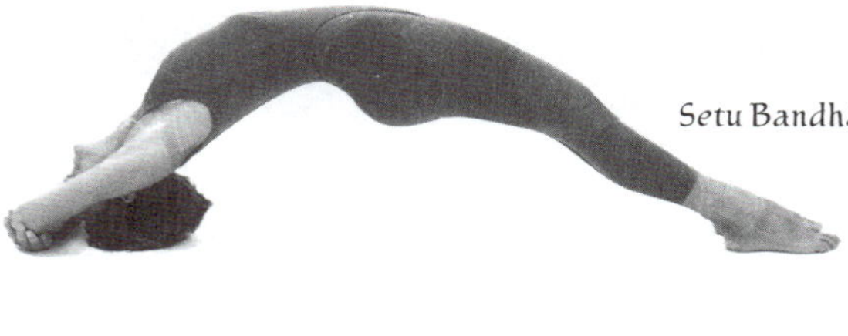
Setu Bandhāsana

♦ GROUP 6

Paryaṅkāsana is the sole member of this group. This fixed-frame posture deeply stretches the front of the thighs. The deep arching of the low back is created by the position of the legs rather than the action of the muscles.

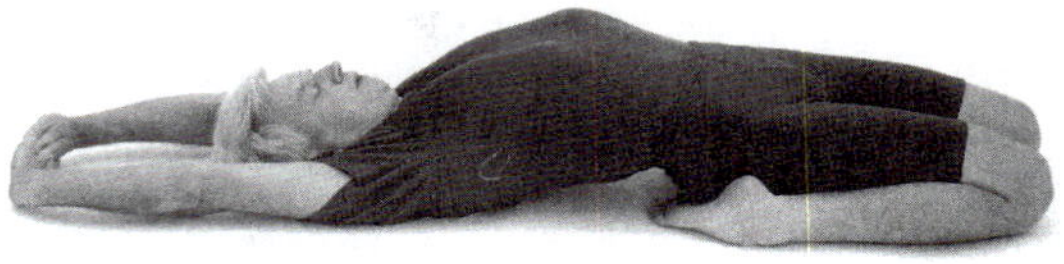

Paryaṅkāsana

Common Release Valves for Backward Bends

1. Excessive arching in the lumbar spine.
2. Collapsing the neck backward from the top of the neck (at the occipital-atlas junction).
3. Leading with the head, initiating the back bend with the musculature of the neck.
4. Shrugging the shoulders toward the ears in postures where the arms are bearing a significant portion of body weight.
5. Rounding the shoulders forward, inhibiting expansion of the upper chest.
6. Hyperflexing the shoulder joints.

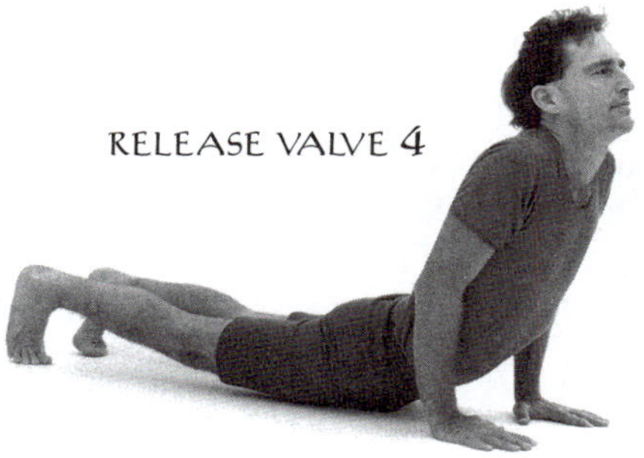

RELEASE VALVE 4

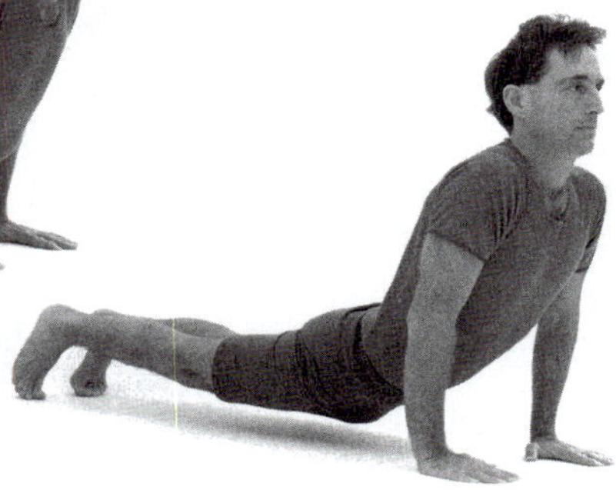

RELEASE VALVE 5

correct

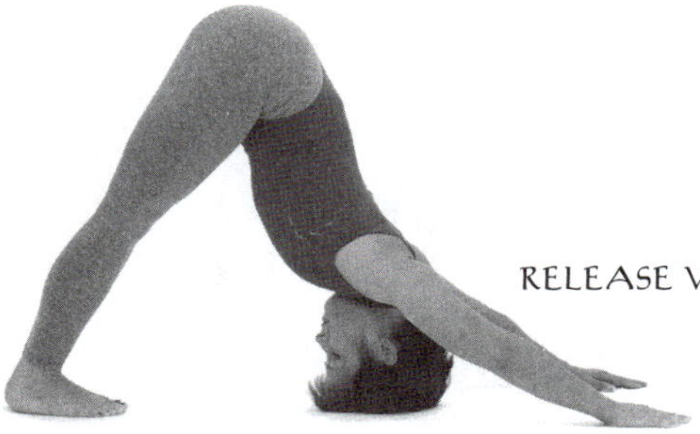

RELEASE VALVE 6

Common Risks

In open- and fixed-frame back bends, there is the risk of lumbo-sacral and cervical strain, and excessive disc compression. Stabilizing the pelvic-lumbar relationship through the abdominal contraction on exhale minimizes this risk. In fixed-frame postures, such as Uṣṭrāsana, Paryaṅkāsana, and Uttānna Pādāsana, where there is a sharper angle between the lumbar spine and the pelvis, the risk is greater. If you have low back pain, your low back is weak, or you are very tight in the front of your thighs and pelvis, these postures should be avoided.

In back bends where the weight of the upper torso is supported on the top of the head, there is increased risk of strain to the cervical muscles and ligaments, as well as excessive disc compression. If your neck is weak, these postures should be avoided.

In Ūrdhva Dhanurāsana, there is risk of strain to the shoulder and wrist joints. Strengthening the shoulders and arms and maximizing the ability to expand the chest and stretch the abdomen will reduce the stress to the joints.

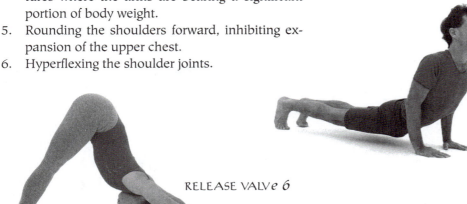

Backward Bending Practice (for Ūrdhva Dhanurāsana)

1.
POSTURE: Vajrāsana.
EMPHASIS: To warm up body. To stretch low back.
TECHNIQUE: Stand on knees with arms over head.

On exhale: Bend forward, sweeping arms behind back, and bringing hands to sacrum, keeping palms up.

On inhale: Return to starting position.

NUMBER: 8 times.
DETAILS: *On exhale:* Bring chest to thighs before bringing buttocks to heels. Rotate arms so palms are up and hands are resting on sacrum. *On inhale:* Expand chest and lift it up off of knees as arms sweep wide.

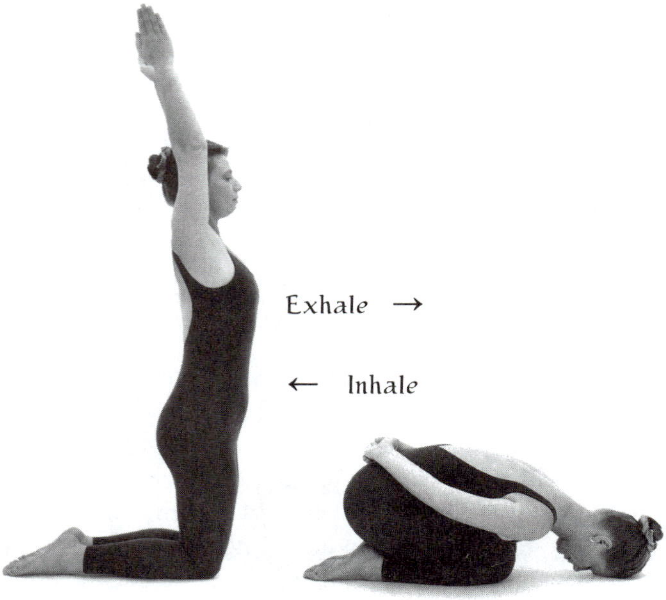

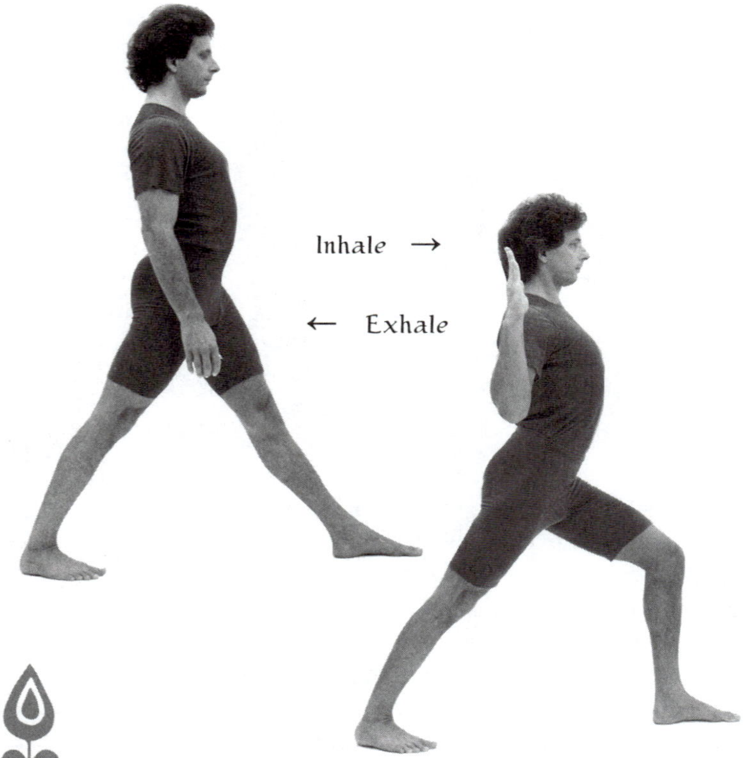

2.
POSTURE: Vīrabhadrāsana.
EMPHASIS: To strengthen muscles of back and legs. To expand chest and flatten upper back. To increase hold after inhalation.
TECHNIQUE: Stand with left foot forward, feet as wide as hips and arms at sides.

On inhale: Simultaneously bend left knee, displace chest slightly forward and hips slightly backward, bringing arms out to sides and shoulders back.

After inhale: Hold breath 2, 4, and 6 seconds, 2 times each, progressively.

On exhale: Return to starting position.

NUMBER: 6 times each side.
DETAILS: *On inhale:* Keep hands and elbows in line with shoulders. Feel opening of chest and flattening of upper back, not compression in low back. Keep head forward. Stay firm on back heel.

3.

Posture: Ekapāda Uṣṭrāsana variation.
Emphasis: To stretch musculature of upper thigh and iliopsoas.
Technique: Stand on right knee, with knee directly below hip, and on left foot, with foot directly below left knee. Hands on left knee.

On inhale: Lift chest upward as you lunge forward, stretching front of body from right thigh to right side of abdomen.

On exhale: Return to starting position.

Repeat 4 times.

Then bend right knee and grasp ankle with both hands. Stay in position 6 breaths.

Repeat on other side.

Details: While staying in the full posture, keep arms straight and push chest forward.

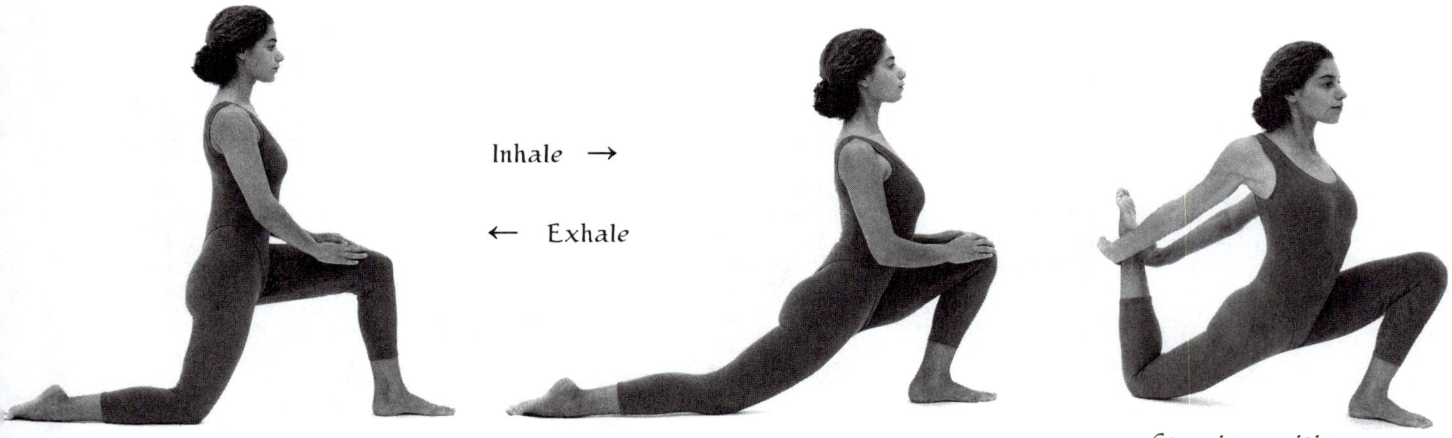

4.

Posture: Ardha Śalabhāsana.
Emphasis: To strengthen and stabilize lower back.
Technique: Lie on stomach, with head to left, and palms on floor by chest.

On inhale: Lift chest and left leg, turning head to center.

On exhale: Lower chest and leg, turning head to right.

Repeat on other side.

Number: 6 times each side, alternately.
Details: *On inhale:* Lift chest slightly before leg, and emphasize chest height. Keep pelvis level.

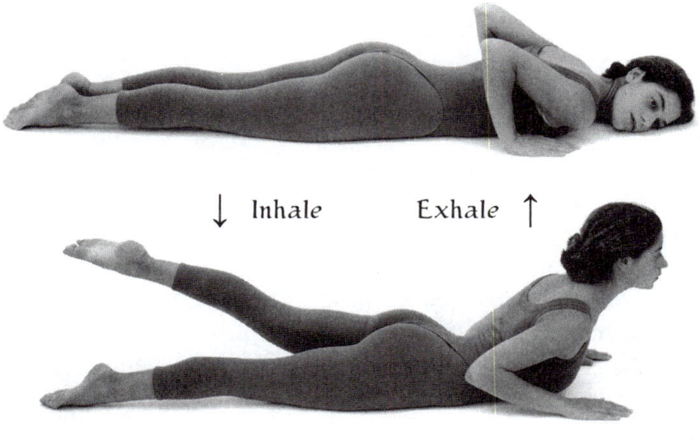

5.

POSTURE: Adho Mukha Śvānāsana/Ūrdhva Mukha Śvānāsana.

EMPHASIS: To prepare shoulders, chest, and abdomen for Ūrdhva Dhanurāsana.

TECHNIQUE: Stand on hands and knees.

On exhale: Push buttocks upward, lifting knees off ground, and pushing chest toward feet. Stay 1 breath.

On inhale: Stretch body forward and arch back. Stay 1 breath.

On exhale: Return to previous position.

Repeat 6 times.

On inhale: Return to starting position.

DETAILS: *On exhale:* Keep knees bent, press chest toward feet, flattening upper back and stretching shoulders. Avoid hyperextension of shoulders. *On inhale:* Stay on toes. Keep shoulders down and back, pushing chest forward and stretching belly. Avoid collapsing pelvis and compressing low back.

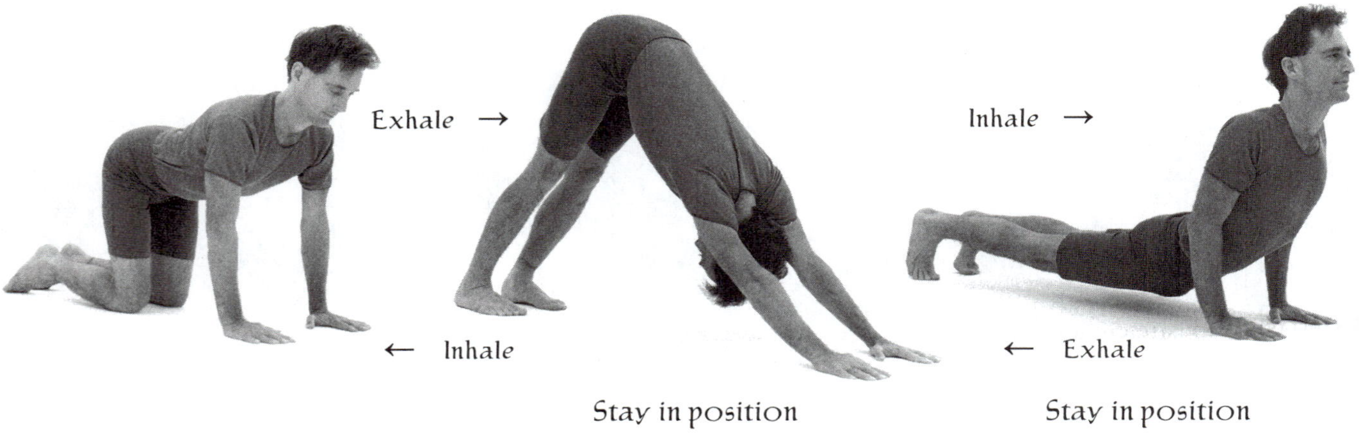
Exhale →
← Inhale
Stay in position
Inhale →
← Exhale
Stay in position

6.

POSTURE: Vajrāsana.

EMPHASIS: To mobilize shoulders, releasing tension after previous posture, and to prepare for the back bend.

TECHNIQUE: Stand on knees with arms over head.

On exhale: Bend forward, sweeping arms behind back, and bringing hands to sacrum, keeping palms up.

On inhale: Return to starting position.

NUMBER: 8 times.

DETAILS: *On exhale:* Bring chest to thighs before bringing buttocks to heels. Rotate arms so palms are up and hands are resting on sacrum. *On inhale:* Expand chest and lift it up off of knees as arms sweep wide.

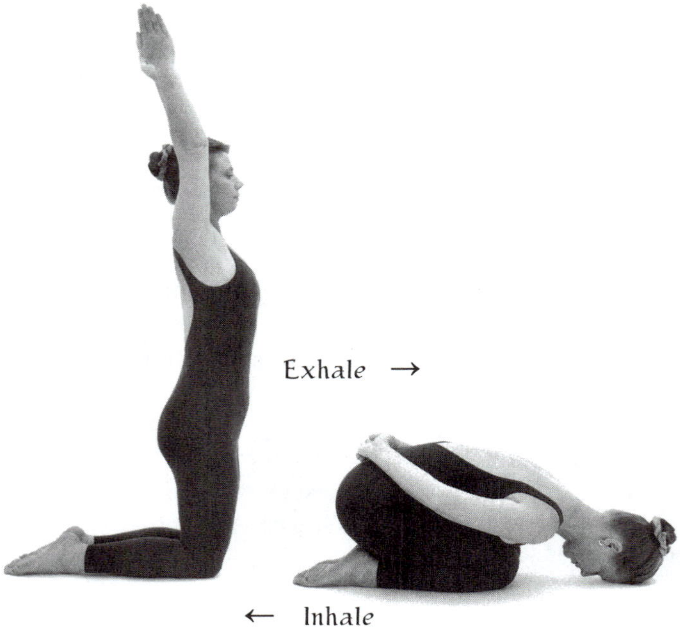
Exhale →
← Inhale

7.

POSTURE: Ūrdhva Dhanurāsana.
EMPHASIS: To deeply stretch the front of torso. To experience a full and deep back bend.
TECHNIQUE: Lie on back with knees bent, feet on floor by buttocks, palms on floor under shoulders with fingers pointing toward feet.

On inhale: Press firmly on arms and feet, raising torso off ground, and create back bend.

Stay in position 6 breaths.

On exhale: Return to starting position.

NUMBER: Stay in full position 6 breaths, repeat 2 times.
DETAILS: *First round:* Work to straighten arms. *Second round:* Work to straighten legs.

8.

POSTURE: Supta Pādāṅguṣṭhāsana.
EMPHASIS: To stretch and relax lower back after back bend.
TECHNIQUE: Lie on back with legs bent, knees lifted toward chest, hands holding thighs behind knee, and arms bent.

On inhale: Extend legs upward, straightening arms.

On exhale: Return to starting position.

NUMBER: 6 times.
DETAILS: *On inhale:* Flex feet as legs are raised upward. Slightly bend knees. Push low back and sacrum downward. Keep chin down.

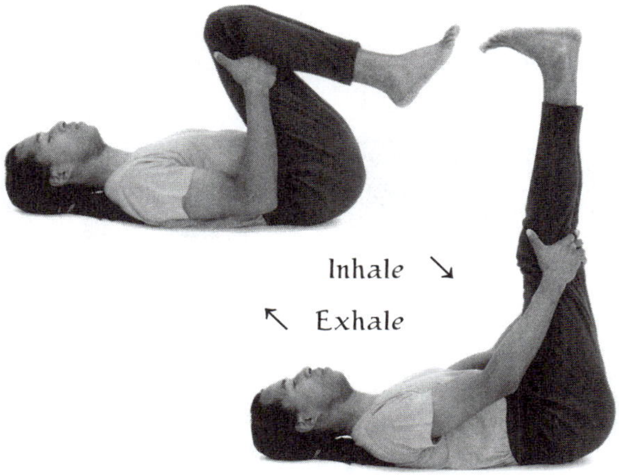

9.

POSTURE: Dvipāda Pīṭham.
EMPHASIS: To relax neck after back bend.
TECHNIQUE: Lie on back with arms down at sides, knees bent, and feet on floor, slightly apart and comfortably close to buttocks.

On inhale: Pressing down on feet and keeping chin down, raise pelvis up toward ceiling, until neck is gently flattened on floor.

On exhale: Return to starting position.

NUMBER: 6 times.
DETAILS: *On inhale:* Lift spine, vertebra by vertebra, from bottom up. *On exhale:* Unwind spine, coming down vertebra by vertebra.

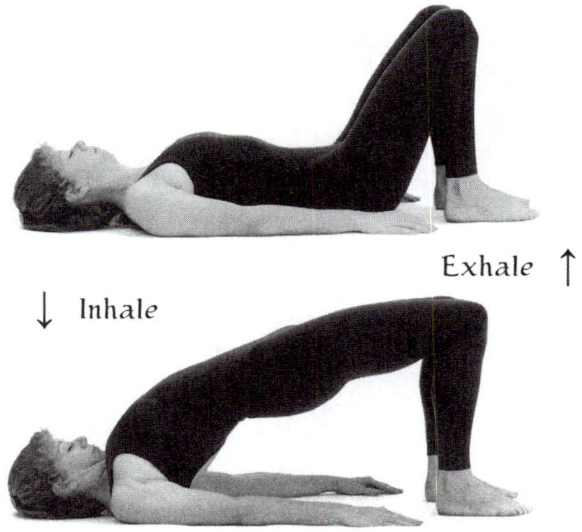

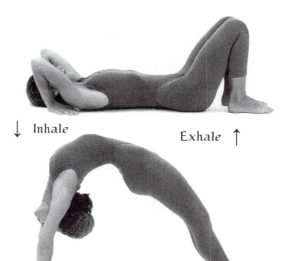

10.

POSTURE: Paścimatānāsana.
EMPHASIS: To stretch back to compensate for back bend.
TECHNIQUE: Sit with legs forward, back straight, and arms raised over head.

On exhale: Bending knees slightly, bend forward, bringing chest to thighs and palms to balls of feet.

On inhale: Return to starting position.

Repeat 6 times.

Then stay in forward-bend position 6 breaths.
DETAILS: *On exhale:* Bend knees to facilitate stretching low back and bring belly and chest to thighs. Move chin down toward throat. *On inhale:* Lift chest up and away from thighs, flattening upper back.

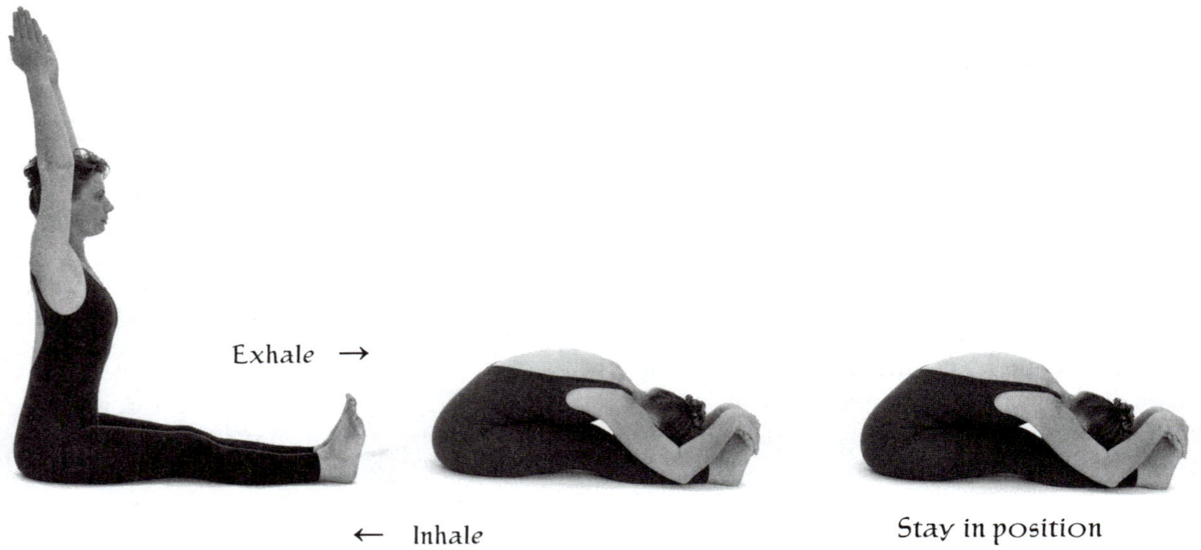

11.

POSTURE: Śavāsana with support.
EMPHASIS: To rest.
TECHNIQUE: Lie flat on back, with arms at sides, palms up, and legs slightly apart. Close eyes. Relax body fully, keeping mind relaxed and alert to sensations in body.
DURATION: Minimum 3 to 5 minutes.

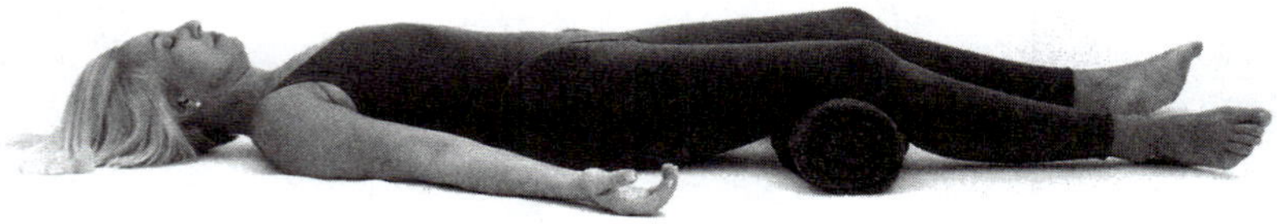

Revolving: An Introduction to Twists

Primary and Secondary Intentions

Twisting postures create rotation between the vertebral bodies of the spine, building strength and flexibility in the deep and superficial spinal and abdominal musculature and maintaining the elasticity of the intervertebral discs and ligaments. Twisting alternately compresses and stretches each hemisphere of the chest, stimulating respiratory function; alternately compresses and stretches the mid-torso, where the kidneys, adrenals, liver, gallbladder, pancreas, spleen, and stomach are located, stimulating their function; and alternately compresses and stretches the intestines, stimulating absorption, digestion, and elimination. In addition, twisting postures adjust the relationship between the shoulder and pelvic girdles and the spine, as well as strengthen and stretch the deep and superficial musculature that bind the head, the shoulders and arms, and the pelvis and legs to the spine. Where there is structural asymmetry in these areas, twisting helps to restore balance.

From a biomechanical perspective, according to the Viniyoga tradition, the *primary intention* of twisting is to rotate the spine.

The *secondary intention* of twisting is to adjust the relationship between the pelvic and shoulder girdles and the spine.

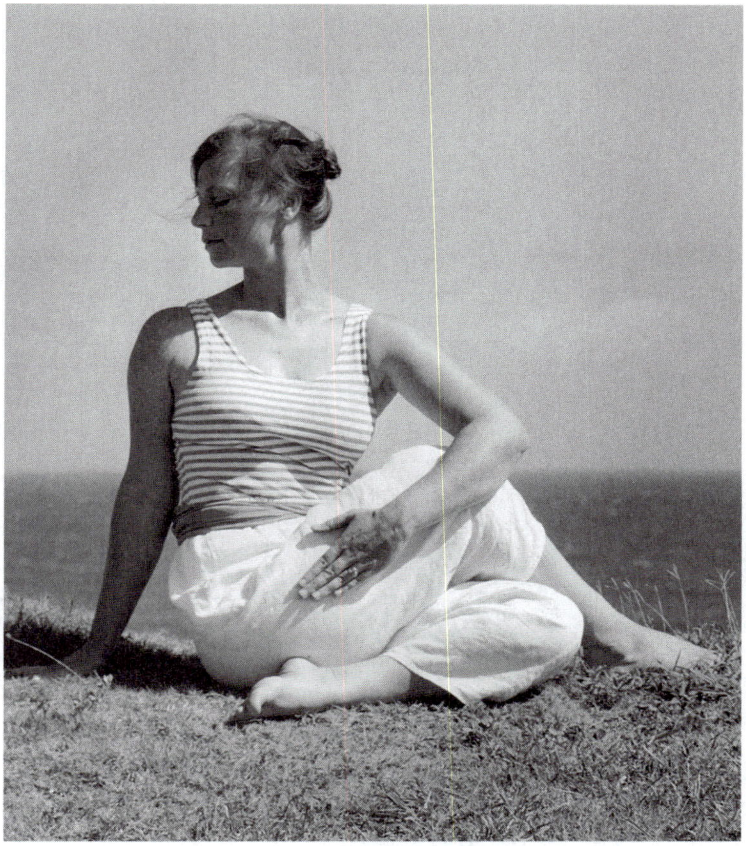

Technique

The key to twisting is the ability to control spinal rotation from the musculature of the abdomen and spine, rather than through the force of leverage generated by the musculature of the shoulders and arms and/or pelvis and legs. In twisting postures, this leverage can be applied, carefully, to augment the rotation of the spine but not to generate it.

The capacity for intervertebral rotation in the lumbar spine is limited. Twisting of the lower abdomen is therefore generated either by stabilzing the pelvis and rotating the spine, by stabilizing the spine and rotating the pelvis, or by rotating both in opposing directions.

The capacity for intervertebral rotation in the thoracic spine is greater than in the lumbar, particularly in the lower thoracic and in the thoraco-lumbar joint (see page 136). Twisting of the mid-torso is therefore generated either by stabilizing the pelvic-lumbar area and rotating the shoulder-thoracic area, by stabilizing the shoulder-thoracic area and rotating the pelvic-lumbar area, or by rotating both in opposing directions.

The cervical spine has the greatest capacity for intervertebral rotation, particularly at the atlas-axis joint (see page 143). Twisting of the neck is generated either by stabilizing the shoulders and rotating the head or by rotating both in opposing directions.

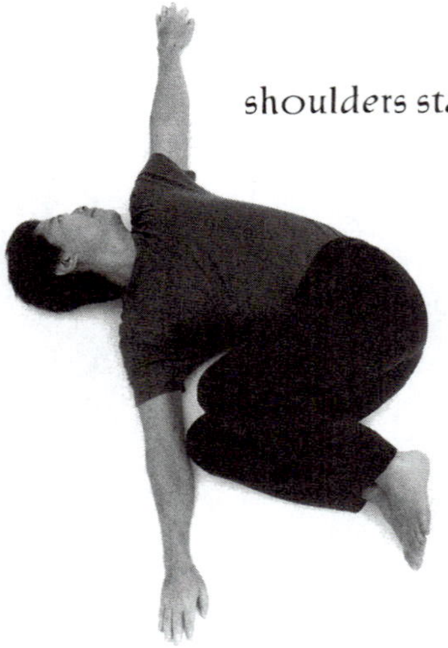
shoulders stable

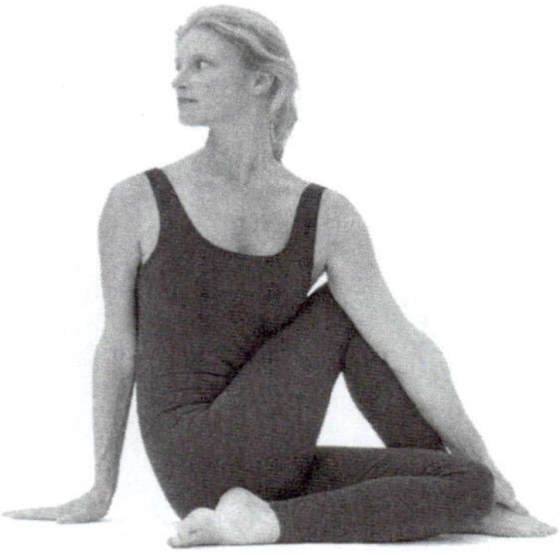
pelvis stable

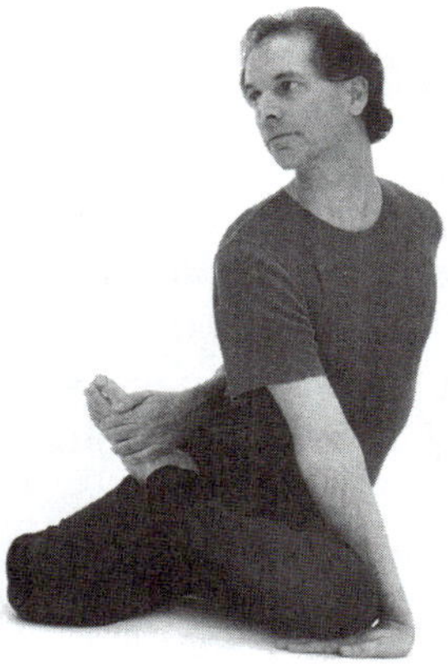
head and shoulders opposed

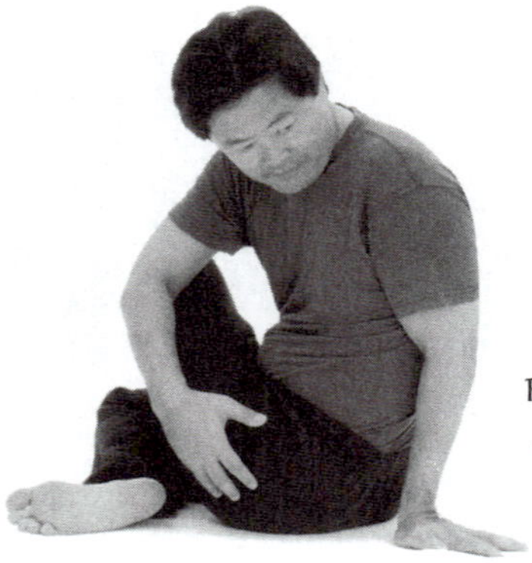
RELEASE VALVE 3, collapsed chest*

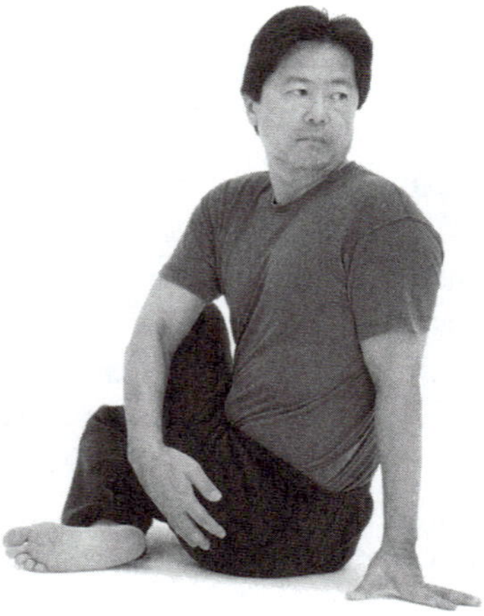
correct

The key to spinal rotation, and therefore to all twisting postures, is the technique of abdominal contraction on exhalation. At the initiation of exhalation, contract the abdominal muscles at their insertion into the pubic bone, to stabilize the pelvic-lumbar relationship, and simultaneously initiate rotation. If you have a deep lumbar curve, pull the pubic bone slightly upward at the beginning of the twist to maximize the vertical extension of the spine. As the twist proceeds, continue the contraction of the abdominal muscles, from the pubic bone to the rib cage, emphasizing trunk rotation.

As with forward bends, the natural curve of the thoracic spine may create the tendency to collapse the rib cage over the belly as you twist. This can be avoided by lengthening between the chest and belly on inhale. With the lengthening of the spine, you will notice a natural "unwinding" of the twist, creating more space between the vertebrae. This will actually allow you to twist more deeply on the subsequent exhale.

* For a list of common release valves for twists, see page 66.

Types of Twists

♦ GROUP 1

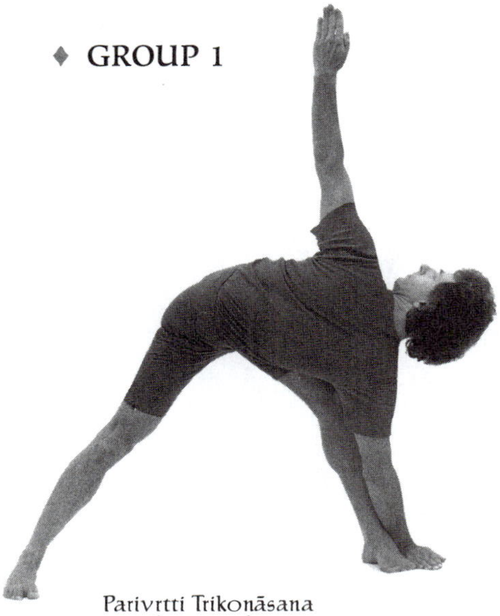
Parivṛtti Trikoṇāsana

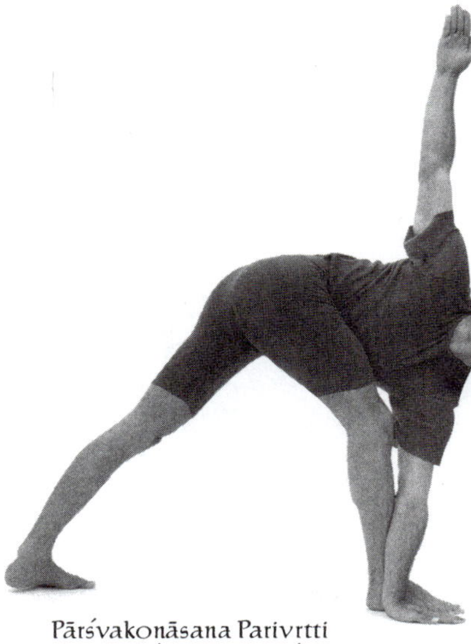
Pārśvakoṇāsana Parivṛtti

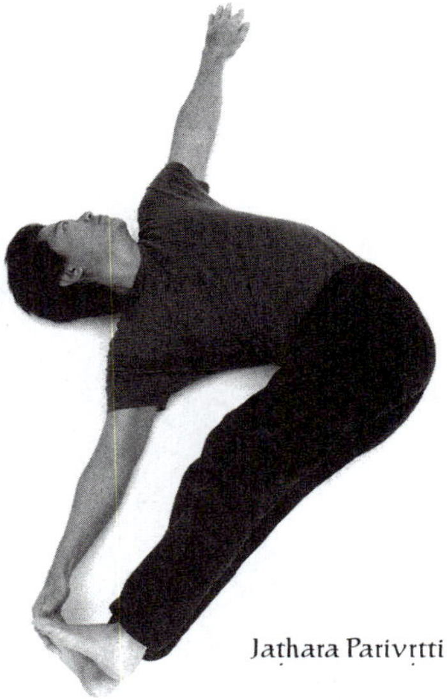
Jaṭhara Parivṛtti

The first group of postures includes standing and supine (on the back) *open-frame* twists, in which the shoulders and arms and the pelvis and legs have relative freedom of movement. These postures stretch and strengthen the large superficial muscles of the spine, shoulders, and pelvis. They also help bring balance to asymmetrical muscular development. If you are tight, muscle-bound, or overweight, you will be able to experience deep twisting in these open-frame postures. Some of these postures can be adapted as *fixed-frame* twists, where the hands hold the feet or the arms wrap around the legs.

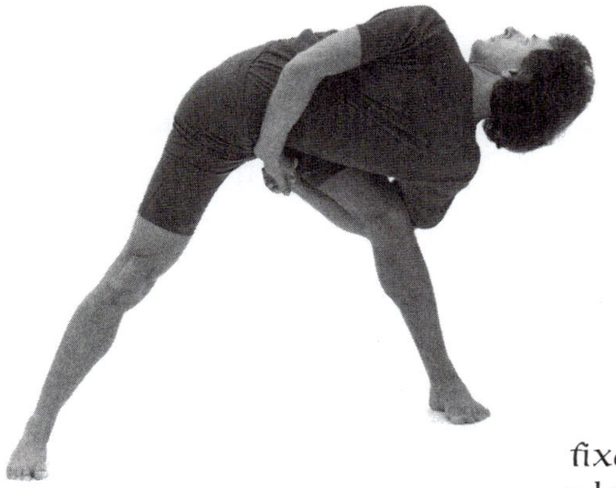
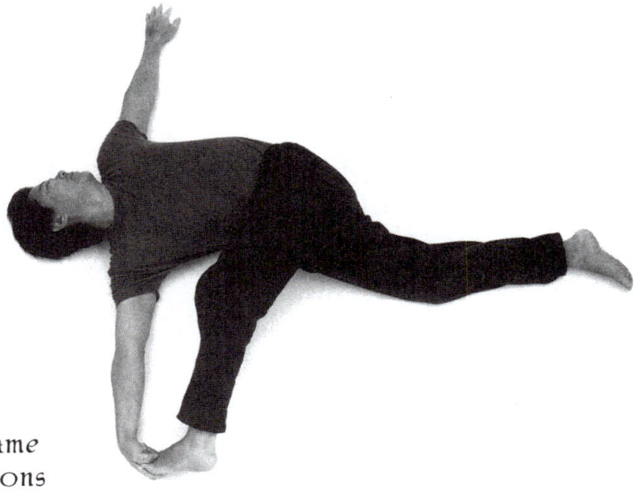
fixed-frame adaptations

In the standing postures, the pelvis is stabilized to emphasize rotation in the spine and shoulders. In the supine postures, the shoulders are stabilized to emphasize rotation in the spine and pelvis.

In these open-frame twists, we can control the location and intensity of the rotation, making these very simple postures profound in their effect. In the standing Parivṛtti Trikoṇāsana, for example, by varying the position of the hand on the floor, we can influence where the primary spinal rotation is experienced. For example, when the hand is midway between the feet, the rotation is felt most between the shoulders, ribs, and upper back; and, as the hand moves progressively toward the opposite foot, the rotation is felt most in the hips, abdomen, and lower back.

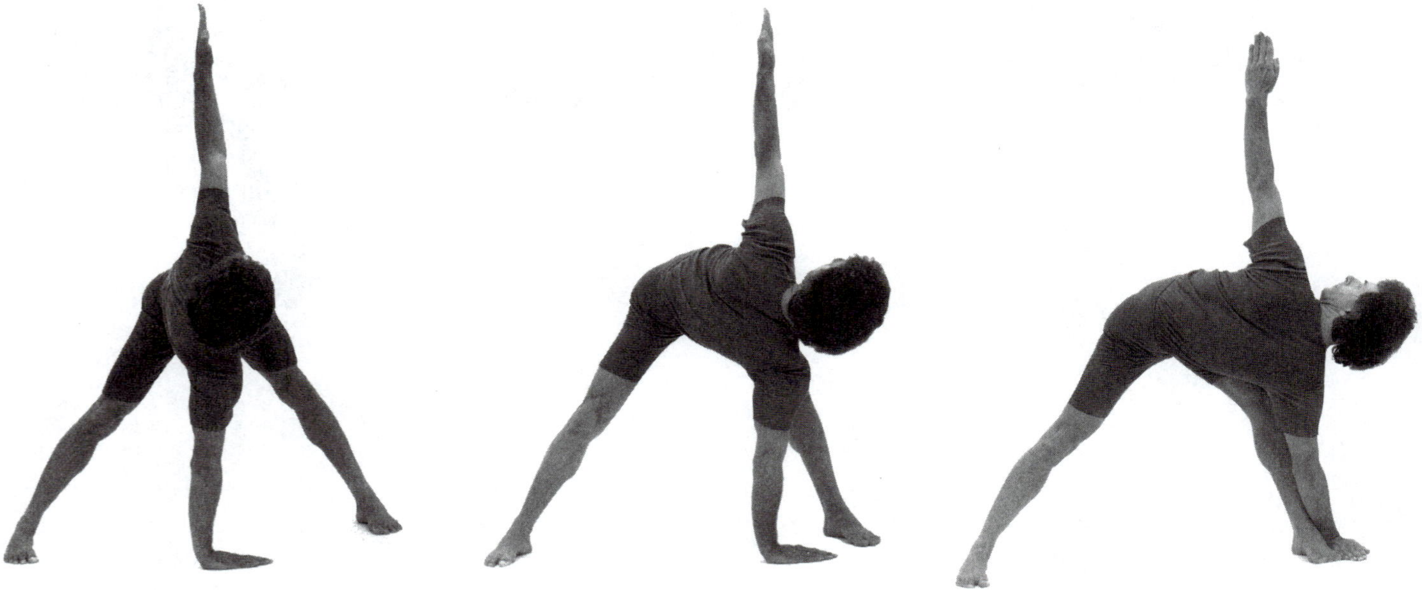

vary arm position

♦ GROUP 2

A) classic postures:

This group of postures includes seated fixed-frame twists in which the arms and legs are used as levers to deepen the spinal torsion. Though the leg positions vary, in all of these postures the pelvis is stabilized and the rotation occurs primarily in the spine and shoulders. Though the arm positions vary, they are used as levers to maximize the rotation of the spine and shoulders. In some postures, in addition to augmenting the rotation of the spine and shoulder girdle, the arms are used to displace one leg in the opposite direction, increasing the stretching of the muscles of that hip. The use of leverage significantly deepens spinal rotation, the activation of the deeper spinal muscles and ligaments, and the stretching of the muscles that bind the shoulders and pelvis to the spine.

In most of these postures, the head rotates in the same direction as the spine and shoulders. In Bhāradvājāsana, the head uniquely rotates in the opposite direction, increasing the stretching of the muscles of the neck. If you can master this special posture, you will discover the truly magical and powerful qualities of balance and integrity that accompany twisting.

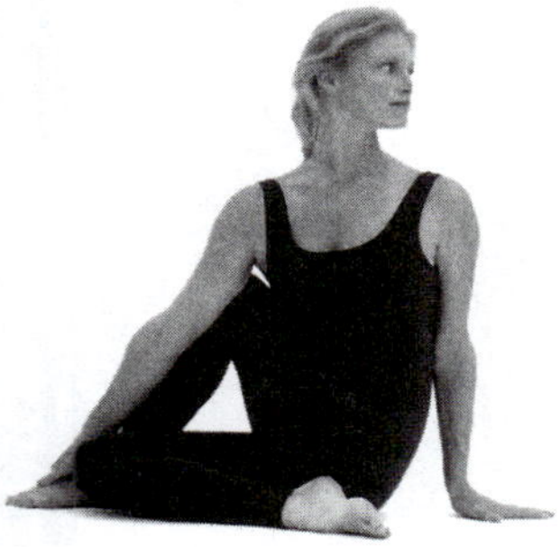

Ardha Matsyendrāsana

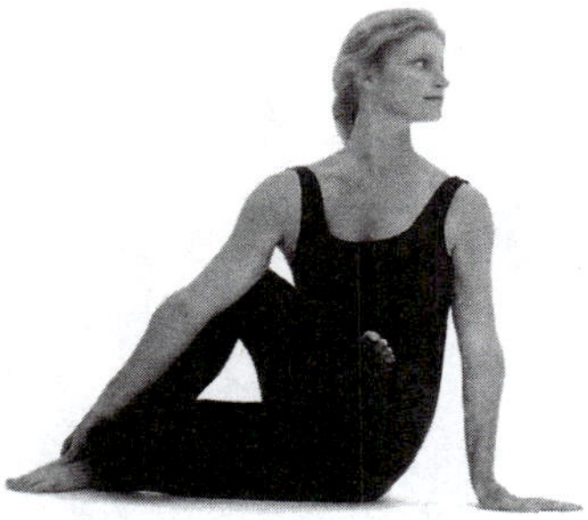

Pūrṇa Matsyendrāsana

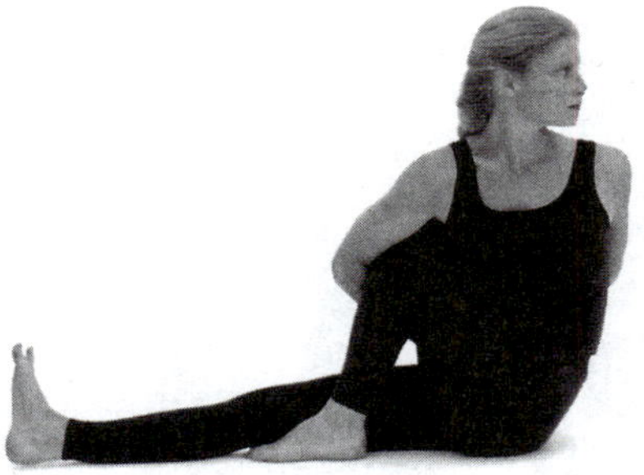

Marīcyāsana Parivṛtti

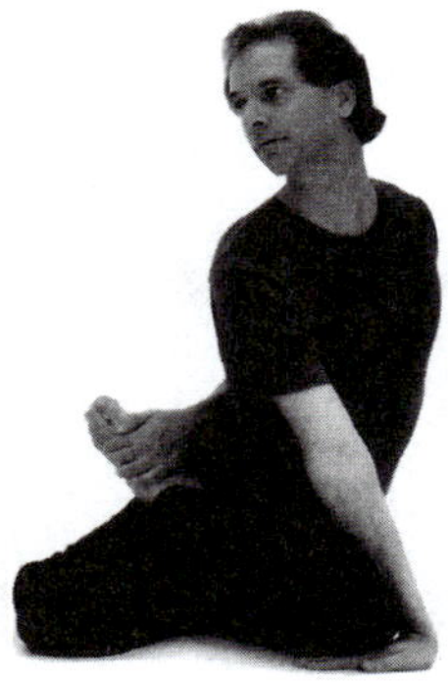

Bhāradvājāsana

B) useful variations:

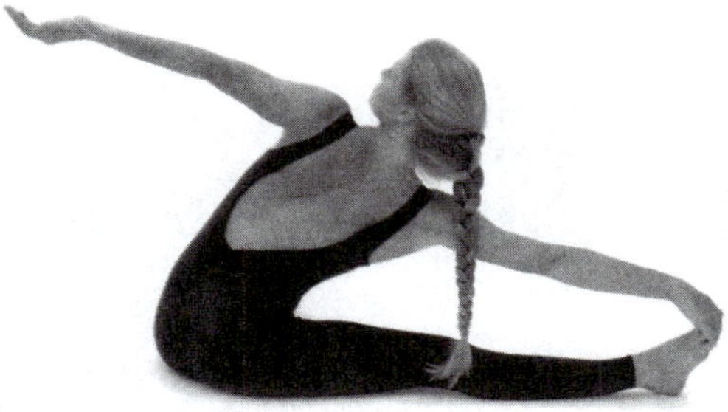

Jānu Śirṣāsana Parivṛtti

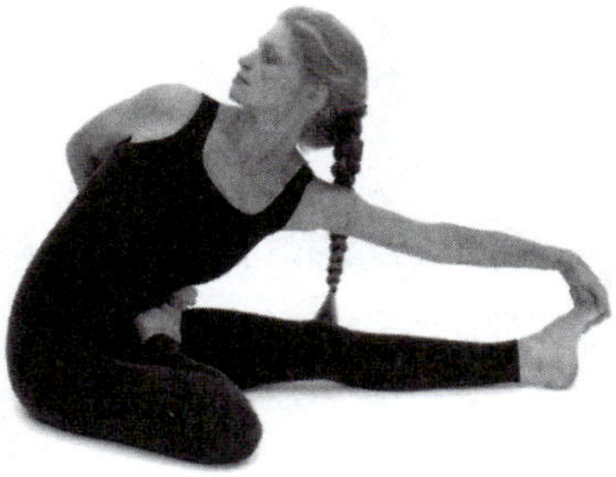

Ardha Baddha Padma Paścimatānāsana Parivṛtti

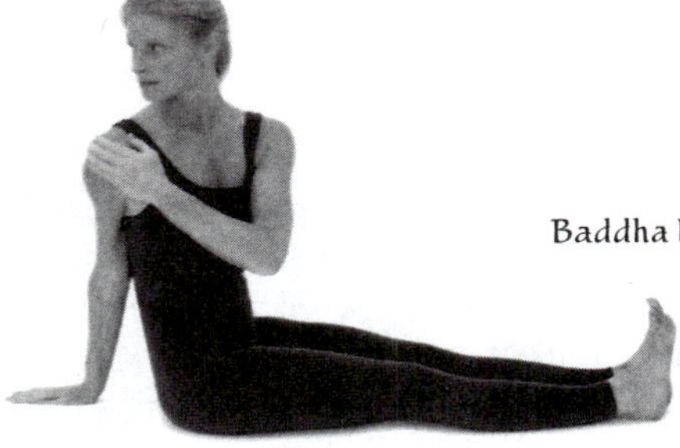

Daṇḍāsana Parivṛtti

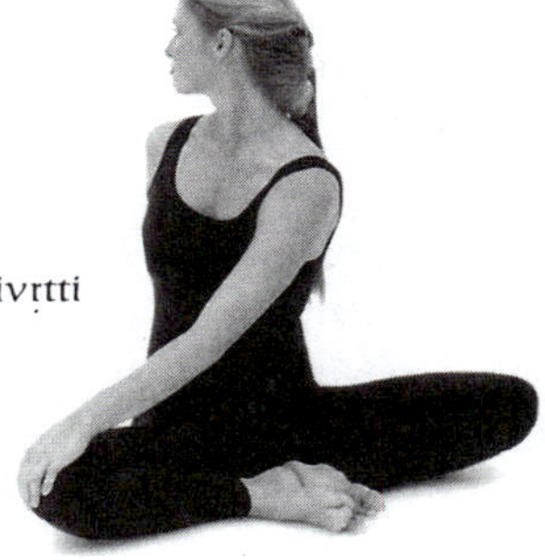

Baddha Koṇāsana Parivṛtti

Common Release Valves for Twists

1. Initiating the action of twisting in the muscles of the shoulder and/or pelvis without sufficiently engaging the abdominal muscles, limiting spinal rotation.
2. Reducing the effects of spinal, shoulder, or pelvic rotation by displacing the stabilized portion of the body in the direction of the twist.

   In standing twists, the displacement of the pelvis or the internal rotation of the opposing thigh, knee, or foot in the direction of the twist reduces hip, spinal, and shoulder rotation. In supine twists, the lifting of the opposing shoulder in the direction of the twist likewise reduces hip, spinal, and shoulder rotation.

   On the other hand, some displacement of the opposing structures may be helpful. If all displacement is blocked, rotation may be so restricted that no benefit is achieved. If you have tight hips, spinal muscles, and shoulders, and insist on restricting all internal rotation of the femur, knee, ankle, and foot in standing postures, you may be unable to create any significant twisting at all. If, in the supine postures, you hold the opposing shoulder firmly down on the floor, you may likewise be unable to effect any significant twisting. Where there is limited mobility, allowing some displacement will enable you to experience the twist and, in fact, achieve more of its benefits.
3. Collapsing the chest over the belly inhibits effective spinal rotation in seated twists.

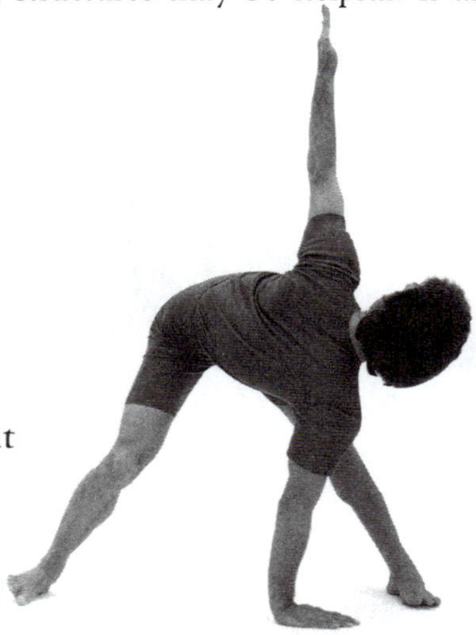

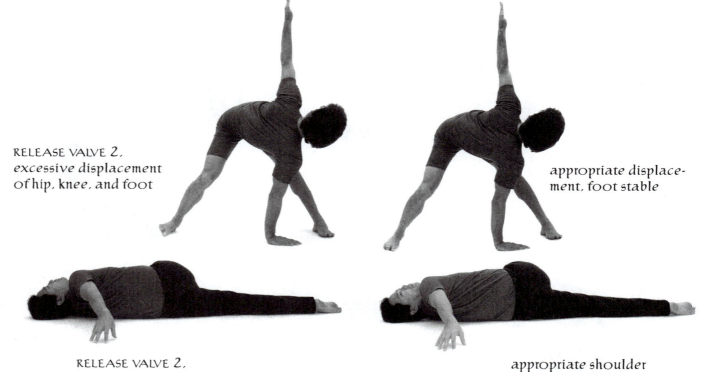

RELEASE VALVE 2, *excessive displacement of hip, knee, and foot*

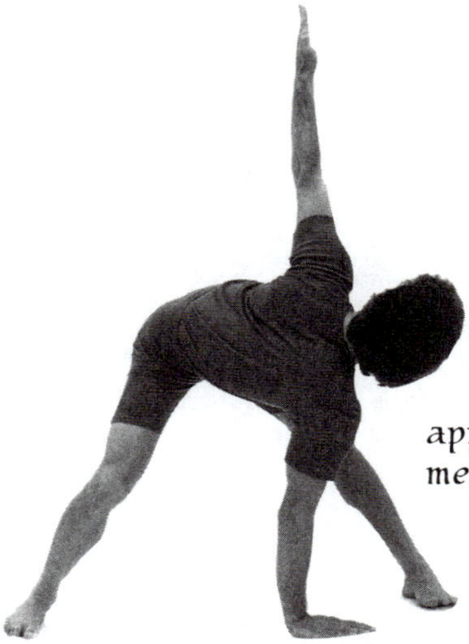

appropriate displacement, foot stable

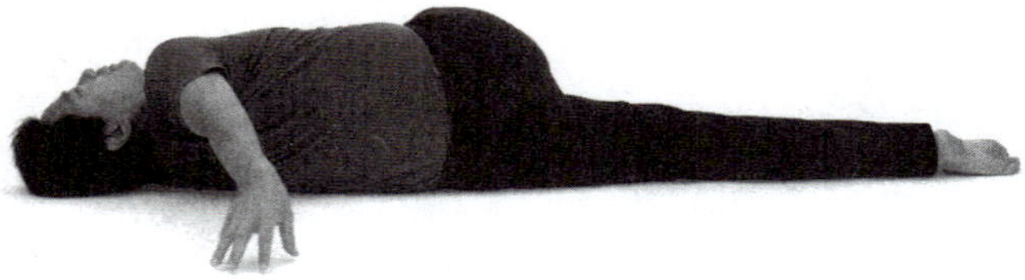

RELEASE VALVE 2, *excessive shoulder displacement*

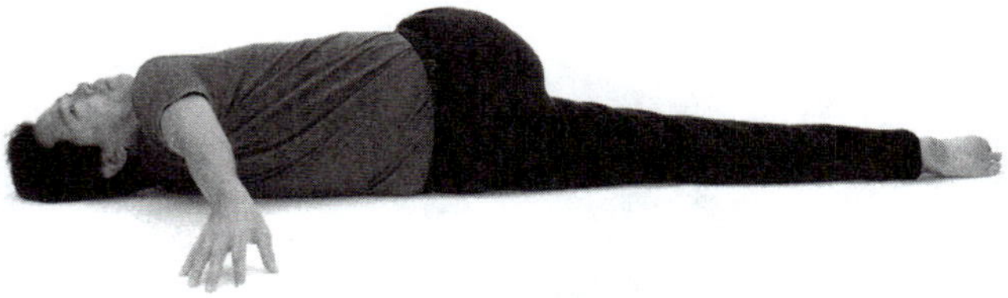

appropriate shoulder displacement

Common Risks

In twisting, the intervertebral discs are compressed. If there are any preexisting conditions of compression in the spine—for example an excessive thoracic and/or lumbar curve or excessive lateral spinal asymmetry—the possibility of injury to the discs increases. Risks can be minimized by adequate preparation, avoiding excessive force when using the arms and legs as levers, and lengthening the spine on inhalation while twisting.

There is also risk, in twisting postures, to the

sacroiliac, hip, and knee joints. This is especially true in standing twists, where these joints are bearing weight, and in fixed-frame seated twists, where the arms and legs are used as levers. To reduce these risks in standing twists, keep the hip, knee, and ankle in vertical alignment, avoiding excessive internal or external rotation. In all twists, generate the rotation from the abdomen, rather than forcing the rotation with the leverage of the arms and legs.

Twisting Practice (for Bhāradvājāsana)

1.

POSTURE: Uttānāsana.
EMPHASIS: To warm up back and legs.
TECHNIQUE: Stand with arms over head.
On exhale: Bend forward, bringing belly and chest toward thighs and bringing hands to feet.
On inhale: return to starting position.
NUMBER: 6 times.
DETAILS: *On exhale:* Bend knees to facilitate stretching of low back. Move chin down toward throat. *On inhale:* Lift chest up and away from thighs, flattening upper back. Keep knees bent until end of movement.

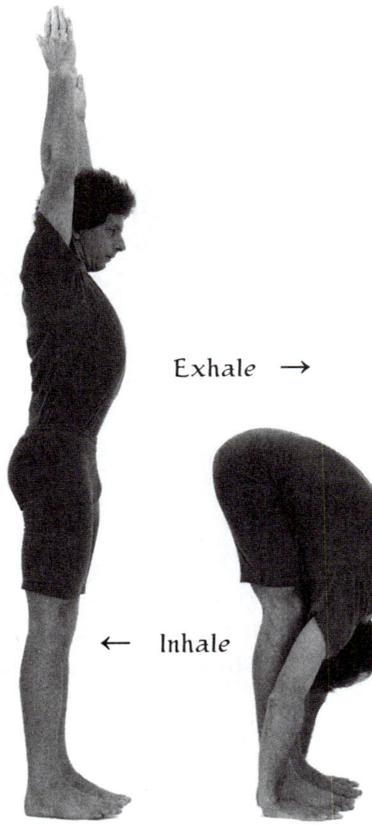

2.

POSTURE: Parivṛtti Trikoṇāsana.
EMPHASIS: To stretch legs, back, and shoulders.
TECHNIQUE: Stand with feet spread wider than shoulders and with arms out to sides and parallel to floor.

On exhale: Bend forward and twist, bringing left hand to floor, pointing right arm upward, and twisting shoulders right. Turn head down toward left hand.

On inhale: Maintaining rotation, and with right shoulder vertically above left, bring right arm up over shoulder and forward, turning head to center and looking at right hand.

On exhale: Return to previous position with right arm pointing upward. Turn head up, looking toward right hand.

On inhale: Return to starting position.

Repeat on other side.

NUMBER: 6 times each side, alternately.
DETAILS: Keep down arm vertically below its respective shoulder, and keep weight of torso off arm. Knees can bend while moving into twist.

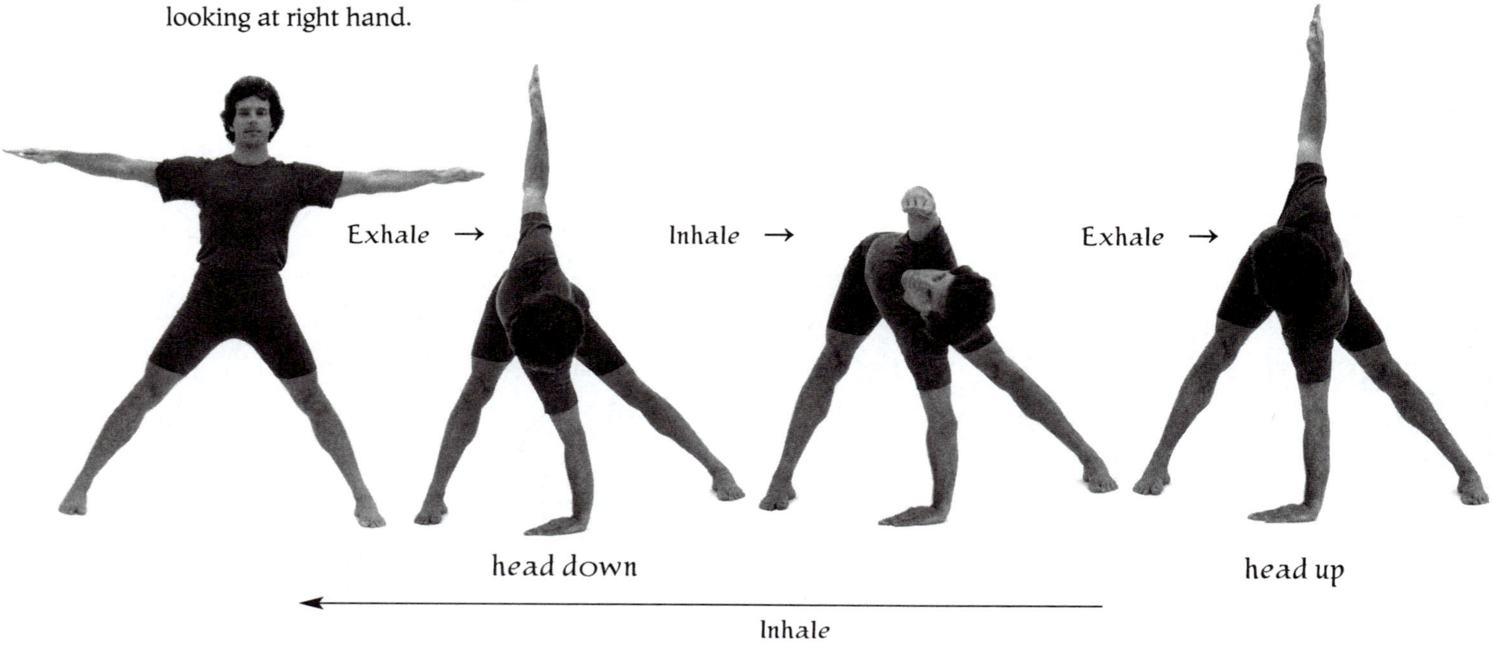

3.

POSTURE: Cakravākāsana.
EMPHASIS: To make transition from standing to supine position. To stretch rib cage on inhale and low back on exhale.
TECHNIQUE: Get down on hands and knees, with shoulders vertically above wrists and with hips above knees.

On inhale: Lift chest up and away from belly.

On exhale: Gently contract belly, round low back, and bring chest toward thighs.

NUMBER: 8 times.
DETAILS: *On inhale:* Lead with chest, keeping chin slightly down. Avoid compressing low back; rather, feel chest expanding. *On exhale:* Round low back without collapsing chest over belly. Avoid increasing curvature of upper back. Let chest lower toward thighs sooner than hips towards heels.

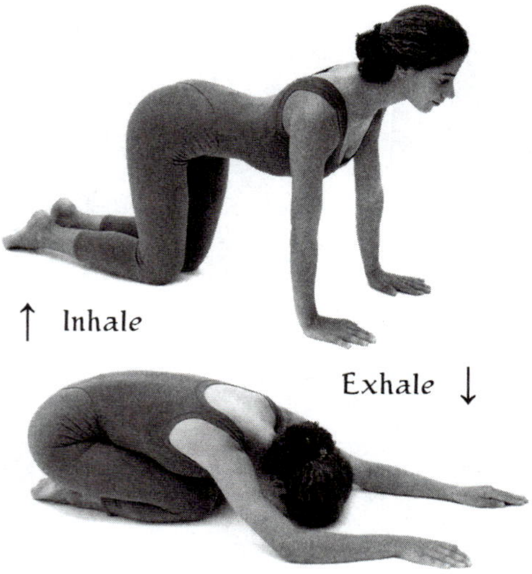

4.

POSTURE: Ekapāda Rājakapotāsana variation.
EMPHASIS: To stretch hip rotator muscles in preparation for Bhāradvājāsana.
TECHNIQUE: Kneel on left knee and extend right leg straight behind you, hands on the floor on either side of right knee. Move right foot forward and toward left hand, displacing left knee further to left.

On inhale: Lift rib cage forward and up, while pulling down and back with hands, pushing chest forward, and flattening upper back.

On exhale: Bend elbows and lower chest toward floor. Stay down 2 breaths.

NUMBER: Repeat 4 times each side.
DETAILS: *On inhale:* Pull down and back with hands, rather than pushing up. Drop shoulders and pull shoulder blades back. *On exhale:* While staying in posture, adjust position of left foot to achieve maximum stretching of left hip.

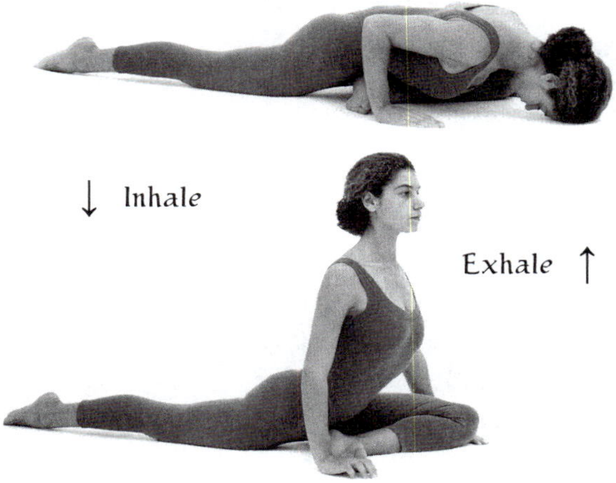

5.

POSTURE: Jaṭhara Parivṛtti.
EMPHASIS: To stretch across hips and back, one side at a time.
TECHNIQUE: Lie flat on back, with arms out to sides, and with left knee pulled up toward chest.

A. *On exhale:* Twist, bringing left knee toward floor on right side of body, while turning head to left.

On inhale: Return to starting position.

Repeat 4 times.

B. Then stay in twist, holding left knee with right hand.

On inhale: With palm up, sweep left arm wide along floor toward ear, turning head to center.

On exhale: Lower arm back to side, turning head to left.

Repeat 6 times.

Repeat on other side.

DETAILS: *On exhale:* When twisting right, keep angles between left arm and torso and between left knee and torso less than ninety degrees.

B: Keep arm that is moving low to floor; palm up on *inhale,* palm down *on exhale.* Hold twisted knee low toward floor.

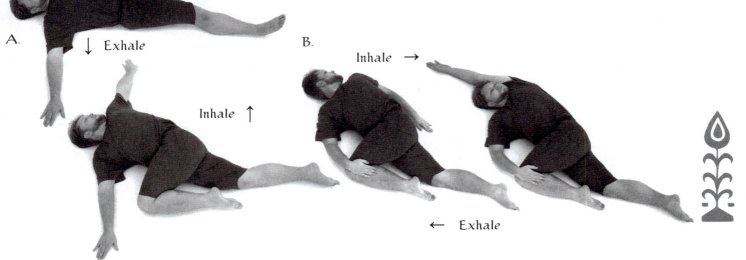

A.

B.

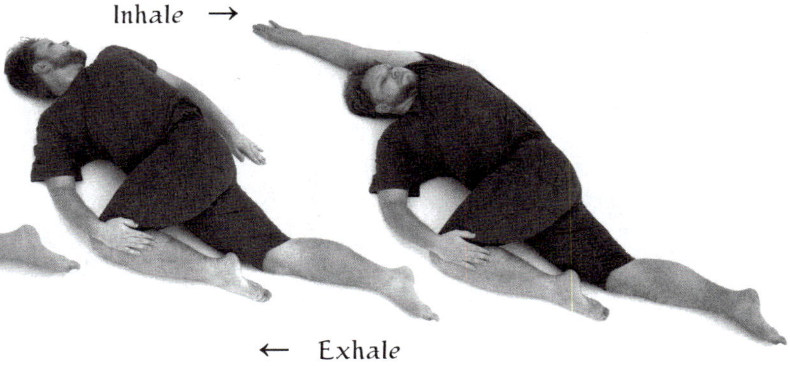

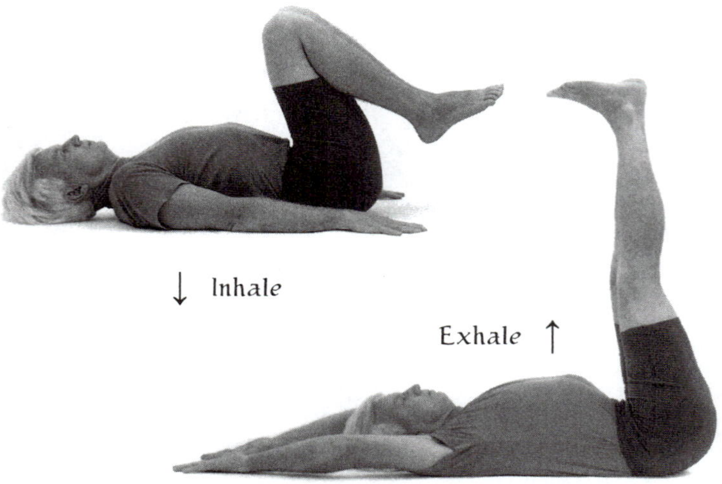

6.

Posture: Ūrdhva Prasārita Pādāsana.
Emphasis: To extend spine and flatten it onto floor. To stretch legs.
Technique: Lie on back with arms down at sides, legs bent and knees held toward chest.

On inhale: Raise arms upward all the way to floor behind head, and raise legs upward toward ceiling.

On exhale: Return to starting position.

Repeat 6 times.

Details: *On inhale:* Flex feet as legs are raised upward. Keep knees slightly bent, and keep angle between legs and torso less than ninety degrees. Push low back and sacrum downward. Bring chin down.

7.

Posture: Bhāradvājāsana.
Emphasis: To experience one of the deepest and most complete spinal twists. To stretch the muscles that bind the head and neck to the spine.
Technique: Sit with the right leg folded back, right foot on the floor to the right of right hip, and the left leg folded with left foot on upper right thigh. Wrap left arm behind back and grasp left foot, and place right palm down on floor on outside of left knee with fingers pointing toward right knee.

On inhale: Extend spine upward.

On exhale: Twist shoulders left and turn head right.

Number: Stay 12 breaths each side.
Details: Lean firmly on right palm, allowing right sit bone to lift off floor. *On exhale:* As you twist shoulders left and turn head right, focus on stretch on left side of neck.

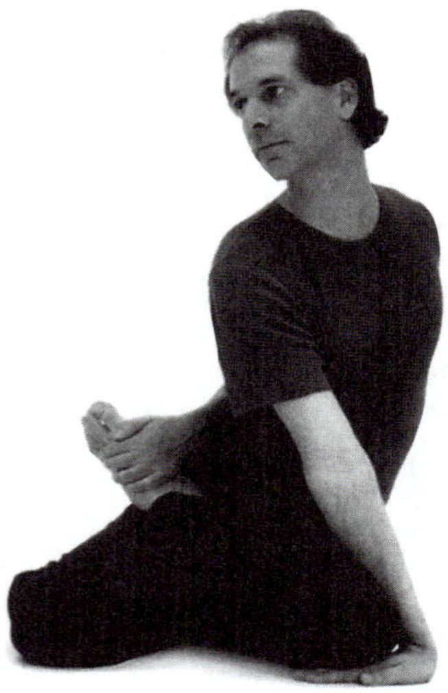

8.

POSTURE: Paścimatānāsana.

EMPHASIS: To stretch back to compensate for twist.

TECHNIQUE: Sit with legs forward, back straight, and arms raised over head.

On exhale: Bending knees slightly, bend forward, bringing chest to thighs, and palms to balls of feet.

On inhale: Return to starting position.

Repeat 4 times.

Then stay in forward bend position 6 breaths.

DETAILS: *On exhale:* Bend knees to facilitate stretching low back and bring belly and chest to thighs. Move chin down toward throat. *On inhale:* Lift chest up and away from thighs, flattening upper back.

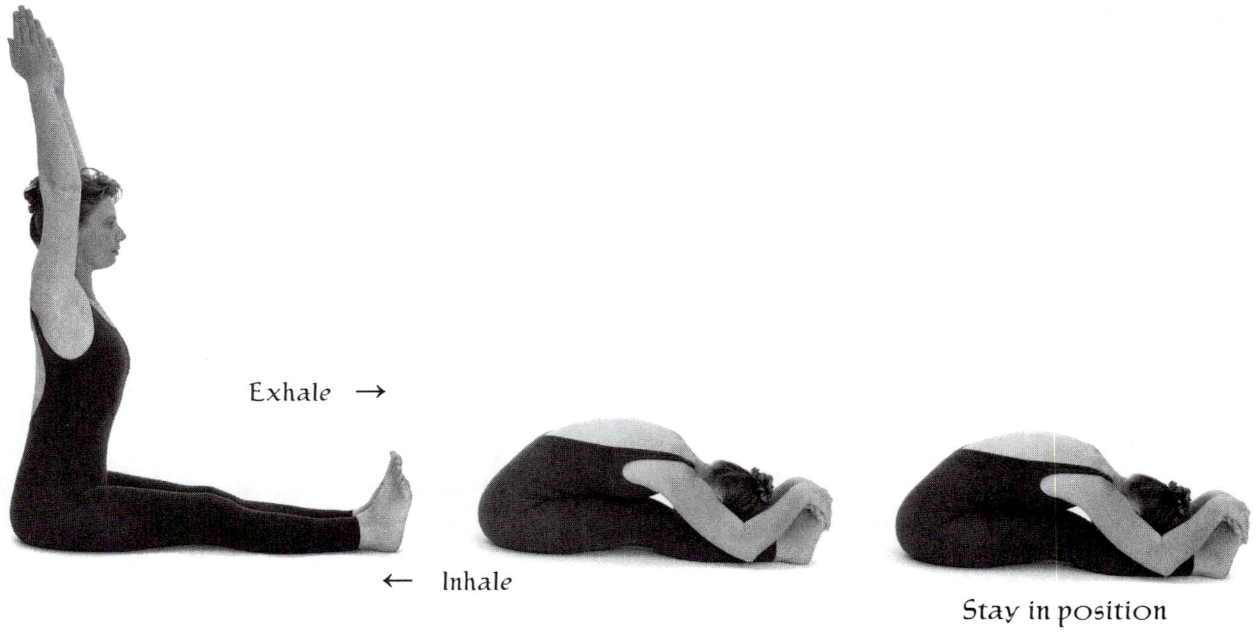

9.

POSTURE: Śavāsana.

EMPHASIS: To rest.

TECHNIQUE: Lie flat on back, with arms at sides, palms up, and legs slightly apart. Close eyes. Relax body fully, keeping mind relaxed and alert to sensations in body.

DURATION: Minimum 3 to 5 minutes.

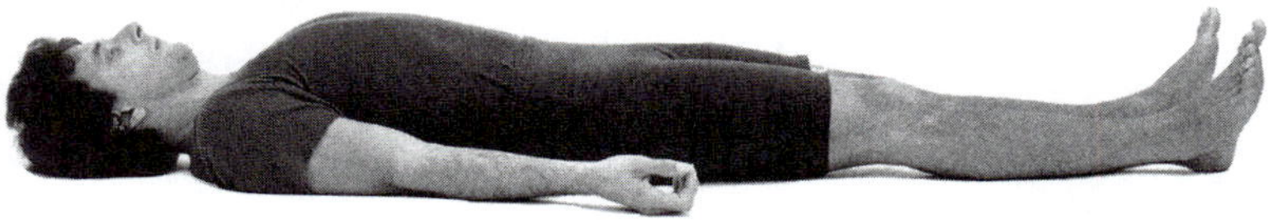

Working the Sides: An Introduction to Lateral Bends

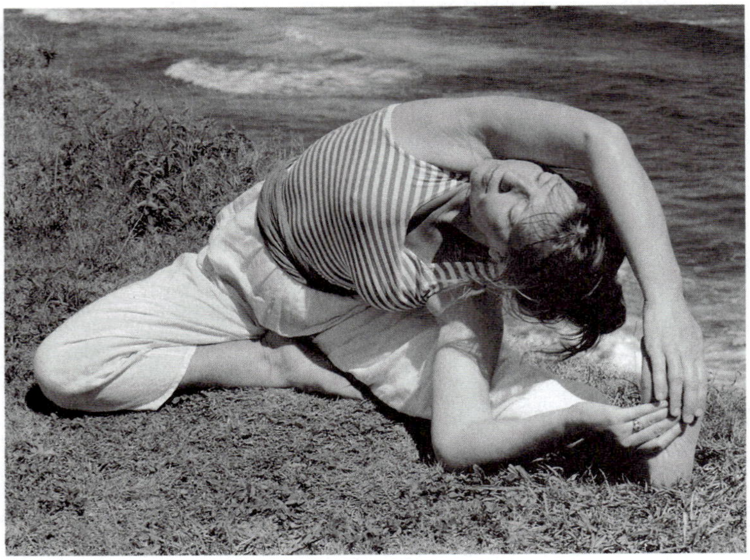

Primary and Secondary Intentions

Lateral bends can be organized into two distinct classes. In the first class, the torso is bent to the side. These postures alternately stretch and compress the deep spinal muscles, the intervertebral ligaments and discs, the intercostal muscles and connective tissues that bind the ribs together, and the deep and superficial muscles that bind the shoulder and pelvic girdles to the spine. They build strength and stability in the musculature of the spine, rib cage, shoulders, and pelvis; they help maintain the elasticity of the rib cage; and they help restore balance to asymmetries of the spine, shoulders, and pelvis. In addition, these postures alternately stretch and compress the lungs and organs of the torso—such as the kidneys, liver, and intestines—and thus stimulate their function.

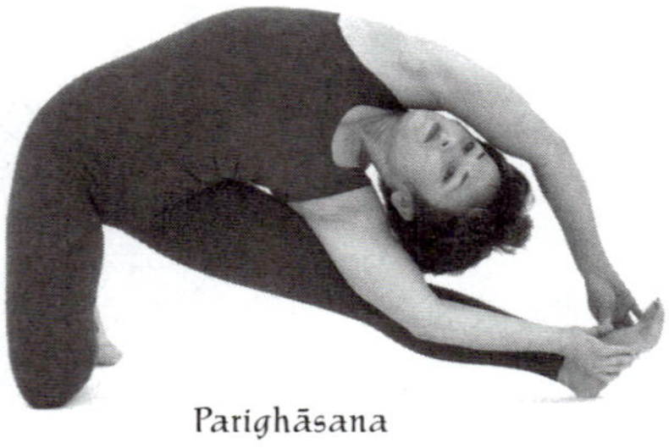

Parighāsana

In the second class of lateral bends, one leg is abducted and rotated outward. These postures stretch the structures of the pelvis, groin, inner thigh, and perineal area, building strength and flexibility in the muscles in these areas. In addition, they increase circulation to the perineal floor and stimulate the function of the reproductive organs. In these effects, they are related to the forward bends with legs spread wide (see Group 4).

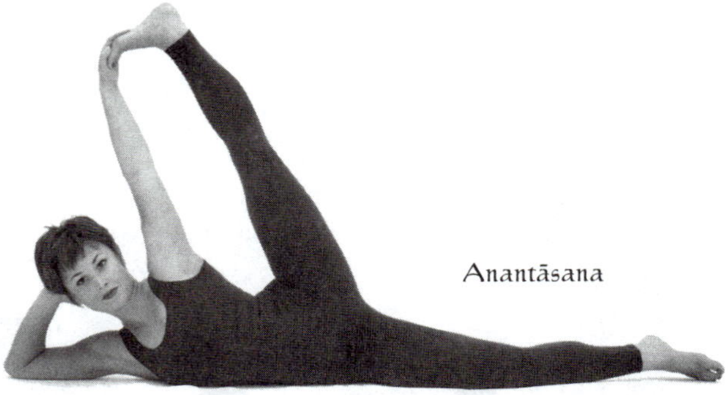

Anantāsana

From a biomechanical perspective, according to the Viniyoga tradition, the *primary intention* of the first class of lateral bends is to laterally stretch the torso from the shoulder to the hip joint, and to laterally flex the spine. The *secondary intention* is to stretch and strengthen the musculature of the shoulder girdle, hip joints, front of the pelvis, and inner thighs.

In the second class of lateral bends, the emphasis is nearly reversed. The *primary intention* is to strengthen and stretch the musculature of the front of the pelvis, hip joints, groin, and inner thighs—these actions are collectively referred to as "pelvic opening." The *secondary intention* is to stretch the lateral portions of the torso and the structures of the shoulder girdle.

Technique

The capacity for pure lateral flexion of the spine is limited and, therefore, is rare in daily activity. Think of pulling over to the curb in your car to talk to a friend on the street. Imagine reaching over to roll down the window on the passenger side with your right hand. The normal tendency is for your hips to displace backward and rotate right as your chest and shoulders displace forward and rotate right. Now imagine keeping your back and shoulders flat against the seat while bending sideways to roll down the window. This is a pure lateral bend.

If you restrict displacement and rotation, you will significantly limit your range of motion, but you will maximize lateral flexion, and herein lies the potential benefit of lateral bends.

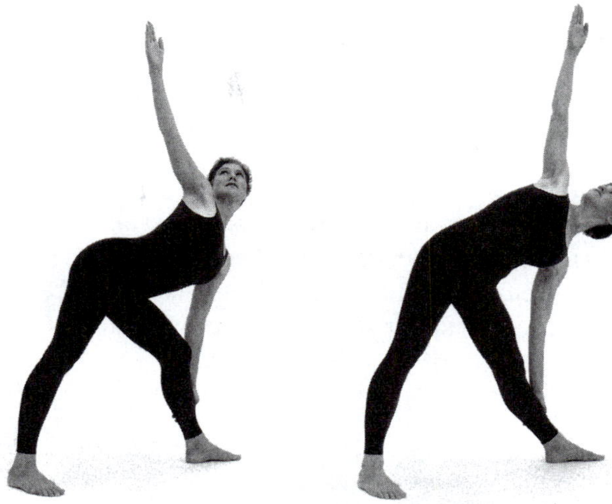

RELEASE VALVES 1, 2, and 5,* pelvis rotated, displaced lumbar arched excessively

correct

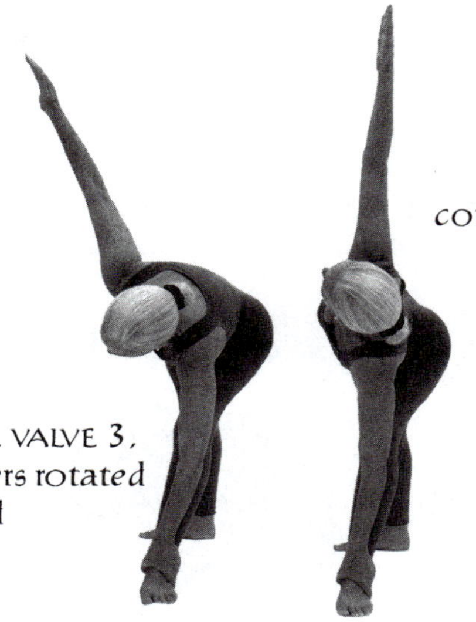

RELEASE VALVE 3, shoulders rotated forward

correct

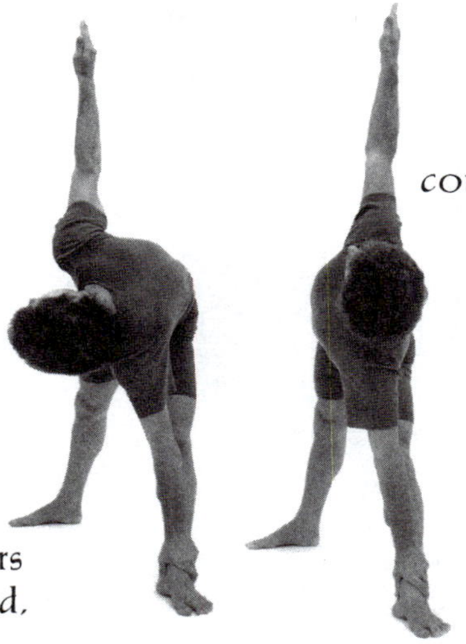

RELEASE VALVES 4 and 6, shoulders displaced forward, chest collapsed

correct

Accordingly, the key to these postures is the ability to control the proportional relationship between pure lateral bending and the natural displacement and rotation described above. And the key to this control is the combined techniques of exhale and inhale.

At the initiation of exhale, contract the abdominal muscles to check the forward rotation of the pelvis, and lengthen the lumbar spine, while simultaneously initiating the lateral bend. If you have a deep lumbar curve, pull the pubic bone slightly upward to check backward displacement of the pelvis. On subsequent exhalations, rotate the top shoulder slightly backward, keeping the shoulders in vertical alignment, to help maintain the lateral quality of the movement. On inhale, lengthen the spine, pull the chest up and away from the belly, pull the shoulders down and back, and flatten the thoracic curve, as in a backward bend. Lengthening the spine creates more space between the vertebrae, increasing the potential for lateral flexion without compressing the intervertebral discs. This action also inhibits the tendency to displace the chest and shoulders forward and helps prevent lateral intervertebral compression. Extending the arm, on the side being stretched, up over the head and forward on inhale increases the stretching of the musculature and connective tissues of the rib cage and torso. To maximize this effect, keep your arm in line with your shoulder and torso.

*For a list of common release valves for forward lateral bends, see page 77.

Types of Lateral Bends

♦ GROUP 1

The first group of postures includes standing and kneeling lateral bends where the primary effect is lateral stretching of the torso and the secondary effect is pelvic opening. In these postures, the pelvis and shoulder girdle are free to rotate and/or displace as the trunk bends laterally. Though this allows for more range of motion, it reduces the lateral stretching. These postures can be practiced either as open- or fixed-frame postures. In fixed-frame variations, the leverage created by the arms blocks the forward rotation and displacement of the shoulders, deepening the lateral stretching of the torso.

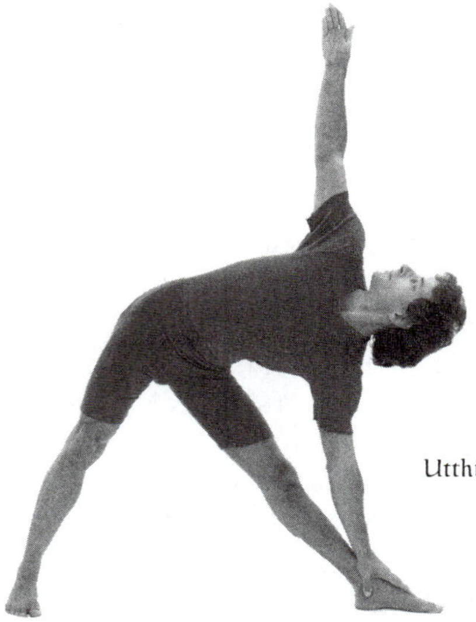

Utthita Trikoṇāsana

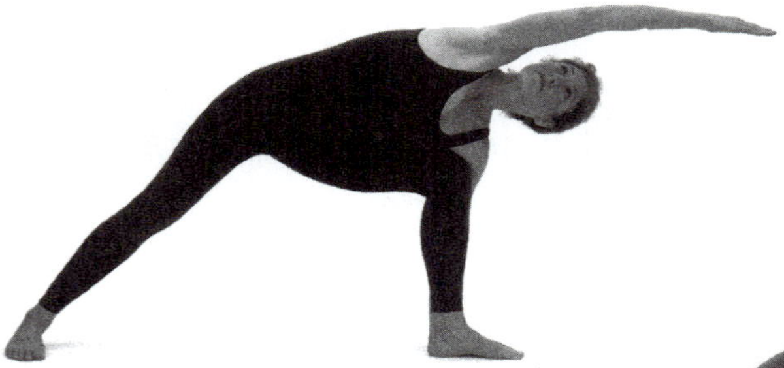

Utthita Pārśva Koṇāsana

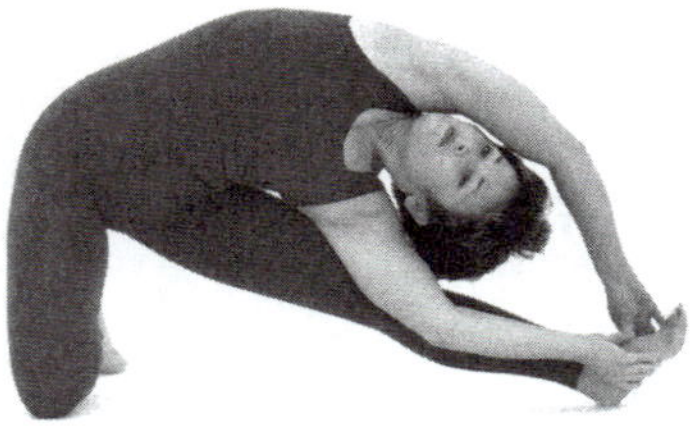

Parighāsana

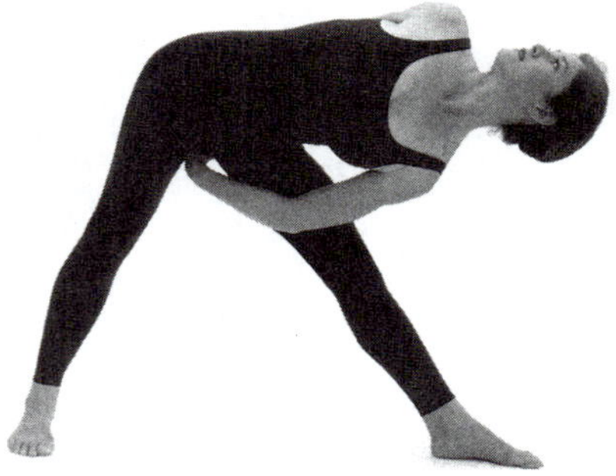

Utthita Trikoṇāsana adaptation

In standing postures, the foot and knee on the side of the bend is turned out at a ninety-degree angle, rotating the leg outward at the hip. The opposite hip and leg remain stabilized in a forward direction. This creates a spreading of the hip bones and a stretching across the front of the pelvis that is similar though less than that created by pelvic openers.

The kneeling lateral bend is the deepest of the lateral stretches. If you can master this posture, you will truly experience the powerful and expanding quality of lateral bends.

♦ GROUP 2

This group includes two postures where the primary effect is lateral stretching of the torso, and where the pelvic opening effect is absent (except in some difficult variations of Vaśiṣṭhāsana). They are both open-frame postures.

In the supine posture, the stretching is primarily in the hip and lower lateral muscles of the torso.

In Vaśiṣṭhāsana, which is also a balance posture, the stretching is primarily in the intercostal muscles and the large latissimus dorsi muscles, which attach from the spine across the ribs to the arm. Further adapations of Vaśiṣṭhāsana can be found ahead in the section on balance.

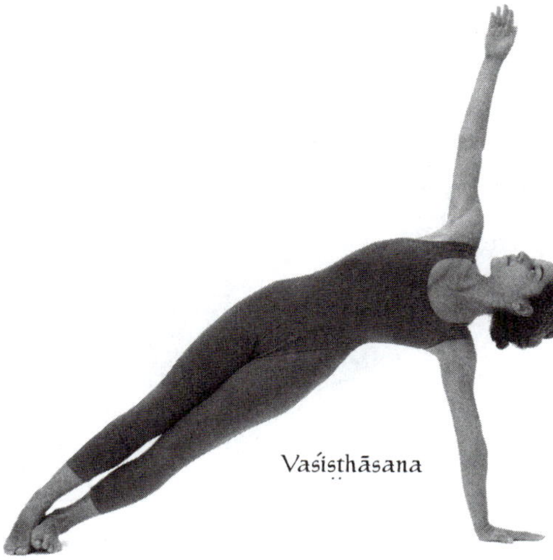

Vaśiṣṭhāsana

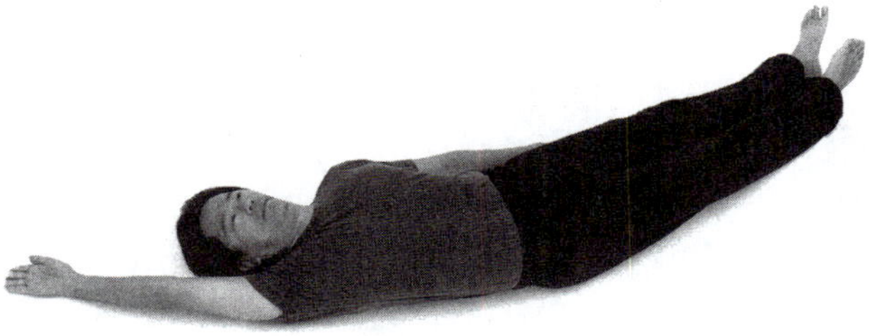

Jaṭhara Parivṛtti, lateral adaptation

♦ GROUP 3

This group of postures includes seated lateral bends, where the primary effect is lateral stretching of the torso. As these postures are seated, the backward displacement of the pelvis is restricted, resulting in a significant forward-bend component. Paścimatānāsana Parivṛtti is a deep, fixed-frame lateral stretch with strong forward bend and twisting elements.

The different leg positions in the three lateral adaptations of the asymmetric forward bends determine the degree of lateral displacement of the pelvis and thus the depth of the lateral stretching of the torso. These postures can be practiced either as open- or fixed-frame postures.

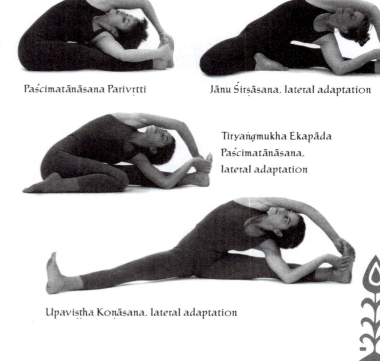

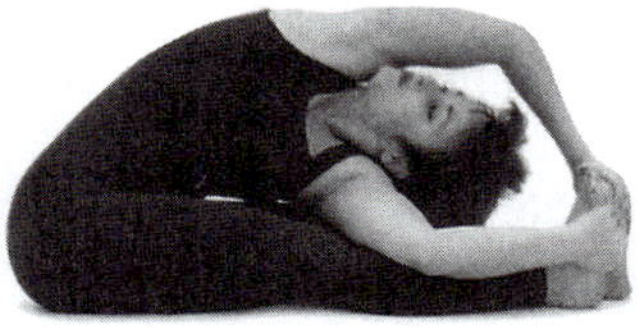

Paścimatānāsana Parivṛtti

Jānu Śirṣāsana, lateral adaptation

Tiryaṅgmukha Ekapāda Paścimatānāsana, lateral adaptation

Upaviṣṭha Koṇāsana, lateral adaptation

♦ GROUP 4

In these two fixed-frame postures, the primary effect is pelvic opening. In these postures, one hand holds the foot on the same side and one arm is used to extend and stretch the same leg. Because excessive stretching may compromise the stability of the hip or sacroiliac joints, we suggest that the primary action be generated by the leg, letting the arm guide rather than pull the leg. In Anantāsana, there is some secondary stretching of the lateral musculature of the lower torso on the opposite side.

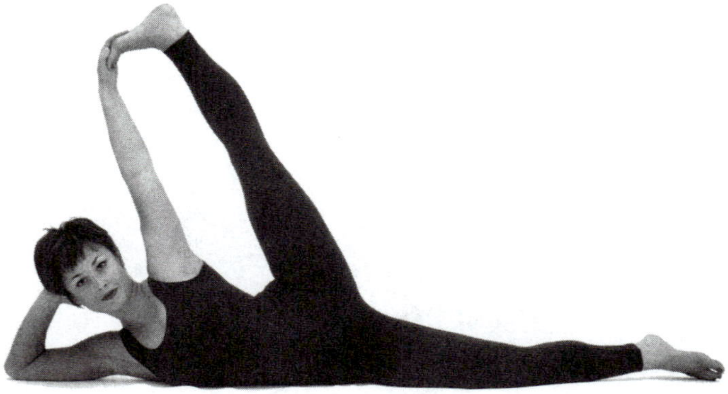

Anantāsana

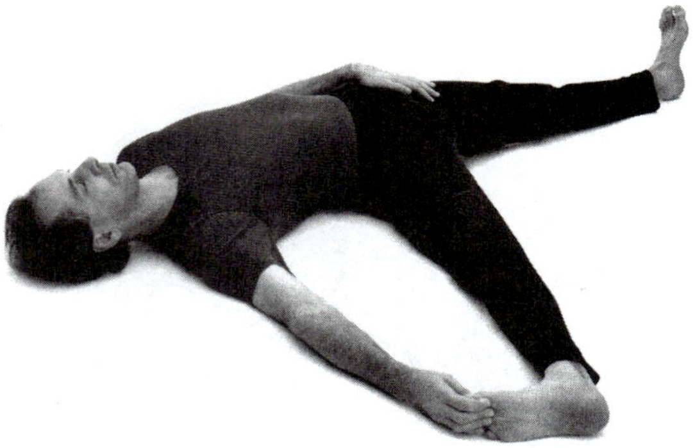

Supta Pārśva Pādāṅguṣṭhāsana

♦ GROUP 5

These two challenging seated postures primarily focus on stretching the deep and superficial muscles that bind the legs to the pelvis. They also stretch deeply the posterior and lateral muscles of the low back. They are particularly risky if there is weakness or instability in the hip or sacroiliac joints. With the leg behind the head, Ekapāda Śirsāsana (not shown) is also risky for the knee and the neck.

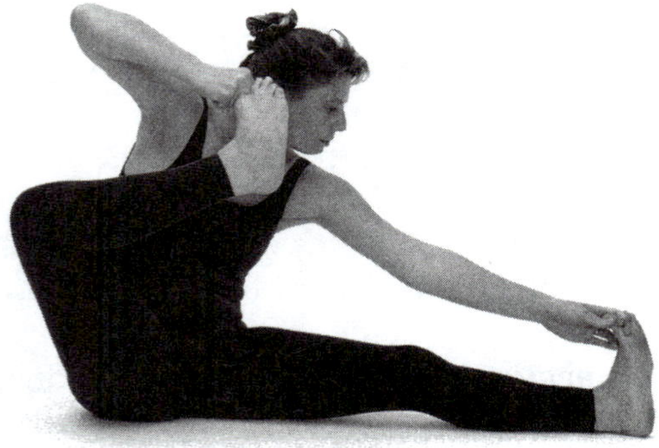

Ākarṇa Dhanurāsana

Common Release Valves for Lateral Bends

1. Rotating the pelvis forward.
2. Displacing the pelvis backward and/or laterally.
3. Rotating the shoulders forward.
4. Displacing the shoulders forward.
5. Excessively arching the lumbar spine.
6. Collapsing the chest over the belly, increasing the thoracic curve.
7. Internally rotating the knee and ankle and/or collapsing the arches.

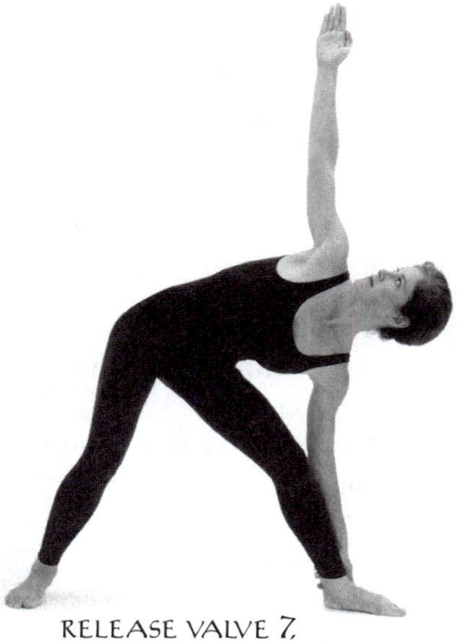

RELEASE VALVE 7
knee rotated internally

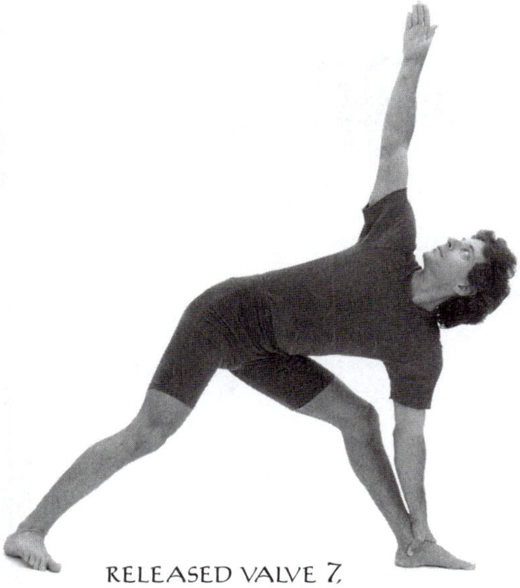

RELEASED VALVE 7
collapsed arch

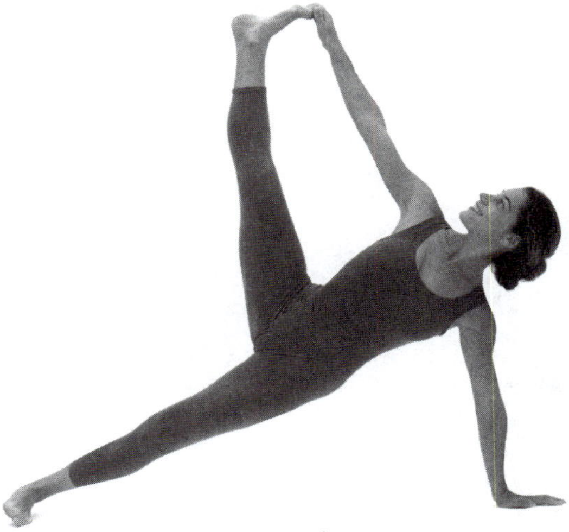

Ekapāda Vasiṣthāsana

Common Risks

In all lateral postures, there is a risk of stress to the sacroiliac, hip, and knee joints. This is especially true in standing and kneeling postures that are weight-bearing, and in standing, kneeling, and seated fixed-frame postures that use the arms as levers to deepen the lateral stretch. Keeping the hip, knee, and ankle in vertical alignment and avoiding excessive internal or external rotation will minimize risks to these joints.

There is a risk of stress to the shoulder joint in fixed-frame standing, kneeling, and seated postures if you strain to grasp the opposite foot with the hand of the extended arm. If you are tight, maintaining the vertical alignment of your shoulders, keeping the extended arm in alignment with the torso, will actually give you a more effective stretch.

The risk of excessive lateral intervertebral compression in both open- and fixed-frame lateral bends is minimized by lengthening the spine on inhale before you bend, and with each successive inhale while in the posture.

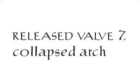

Lateral Bending Practice (for Parighāsana)

1.
POSTURE: Vajrāsana.
EMPHASIS: To warm up body, gently stretching back, one side at a time.
TECHNIQUE: Stand on knees with left arm over head and right arm folded behind back.

On exhale: Bend forward, pushing left arm forward and bringing chest to thighs and hand and forehead to floor.

On inhale: Return to starting position.

NUMBER: 4 times each side, one side at a time.
DETAILS: *On exhale:* Bring chest to thighs before bringing buttocks to heels. *On inhale:* Lift chest and arm, flattening upper back upon return.

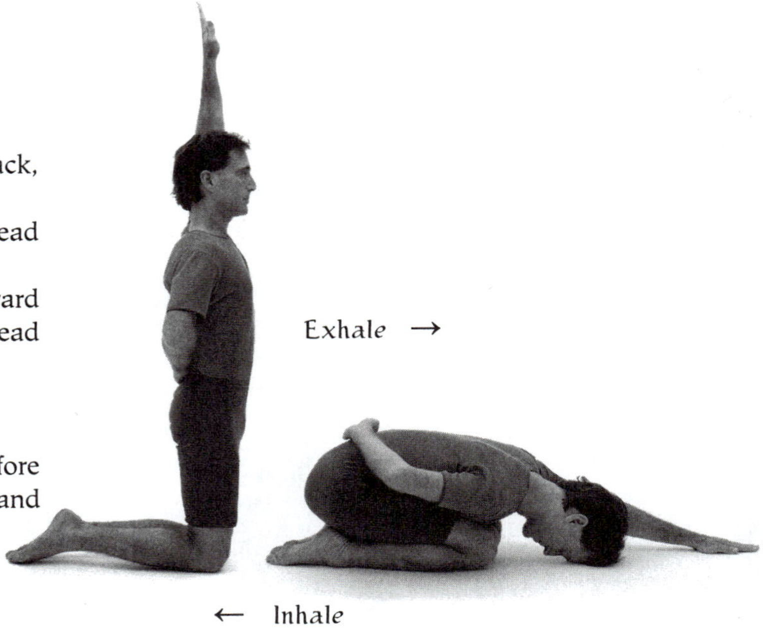

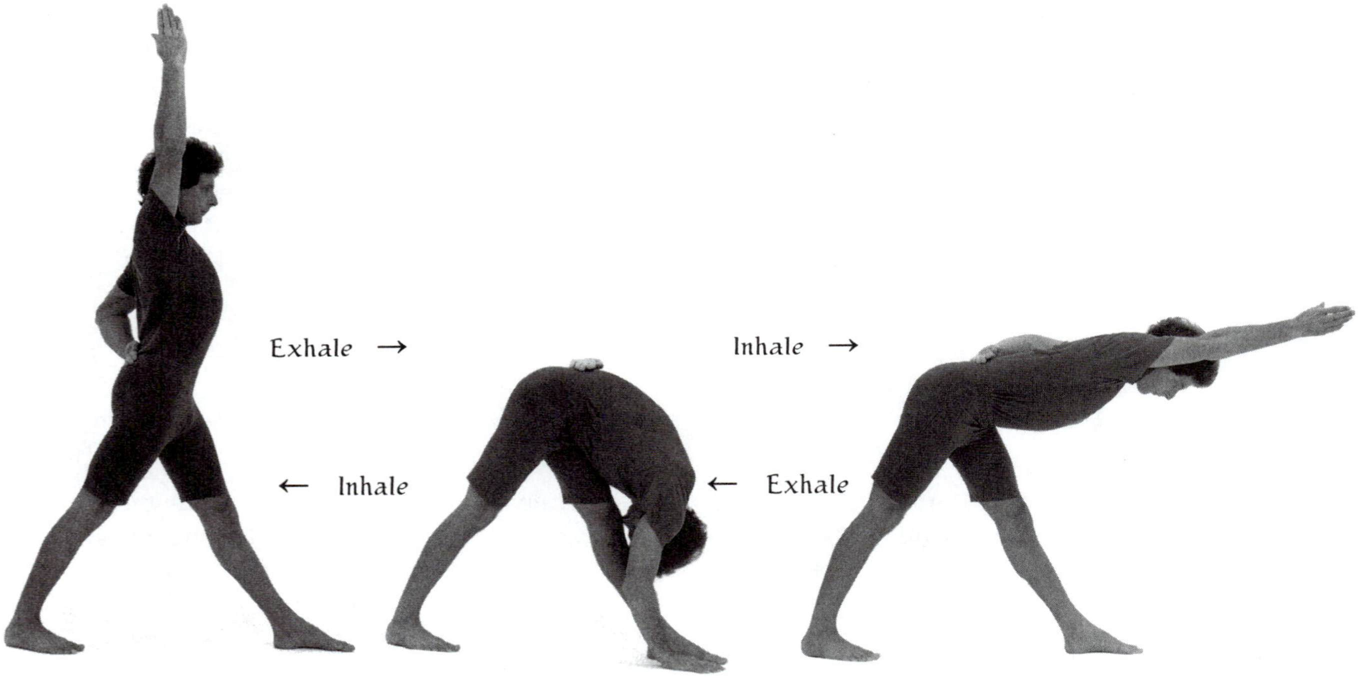

2.
POSTURE: Ardha Pārśvottānāsana.
EMPHASIS: To stretch and strengthen low back, one side at a time.
TECHNIQUE: Stand with left foot forward, right foot turned slightly outward, right arm over head, and left arm folded behind back.

On exhale: Bend forward, flexing left knee, bringing chest toward left thigh, and right hand to left foot.

On inhale: Lift chest and arm until torso is parallel to ground.

On exhale: Return to forward bend position.

On inhale: Return to starting position.

NUMBER: 4 times each side.
DETAILS: Stay stable on back heel and keep shoulders level throughout movement.

3.

POSTURE: Utthita Trikoṇāsana.
EMPHASIS: To laterally stretch torso and rib cage.
TECHNIQUE:

A: Stand with feet spread wider than shoulders, left foot turned out at a ninety-degree angle to right foot, left arm over head, and right arm straight down at waist and slightly rotated externally.

On exhale: Keeping shoulders in same plane as hips, bend laterally, lowering left shoulder and bringing left hand below left knee while turning head down toward left hand.

On inhale: Return to starting position.

Repeat.

B: With left hand down along left leg:

On inhale: Bring right arm up and forward while turning head forward toward right hand.

On exhale: Return right hand to starting position while turning head down toward left hand.

Repeat.

C: With left hand down along left leg, wrap right arm behind back and left arm under inside of left leg. Clasp hands behind back and turn head down toward left foot.

NUMBER: Repeat A four times, then B four times, and then stay in C six breaths. Repeat on other side.

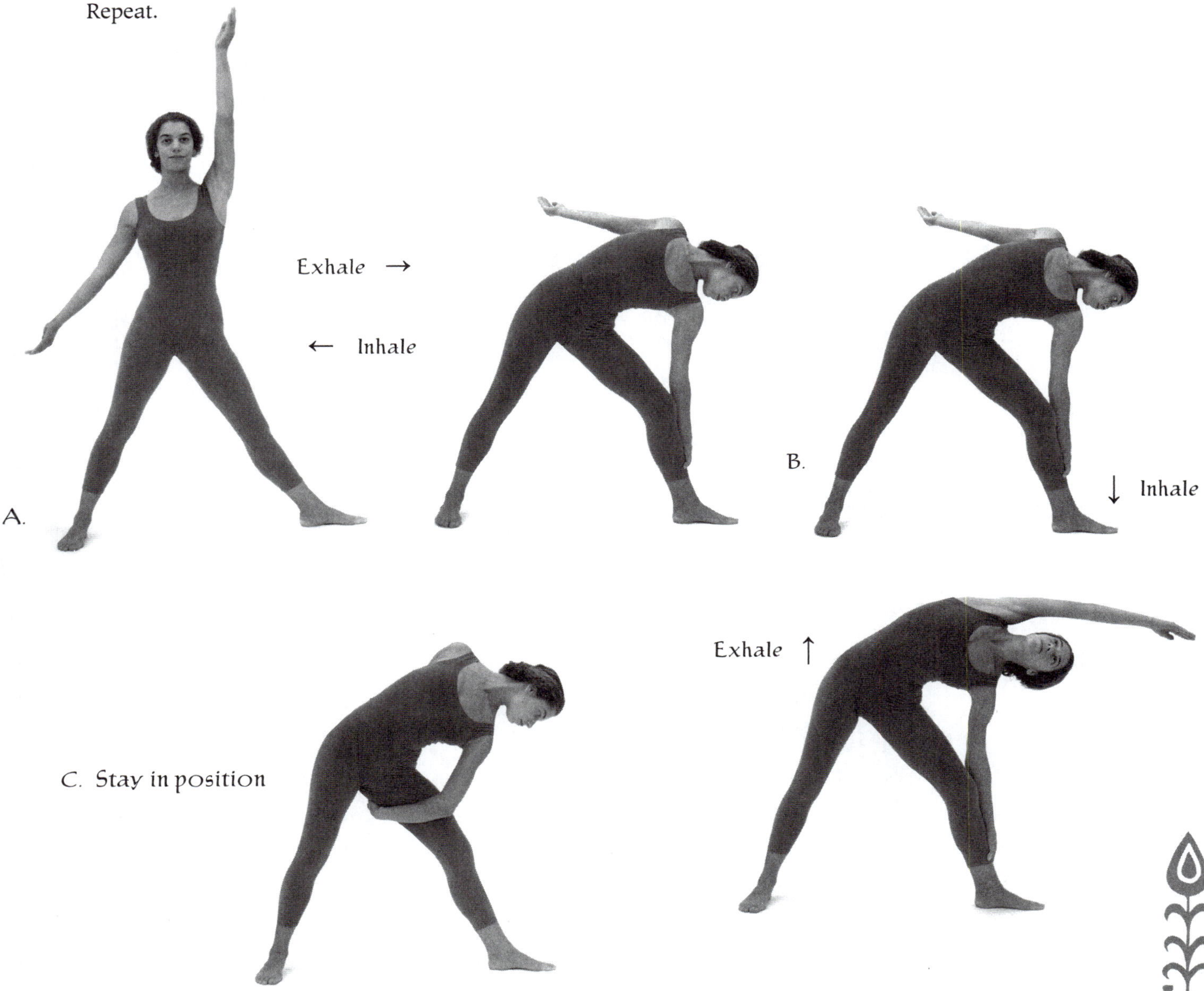
A.
Exhale →
← Inhale
B.
↓ Inhale
Exhale ↑
C. Stay in position

4.

POSTURE: Vajrāsana.
EMPHASIS: To stretch back symmetrically. To transition from standing to supine position.
TECHNIQUE: Stand on knees with arms over head.

On exhale: Bend forward, sweeping arms behind back, bringing hands to sacrum, palms up.

On inhale: Return to starting position.

NUMBER: 8 times.
DETAILS: *On exhale:* Bring chest to thighs before bringing buttocks to heels. Rotate arms so palms are up and hands are resting on sacrum. *On inhale:* As arms sweep wide, open chest, pull shoulder blades back, and flatten upper back.

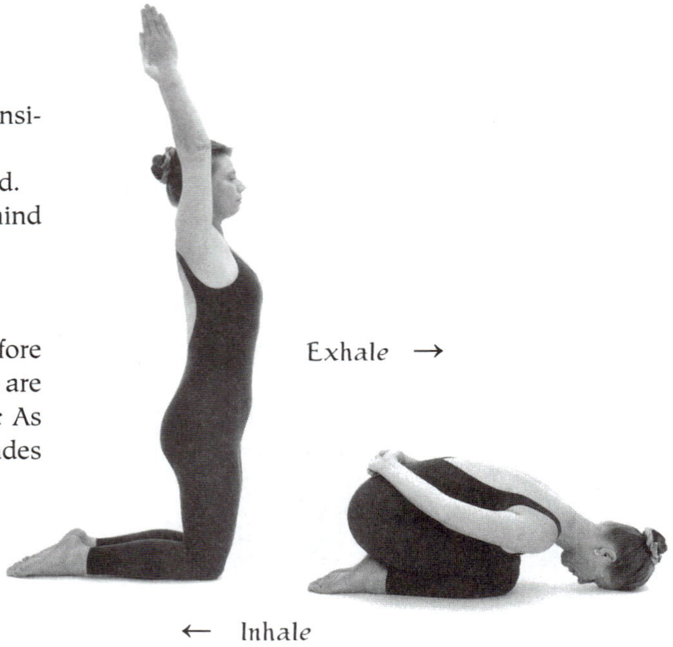
Exhale →
← Inhale

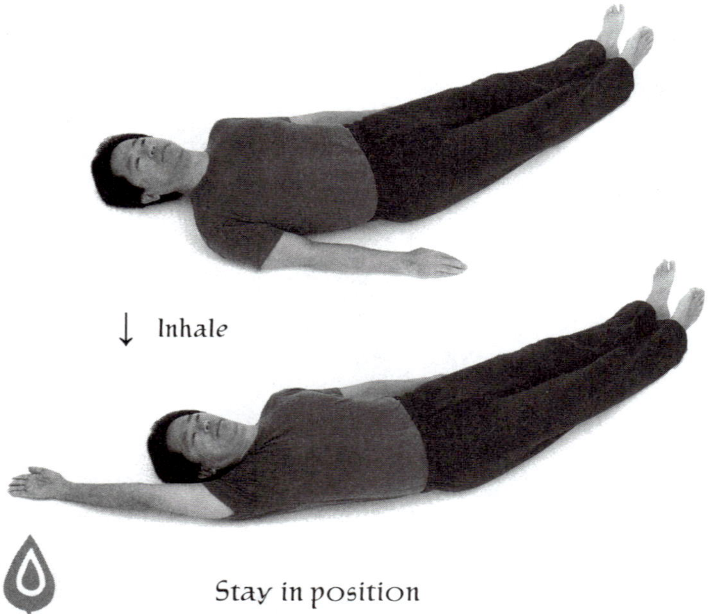
↓ Inhale
Stay in position

5.

POSTURE: Jaṭhara Parivṛtti variation.
EMPHASIS: To gently stretch torso laterally.
TECHNIQUE: Lie on back with legs straight, and arms flat and at a small angle from sides.

Walk both feet in small increments to left until right side of lower torso and hip are gently stretched. Raise right arm up over head.

Stay and breathe deeply, gently protruding belly *on inhale.*

Return to starting point.

Repeat on other side.

NUMBER: Stay 8 deep breaths each side.
DETAILS: Go only as far with legs as allows low back and hips to stay stable on floor. Avoid increasing arch of low back.

6.

POSTURE: Ūrdhva Prasārita Pādāsana, one side at a time.
EMPHASIS: To gently stretch low back and to stretch legs, emphasizing one side at a time.
TECHNIQUE: Lie on back with both knees lifted toward chest, feet off floor.

On inhale: Extend left leg upward, raising right arm up and over head to floor behind you.

On exhale: Return to starting position.

Repeat on other side.

NUMBER: 6 times each side, alternately.
DETAILS: *On inhale:* Flex foot as leg is raised upward. Knee can remain slightly bent. Low back and sacrum push downward. Chin is down.

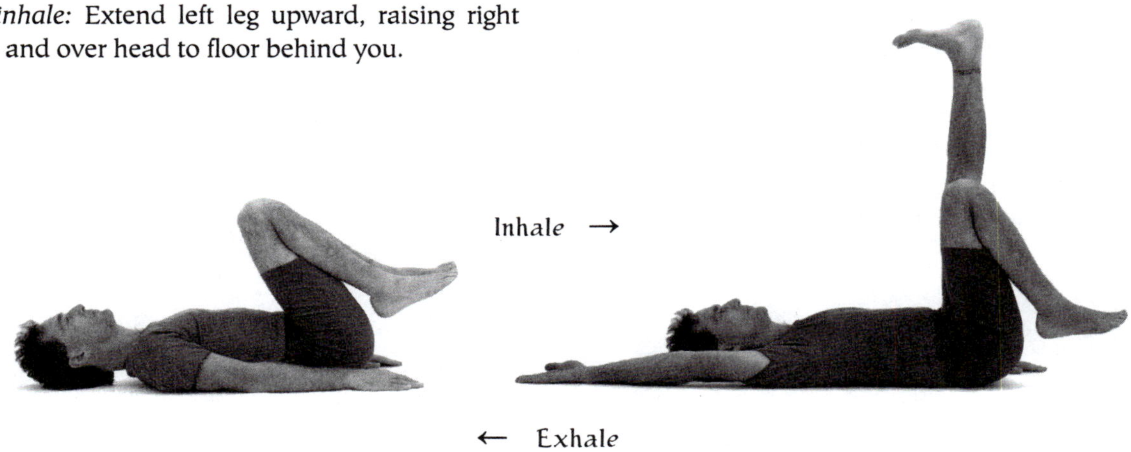

7.

POSTURE: Paścimatānāsana.
EMPHASIS: To stretch back. To prepare for Jānu Śirṣāsana Parivṛtti.
TECHNIQUE: Sit with legs forward, back straight, and arms raised over head.

On exhale: Bending knees slightly, bend forward, bringing chest to thighs, and palms to balls of feet.

On inhale: Return to starting position.

Repeat 6 times.

DETAILS: *On exhale:* Bend knees to facilitate stretching low back and bring belly and chest to thighs. Move chin down toward throat. *On inhale:* Lift chest up and away from thighs, flattening upper back.

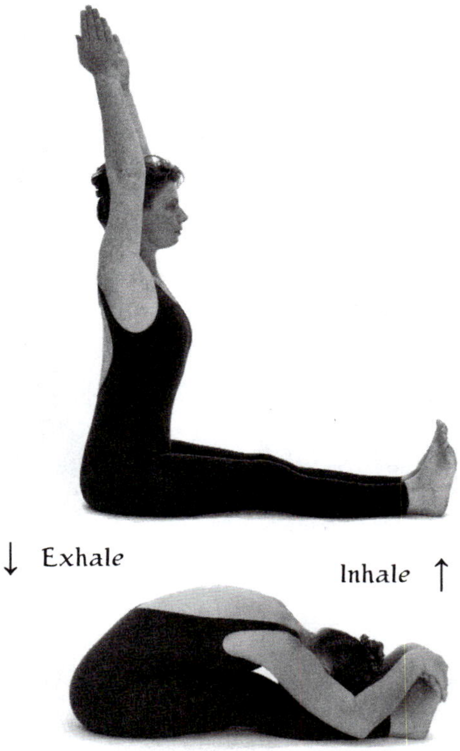

8.

POSTURE: Jānu Śirṣāsana Parivṛtti.

EMPHASIS: To deeply stretch lateral portion of torso, one side at a time. To prepare for Parighāsana.

TECHNIQUE: Sit with right leg folded in, heel to groin, left leg extended forward at an angle, left arm overhead, and right arm bent as shown.

On exhale: Bending left knee slightly, bend laterally, bringing left hand toward left foot, keeping shoulders twisted so right shoulder is vertically above left, and turning head down toward left knee. Place right palm above right shoulder.

On inhale: Extend right arm forward, stretching right side of torso, and look toward right hand.

On exhale: Bend right arm again, turning head down toward knee.

Repeat 4 times.

Then stay in the full stretch 4 breaths.

Repeat on other side.

DETAILS: Bend left knee enough to comfortably lower left shoulder toward knee. Rotate left hand externally to grasp inside arch of left foot. Keep shoulders in vertical alignment. In full position, if possible, grasp left foot with right hand.

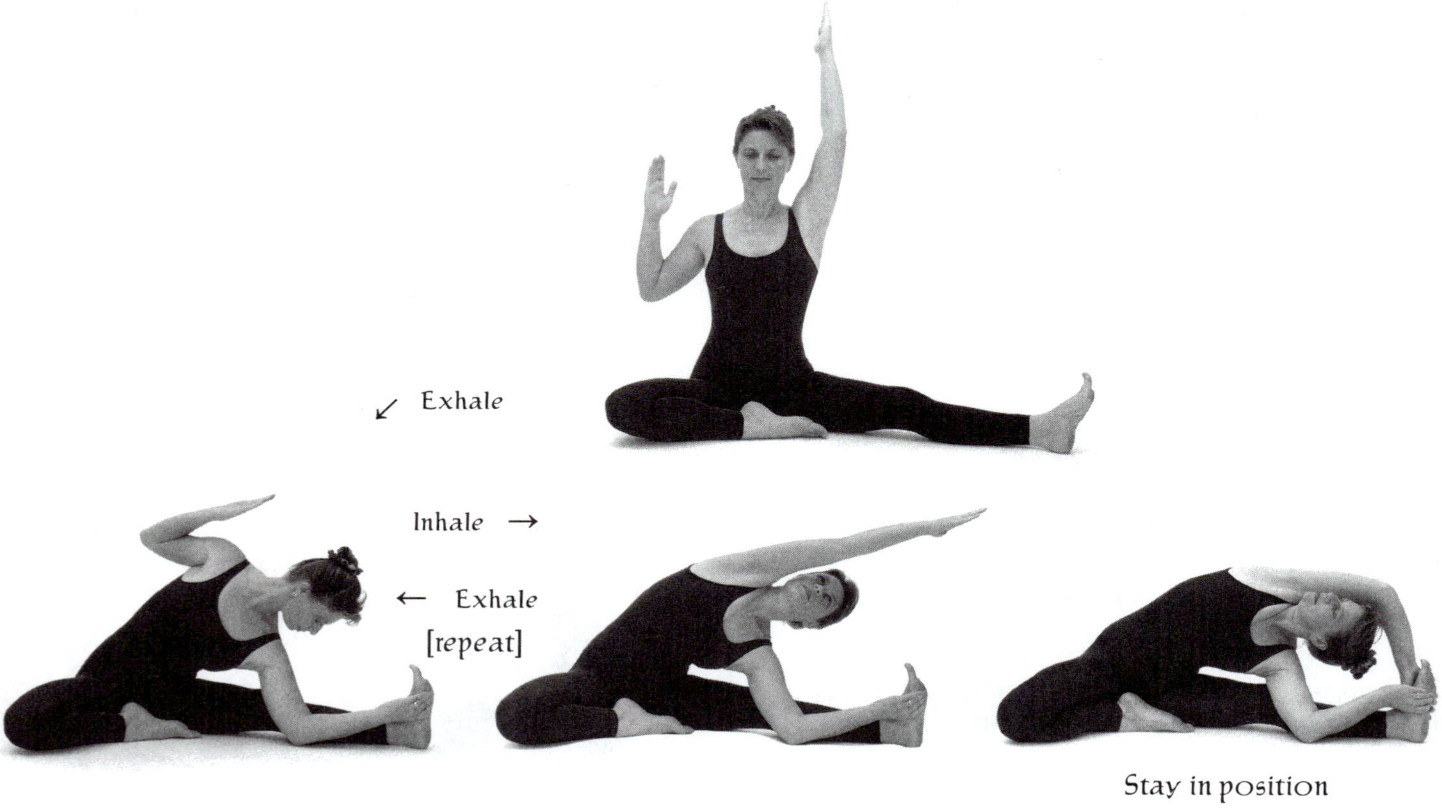

9.

POSTURE: Parighāsana.
EMPHASIS: To deeply stretch lateral portion of torso, one side at a time. To experience one of the deepest lateral bends.
TECHNIQUE: Stand on right knee with left leg straight and extended out to left side and left arm over head.

On exhale: Bend laterally, placing left hand on left foot, keeping shoulders twisted so right shoulder is vertically above left, and turning head up over the right shoulder. Place right palm above right shoulder.

On inhale: Extend right arm forward, stretching right side of torso, and look toward right hand.

On exhale: Bend right arm again, turning head up over the right shoulder.

Repeat 4 times.

Then stay in the full stretch 6 breaths.

Repeat on other side.

DETAILS: Rotate left hand externally to grasp inside arch of left foot. Keep shoulders in vertical alignment. In full position, if possible, grasp left foot with right hand.

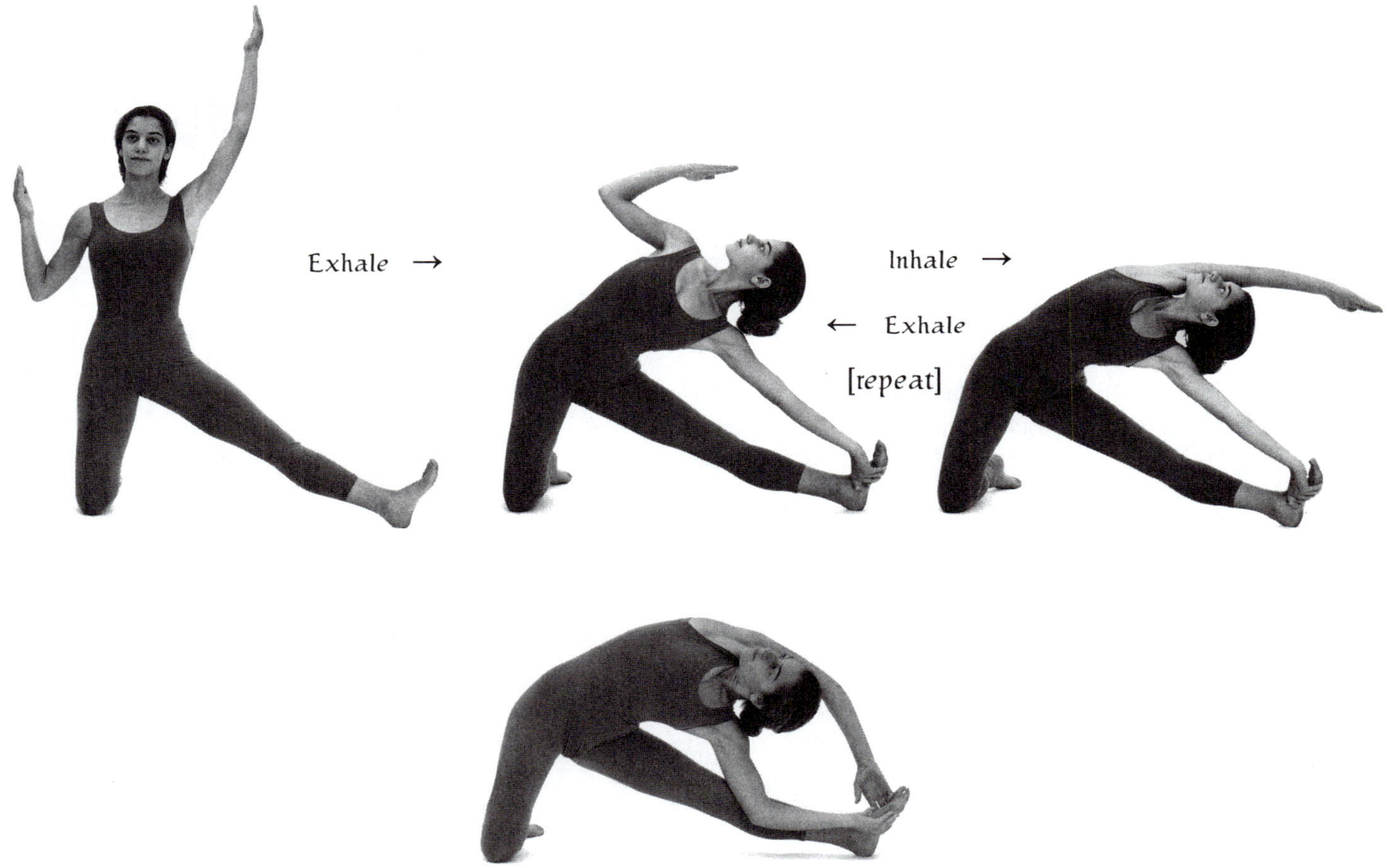

Stay in position

10.

Posture: Vajrāsana.
Emphasis: To stretch back symmetrically after deep lateral bend.
Technique: Stand on knees with arms over head.
On exhale: Bend forward, sweeping arms behind back, bringing hands to sacrum, palms up.
On inhale: Return to starting position.
Number: 8 times.
Details: *On exhale:* Bring chest to thighs before bringing buttocks to heels. Rotate arms so palms are up and hands are resting on sacrum. *On inhale:* As arms sweep wide, open chest, pull shoulder blades back, and flatten upper back.

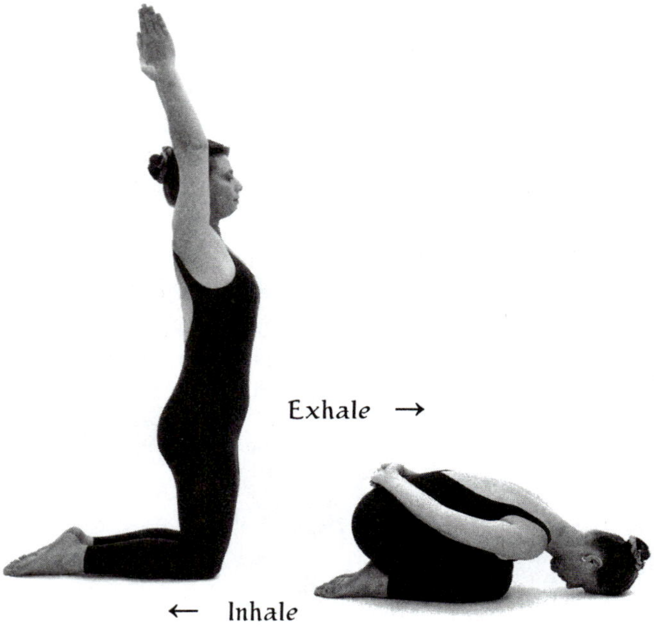

11.

Posture: Śavāsana.
Emphasis: To rest.
Technique: Lie flat on back, with arms at sides, palms up, and legs slightly apart. Close eyes. Relax body fully, keeping mind relaxed and alert to sensations in body.
Duration: Minimum 3 to 5 minutes.

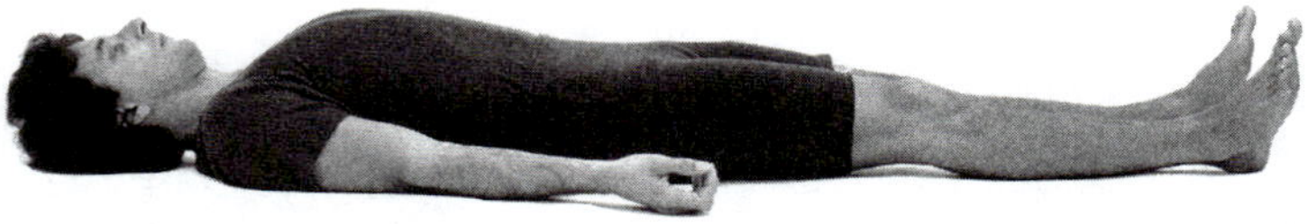

Lengthening the Core: An Introduction to Extension

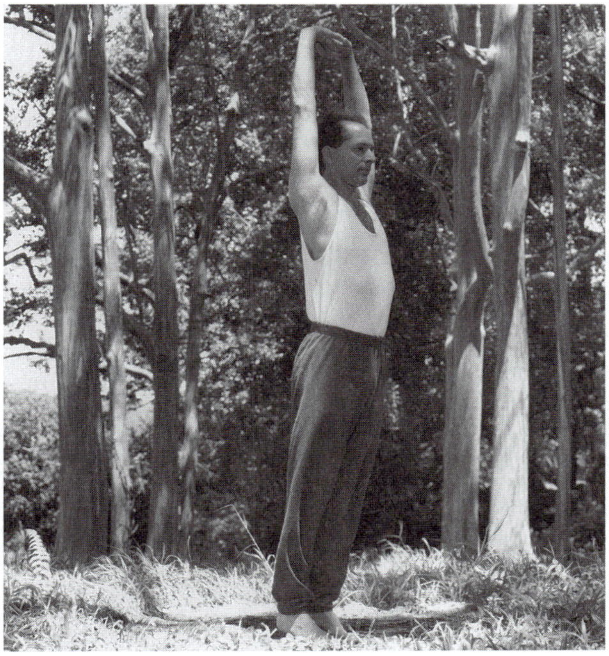

Primary and Secondary Intentions

In anatomical parlance, extension refers to moving the spine, arms, or legs backward, or staightening them from a flexed position. In the context of this study, however, extension refers to lengthening and straightening the spine, creating maximum space between the vertebral bodies and integrating the spinal curves. Lengthening the spine enables us to move more deeply in forward bends, back bends, twists, and lateral bends, and their practice results in a more naturally lengthened spine. Thus, from a biomechanical perspective, extension is both the means and the goal of āsana practice. In this sense, all postures can be considered extension postures.

In this category, then, we find postures in which the most significant movement of the spine is extension, and any forward, backward, twisting, or lateral movement is minimized. Though movement in these postures is limited, they build strength and elasticity in the superficial and deep musculature, ligaments, and connective tissues of the spine and rib cage. They also strengthen the diaphragm and abdominal muscles. Through these combined effects, extension postures help us improve our postural alignment and overall structural integration. Improved postural alignment reduces stress to the musculature and organs of the torso and improves digestion, respiration, and circulation.

Some extension postures also stretch the arms and/or legs away from the torso, facilitating the extension of the spine, stretching and strengthening the muscles and ligaments that bind them to the spine, creating more space in the shoulder and hip joints. This action also improves peripheral circulation.

Extension postures are at the same time the simplest and most challenging of all postures. Try sitting still with a focused mind and an extended spine, following the movement of inhale and exhale, for several minutes.

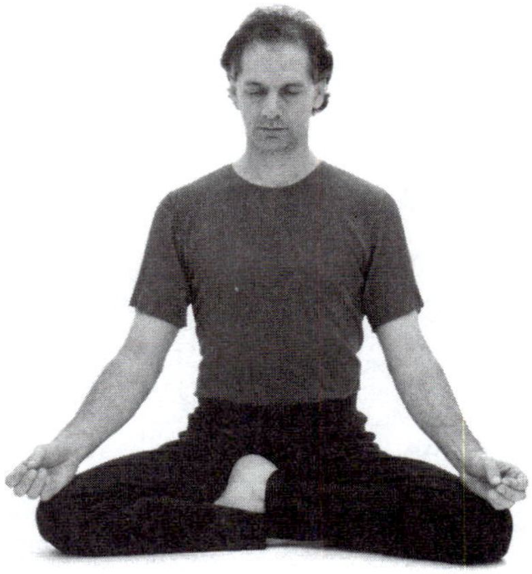

Siddhāsana

After some time you may begin to feel resistance, tightness, and discomfort in your back, neck, shoulders, hips, and/or knees. The discomforts experienced in this simple extension posture reveal imbalances in your structure. In this sense, simple extension postures can be used as diagnostic tools, giving direction to the use of forward bends, back bends, twists, and lateral bends in āsana practice. A sign of progress is the ability to remain in simple extension postures for longer periods of time with less stress. Then more attention can be given to subtler aspects of the spine, breath, and energy, and to experiencing the centering and stilling qualities of extension postures.

From a biomechanical perspective, the *primary intention* in extension postures is to bring the spine to maximum vertical alignment, integrating the spinal curves without strain or compression.

The *secondary intention* is to extend the arms and legs, augmenting the extension of the spine, creating space in the shoulder and hip joints and improving circulation.

The natural curvatures of the spine serve an important biomechanical purpose, and, therefore, a straight spine is neither possible nor desirable. Beyond these natural curves, however, we all have some irregularities in our spine. One or another of the curves may be exaggerated or flattened, in any combination. Besides irregularities of the natural spinal curves, there is also almost always some degree of lateral asymmetry. These spinal conditions are accompanied by asymmetrical conditions in the deep and superficial musculature and ligaments of the torso, shoulder, and pelvic girdles.

The spinal curves move in reciprocal relation to each other. Theoretically, lengthening the cervical spine should lengthen the thoracic spine, which should, in turn, lengthen the lumbar spine. In practice, however, lengthening the thoracic curve often increases the lumbar curve, and flattening the lumbar curve often increases the thoracic curve.

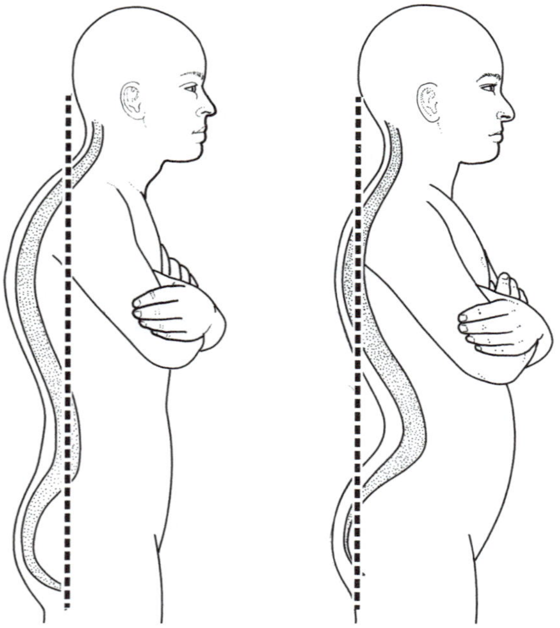

Thoracic kyphosis
Excessive curvature
of the upper back

Lumbar lordosis
Excessive curvature
of the lower back

Technique

The key to integrating the spinal curves, and therefore the key to extension postures, is the combined techniques of inhale and exhale. Initiate the inhale in the upper portion of the chest, emphasizing the natural lifting and expansion of the rib cage that takes place as the lungs fill with air. Tuck the chin slightly in and displace the head slightly backward, to lengthen the neck, as the chest expands and upper ribs lift forward and up. At the same time, the upper thoracic spine begins to straighten. Let the upward and outward movement of the ribs move successively from rib to rib, from the top downward, until the entire rib cage is fully expanded. As this happens, the thoracic spine lengthens vertebra by vertebra, from the top down. If your thoracic curve is exaggerated, displace your chest slightly forward to flatten the curve as you lift and lengthen the spine. If, on the other hand, your thoracic spine is flattened, focus on extending the spine without pushing your chest forward. As the air is drawn into the lungs, follow the downward movement of the diaphragm to the abdomen and lengthen the lumbar spine. If your lumbar curve is reversed, rotate your pelvis forward to regain the natural curve and facilitate the lengthening of the spine. If your lumbar curve is exaggerated, use the abdominal contraction, at the initiation of exhale, to pull the pubic bone upward and to flatten the lumbar spine. On exhale, as the diaphragm moves upward, keep the chest lifted, pull the shoulders down and back, and increase the extension of the spine. Maintain a partial contraction of the lower abdomen through successive inhales, stabilizing the lumbar-pelvic relationship, increasing the lift of the rib cage, and furthering the extension of the spine.

Types of Extension Postures

♦ GROUP 1

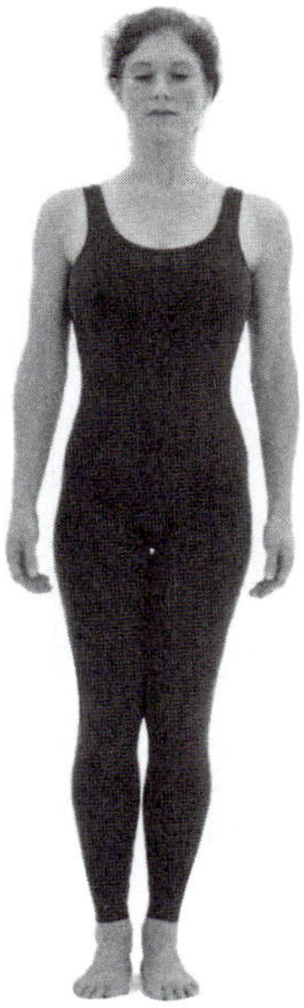

Samasthiti

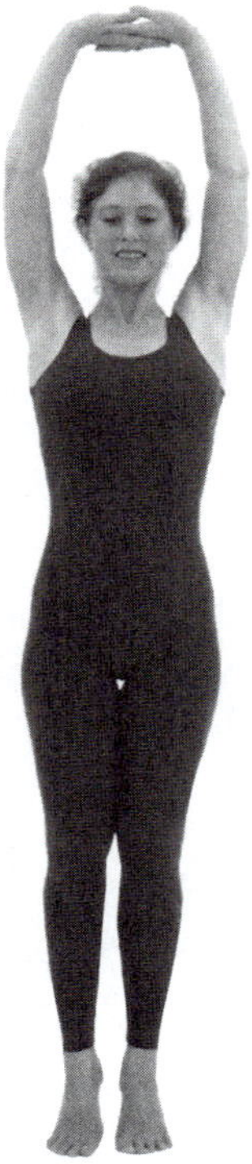

Tadāsana

The first group includes postures where the torso and legs are flat and extended. The first two are standing postures. Raising the heels up off the ground gives Tāḍāsana some of the qualities of a balance posture. The next two are supine postures. The intention of Śavāsana is to deeply rest, and, therefore, the challenge is to simply "let go" of doing, rather than extending the spine. Taḍākamudrā incorporates a special technique of pulling the belly in and up, while expanding and lifting the rib cage and holding the breath out after exhale. In Caturaṅga Daṇḍāsana, the only fixed-frame posture of this group, the legs and torso are held parallel above the ground on the hands and balls of the feet. This requires strength in the belly and low back as well as in the legs and shoulders.

torso collapsed

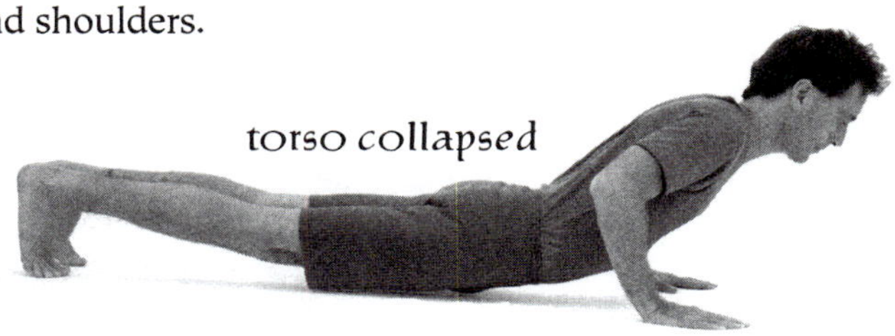

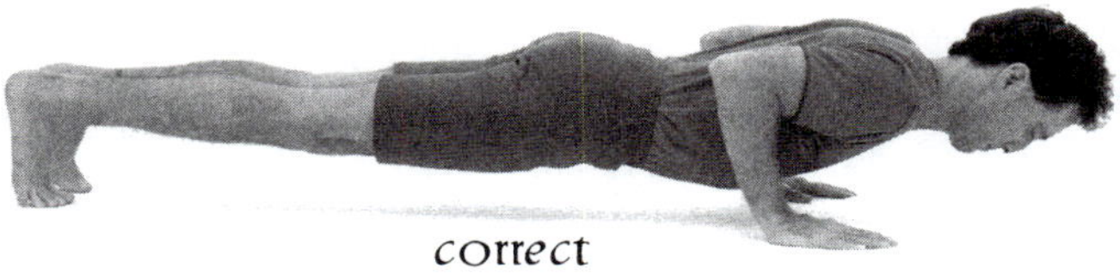

correct

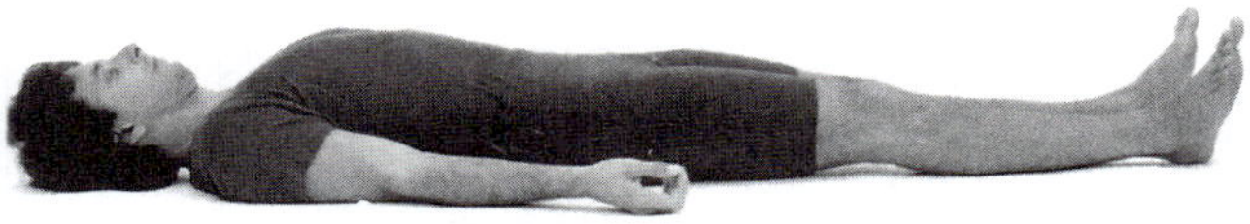

Śavāsana

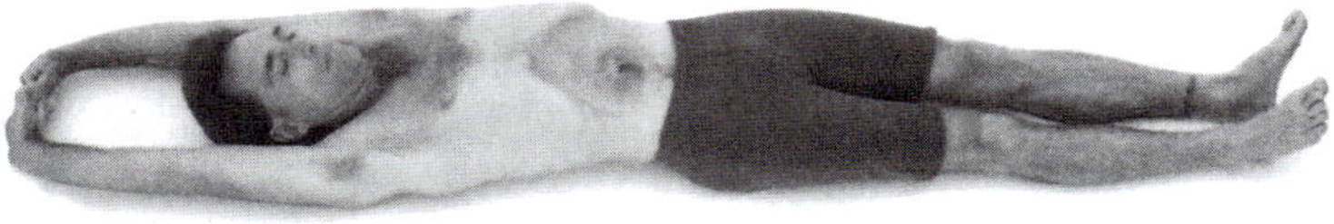

Taḍākamudrā

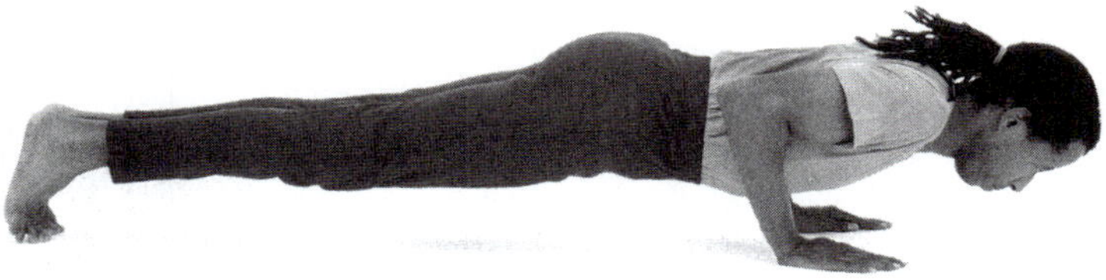

Caturaṅga Daṇḍāsana

♦ GROUP 2

Adho Mukha Śvānāsana, Daṇḍāsana, and Ūrdhva Prasārita Pādāsana have nearly identical forms, with different bases, though only Adho Mukha Śvānāsana is fixed-frame. In all of these postures, the torso is held at ninety degrees to the legs, giving the postures a quality of forward bending. At the same time, the chest is lifted up and away from the belly, stretching in the front of the abdomen, giving them a quality of back bending.

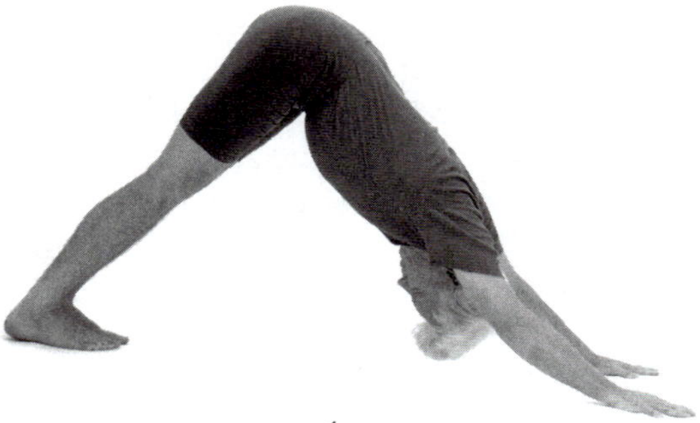

Adho Mukha Śvānāsana

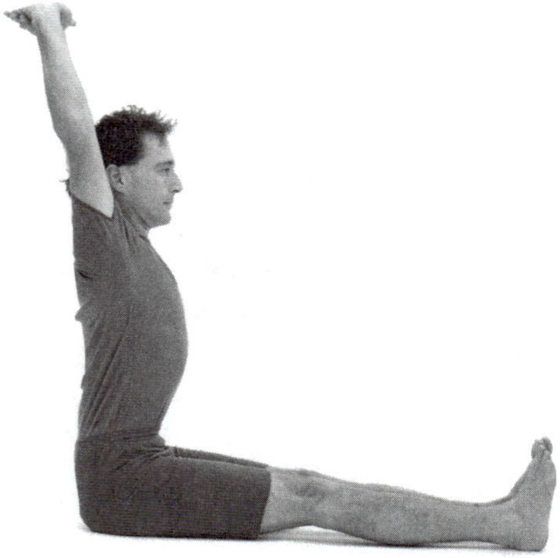

Daṇḍāsana

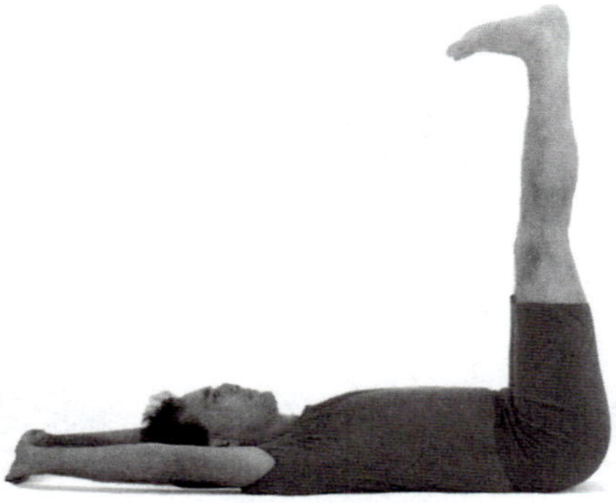

Ūrdhva Prasārita Pādāsana

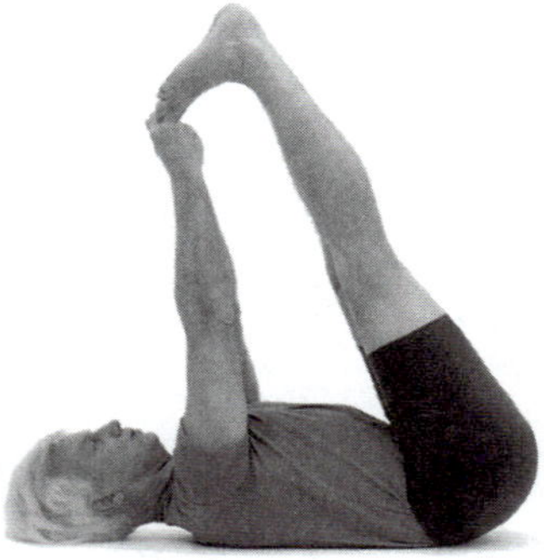

Supta Pādāṅguṣṭhāsana

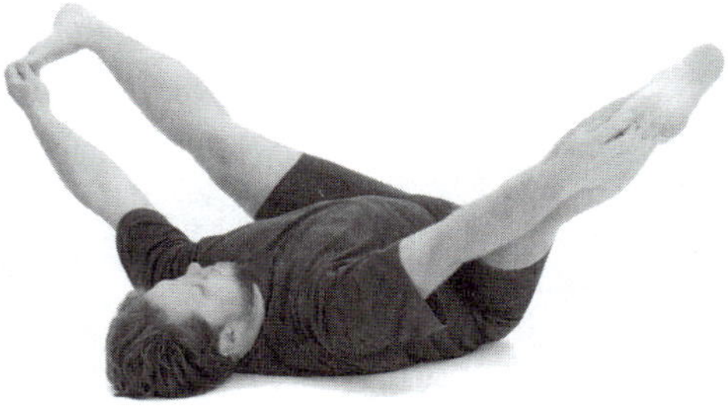

Supta Prasārita Pādāṅguṣṭhāsana

In the supine postures, extending the arms and legs and flattening the cervical and lumbar spine into the floor makes these simple postures surprisingly effective. To get maximum extension in the spine, keep the legs at ninety degrees or less to the torso, even if the knees have to be bent, and push the lumbosacral spine down.

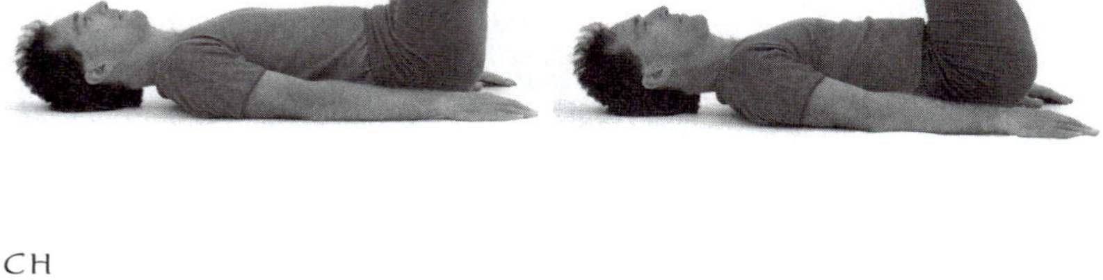

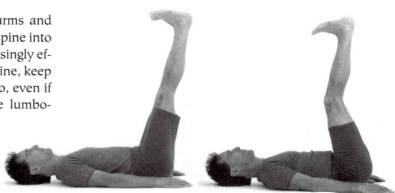

These postures include two classical fixed-frame variations in which the hands hold the feet. In the second, Supta Prasārita Pādāṅguṣṭhāsana, the legs are spread wide, stretching the insides of the thighs and perineal floor.

In Adho Mukha Śvānāsana and Daṇḍāsana either excessive tightness or looseness in the hips and/or shoulders, as well as excessive or flattened curvature in the lumbar and/or cervical spine will complicate and inhibit extension. Adho Mukha Śvānāsana is one of the more complex postures, due to the variety of angles possible at the ankle, knee, hip, and shoulder joints. In this posture, integrating the spinal curves and extending the spine is challenging and requires sensitivity and control. The shoulder joints may be strained in this position. In Daṇḍāsana, extension requires strength in the thighs, abdomen, and low back. The lumbo-sacral spine may be strained in this posture.

♦ GROUP 3

These seated fixed-frame postures are challenging. Mahāmudrā is considered, in the Viniyoga tradition, to be the most extraordinary of postures. In it are contained elements of forward bending, backward bending, twisting, and lateral bending. If you practice Mahāmudrā, you will experience the powerful, integrating, and stilling quality of extension postures. Baddha Koṇāsana, with the soles of the feet together, blocks the forward rotation of the hips, making full extension of the spine very challenging. It strongly stretches the inner thighs and groin.

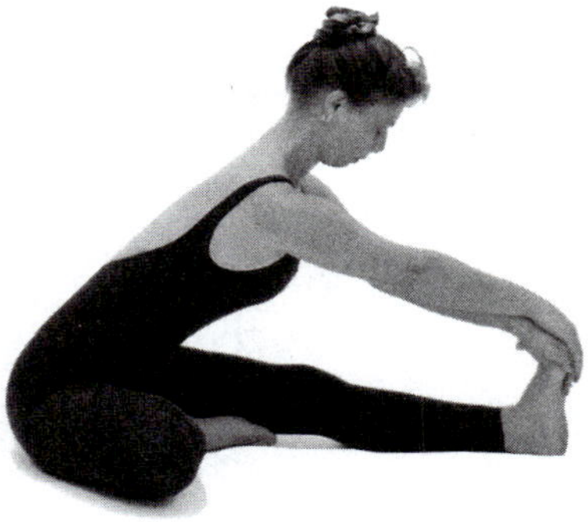

Mahāmudrā

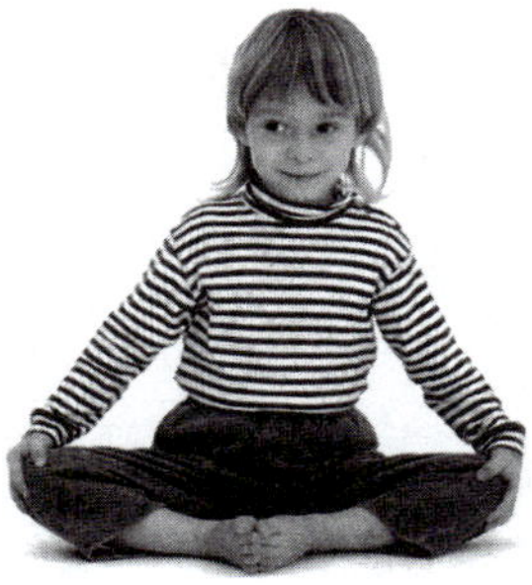

Baddha Koṇāsana

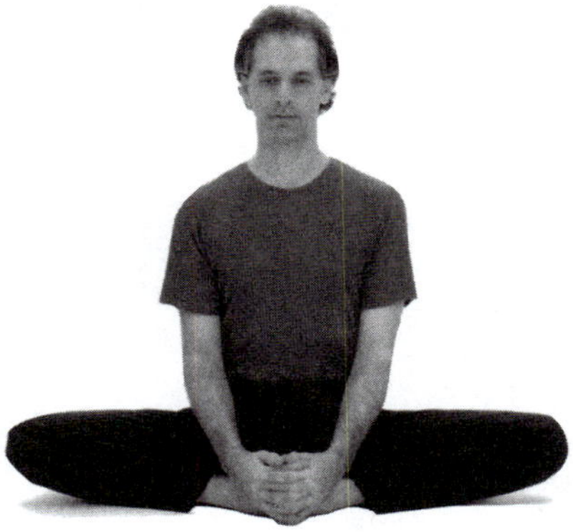

Baddha Koṇāsana

♦ GROUP 4

The postures in this group are the classic seated meditation postures. Though extension is their primary characteristic, these postures are distinctly different from other āsanas. Their intention is to provide a balanced position in which the spine can be held in an extended position for long periods of time with minimum effort, so that the attention is freed from structural tensions and can focus on subtler aspects of the breath and meditation.

Padmāsana, the classic mediation posture, and Gomukhāsana involve significant external rotation of the legs at the hip joints and some torque of the knees. In Vīrāsana, the legs are inwardly rotated at the hip joints, and there is also some torque in the knees. In Vajrāsana, there is a tendency toward increased forward rotation of the pelvis.

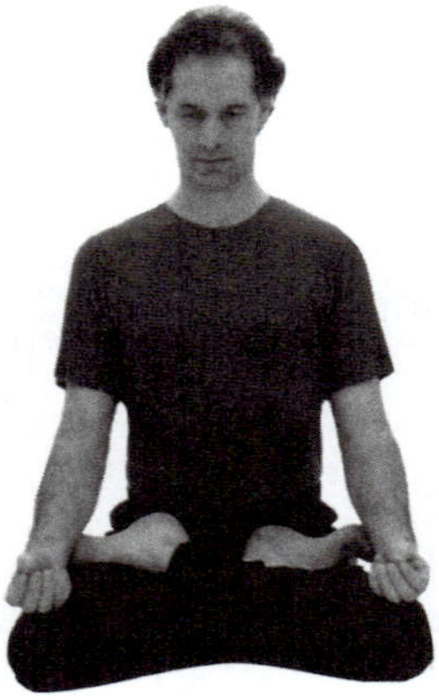

Padmāsana

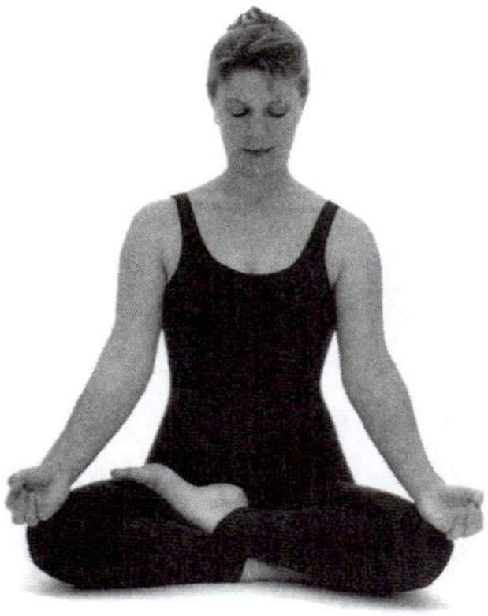

Brahmāsana

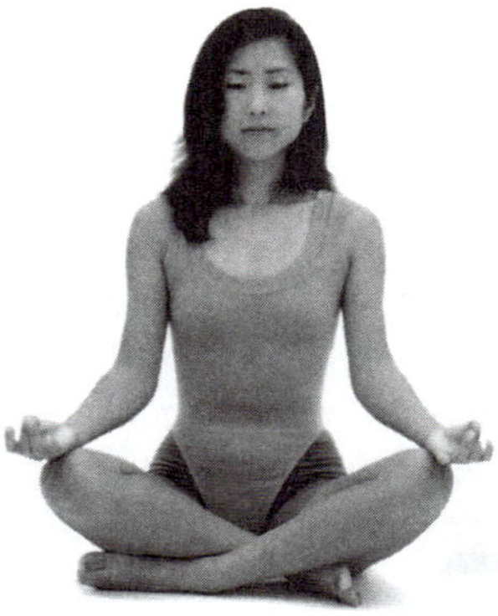

Sukhāsana

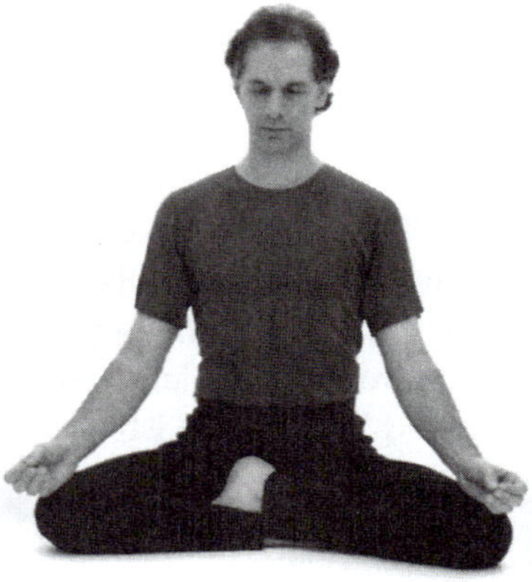

Siddhāsana

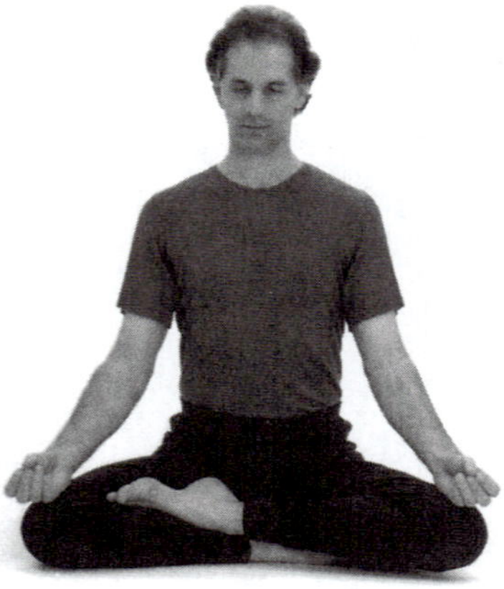

Svastikāsana

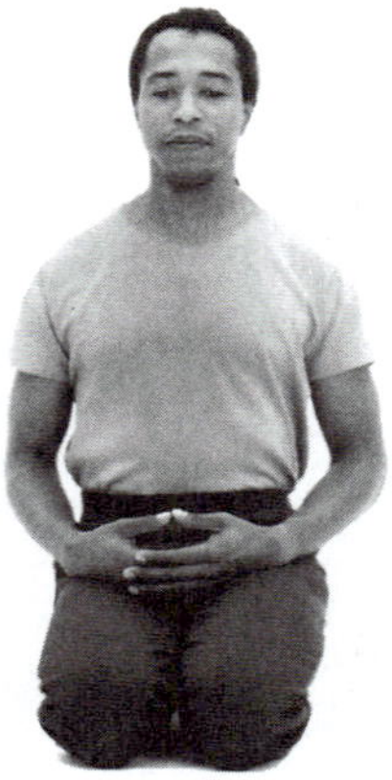

Vajrāsana

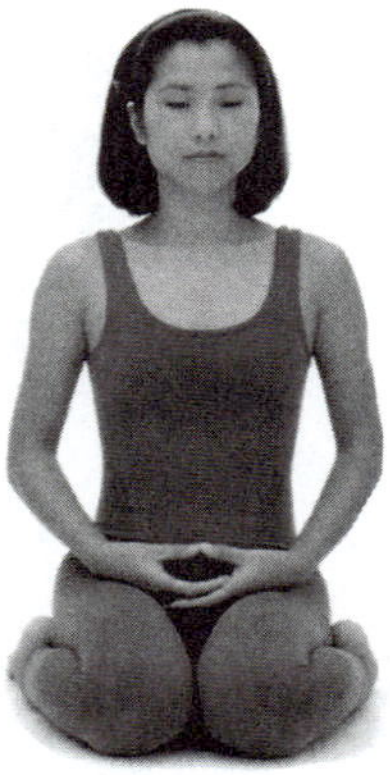

Vīrāsana

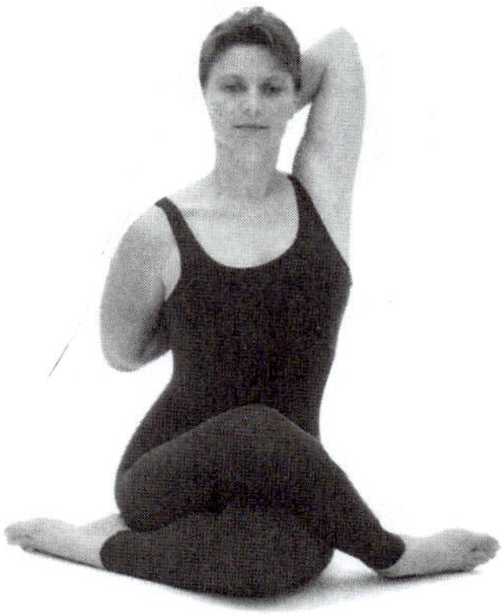

Gomukhāsana

Common Release Valves for Extensions

1. Rotating the pelvis excessively forward or backward.

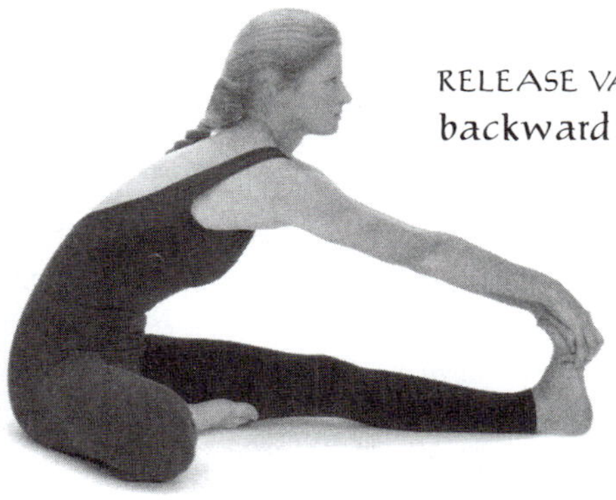

RELEASE VALVE 1, backward rotation

2. Collapsing the chest over the belly.
3. Jutting the chin forward, or collapsing the head backward.
4. Rounding the shoulders forward.
5. Hyperflexing the shoulders in Adho Mukha Śvānāsana (see the following page).

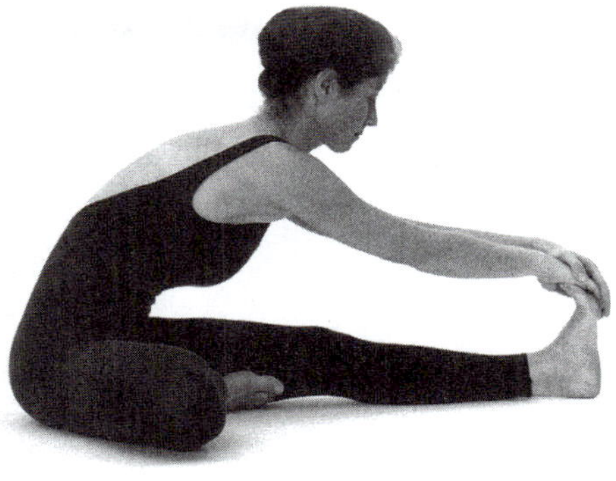

RELEASE VALVE 2

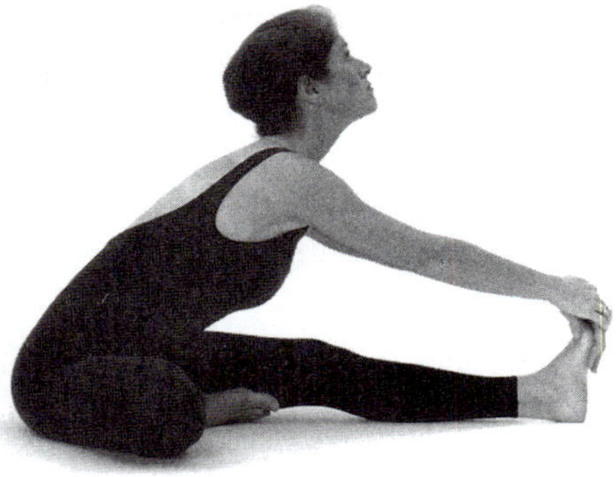

RELEASE VALVE 3

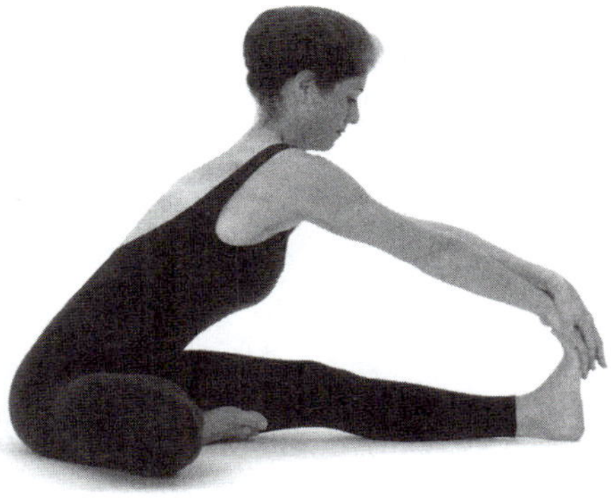

RELEASE VALVE 4

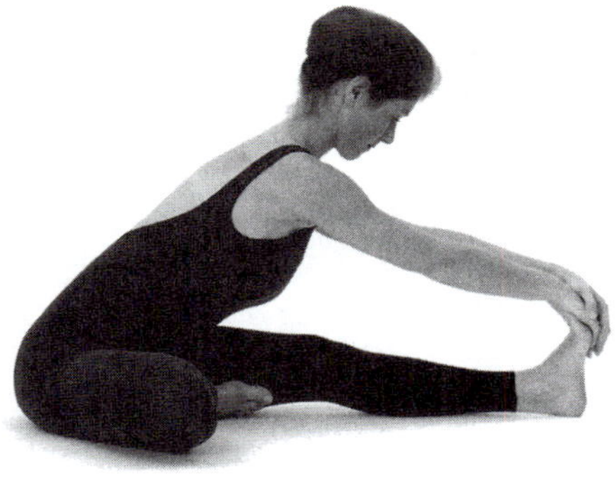

correct

Common Risks

In seated extension postures, there is risk of strain to the musculature of the lumbo-sacral spine, strain to the sacroiliac ligaments, and excessive intervertebral disc compression. Where the hips are rotated externally or internally, there is risk of strain to the hips and knee joints. There is also the possibility of strain to the musculature of the upper back, shoulders, and neck. In Adho Mukha Śvānāsana, there is added risk of strain to the shoulder joints.

Risks can be minimized by initiating movement from the deeper musculature with the breath and by avoiding forcing the spine with other muscles. This is especially true in fixed-frame postures. Extra caution should be taken to avoid excessive force to the shoulders in Adho Mukha Śvānāsana and to the hips and knees in some of the seated meditation postures.

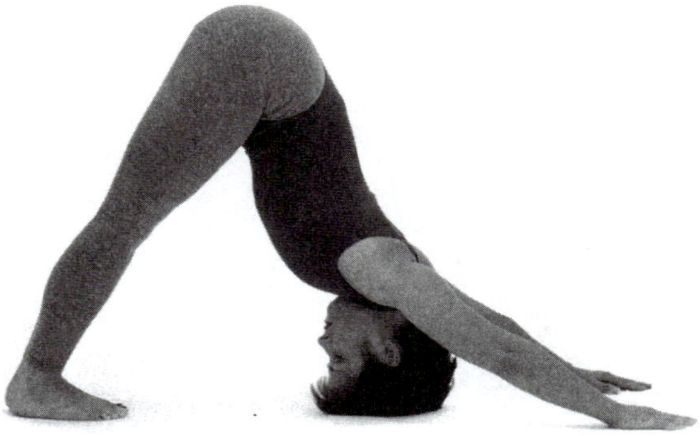

RELEASE VALVE 5

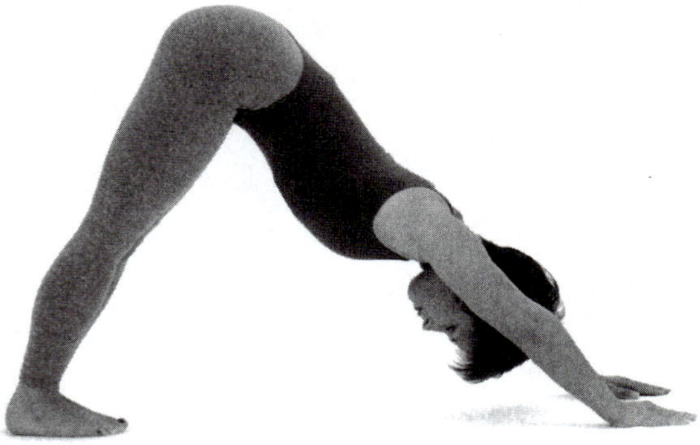

correct

Extension Practice (for Mahāmudrā)

1.

POSTURE: Ardha Pārśvottānāsana.
EMPHASIS: To stretch and strengthen low back, one side at a time.
TECHNIQUE: Stand with left foot forward, right foot turned slightly outward, both arms over head.
On exhale: Bend forward, flexing left knee, bringing chest toward left thigh, and hands to either side of left foot.
On inhale: Lift chest and arms until torso is parallel to ground.
On exhale: Return to forward bend position.
On inhale: Return to starting position.
NUMBER: 4 times each side.
DETAILS: Stay stable on back heel and keep shoulders level throughout movement.

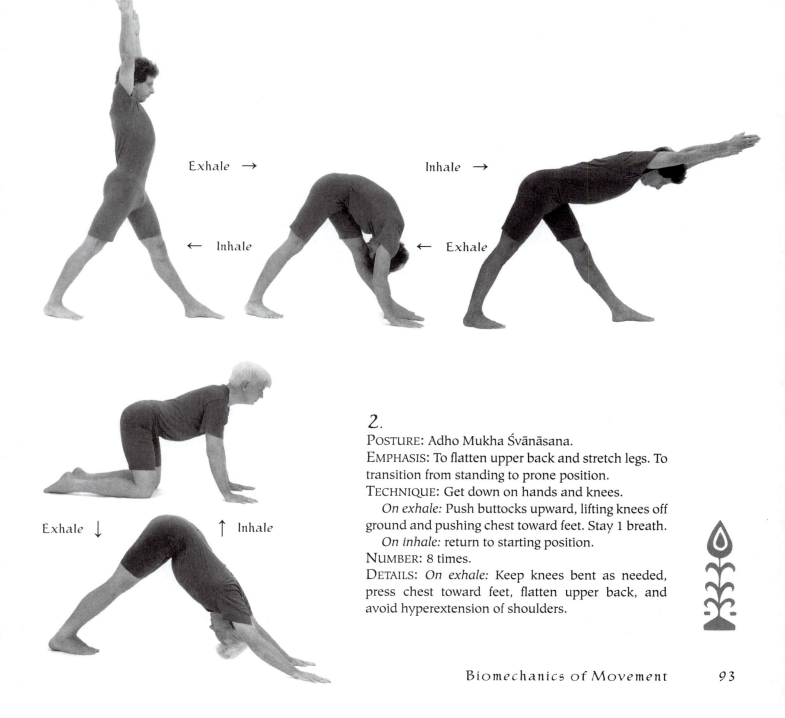

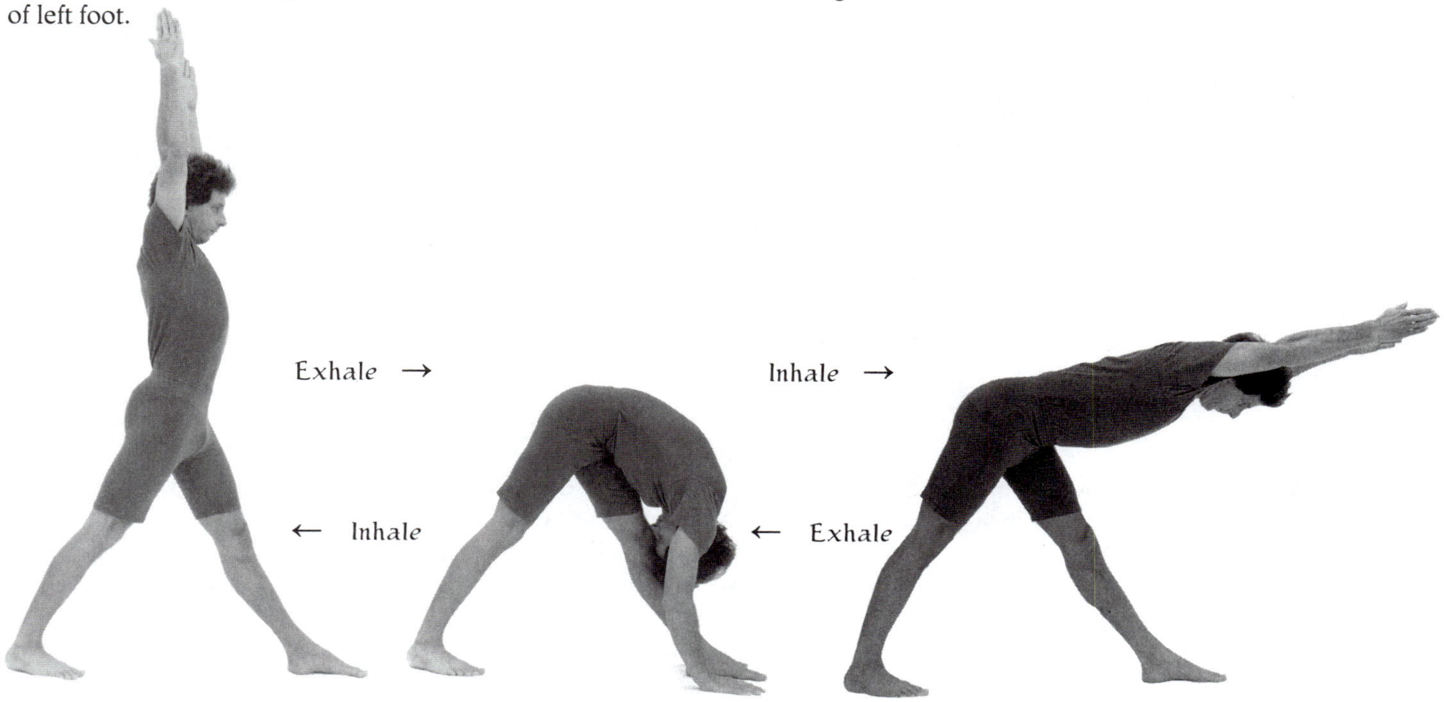
Exhale →
← Inhale
Inhale →
← Exhale

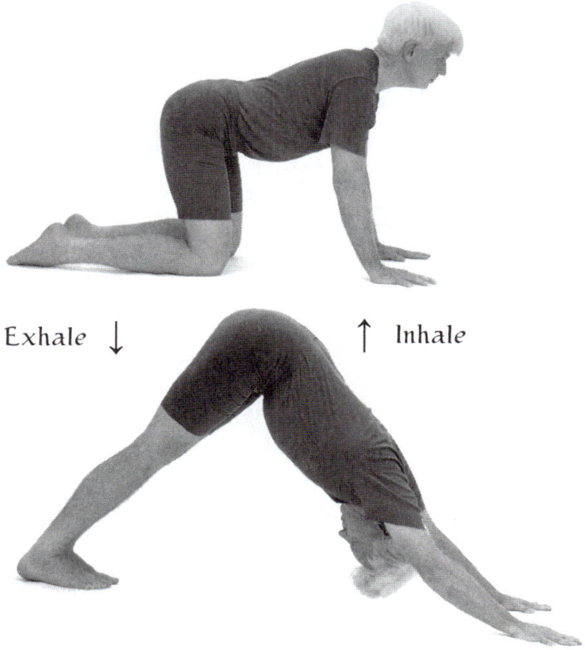
Exhale ↓
↑ Inhale

2.

POSTURE: Adho Mukha Śvānāsana.
EMPHASIS: To flatten upper back and stretch legs. To transition from standing to prone position.
TECHNIQUE: Get down on hands and knees.
On exhale: Push buttocks upward, lifting knees off ground and pushing chest toward feet. Stay 1 breath.
On inhale: return to starting position.
NUMBER: 8 times.
DETAILS: *On exhale:* Keep knees bent as needed, press chest toward feet, flatten upper back, and avoid hyperextension of shoulders.

3.

Posture: Ardha Śalabhāsana.
Emphasis: To strengthen lower back. To prepare for Mahāmudrā.
Technique: Lie on stomach, with head facing left, and palms on floor by chest.

On inhale: Lift chest and left leg, turning head to center.

On exhale: Lower chest and leg, turning head to right side.

Repeat on other side.

Number: 6 times each side, alternately.
Details: *On inhale:* Lift chest slightly before leg, and emphasize chest height. Keep pelvis level.

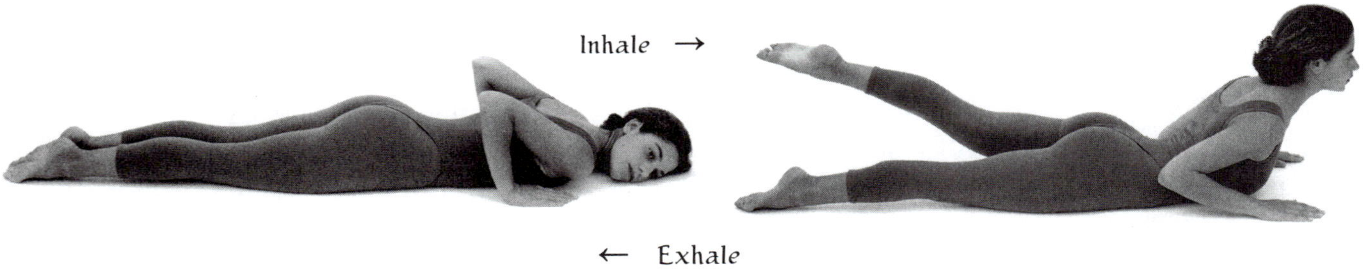

4.

Posture: Supta Pādāṅguṣṭhāsana.
Emphasis: To stretch legs and back in preparation for Mahāmudrā.
Technique: Lie on back with legs bent, knees lifted toward chest, hands holding toes of feet.

On inhale: Extend legs upward, straightening arms.

On exhale: Return to starting position.

Number: 6 times.
Details: *On inhale:* Flex feet as legs are raised upward. Bend knees slightly. Push low back and sacrum downward. Keep chin down.

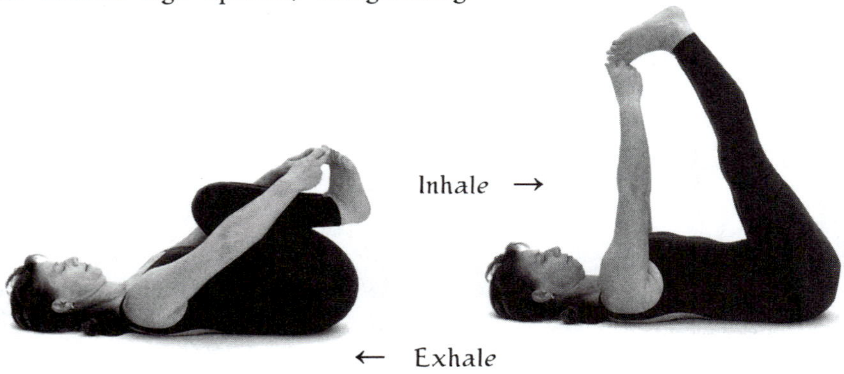

5.

POSTURE: Jaṭhara Parivṛtti.

EMPHASIS: To twist and compress belly. To stretch legs. To facilitate exhalation.

TECHNIQUE:

A: Lie flat on back, with arms out to sides, and with left knee pulled up toward chest.

On exhale: Twist, bringing left knee toward floor on right side of body while turning head to left.

On inhale: Return to starting position.

Repeat 4 times.

B: Then stay in twist, holding left foot with right hand.

On inhale: Extend left leg.

On exhale: Bend left leg.

Repeat 4 times.

C: Then stay in full twist 4 breaths.

Repeat A, B, and C on other side.

DETAILS: B: *On inhale,* straighten leg from hip, using hand to guide foot.

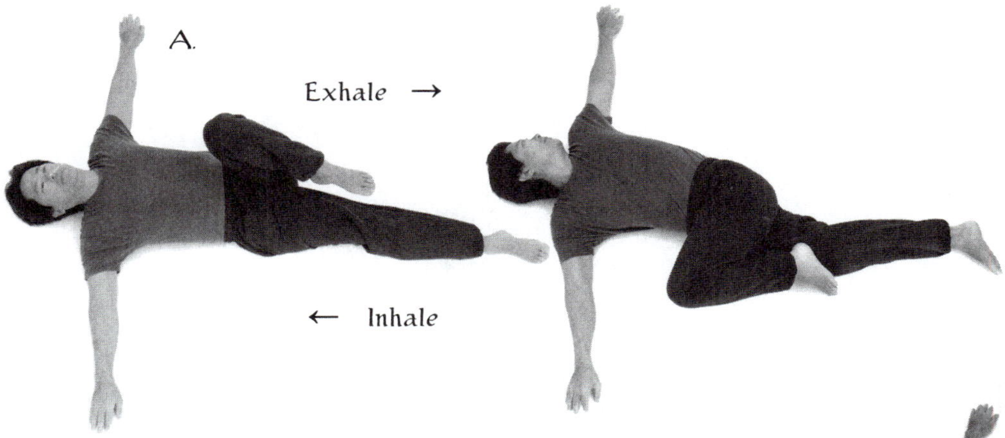

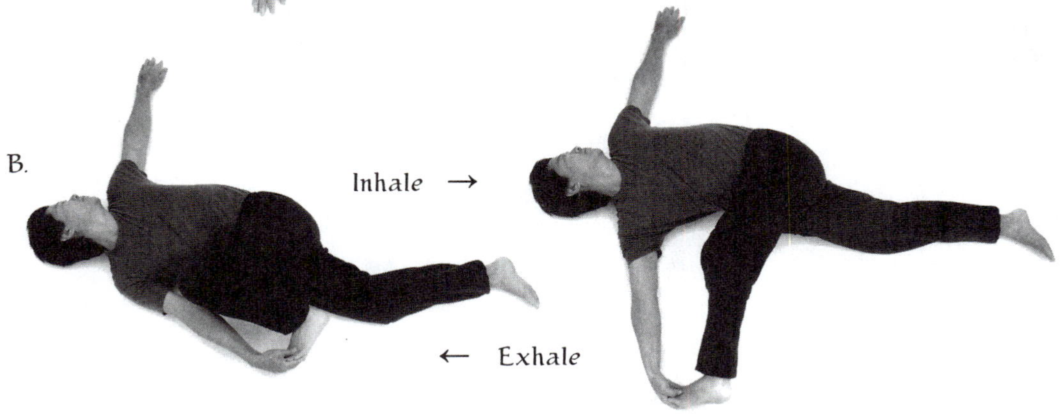

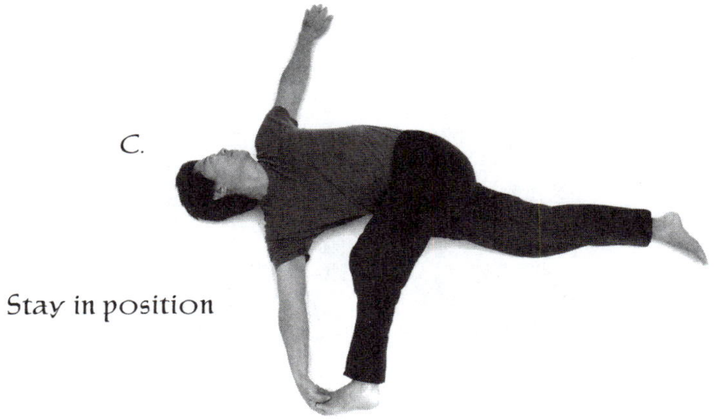

6.

POSTURE: Jānu Śirṣāsana and Mahāmudrā combination.

EMPHASIS: Jānu Śirṣāsana: to stretch lower back and legs; to prepare for Mahāmudrā; after Mahāmudrā, to relax back and rest.

Mahāmudrā: to strengthen musculature of torso; to deepen breathing capacity; to experience one of the deepest extension postures.

TECHNIQUE: Sit with right leg folded in, heel to groin, left leg extended forward and arms over head.

On exhale: Bend forward, bringing belly and chest toward left leg and bringing hands to left foot.

On inhale: Return to starting position.

Repeat 4 times.

Then: *On inhale:* Extend spine upward, expanding chest, flattening upper back, and lengthening front of torso. Hold breath after inhale one half the length of inhale.

On exhale: Maintain posture while pulling upward from perineal floor and pulling belly firmly in. Sustain for one half the length of exhale.

Repeat 8 times.

Then stay down in forward bend position for 4 breaths.

Repeat on other side.

DETAILS: While in Mahāmudrā: *On inhale,* lift chest slightly, extending spine; *on exhale,* tighten belly, maintaining extended spine.

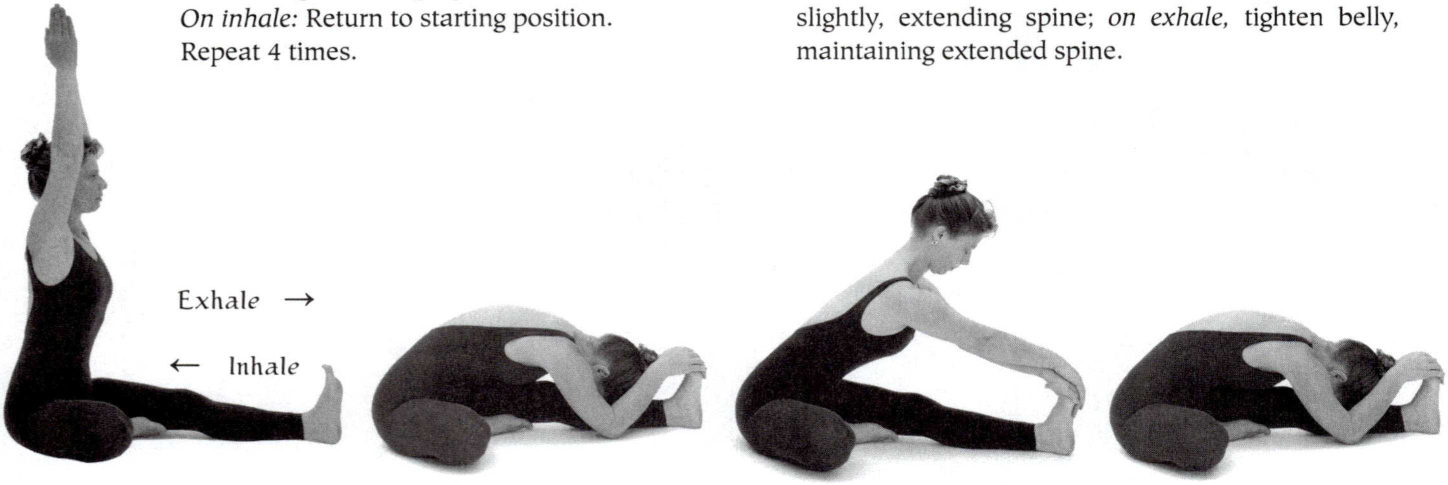

Stay in position

Stay in position

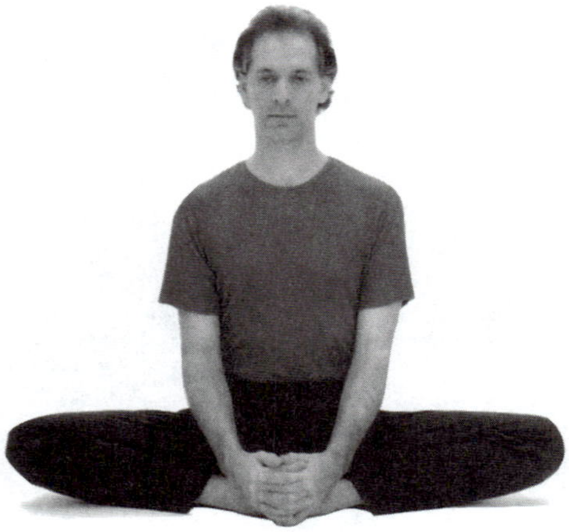

7.

POSTURE: Baddha Koṇāsana.

EMPHASIS: To stretch area of inner thighs and groin. To balance hips after Mahāmudrā.

TECHNIQUE: Sit with soles of feet together, heels close to groin.

On inhale: Holding feet with both hands, extend spine upward, flattening upper back.

On exhale: Pull upward from perineal floor, and pull belly firmly in.

Repeat 8 times.

DETAILS: *On inhale:* Expand chest, then gradually release first belly and then perineal floor.

8.

POSTURE: Dvipāda Pīṭham.

EMPHASIS: To relax upper and lower back, and to stretch between belly and thighs.

TECHNIQUE: Lie on back with arms down at sides, knees bent, feet on floor, slightly apart and comfortably close to buttocks.

On inhale: Press down on feet, raising pelvis up toward ceiling, keeping chin down, until neck is gently flattened on floor.

On exhale: Return to starting position.

NUMBER: 6 times.

DETAILS: *On inhale:* Lift spine, vertebra by vertebra, from bottom up. *On exhale:* Unwind spine, coming down vertebra by vertebra.

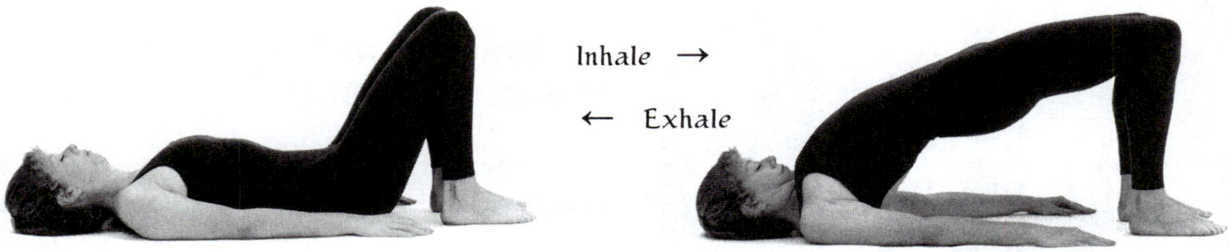

9.

POSTURE: Śavāsana.

EMPHASIS: To rest.

TECHNIQUE: Lie flat on back, arms at sides, palms up, and legs slightly apart. Close eyes. Relax body fully, keeping mind relaxed and alert to sensations in body.

DURATION: Minimum 3 to 5 minutes.

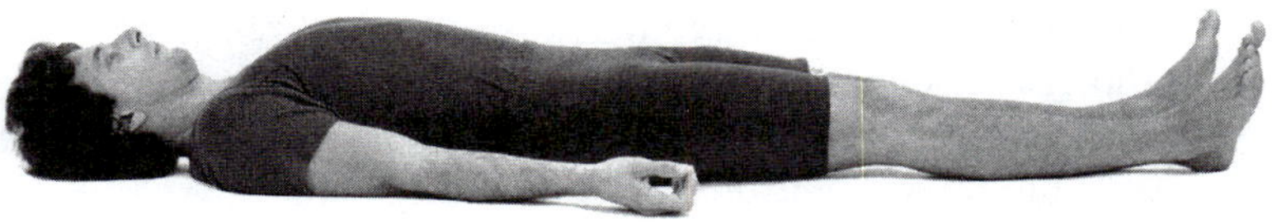

Active Reversal: An Introduction to Inversion

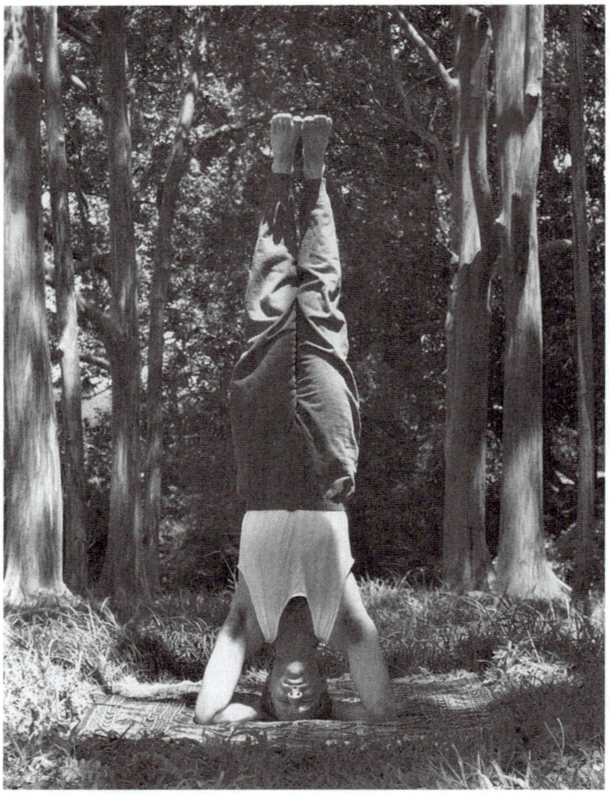

Primary and Secondary Intentions

The ancient yogis recognized the value of turning the body upside down, thereby tonifying the vital organs, stimulating the endocrine glands, and promoting the balanced and efficient functioning of our entire physiology. They called this process and effect *viparīta karaṇī*, "active reversal." Inversion postures also build strength and elasticity in the superficial and deep musculature, ligaments, and connective tissues of the spine and rib cage; and they strengthen the diaphragm and abdominal muscles, as well as the muscles that bind the shoulder and pelvic girdles to the spine. Like extension postures, inversions help improve our posture and overall structural integration, reducing stress to the musculature and organs of the torso, and improving digestion, respiration, and circulation.

From a biomechanical perspective, according to the Viniyoga tradition, the *primary intention* in inversion postures is to achieve the active reversal effect. The *secondary intention* in inversion postures is to strengthen the musculature of the torso, improving the functional integration of the spinal curves and deepening the respiratory rhythms.

Techniques and Types of Inversion Postures

Any posture in which the legs are raised above the head or in which the head moves below the waist provides some *viparīta* effect. The supine extension postures with legs raised, as well as the standing forward bends, the downward dog posture, and the arm balances give some of the inversion effect. The postures in which inversion is the primary effect, however, are limited to headstand (Śīrṣāsana) and its variations, and shoulder stand (Sarvāṅgāsana) and its variations.

The key to achieving the active reversal effect is the ability to remain in the inverted posture for a length of time without stress to the structure. To minimize stress, we have to be able to bring the natural curves of the spine, as well as any lateral curves, into maximum vertical alignment, relative to the different base in each posture. The keys to achieving vertical alignment are the combined techniques of inhale and exhale.

In headstand, the base is the top of the head, forearms, and hands. Ideally, approximately thirty percent of the weight of the torso and legs is transferred directly through the neck to the top of the head, with the remaining seventy percent transferred through the shoulders and arms. As the rib cage expands on inhale, lift the shoulders away from the head, lengthening the neck; lift the pelvis away from the rib cage, lengthening the torso; and lift the legs away from the pelvis. On exhale, use the abdominal contraction to influence the lumbar-pelvic relationship, minimizing lumbar lordosis and controlling the position of the legs. The greater the vertical alignment in this posture, the more effortless it becomes.

In shoulder stand, the base is formed by the upper back, shoulder girdle, neck, and head. Classically, the torso is raised as high as possible from the shoulders, with the spine and legs held in vertical alignment above the shoulders. In the Viniyoga tradition, however, we recommend maintaining a slight angle between the pelvis and legs. This adaptation, along with the classic variation of shoulder stand—also called Viparīta Karaṇī—sacrifices some inversion quality but minimizes the risk of hyperextension to the neck and upper back. The shoulder stands also strengthen the musculature of the legs, low back, and abdomen. While practicing these postures, on inhale, lengthen the spine and extend the legs away from the pelvis; on exhale, contract the belly and stabilize the position of the legs.

In both headstand and shoulder stand, the classic positions of the arms and hands stabilize the base and support the posture. In both postures, the position of the arms and hands can be modified, changing the character of the base. These variations generally require more strength in the torso than the classical positions, reduce the stability of the base, and therefore increase risks. They are collectively termed *nirālamba,* "without support."

In addition, a full range of movement can be practiced from headstand and shoulder stand, including forward bends, back bends, twists, and lateral bends. These variations require greater strength and stability than the basic postures, and their practice increases risk of strain and injury.

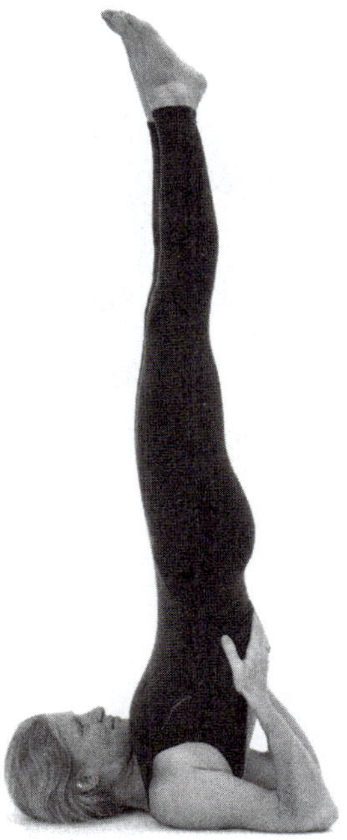

Classic Sarvāṅgāsana

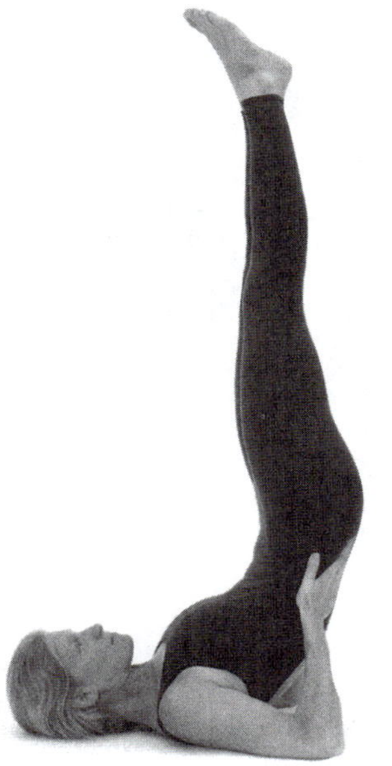

Viparīta Karaṇī

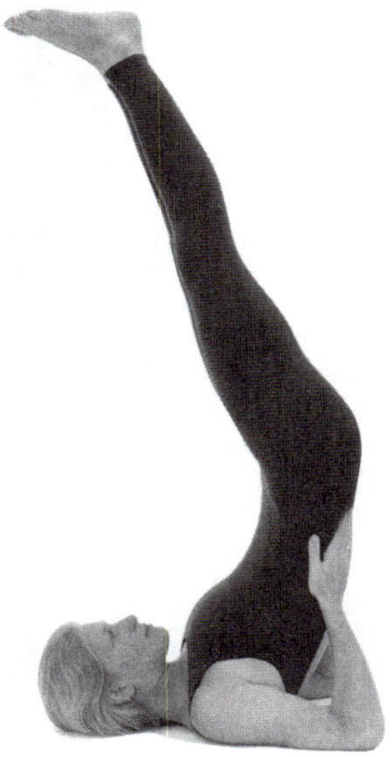

Viniyoga adaptation

Forward bend variations include a variety of postures in which the legs are lowered toward the floor. These postures strengthen the entire torso, especially the low back and abdomen. Most of these variations involve a considerable displacement of weight away from the line of the center of gravity, placing additional stress on the neck and shoulders. In addition, inverted forward bends stretch the muscles of the back and legs and, as with other forward bends, they compress the abdominal organs and stretch the kidney/adrenal area.

♦ **Śīrṣāsana:**

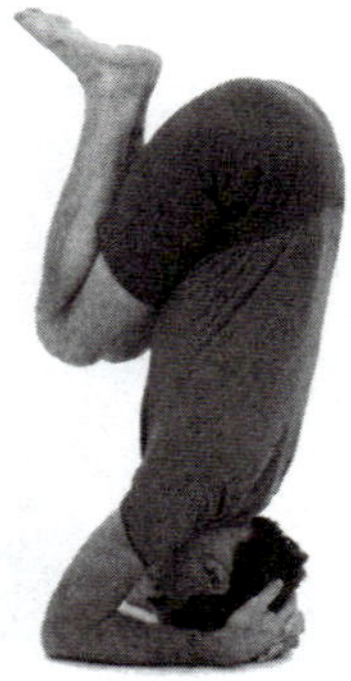
Ākuñcanāsana

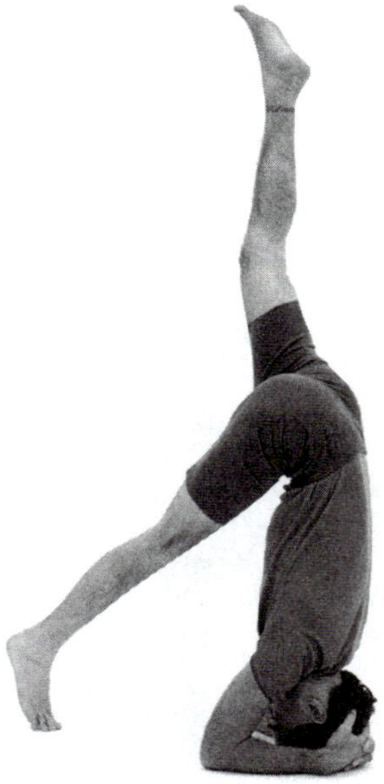
Ekapāda Viparīta Karaṇī

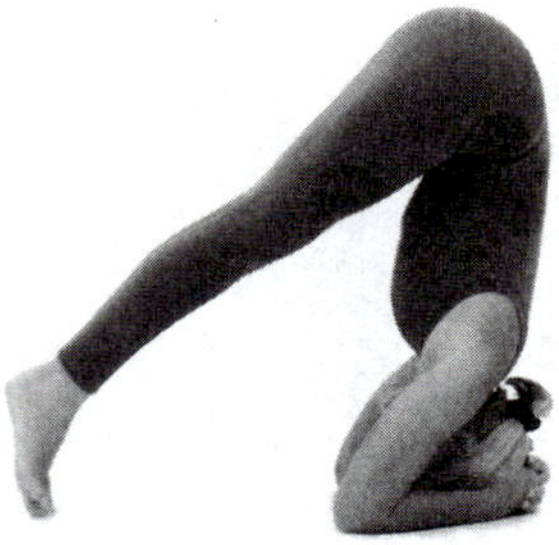
Dvipāda Viparīta Karaṇī

♦ **Sarvāṅgāsana:**

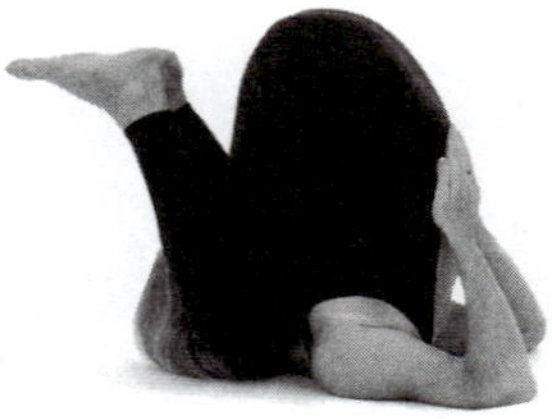
Ākuñcanāsana

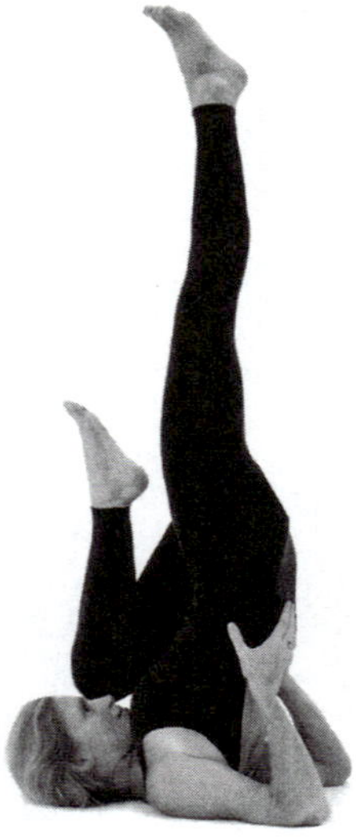
Ekapāda Ākuñcanāsana

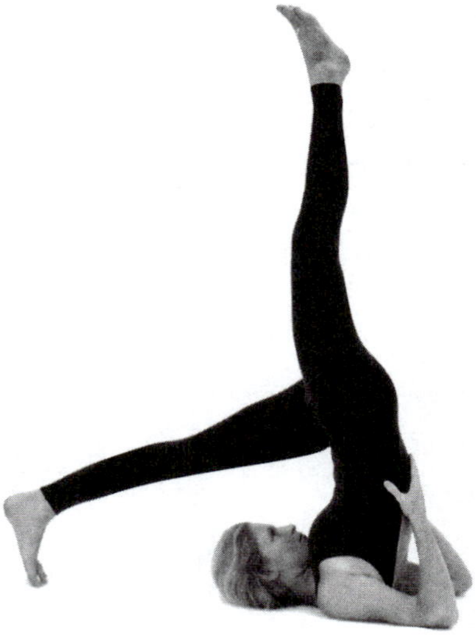
Ekapāda Sarvāṅgāsana

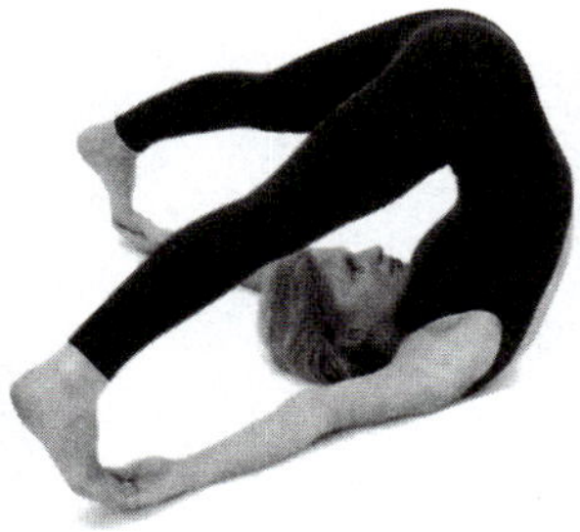
Supta Koṇāsana

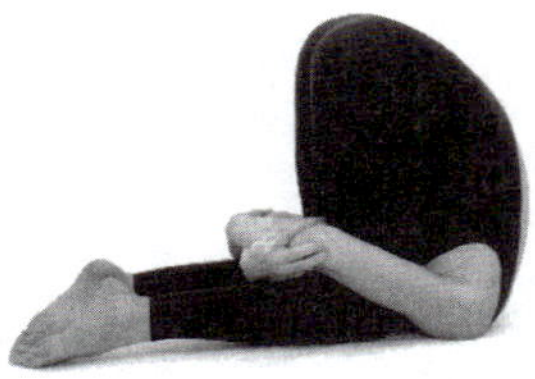

Karṇapīḍāsana

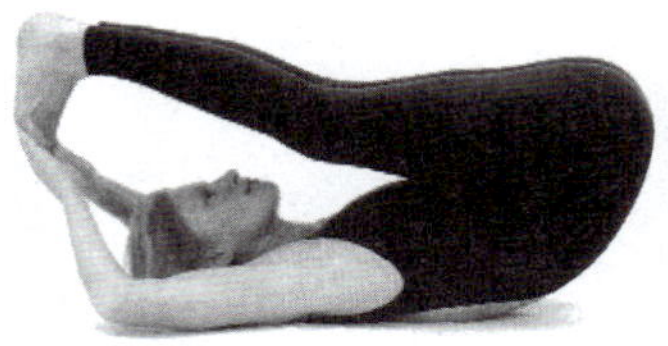

Ūrdhva Mukha Paścimatānāsana

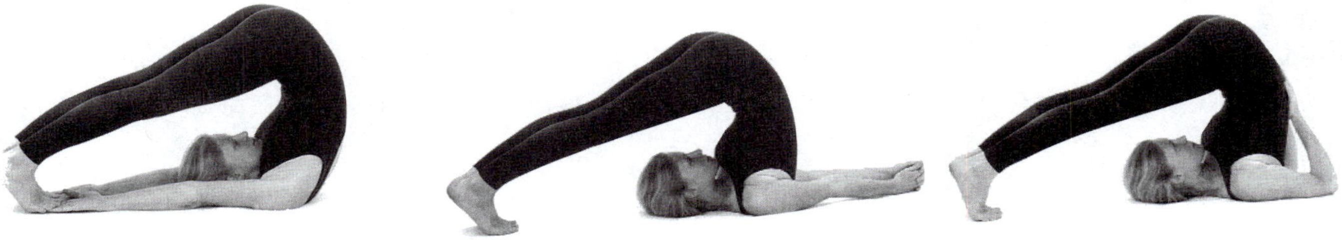

Halāsana variations

Backward bend variations are perhaps the most challenging. In these variations, the torso is arching backward with one or both legs lowered to the floor. These variations build strength, particularly in the abdominal and psoas muscles, which are responsible for controlling the lowering of the pelvis and the legs. They also stretch the intercostal, diaphragm, abdominal, and psoas muscles. As with other back bends, they stretch the abdominal organs and gently compress the kidney/adrenal area.

♦ **Śīrṣāsana:**

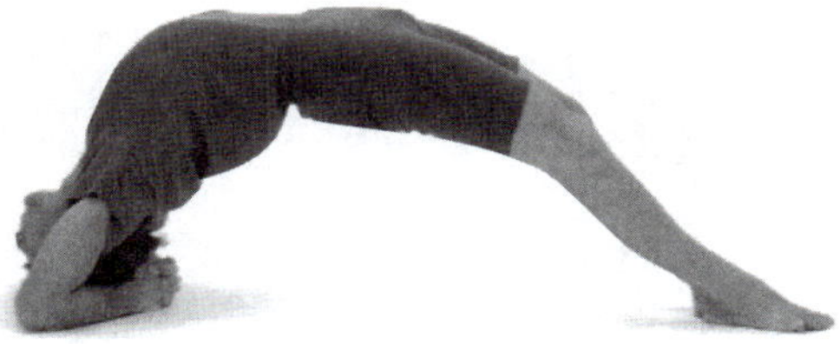

Viparīta Daṇḍāsana

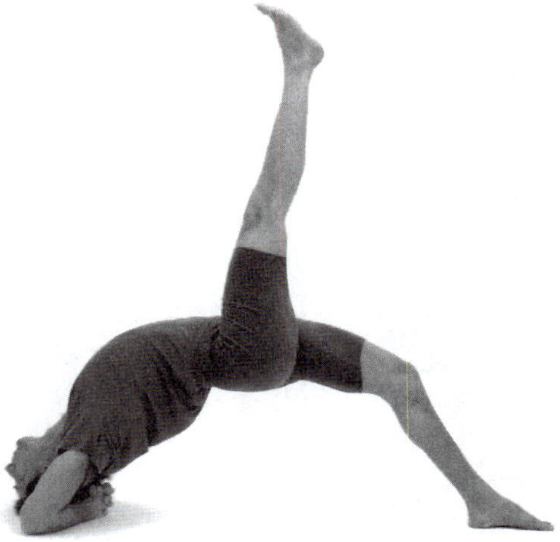

Ekapāda Viparīta Daṇḍāsana

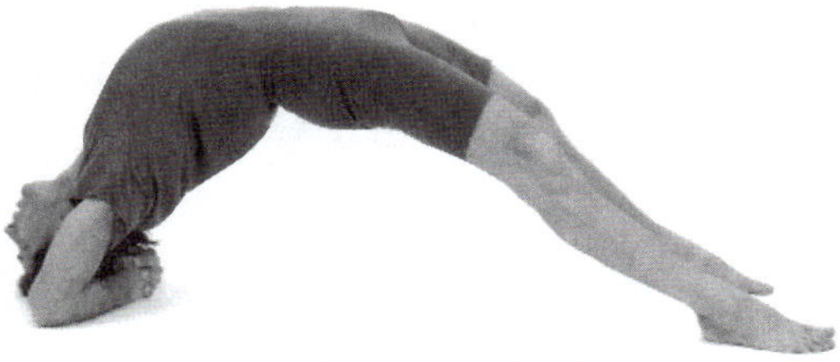

Prasarīta Pāda Viparīta Daṇḍāsana

♦ **Sarvāṅgāsana:**

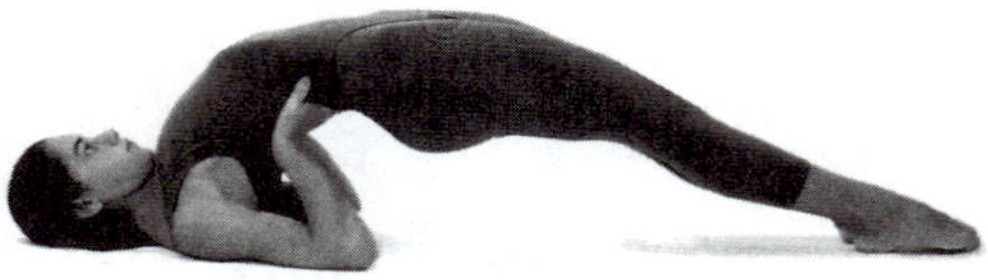

Uttāna Mayūrāsana

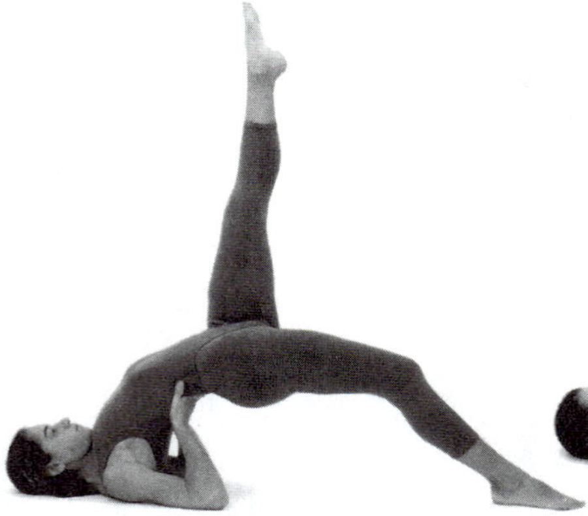

Ekapāda Uttāna Mayūrāsana

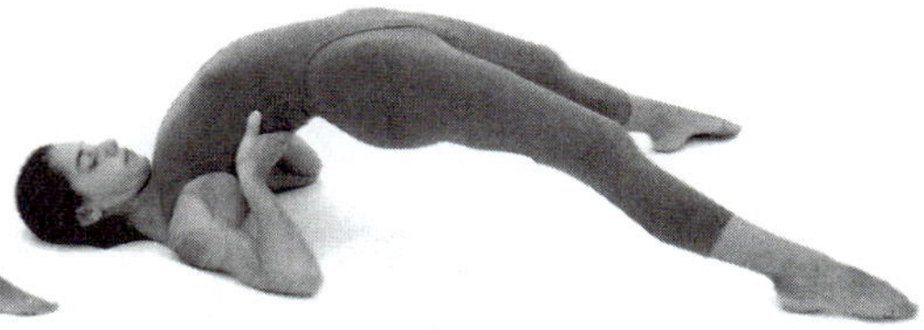

Prasarīta Pāda Uttāna Mayūrāsana

Twisting variations of inversion include postures in which the legs are straight or bent and the torso remains in an extended position, and postures in which one or both legs are twisted and lowered into a forward bend position. These variations strengthen and stretch the musculature of the torso and, alternately, stretch and compress the abdominal organs.

♦ **Śīrṣāsana:**

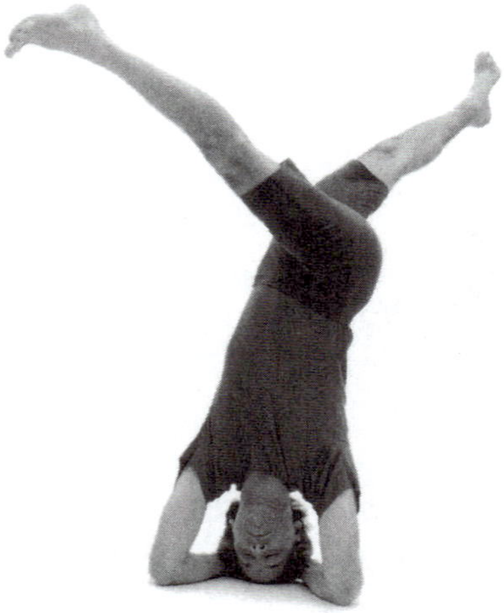

Viparīta Koṇāsana Parivṛtti

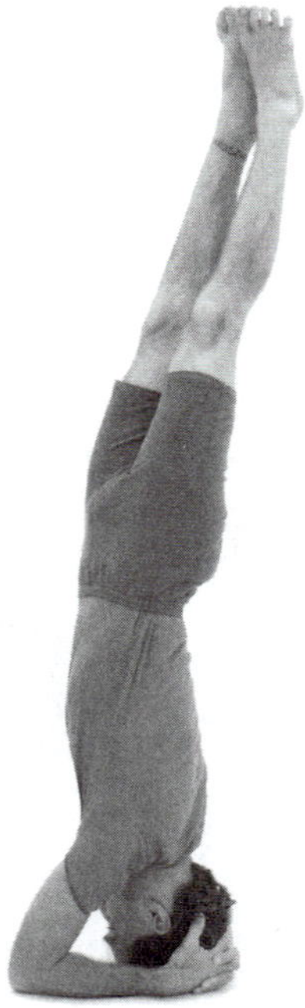

Śirṣāsana Parivṛtti

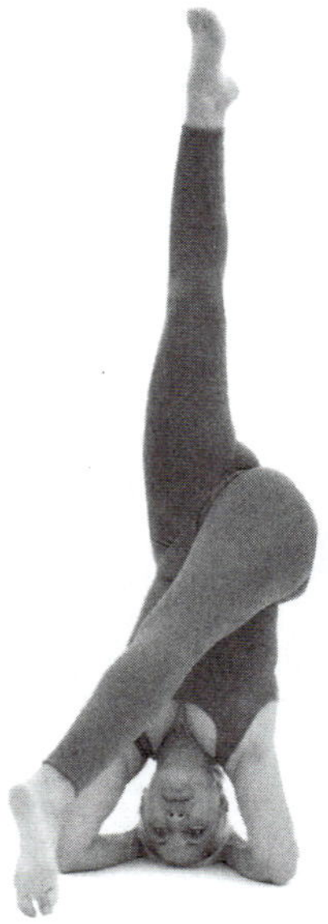

Ekapāda Viparīta Karaṇī Parivṛtti

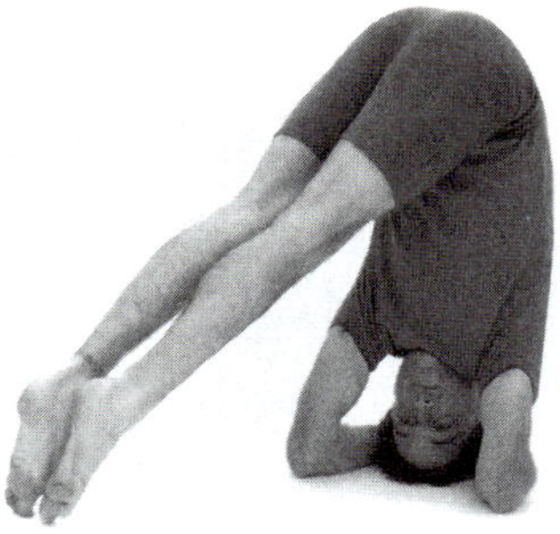

Dvipāda Viparīta Karaṇī Parivṛtti

♦ **Sarvāṅgāsana:**

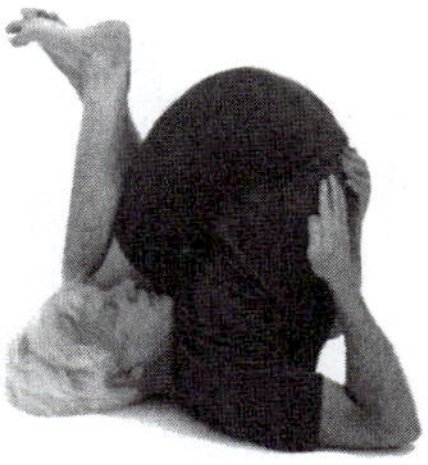

Ākuñcanāsana Parivṛtti

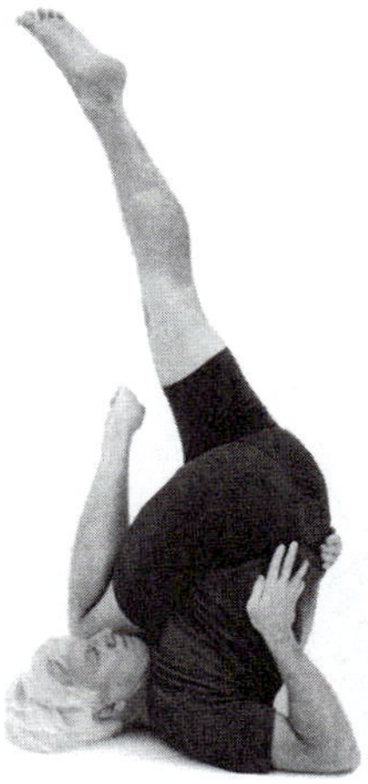

Ekapāda Ākuñcanāsana Parivṛtti

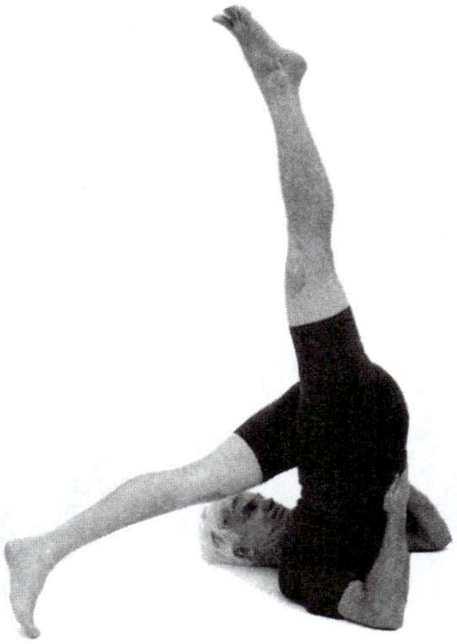

Ekapāda Sarvāṅgāsana Parivṛtti

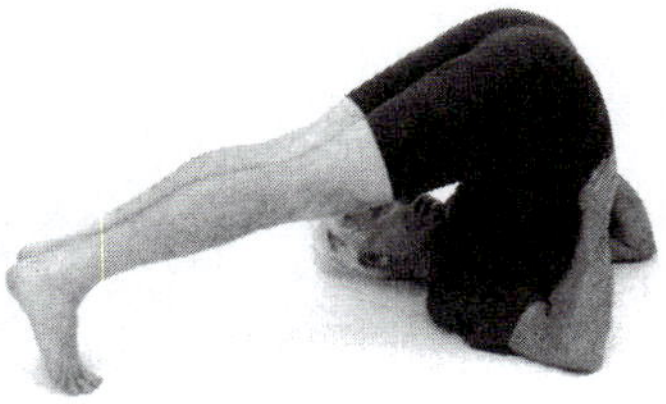

Halāsana Parivṛtti

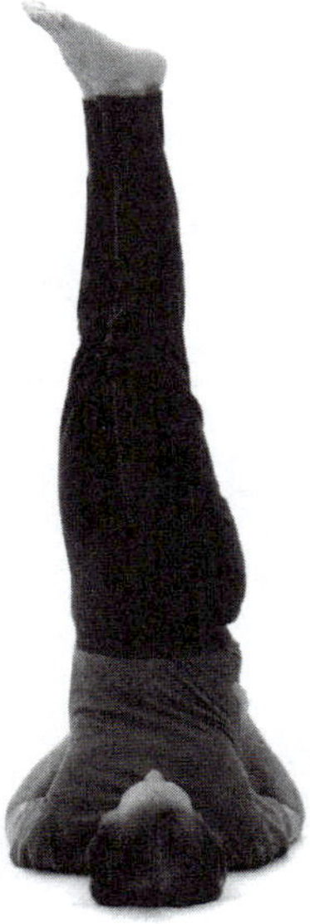

Sarvāṅgāsana Parivṛtti

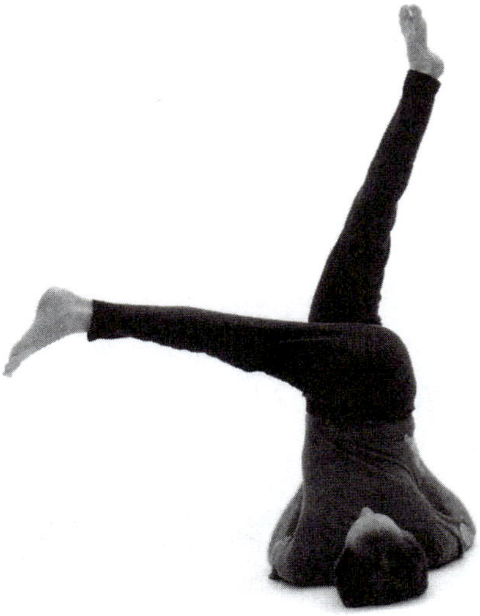

Ūrdhva Koṇāsana Parivṛtti

Pelvic opening variations of inversions include postures in which straight or bent legs are spread wide while the torso remains in an extended vertical position, and postures in which one or both legs are rotated in a semicircle from forward to lateral to vertical position. These variations stretch and strengthen muscles of the hips, groin, inner thighs, and perineal area. In addition, they increase circulation to the perineal floor and stimulate the function of the reproductive organs.

- **Śīrṣāsana:**

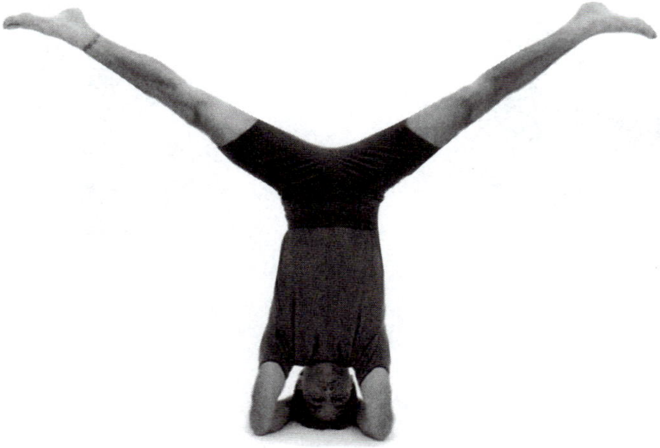

Ūrdhva Koṇāsana

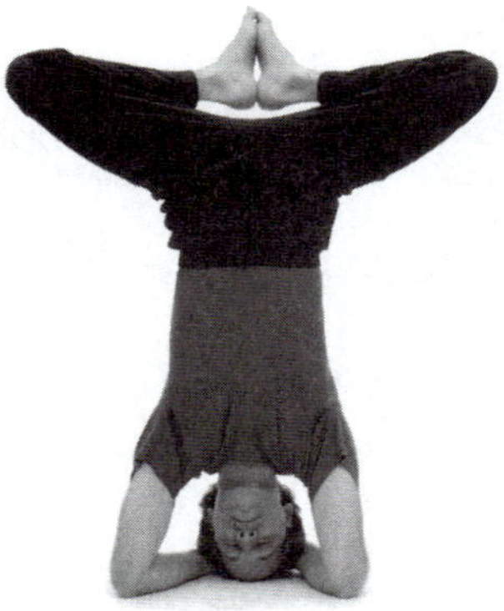

Ūrdhva Baddha Koṇāsana

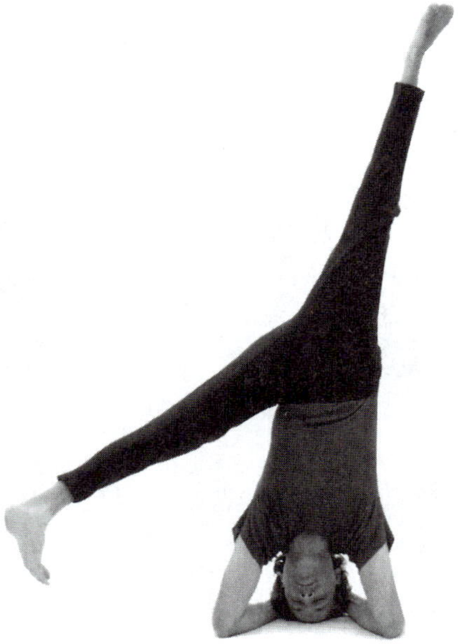

Pārśva Pāda Sarvāṅgāsana

- **Sarvāṅgāsana:**

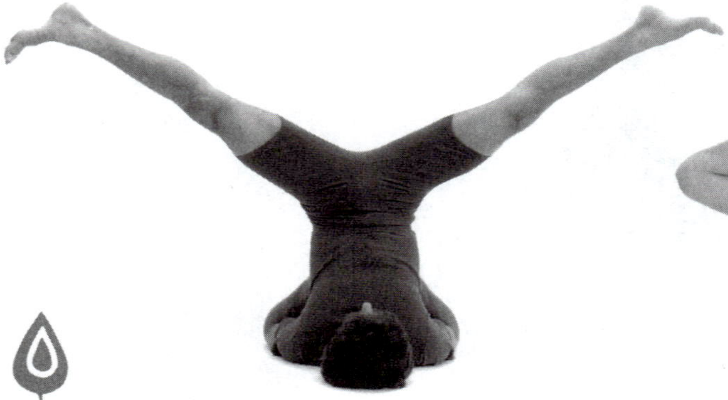

Ūrdhva Koṇāsana

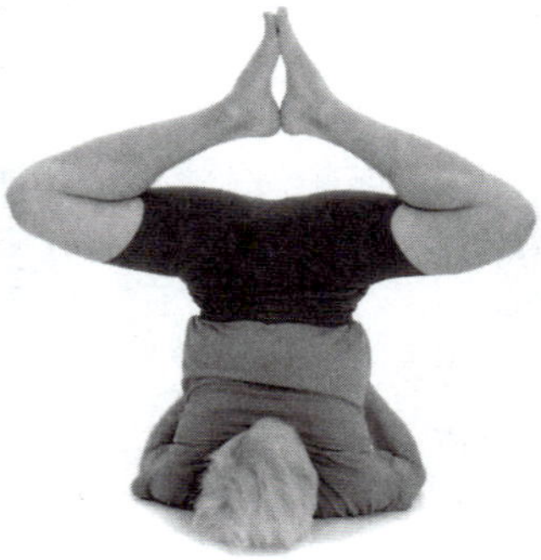

Ūrdhva Baddha Koṇāsana

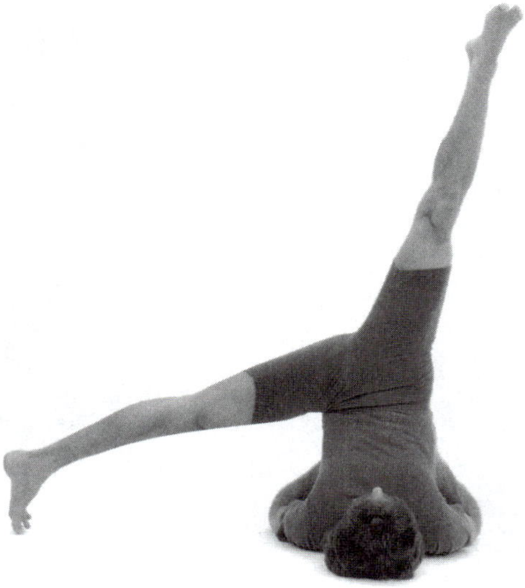

Pārśva Pāda Sarvāṅgāsana

Extension variations of inversion include various ways to modify the base of support. These positions demand greater strength, balance, and mental focus.

- **Śīrṣāsana:**

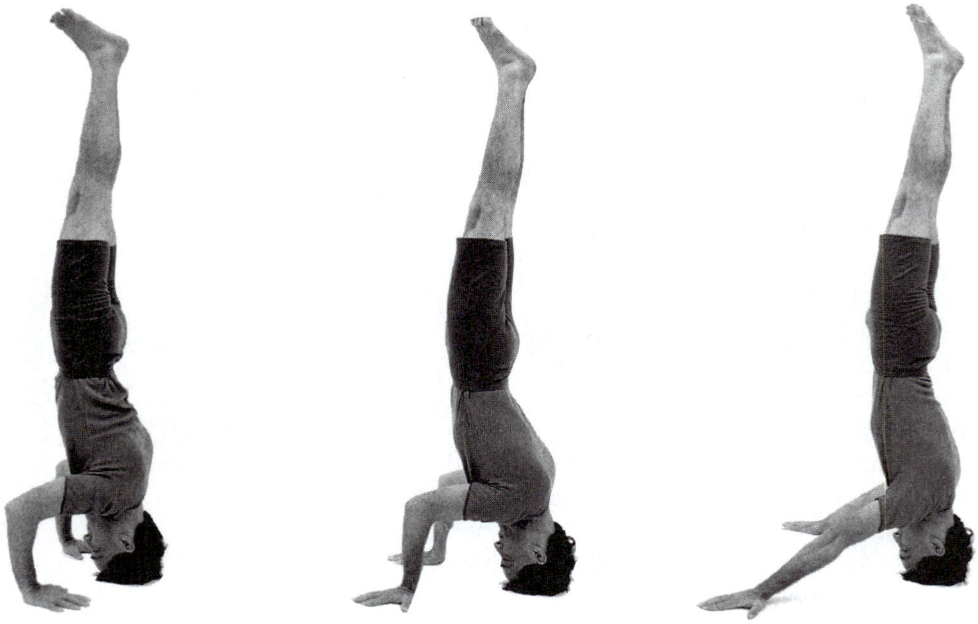

Niralāmba Śīrṣāsana variations

- **Sarvāṅgāsana:**

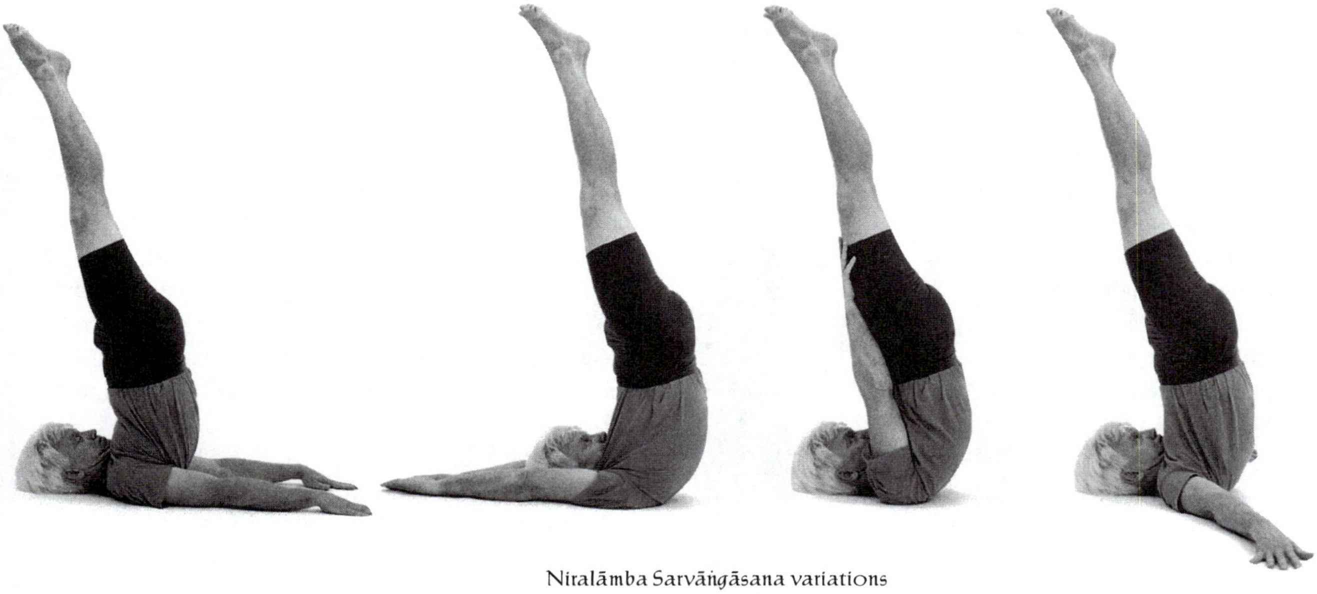

Niralāmba Sarvāṅgāsana variations

Common Release Valves and Risks

The vertebral column is like a pyramid. At the top of the spine, the vertebrae and discs support only the weight of the head, and are therefore relatively small and light. The vertebral structures, ligaments, and muscles of the cervical spine give the head great mobility and relatively less stability. Moving downward, the vertebrae and discs become progressively larger in order to support the increased weight. The vertebral structures, ligaments, and muscles of the lumbosacral spine give the pelvis great stability and relatively less mobility.

The vertebral canal, the space between the vertebrae and the spinous processes through which the spinal cord passes, is like an inverted pyramid, larger at the top and smaller at the bottom. This is due to the fact that the spinal cord, the bundle of central nerves that passes along the spine, is thicker at the top than at the base. In inverted postures, therefore, the greatest demands are placed upon the most fragile and least stable portion of the spine.

The most significant risk in inversion postures, therefore, is strain to the muscles, ligaments, and nerves of the neck, as well as excessive intervertebral disc compression. There is also risk of strain to the muscles and ligaments of the lumbar spine, as well as risk of excessive intervertebral disc compression. This risk is cumulative, and problems often only become manifest years into a practice! Proper sequencing, including preparation and compensation, and establishing the maximum vertical alignment while in the postures, will minimize these risks.

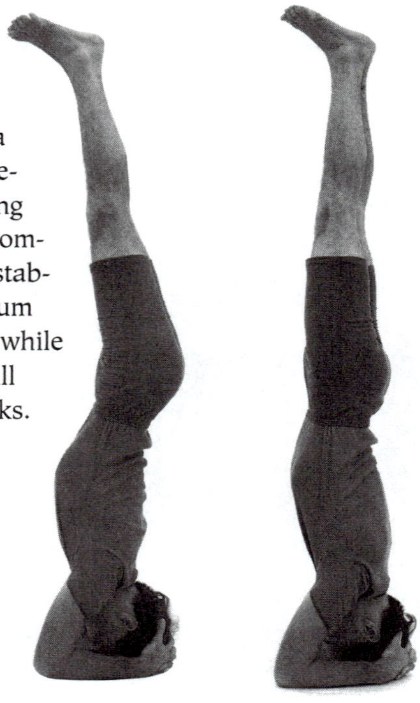

misalignment correct

The use of leg or arm variations substantially increases the risk to the neck and shoulders as well as to the lumbo-sacral area. As the weight of the hips displaces backward or laterally, in forward bend, back bend, and twist variations, there is a tendency to contract the neck and shoulder muscles to stabilize the position. This increases the risk of muscle strain and excessive intervertebral disc compression.

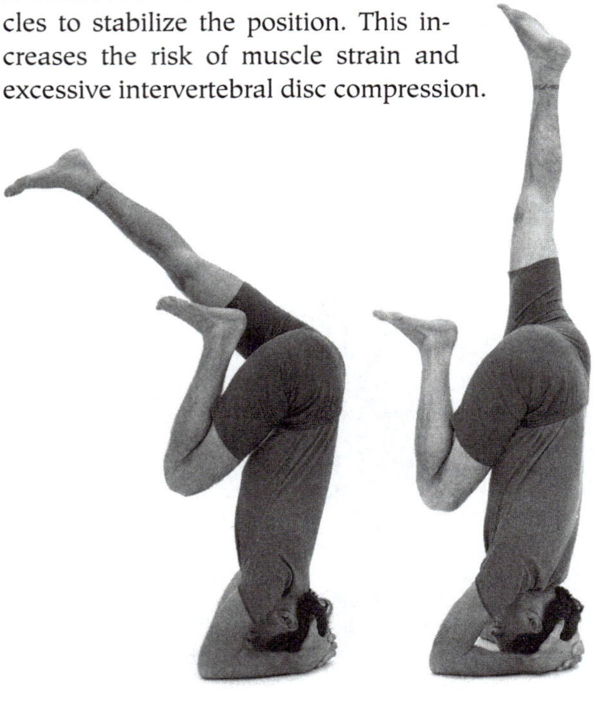

displaced weight correct

It is important to remember that the benefits of inversion postures do not necessarily warrant the risks. The benefit/risk ratio must be considered based on your current condition. A certain degree of strength, stability, and functional integration in the neck and shoulders as well as in the low back and pelvis are a prerequisite.

The principles of preparation, counterpose, and intelligent sequencing are essential for the safe use of inversion postures. Your body must be prepared over time, through carefully planned developmental work. Attention must also be given to proper compensation, for no matter how well prepared you are, there is going to be residual stress that requires compensation.

Headstand, in particular, requires a high degree of strength, stability, and functional integrity in the neck and shoulders, the upper and lower back, the pelvic girdle, and the legs. In order to practice Śīrṣāsana safely, your whole body must be developed. The variations of headstand require an even greater degree of preparation and should not be practiced casually. Commitment to long-term preparation as well as an awareness of current conditions is required. And even if you have this commitment, you must respect the actual condition of the neck, which can change from day to day, each time you practice. If, during preparation for headstand, you find stiffensss or pain in your neck, it is better not to do it that day.

Contraindications to Headstand and Shoulder Stand

1. Severe structural asymmetries or severe scoliosis
2. Weakness, strain, or stiffness in the neck, shoulders, or upper back
3. Chronic forward thrust of the neck
4. Flattened cervical spine (in shoulder stand)*
5. Long neck and weak upper back
6. Small upper torso and large lower torso
7. Severe lumbar lordosis
8. Any disc problems
9. High blood pressure
10. Glaucoma
11. Obesity
12. Head cold or sinus blockage
13. During menstruation
14. During pregnancy

*The use of a pad under the shoulders, wide enough to support the elbows, is useful if this condition is not too severe. The pad elevates the shoulders, allowing the normal curve of the neck to be retained. The use of a pad does, however, reduce the stretch of the upper back.

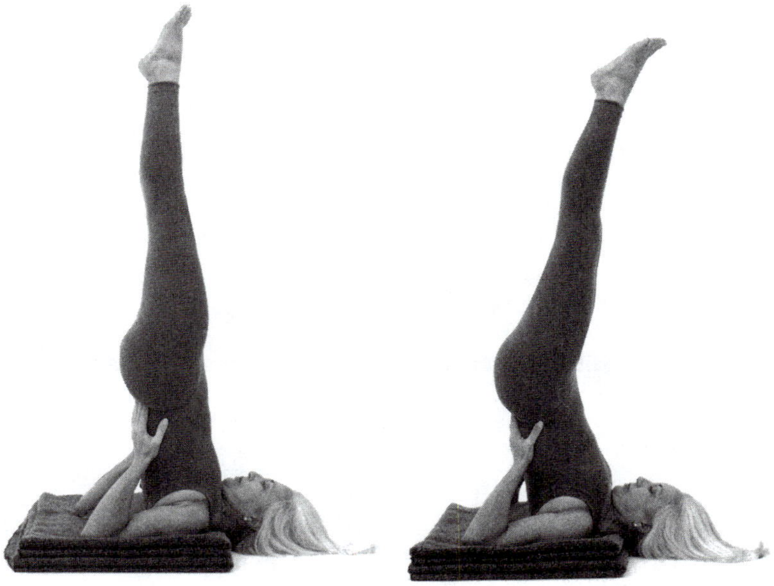

Inversion Practice (for Ekapāda Viparīta Karaṇī)

1.

POSTURE: Ardha Uttānāsana.
EMPHASIS: To warm up the back muscles in preparation for headstand.
TECHNIQUE: Stand with arms over head.

On exhale: Bend forward, bringing belly and chest toward thighs, and hands to feet.

On inhale: Lift chest and arms until parallel to ground. Hold breath 4 seconds.

On exhale: Return to forward bend position.

On inhale: Return to starting position.

NUMBER: 6 times.

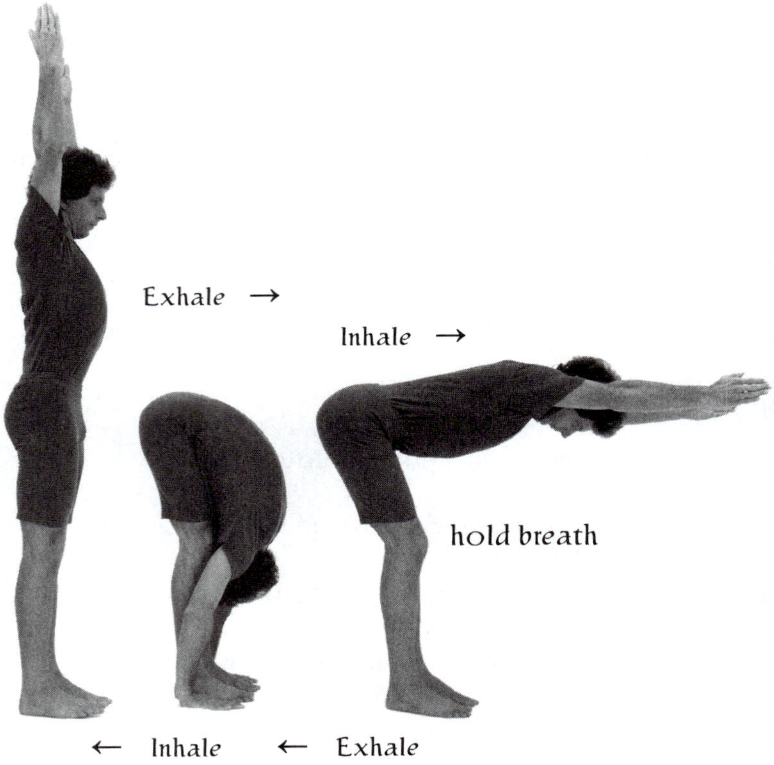
Exhale →
Inhale →
hold breath
← Inhale
← Exhale

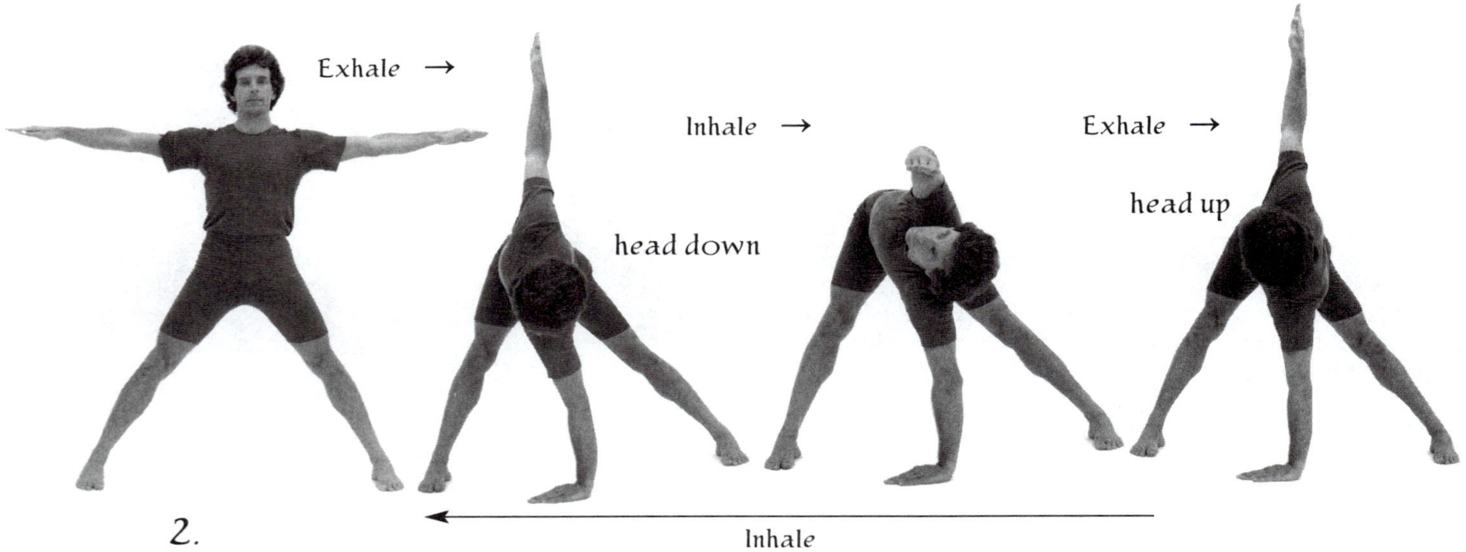
Exhale →
Inhale →
Exhale →
head down
head up
Inhale

2.

POSTURE: Parivṛtti Trikoṇāsana.
EMPHASIS: To stretch legs, back, and shoulders. To warm up neck for headstand.
TECHNIQUE: Stand with feet spread wider than shoulders and with arms out to sides and parallel to floor.

On exhale: Bend forward and twist, bringing left hand to floor, pointing right arm upward and twisting shoulders right. Turn head down toward left hand.

On inhale: Maintaining rotation, and with right shoulder vertically above left, bring right arm up over shoulder and forward, turning head to center and looking at right hand.

On exhale: Return to previous position with right arm pointing upward. Turn head up, looking toward right hand.

On inhale: Return to starting position.

Repeat on other side.

NUMBER: 6 times each side, alternately.
DETAILS: Keep down arm vertically below its respective shoulder, and keep weight of torso off arm. Knees can bend while moving into twist.

3.
POSTURE: Cakravākāsana.
EMPHASIS: To make transition from standing to supine position. To stretch rib cage on inhale and low back on exhale.
TECHNIQUE: Get down on hands and knees, with shoulders vertically above wrists and with hips above knees.

On inhale: Lift chest up and away from belly.

On exhale: Gently contract belly, round low back, and bring chest toward thighs.

NUMBER: 8 times.
DETAILS: *On inhale:* Lead with chest, keeping chin slightly down. Avoid compressing low back; rather, feel chest expanding. *On exhale:* Round low back without collapsing chest over belly. Avoid increasing curvature of upper back. Let chest lower toward thighs sooner than hips toward heels.

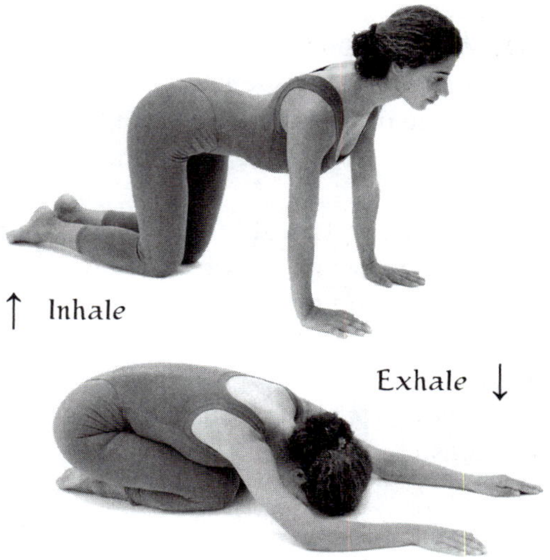
↑ Inhale
Exhale ↓

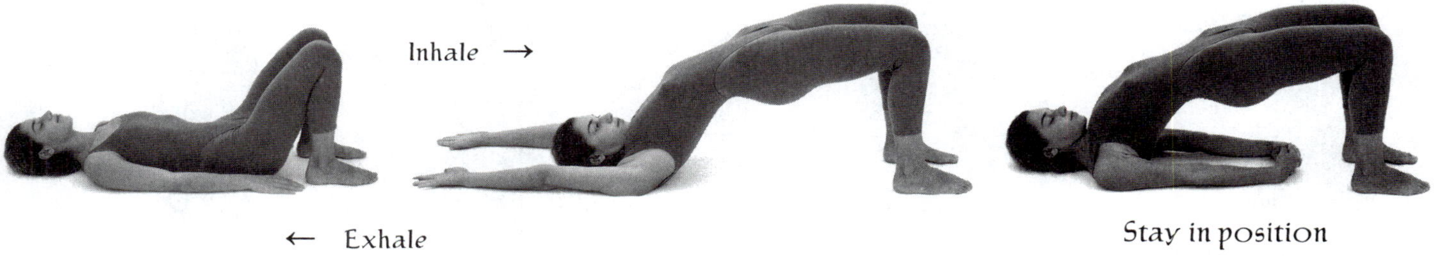
Inhale →
← Exhale
Stay in position

4.
POSTURE: Dvipāda Pīṭham.
EMPHASIS: To stretch upper back and neck in preparation for headstand.
TECHNIQUE:

A: Lie on back with arms down at sides, knees bent, and feet on floor, slightly apart and comfortably close to buttocks.

On inhale: Pressing down on feet and keeping chin down, raise pelvis until neck is gently flattened on floor, while raising arms up overhead to floor behind.

On exhale: Return to starting position.

B: Stay up in position, fingers interlocked on floor under pelvis, gently pulling shoulders together and stretching upper back and neck.

NUMBER: A, four times; B, stay four breaths.
DETAILS: *On inhale:* Lift spine, vertebra by vertebra, from bottom up. *On exhale:* Unwind spine, coming down vertebra by vertebra.

5.

POSTURE: Śīrṣāsana with Viparīta Koṇāsana and Viparīta Baddha Koṇāsana.
EMPHASIS: To strengthen musculature of back and shoulders. To stretch the inner thighs and perineal floor. To experience a headstand variation.
TECHNIQUE:

Śīrsāsana: From hands and knees, interlock fingers with elbows forearm's length apart. Cupping head in hands, stand on toes, lifting knees off floor. Walk forward with toes until hips are vertically above shoulders.

On inhale: Lift legs to vertical position.

Stay 8 breaths.

Viparīta Koṇāsana and Viparīta Baddha Koṇāsana, from headstand:

On inhale: Spread legs as wide as possible.

Stay in position 4 breaths.

On inhale: Return to headstand.

On exhale: Bend knees, placing soles of feet together.

Stay in position 4 breaths.

On inhale: Return to headstand.

DETAILS: Position should be comfortable. If there is neck stress, come down. In both variations, keep legs on same vertical plane.

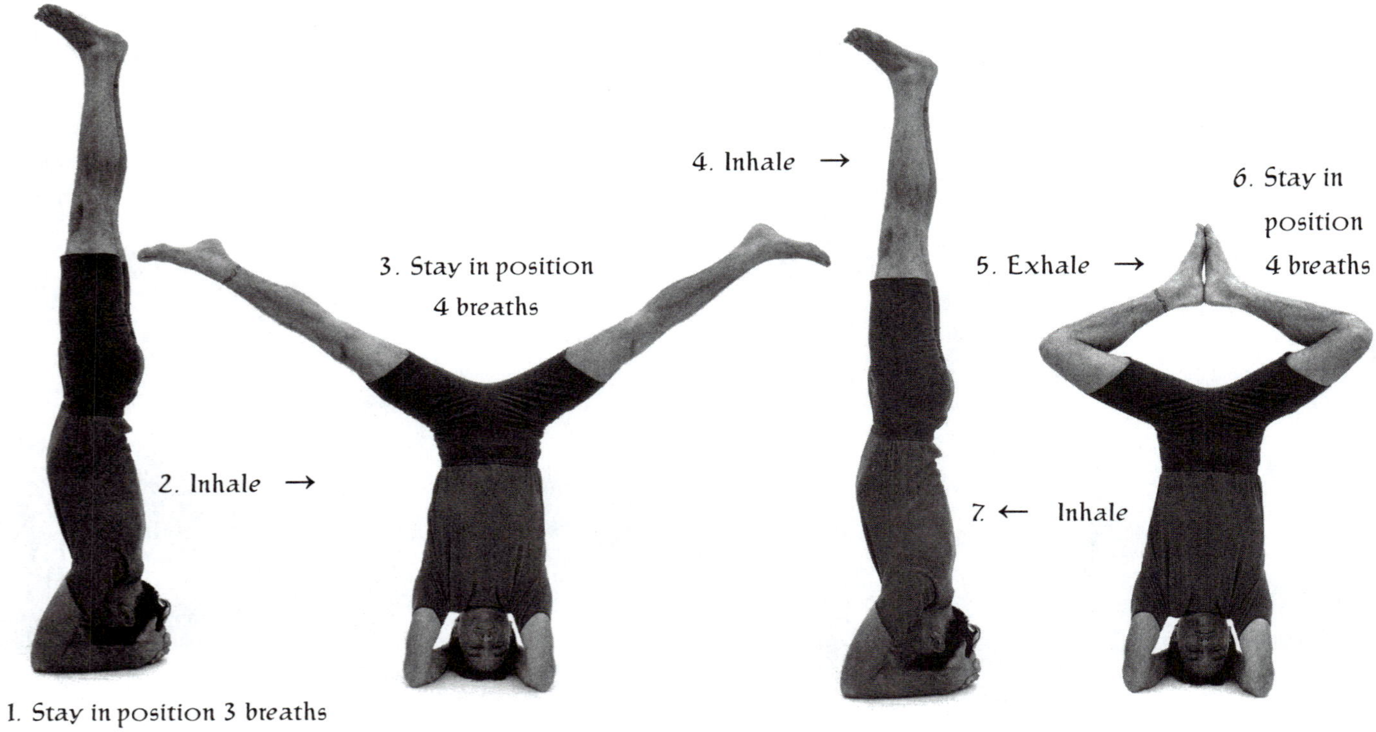
4. Inhale →
6. Stay in position 4 breaths
3. Stay in position 4 breaths
5. Exhale →
2. Inhale →
7. ← Inhale
1. Stay in position 3 breaths

6.

POSTURE: Sarvāṅgāsana and Ekapāda Akuñcānāsana/Ekapāda Sarvāṅgāsana combination.
EMPHASIS: Sarvāṅgāsana: To stretch upper back and neck to counter effects of headstand. Combination: To strengthen musculature of low back.
TECHNIQUE:

Sarvāṅgāsana: Lie on back.

On exhale: Flip legs up over head, lifting buttocks and lower to middle back off floor, and place palms on middle of back.

On inhale: Raise legs upward.

Stay and breathe deeply 12 breaths.

Combination, from shoulderstand:

On exhale: Lower right knee toward chest, keeping right heel toward right buttock.

On inhale: Stay in position.

On exhale: Lower left leg straight until left foot touches floor.

On inhale: Return to previous position, keeping right knee stable by the chest. Repeat 6 times each side, one side at a time.

DETAILS: Place hips vertically above elbows, rather than shoulders, and feet slightly beyond head. Make inhale and exhale equal and at a comfortable maximum length.

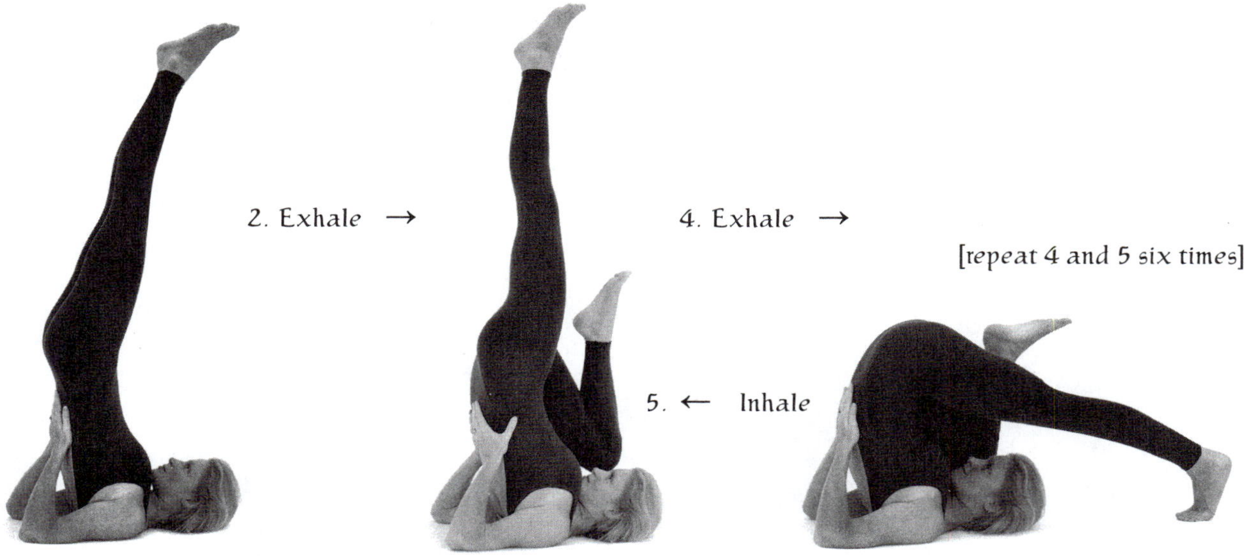
2. Exhale →
4. Exhale →
[repeat 4 and 5 six times]
5. ← Inhale

1. Stay in position 12 breaths

3. Inhale in position

7.

POSTURE: Ardha Śalabhāsana.

EMPHASIS: To arch upper back and neck while mobilizing arms.

TECHNIQUE: Lie on stomach, with head turned to right, hands crossed over sacrum, and palms up.

On inhale: Lift chest, right arm, and left leg, turning head to center.

On exhale: Lower chest and leg while sweeping arm behind back and turning head to left.

Repeat on other side.

NUMBER: 6 times each side, alternately.

DETAILS: *On inhale:* Lift chest slightly before leg, and emphasize chest height. Keep pelvis level. *On exhale:* Turn head opposite arm being lowered.

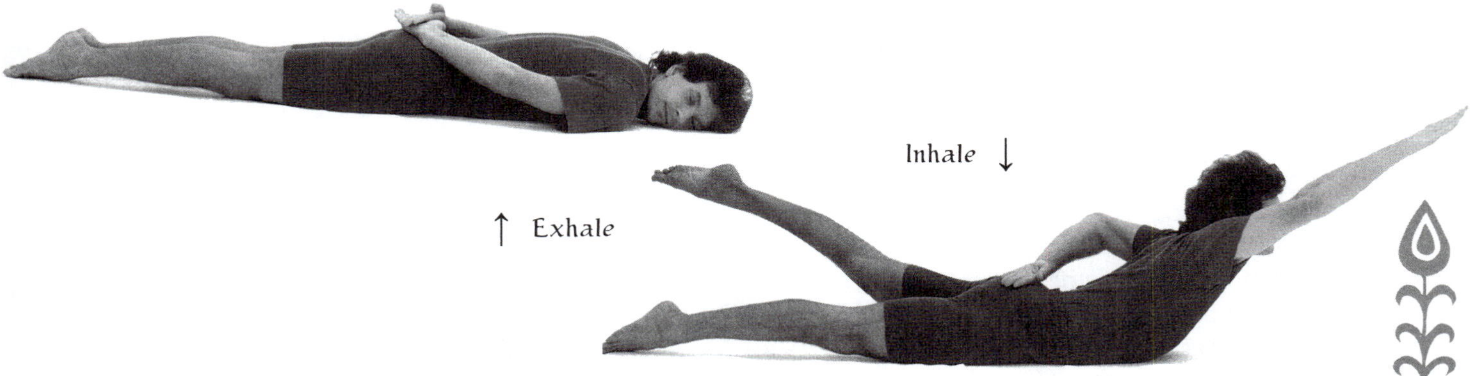
Inhale ↓
↑ Exhale

8.

POSTURE: Ūrdhva Prasārita Pādāsana.
EMPHASIS: To extend spine and flatten it onto floor. To stretch legs.
TECHNIQUE: Lie on back with arms down at sides, legs bent, and knees in toward chest.

On inhale: Raise arms upward all the way to floor behind head, and raise legs upward toward ceiling.

Stay in stretch 2 full breaths.

On exhale: Return to starting position.

NUMBER: 4 times.
DETAILS: *On inhale:* Flex feet as legs are raised upward. Bend knees slightly, keeping angle between legs and torso less than ninety degrees. Push low back and sacrum downward. Bring chin down. While staying in position: *On exhale,* flex knees and elbows slightly; *on inhale,* extend arms and legs straighter.

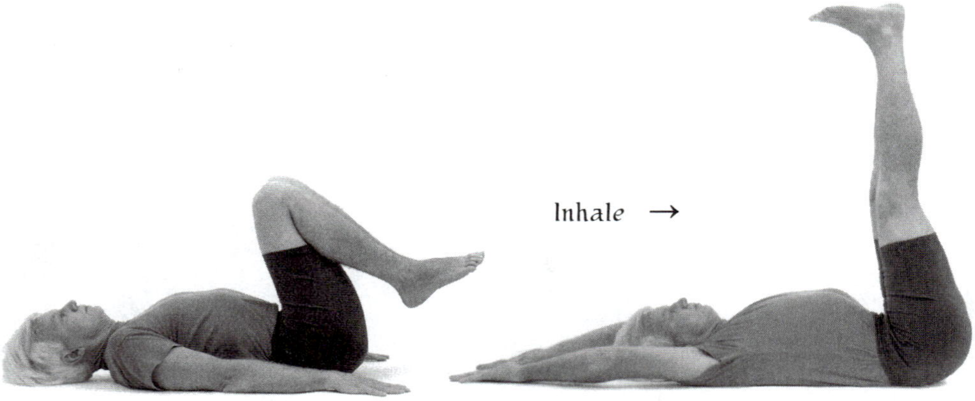

9.

POSTURE: Marīcyāsana.
EMPHASIS: To stretch muscles between shoulder blade and spine, and from shoulders to neck. To help balance neck and shoulders after headstand.
TECHNIQUE: Sit with left leg extended forward, right knee bent with heel close to sit bone and knee toward chest. Wrap right arm, from inside of right thigh, around outside of right thigh and behind back. Wrap left arm behind back and grasp left wrist with right hand.

On inhale: Lift chest and flatten upper back, bringing left shoulder forward and keeping it as level with right shoulder as possible.

On exhale: Bend forward, bringing chest down toward left leg.

Repeat 6 times.

Wait, in a symmetric position, feeling a quality of space in right shoulder.

Repeat on other side.

DETAILS: Allow right sit bone to come off floor when bending forward. Allow left knee to bend on exhale.

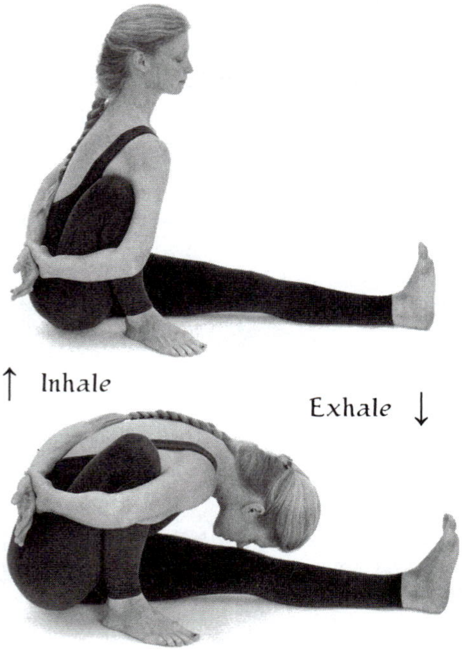

10.

POSTURE: Ardha Matsyendrāsana.
EMPHASIS: To twist spine. To help balance neck and shoulders after headstand.
TECHNIQUE: Sit with left leg bent, left foot by right hip, and right knee straight up, right foot crossing over on outside of left knee, right arm behind back with palm down on floor by sacrum, and left arm across outside of right thigh, left arm on the outside of right leg and left hand in the arch of right foot.

On inhale: Extend spine upward.

On exhale: Twist torso and look over right shoulder.

NUMBER: 8 times each side.
DETAILS: *On exhale:* control torsion from deep in belly, using arm leverage only to augment twist. *On inhale:* subtly untwist body to facilitate extension of spine.

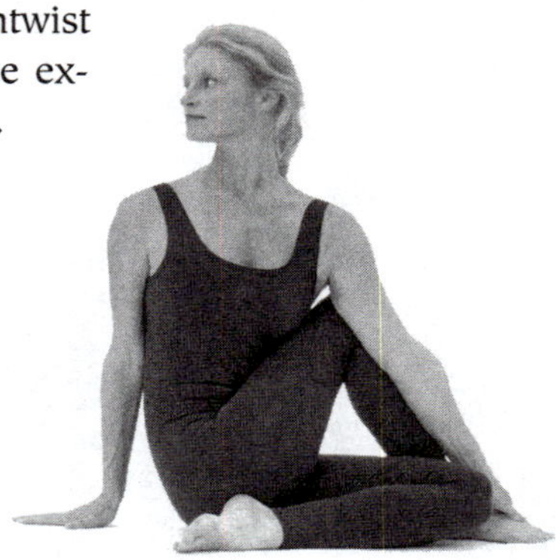

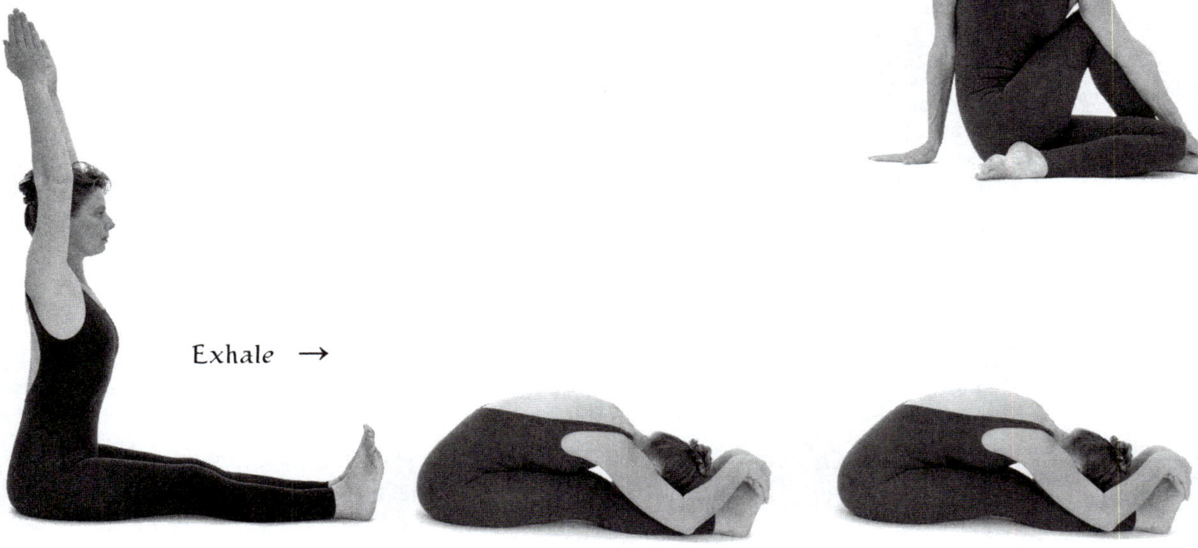

11.

POSTURE: Paścimatānāsana.
EMPHASIS: To stretch back symmetrically after twists.
TECHNIQUE: Sit with legs forward, back straight, and arms raised over head.

On exhale: Bending knees slightly, bend forward, bringing chest to thighs, and palms to balls of feet.

Hold after exhale 4 to 6 seconds.

On inhale: Return to starting position.

Repeat 4 times.

Then stay in forward bend position 4 breaths.

DETAILS: *On exhale:* Bend knees to facilitate stretching low back, and bring belly and chest to thighs. Move chin down toward throat. Feel like diaphragm moves up while holding after exhale. *On inhale:* Lift chest up and away from thighs, flattening upper back.

12.

POSTURE: Śavāsana.
EMPHASIS: To rest.
TECHNIQUE: Lie flat on back, with arms at sides, palms up, and legs slightly apart. Close eyes. Relax body fully, keeping mind relaxed and alert to sensations in body.
DURATION: Minimum 3 to 5 minutes.

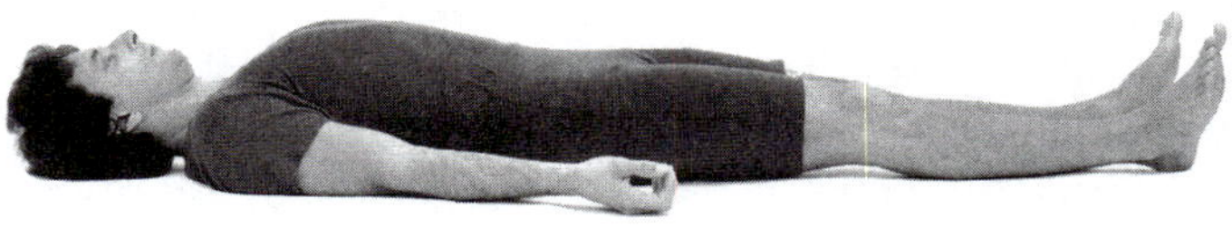

Accomplishing the Peculiar: An Introduction to Balance

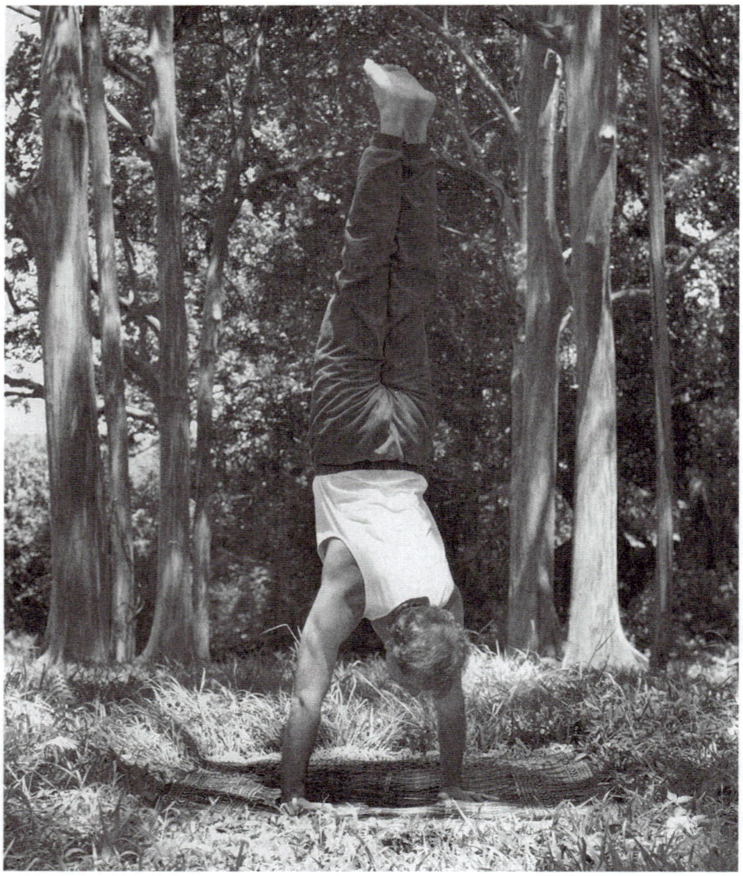

Primary and Secondary Intentions

The ancient yogis knew the value of balance postures for strengthening the body and improving its structural integration and for developing mental stability and focused attention. They called these postures "peculiar" accomplishments. Balance postures can be organized into two distinct classes. The first class of balance postures, which we will call leg balances, are practiced while standing on the toes or on one foot. In addition to developing a focused mind and improving the body's overall strength and structural integration—particularly of the feet, legs, and hips—leg balances help us refine the way we hold and move our body weight. The second class of balance postures, which we will call arm balances, are practiced while standing on the hands, or forearms and hands. In addition to the general benefits already described, arm balances emphasize strengthening the muscles of the arms and shoulders, as well as the low back, abdomen, and pelvis. All balance postures give us a sense of increased mastery over our body, promote a feeling of lightness and well-being, and tend to boost our self-confidence.

The *primary intention* in balance postures is to establish and maintain a "peculiar" position for a period of time without stress or strain and, through this accomplishment, to develop a focused and stable mind.

The *secondary intention* in balance postures is variable, depending on the posture, but usually involves increasing the overall structural integrity and strength of the body.

Technique and Types of Balance Postures

In a practical sense, from a mechanical perspective, the structure of the body is a weight support and transference mechanism. The weight of the body is transferred through the structure to the base of support, which varies depending on our position, and then to the earth. When we are standing, the bodily base of support is the feet; when we are sitting, the base is the buttocks and legs; and when we are lying down, the base is the full length of the body. In general, the larger the base, the greater stability. Thus lying postures, for example, are typically more stable than seated postures, which are typically more stable than standing postures.

When the weight of the body is aligned vertically above a broad and stable base of support, there is maximum stability. In balance postures, the base is characteristically smaller and relatively unstable. Stability is further compromised because, in most balance postures, the weight of the body is not in vertical alignment above the base. In leg balance postures, the lifted leg is extended in front, behind, or to the side of the line vertically above the supporting foot. In arm balance postures, the torso and legs are also extended in front, behind, or to the side of the supporting hands, or forearms and hands.

The key to accomplishing balance postures, then, is the ability to achieve equilibrium on an unstable base, using the displaced body weight as a counterbalance. If we have excessively tight ligaments and/or muscles, it will be difficult to move the body weight sufficiently to create the counterbalancing effect necessary to maintain the postures. If, on the other hand, we have excessively loose ligaments and/or muscles, it will be difficult to stabilize the joints through which the body weight is transferred, and therefore difficult to maintain the postures. Through the use of āsana practice in general, we can develop the strength, flexibility, and stability necessary to maintain the more challenging balance postures.

While in these postures, the combined techniques of inhale and exhale help us to make the subtle adjustments of the torso, arms, and legs that are necessary to achieve balance. In addition, the eyes are a key to our ability to maintain equilibrium and should be focused on a point out in front of us. In addition to facilitating spacial awareness, this technique will also help to keep the mind present and free from distraction.

Whether on one foot, both toes, the hands, or the hands and forearms, in addition to the primary balance component, these postures involve elements of forward bending, back bending, twisting, lateral bending, extension, and/or inversion.

Leg Balances

♦ GROUP 1

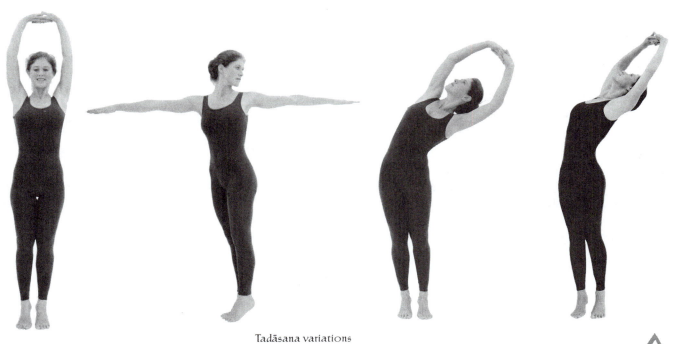

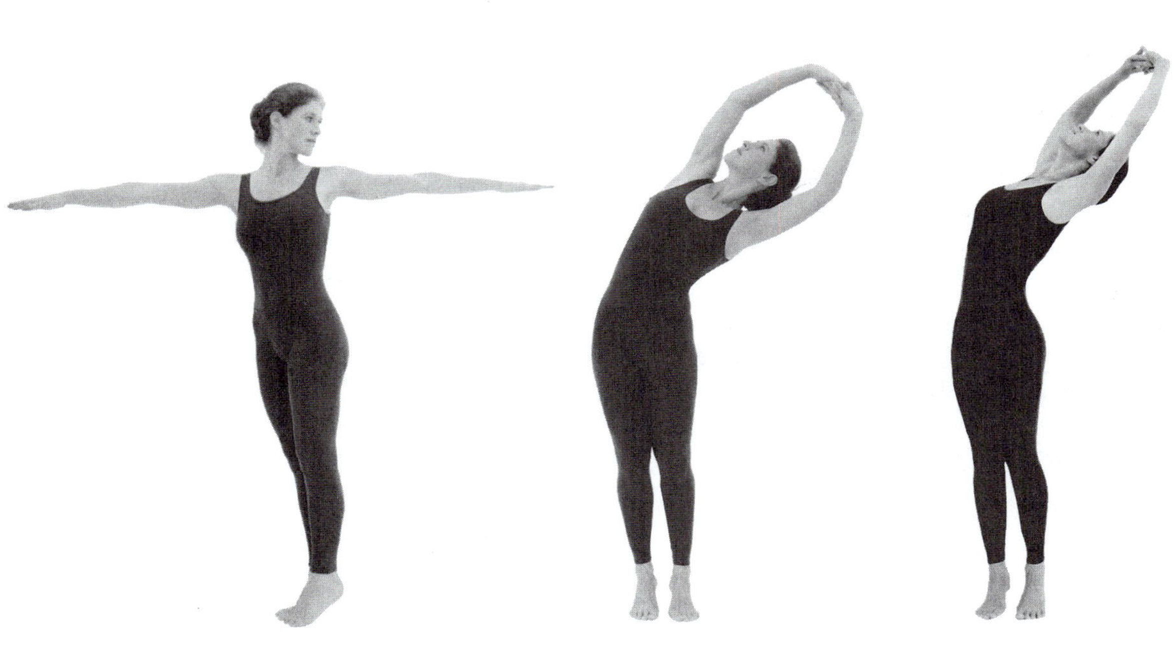

Taḍāsana variations

Taḍāsana is grouped as an extension posture. When adapted to include a back bending, twisting, or lateral bending component, the adaptations require significant weight distribution and, therefore, become primarily balance postures. These postures are particularly useful for strengthening the feet and lower legs.

♦ GROUP 2

This group of postures includes leg balances with the spine extended upward. Utthita Pārśva Pādāṅguṣṭhāsana has elements of pelvic opening.

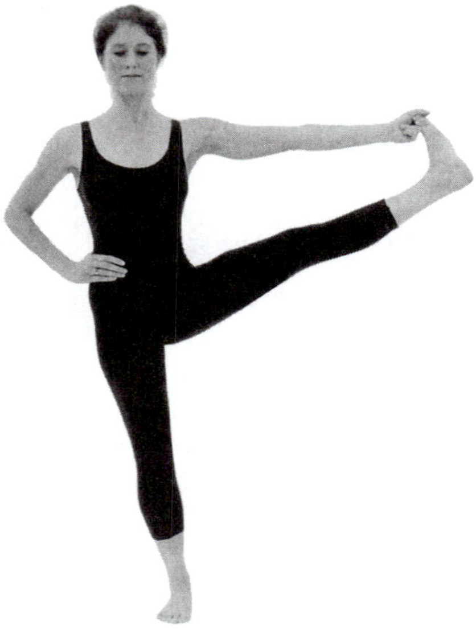

Utthita Pārśva Pādāṅguṣṭhāsana

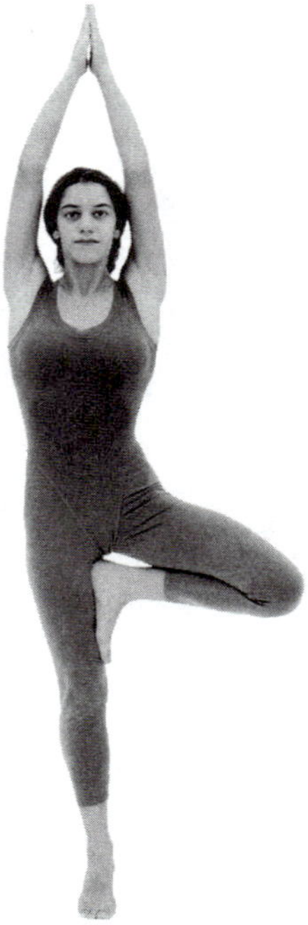

Bhagīrathāsana

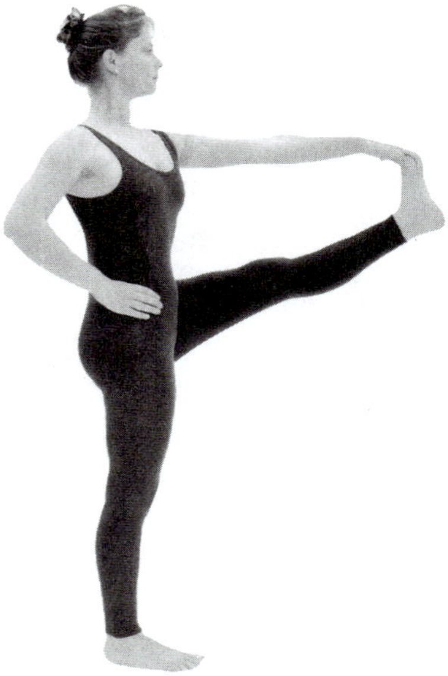

Utthita Eka Pādāṅguṣṭhāsana

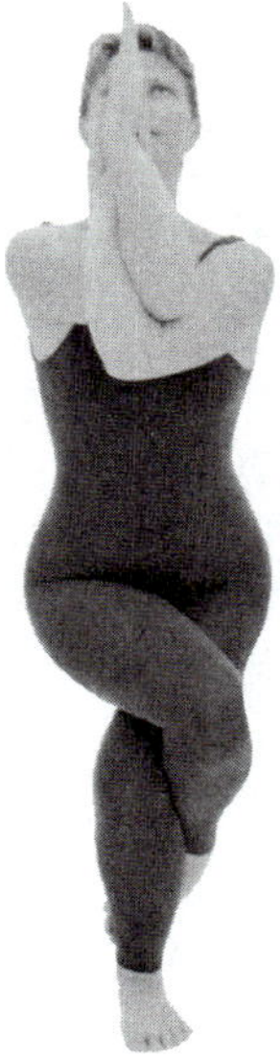

Garuḍāsana

♦ GROUP 3

This group of postures includes leg balances with a forward bend component.

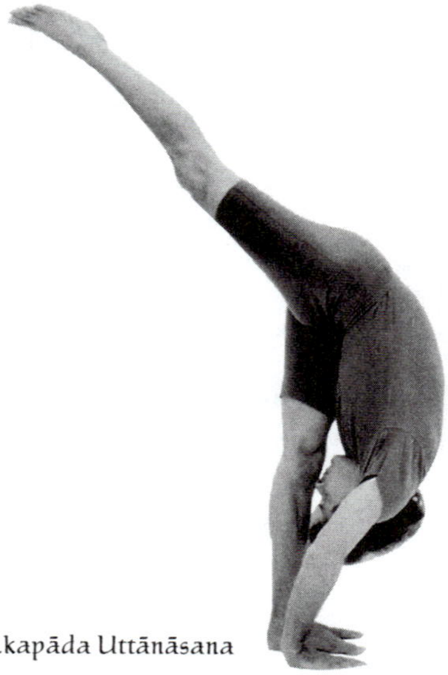

Ekapāda Uttānāsana

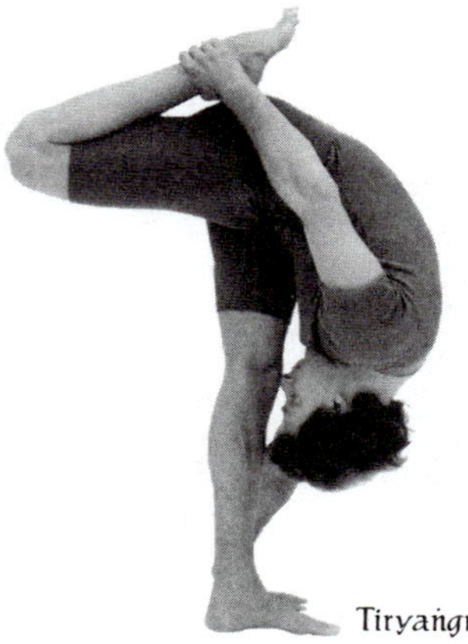

Tiryaṅgmukha Ekapāda Uttānāsana

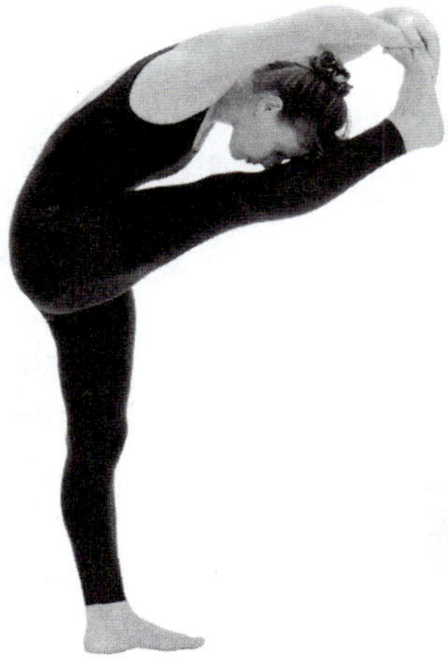
Utthita Pāda Paścimatānāsana

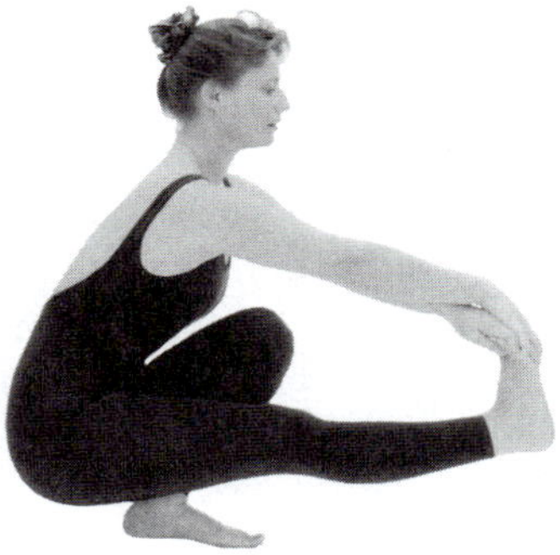
Ekapāda Utkaṭāsana

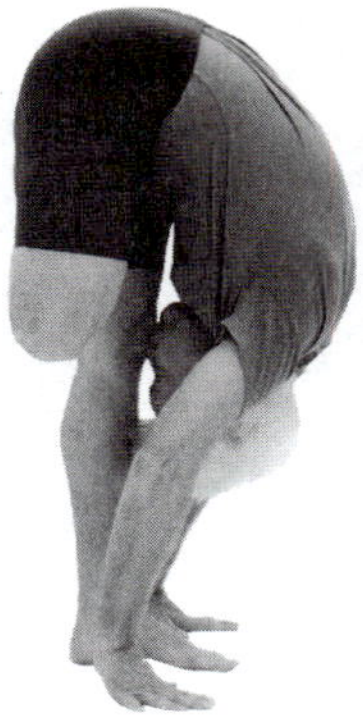
Ardha Padma Uttānāsana

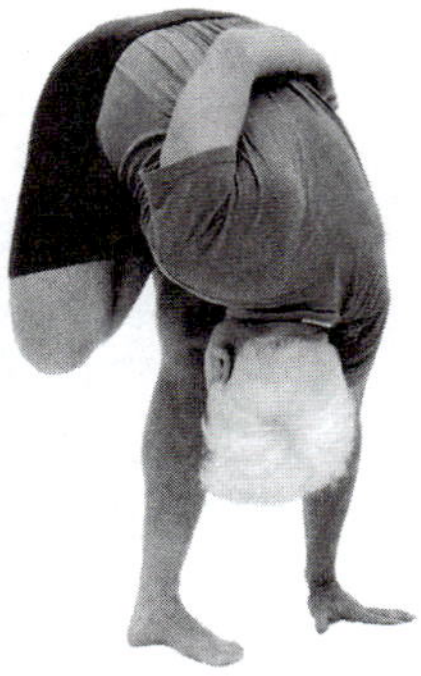
Ardha Baddha Padma Uttānāsana

♦ GROUP 4

This group of postures includes leg balances with a back bend component. The Vīrabhadrāsana variation is particularly useful for developing strength and stability in the hips.

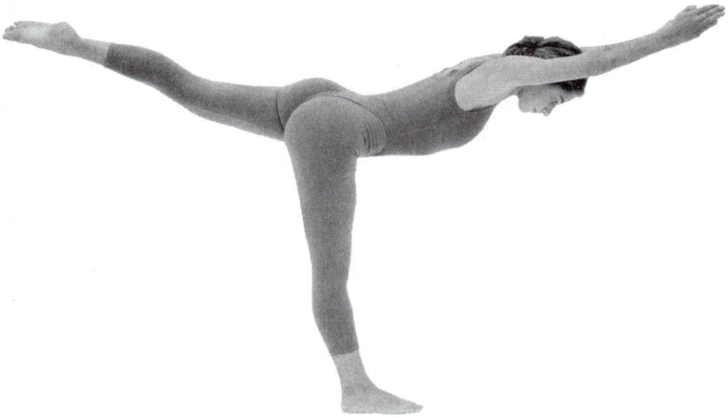
Vīrabhadrāsana

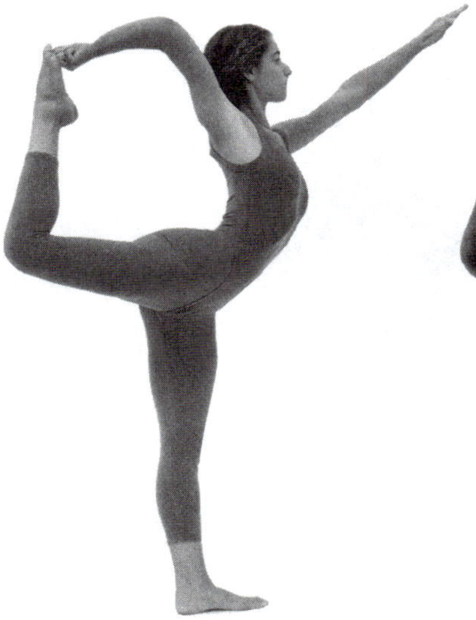
Natarājāsana variation

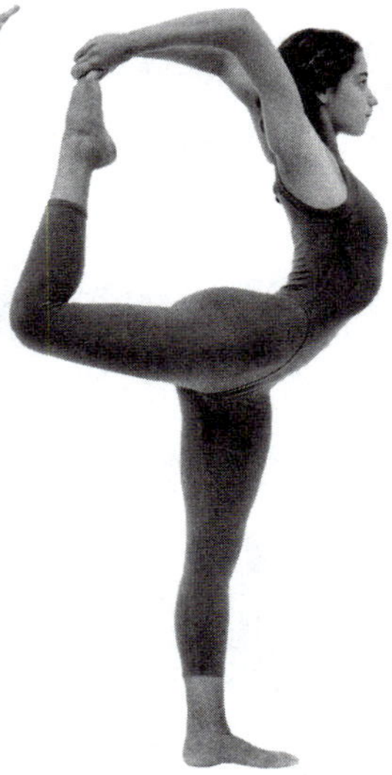
Naṭarājāsana variation

Arm Balances

♦ GROUP 1

This group of postures includes inverted arm balances, which are classically moved into from an adaptation of headstand. They all have a forward bend component, and three have an additional twisting component. They require—and develop—upper body strength, good functional integrity between the upper and lower torso and between the pelvis and legs, strength in the abdomen and low back, and stability in the shoulder, elbow, and wrist joints.

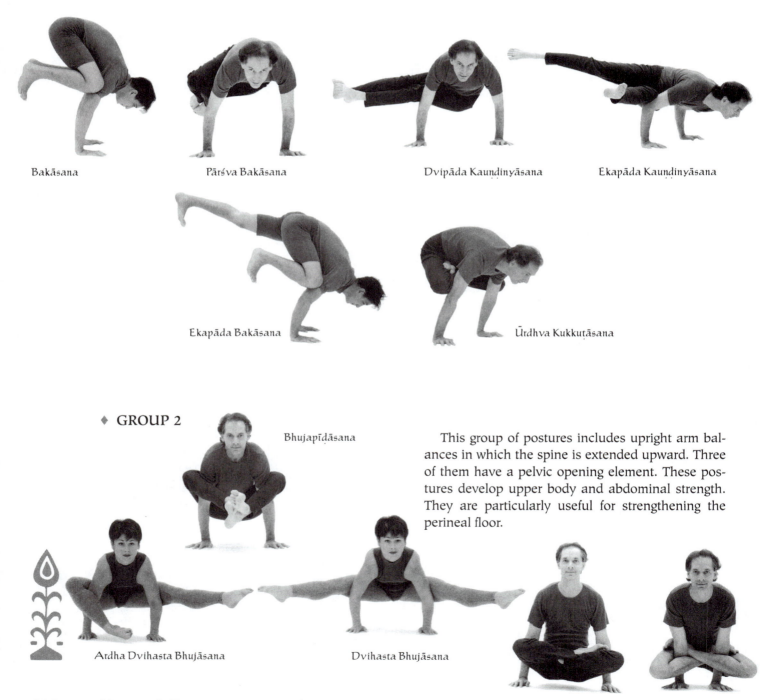

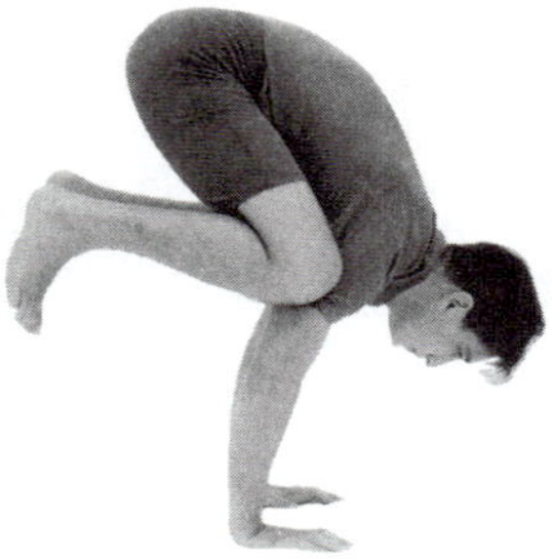
Bakāsana

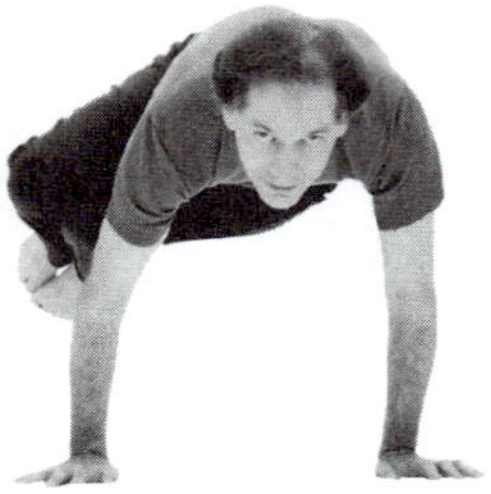
Pārśva Bakāsana

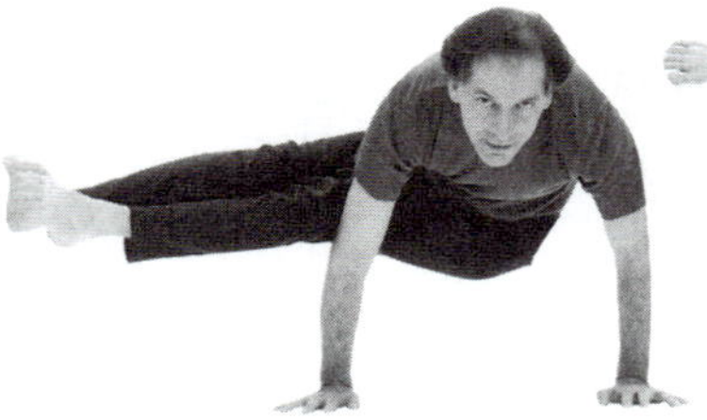
Dvipāda Kauṇḍinyāsana

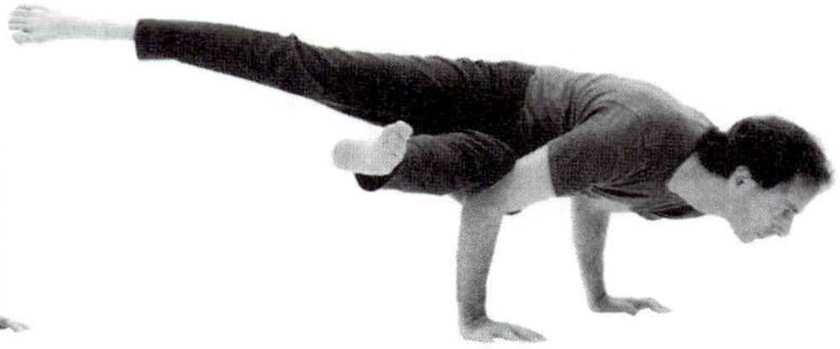
Ekapāda Kauṇḍinyāsana

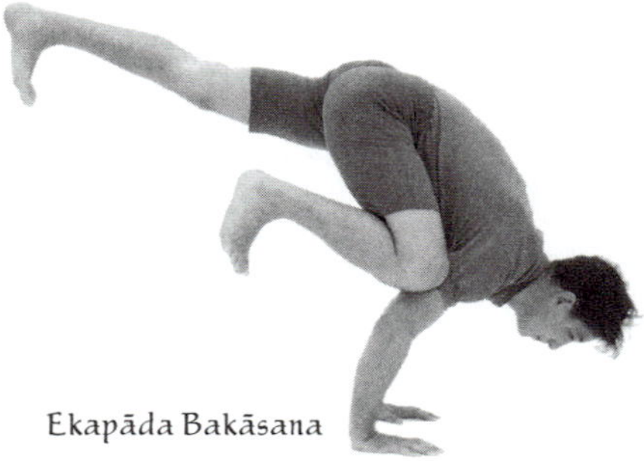
Ekapāda Bakāsana

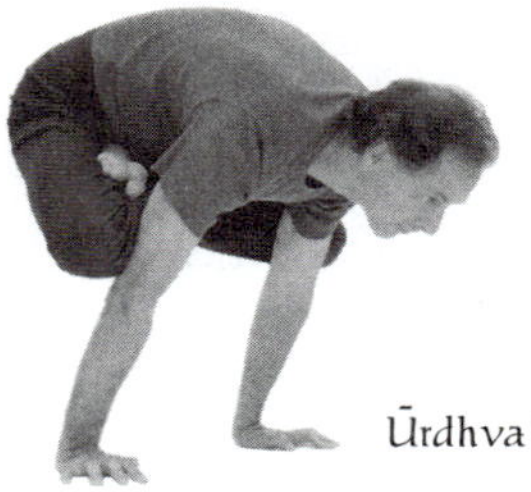
Ūrdhva Kukkuṭāsana

♦ GROUP 2

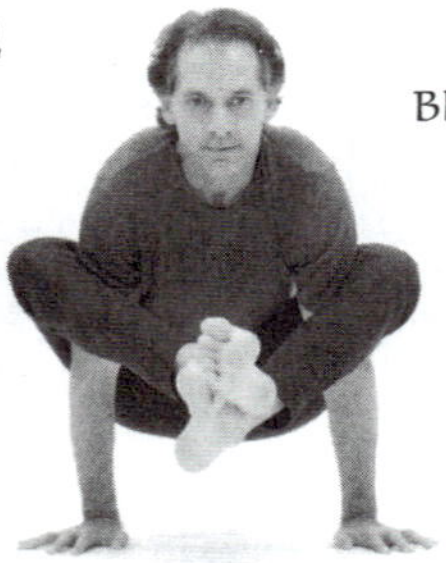
Bhujapīḍāsana

This group of postures includes upright arm balances in which the spine is extended upward. Three of them have a pelvic opening element. These postures develop upper body and abdominal strength. They are particularly useful for strengthening the perineal floor.

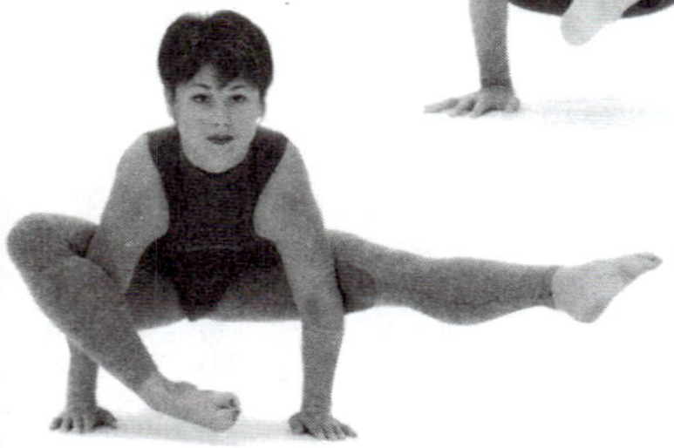
Ardha Dvihasta Bhujāsana

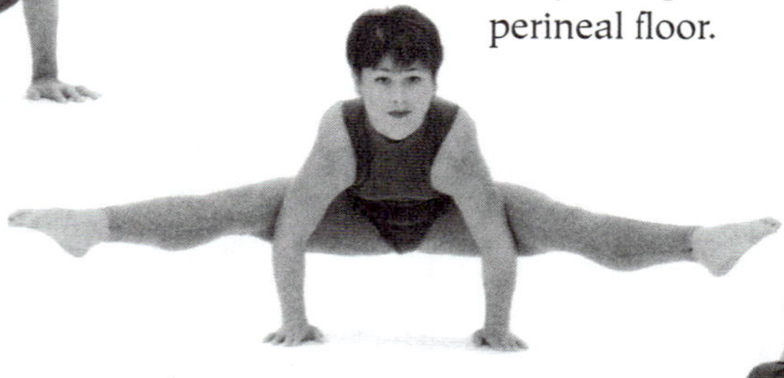
Dvihasta Bhujāsana

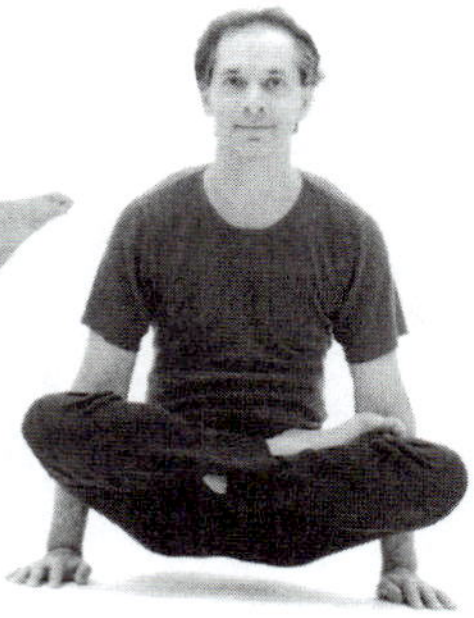
Lolāsana

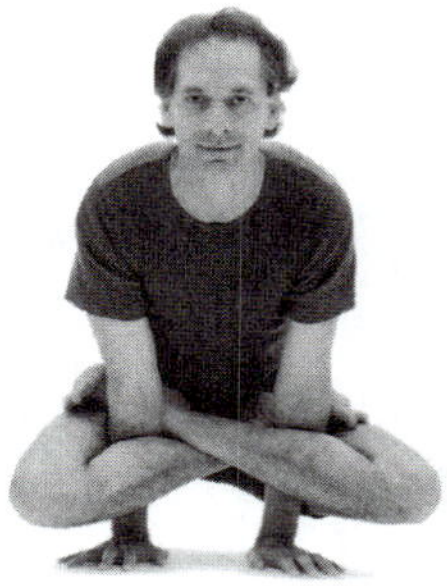
Kukkuṭāsana

♦ GROUP 3

This group of postures includes inverted arm balances with a back bend component. Like all arm balances, they require a strong and well-integrated structure. The handstand and forearm stand postures have a strongly energizing effect.

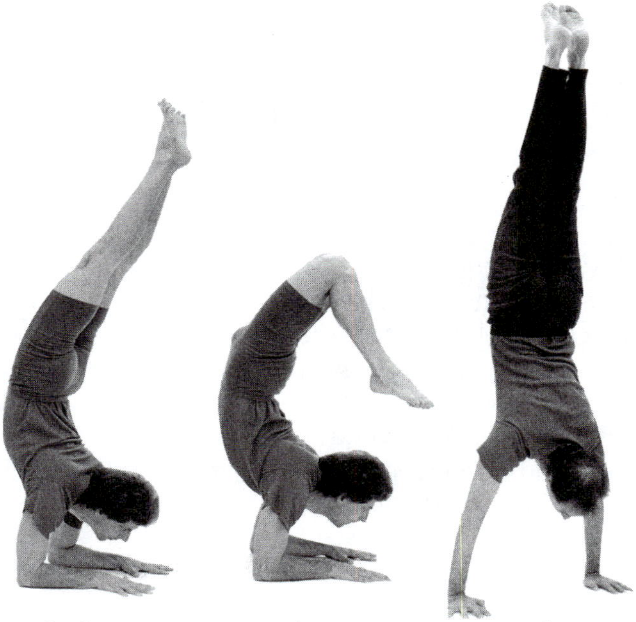

Piñchamayūrāsana Vṛścikāsana Vṛkṣāsana

♦ GROUP 4

Mayūrāsana is the only balance posture in this group. Because of the pressure of the upper arms and elbows on the abdomen, this posture stimulates the organs and improves their function.

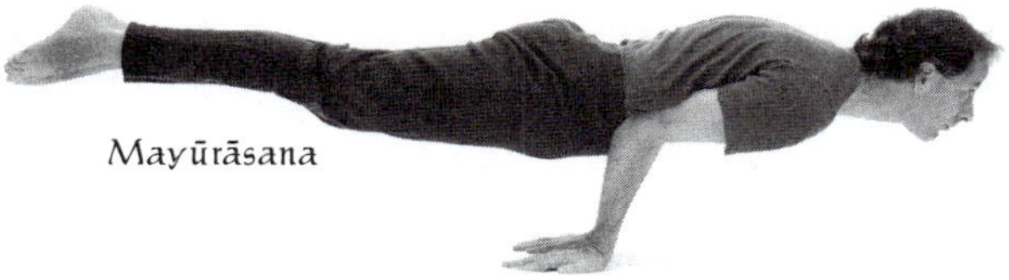

Mayūrāsana

Common Release Valves

Leg Balances

1. Lateral or backward displacing of the hips.
2. Collapsing of the chest over the belly.
3. Twisting of the torso.
4. Inward or outward rotating of the supporting leg.
5. Jutting the chin forward, or collapsing the head backward at the occipital/atlas junction.

Arm Balances

1. Collapsing the chest over the belly, increasing the thoracic kyphosis (except in inverted back bend series).
2. Elevating the shoulders toward the ears—upright series.
3. Sinking of the pelvis into the arms—inverted forward bend and twist series.
4. Increasing excessively the lumbar curve—inverted back bend series.

Common Risks

The most common risks in leg balances are compression or strain in the low back and shear stress in the hip, knee, ankle, or sacroiliac joints. Stress or strain may also occur in the neck and shoulders as muscles in those areas contract excessively in the effort to achieve balance. In arm balances there is significant risk to the wrists, elbows, shoulders, neck, and upper back. Bending backward in arm balances also creates risk of excessive compression in the low back. In leg balances, the risks can be minimized by adequately preparing the body for the postures and avoiding any force when the position involves the use of the arms to leverage the position of the lifted leg. In arm balance postures, adequate preparation will also help minimize risk. These postures are contraindicated if you have weaknesses or injuries in the wrist, elbow, or shoulder joints.

Balance Practice (for Vīrabhādrasana Variation and Bakāsana)

1.

POSTURE: Vajrāsana.
EMPHASIS: To warm up body. To mobilize rib cage to support respiration. To stretch low back.
TECHNIQUE: Stand on knees with arms over head and head turned to center.

On exhale: Bend forward, sweeping arms behind back and bringing hands to sacrum, keeping palms up, and turn head to the right.

On inhale: Return to starting position.

NUMBER: 8 times.
DETAILS: *On exhale:* Turn head to alternate sides on successive exhales. Bring chest to thighs before bringing buttocks to heels. Rotate arms so palms are up and hands are resting on sacrum. *On inhale:* Expand chest and lift it up off of knees as arms sweep wide.

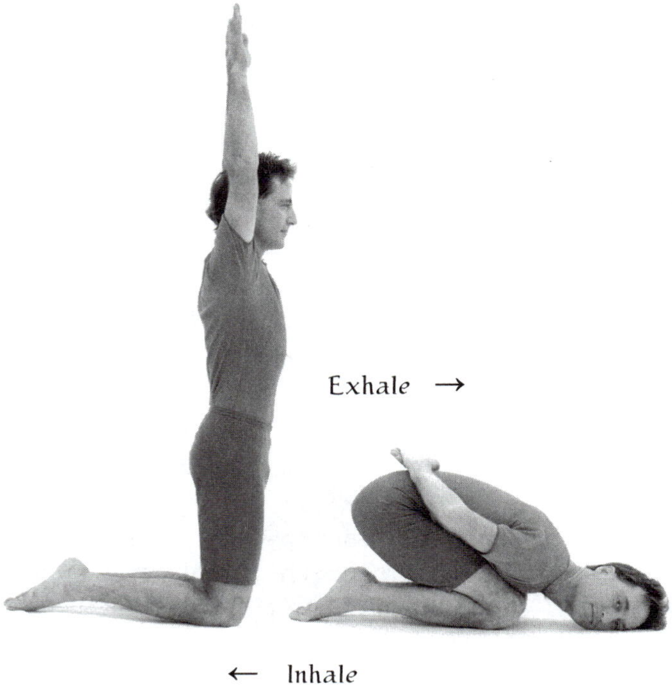

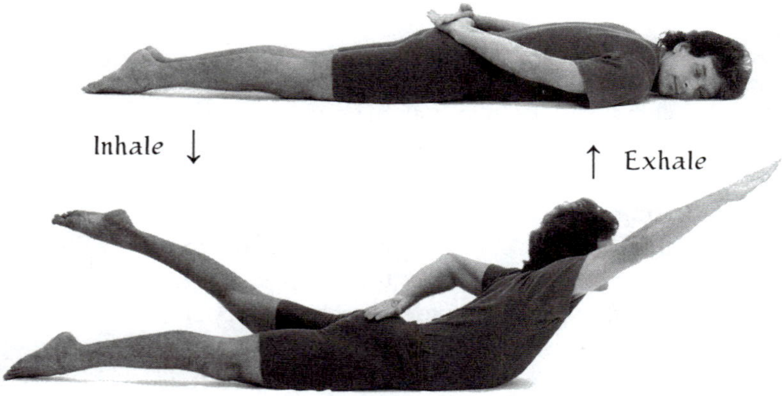

2.

POSTURE: Ardha Śalabhāsana.
EMPHASIS: To strengthen lower back. To stabilize hips in preparation for Vīrabhadrāsana.
TECHNIQUE: Lie on stomach, with head to right, crossing hands over sacrum and turning palms up.

On inhale: Lift chest, right arm and left leg, turning head to center.

On exhale: Lower chest and leg while sweeping arm behind back and turning head to left.

Repeat on other side.

NUMBER: 6 times each side, alternately.
DETAILS: *On inhale:* Lift chest slightly before leg, and emphasize chest height. Keep pelvis level.

3.

Posture: Cakravākāsana.
Emphasis: To stretch low back after back bend. To transition from prone to standing position.
Technique: Get down on hands and knees, with shoulders vertically above wrists and with hips above knees.

On inhale: Lift chest up and away from belly.

On exhale: Gently contract belly, round low back, and bring chest toward thighs.

Number: 8 times.
Details: *On inhale:* Lead with chest, keeping chin slightly down. Avoid compressing low back; rather, feel chest expanding. *On exhale:* Round low back without collapsing chest over belly. Avoid increasing curvature of upper back. Let chest lower toward thighs sooner than hips toward heels.

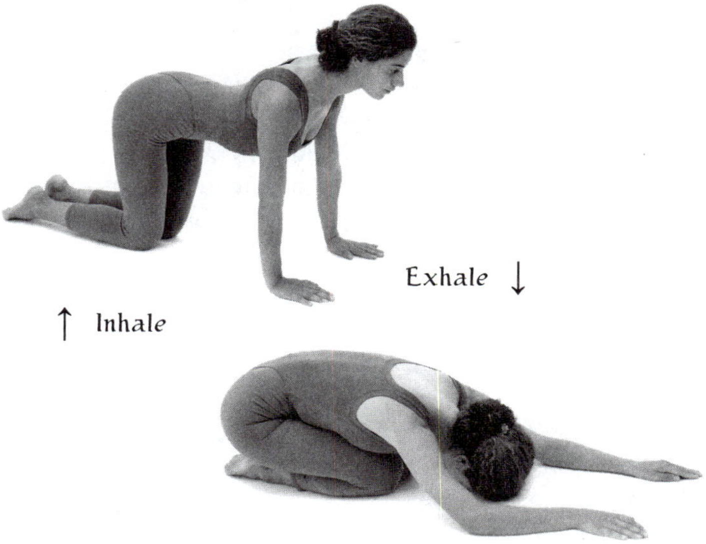

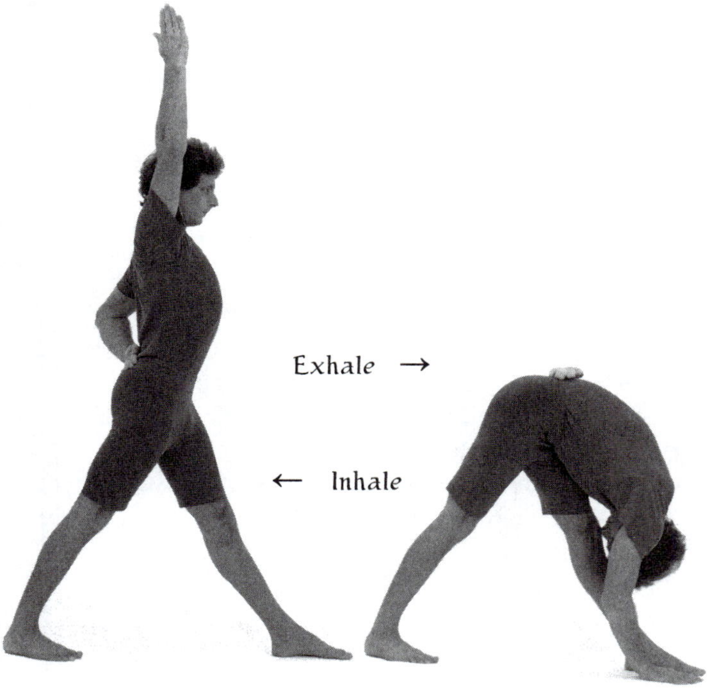

4.

Posture: Ardha Pārśvottānāsana.
Emphasis: To asymmetrically stretch and strengthen back and legs. To prepare for Vīrabhadrāsana.
Technique: Stand with left foot forward, right foot turned out a bit less than forty-five degrees, left arm folded behind back, and right arm raised over head.

On exhale: Bend forward, bringing belly and chest toward left thigh and right hand toward left foot.

On inhale: Return to starting position.

Repeat on other side.

Number: 8 times each side, one side at a time.
Details: *On exhale:* Keep back heel firmly down on floor. Bend front knee slightly. *On inhale:* Lift chest first, letting arms and head follow.

5.

POSTURE: Vīrabhadrāsana Variation.
EMPHASIS: To strengthen legs, hips, and back. To focus attention and increase balance. To experience a standing balance posture.
TECHNIQUE: Stand with arms over head.

On exhale: Bend forward, extending arms forward and lifting right leg behind, until torso and right leg are parallel to floor.

On inhale: Return to starting point.

Repeat 4 times.

Then stay in balance position 6 breaths.

Repeat on other side.

DETAILS: *On inhale:* Arch back and lift right leg. Keep arms level with ears.

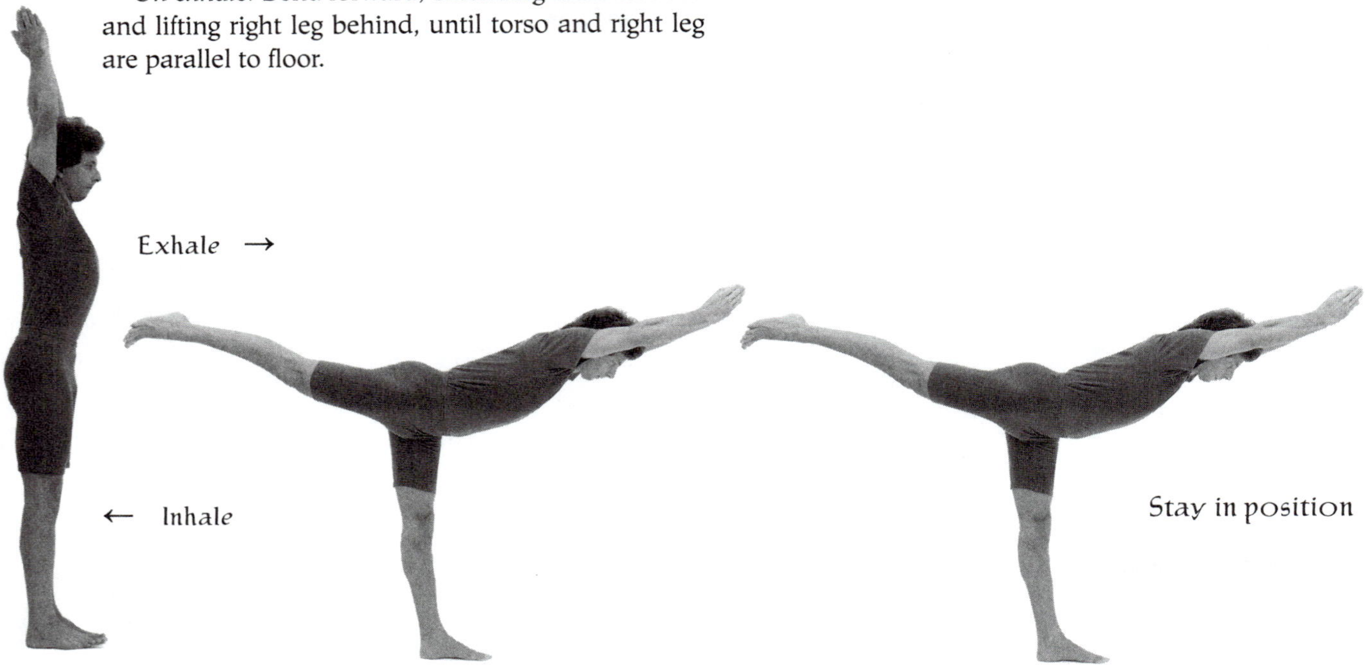

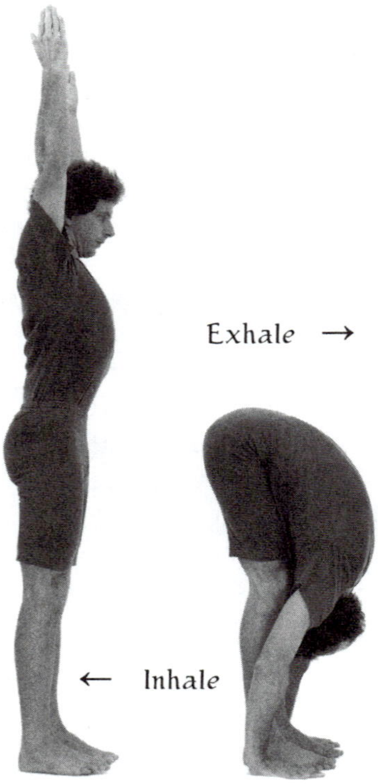

6.

POSTURE: Uttānāsana.
EMPHASIS: To stretch and relax low back.
TECHNIQUE: Stand with arms over head.

On exhale: Bend forward, bringing belly and chest toward thighs and bringing hands to feet. Stay in forward bended position 6 breaths.

On inhale: return to starting position.

Repeat 6 times.

DETAILS: *On exhale:* Bend knees to facilitate stretching of low back. Move chin down toward throat. *On inhale:* Lift chest up and away from thighs, flattening upper back. Keep knees bent until end of movement.

7.

POSTURE: Parivṛtti Trikoṇāsana.

EMPHASIS: To loosen back and shoulders. To release tension in neck from Vīrabhadrāsana. To help prepare shoulders for Bakāsana.

TECHNIQUE: Stand with feet spread wider than shoulders and with arms out to sides and parallel to floor.

On exhale: Bend forward and twist, bringing left hand to floor, pointing right arm upward and twisting shoulders right. Turn head down toward left hand.

On inhale: Maintaining rotation, and with right shoulder vertically above left, bring right arm up over shoulder and forward, turning head to center and looking at right hand.

On exhale: Return to previous position with right arm pointing upward. Turn head up, looking toward right hand.

On inhale: Return to starting position.

Repeat on other side.

NUMBER: 6 times each side, alternately.

DETAILS: Keep down arm vertically below its respective shoulder, and keep weight of torso off arm. Knees can bend while moving into twist.

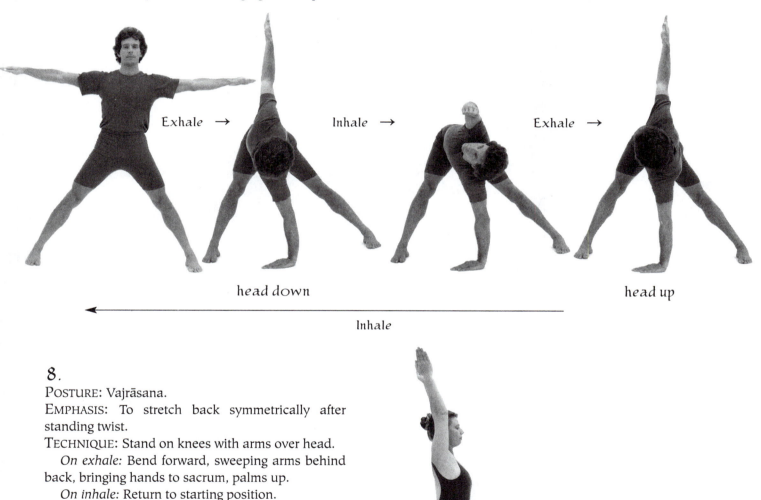

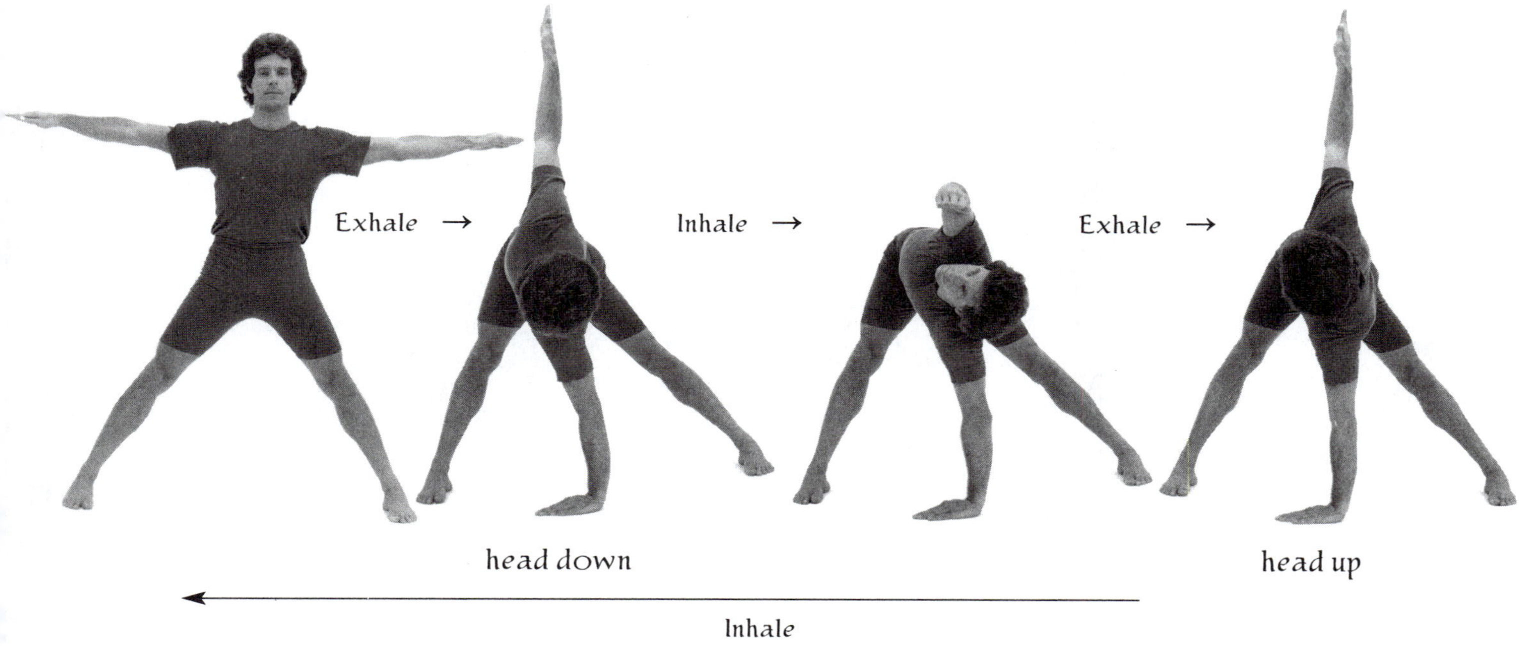
Exhale →
Inhale →
Exhale →
head down
head up
Inhale

8.

POSTURE: Vajrāsana.

EMPHASIS: To stretch back symmetrically after standing twist.

TECHNIQUE: Stand on knees with arms over head.

On exhale: Bend forward, sweeping arms behind back, bringing hands to sacrum, palms up.

On inhale: Return to starting position.

NUMBER: 8 times.

DETAILS: *On exhale:* Bring chest to thighs before bringing buttocks to heels. Rotate arms so palms are up and hands are resting on sacrum. *On inhale:* As arms sweep wide, open chest, pull shoulder blades back, and flatten upper back.

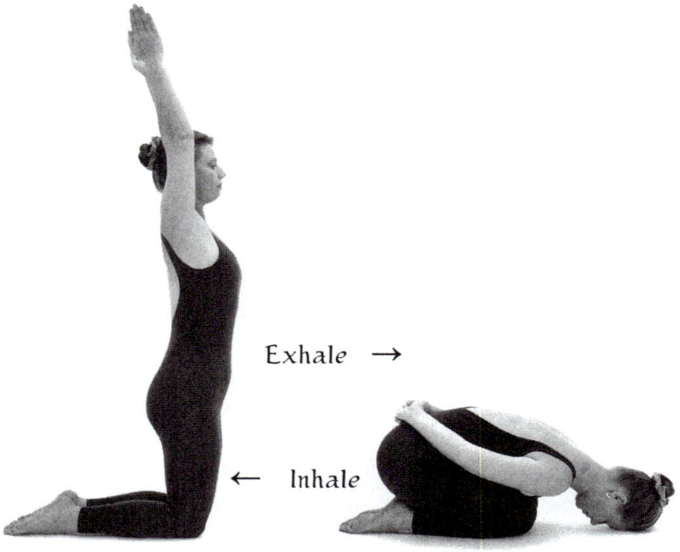
Exhale →
← Inhale

9.

POSTURE: Bakāsana.
EMPHASIS: To strengthen arms, shoulders, back, and abdomen. To experience an arm balance posture.
TECHNIQUE: From hands and knees, place head on floor, forming an equilateral triangle with hands. Stand on toes, lifting knees off floor. Walk forward with toes until hips are vertically above shoulders. Lift legs to vertical position.

On exhale: Lower legs until knees rest on upper arms near arm pits.

On inhale: Press on hands, straightening arms, lifting head up off floor, and holding hips higher than shoulders.

Stay in position as long as comfortable.

On exhale: Return to second position.

On inhale: Return to starting position.

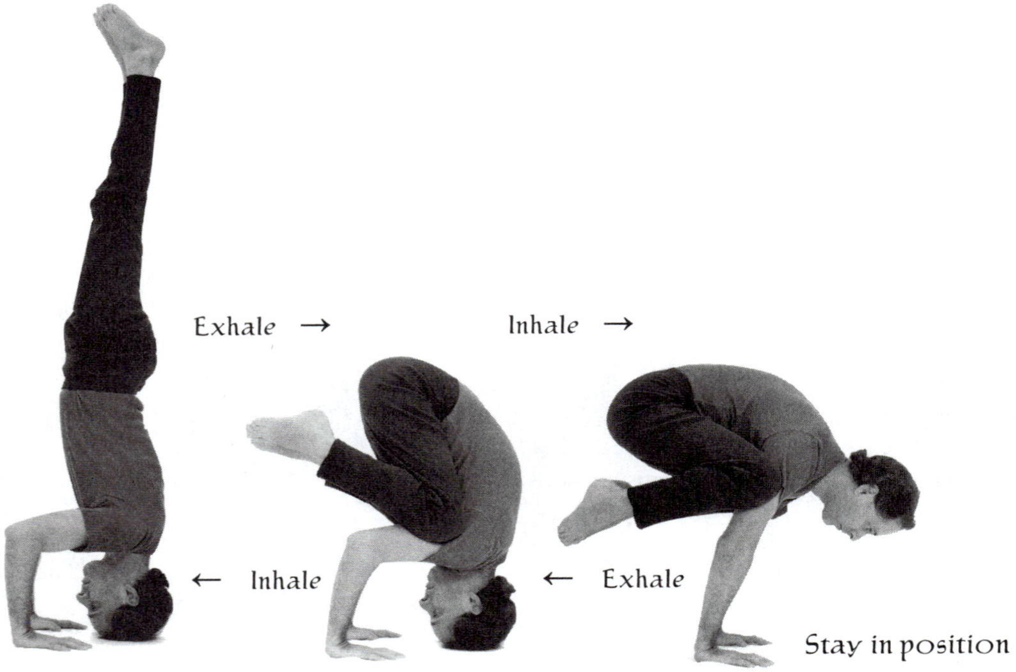
Exhale →
Inhale →
← Inhale
← Exhale
Stay in position

10.

POSTURE: Dvipāda Pīṭham.
EMPHASIS: To relax back and neck after Bakāsana.
TECHNIQUE: Lie on back with arms down at sides, knees bent, and feet on floor, slightly apart and comfortably close to buttocks.

On inhale: Pressing down on feet and keeping chin down, raise pelvis up toward ceiling, until neck is gently flattened on floor.

On exhale: Return to starting position.

NUMBER: 6 times.
DETAILS: *On inhale:* Lift spine, vertebra by vertebra, from bottom up. *On exhale:* Unwind spine, coming down vertebra by vertebra.

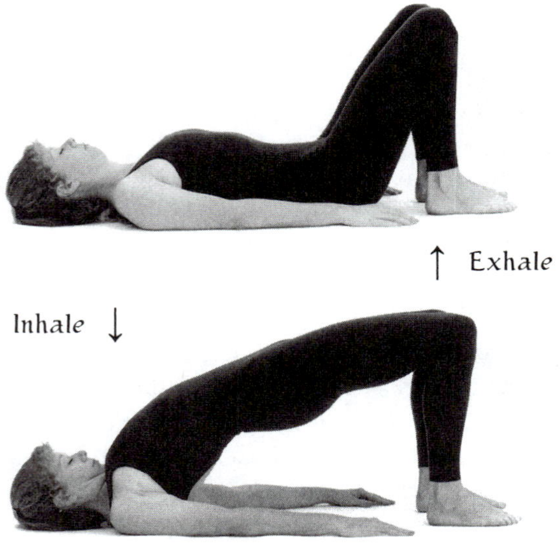
↑ Exhale
Inhale ↓

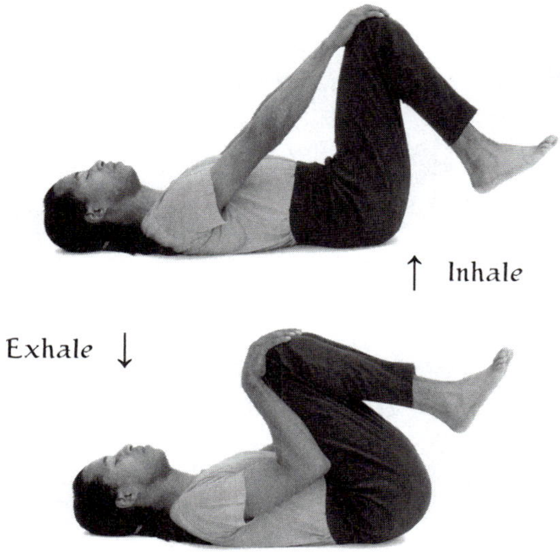

11.

POSTURE: Apānāsana.
EMPHASIS: To relax low back.
TECHNIQUE: Lie on back with both knees bent toward chest and with feet off floor. Place each hand on its respective knee.

On exhale: Pull thighs gently but progressively toward chest.

On inhale: Return to starting position.

NUMBER: 8 times.
DETAILS: *On exhale:* Pull gently with arms, keeping shoulders down on floor and relaxed. Press low back down into floor, dropping chin slightly toward throat. Progressively lengthen exhale with each successive repetition.

12.

POSTURE: Śavāsana.
EMPHASIS: To rest.
TECHNIQUE: Lie flat on back, with arms at sides, palms up, and legs slightly apart. Close eyes. Relax body fully, keeping mind relaxed and alert to sensations in body.
DURATION: Minimum 3 to 5 minutes.

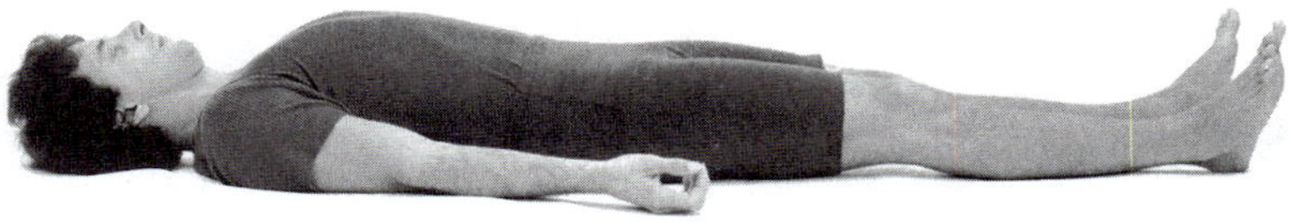

Part II

YOGA:
A
Therapeutic
Approach

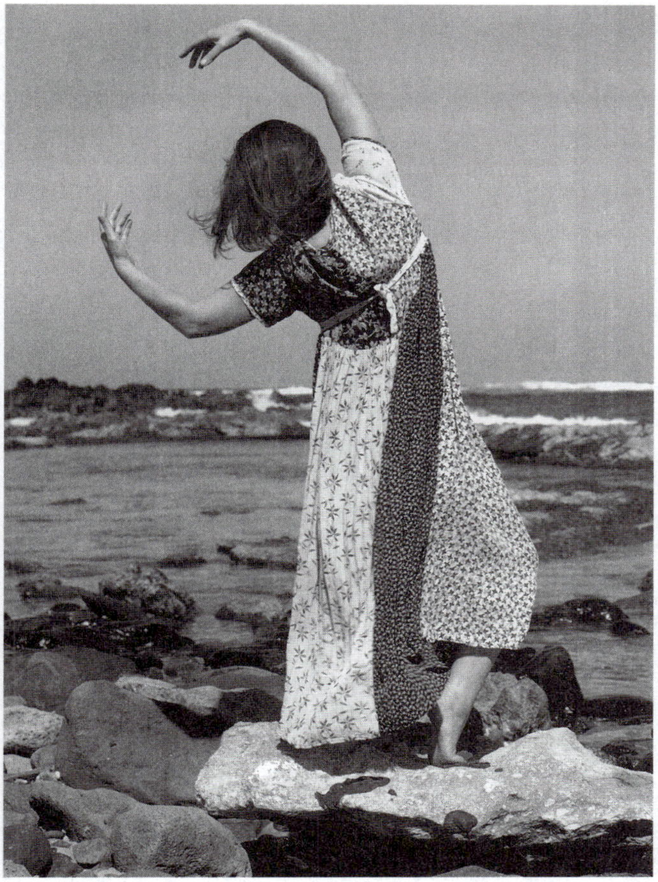

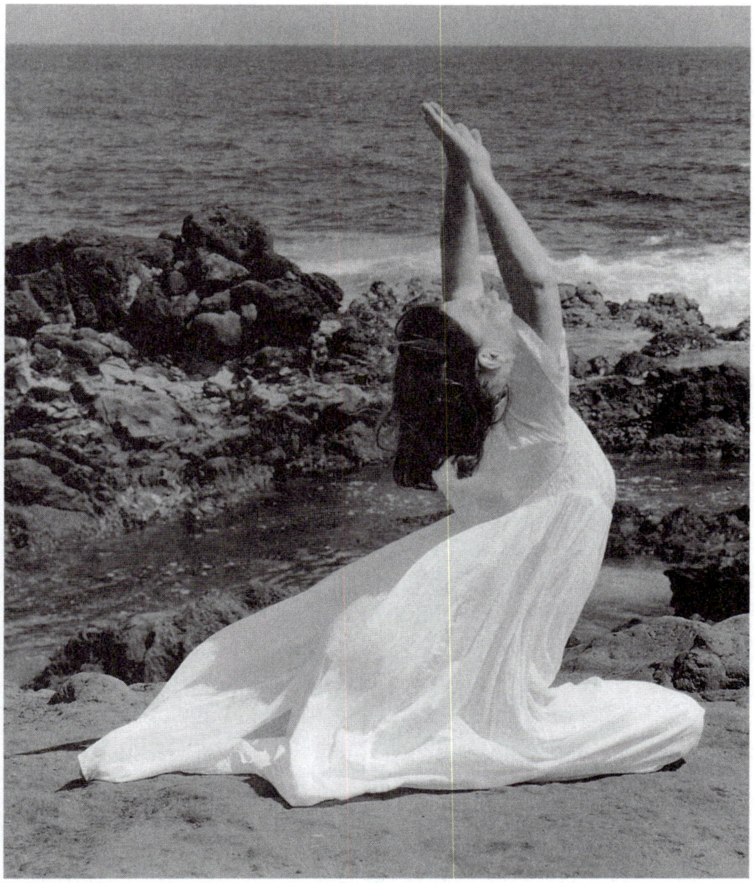

Yoga Cikiṭsa: An Introduction to Yoga Therapy

Duḥkha Saṃyoga Viyoga Yogaha—
"Yoga is separating from identification with suffering"

The Yoga therapy presented in this book derives from an ancient tradition called *Yoga cikiṭsa* (*cikiṭsa* can be translated as therapy). This form of Yoga therapy is based on the ancient principles of *cikiṭsa krama* (therapeutic orientation), which derive from the Yoga tradition of Patañjali and the Āyurvedic system of health, both of which, in turn, derive from the Sankhya and Upaniṣadic traditions of Vedic India.

Yoga cikiṭsa is a remedial tradition, founded on a recognition that our physical condition, emotional states, attitudes, dietary and behavioral patterns, lifestyle and personal associations, and the environment in which we live and work are all intimately linked to each other and to the state of our health.

According to Yoga theory, we live within a framework of constant change (*pariṇāma*), and, within this framework, develop conditioned patterns (*saṃskāras*) that are present in every dimension of our lives and that influence our perceptions, thoughts, attitudes, and behavior at every level. The good news is that because nothing is static, our condition will inevitably change. The salient question is, will it change for better or for worse? Our challenge is to influence the direction of change for the better. This challenge is complicated by those patterns, often operating beneath the level of our conscious awareness, that influence our action. We may heal the body through some medical or alternate healing modality, but, unless there is transformation at the level of our deep patterns, we may end up re-creating the same or similar conditions again.

Yoga cikiṭsa is the art of tapping the resources deep within us to heal ourselves. The belief that healing is a natural process goes along with a recognition that our attitudes and behavior can create conditions in our system—structurally, physiologically, and psychologically—that inhibit that natural process. The allopathic physician's orientation is to treat the disease; the Yoga orientation is to treat the *person*. In Yoga therapy, therefore, we are first and foremost seeking to change attitudes and actions that inhibit the natural healing process. The ideal is to develop the mind so that it can lead us on a path to improve the quality of life. In fact, according to the ancient teachings, the main goal of Yoga is to influence the state of mind. My teacher has said that Yoga cikiṭsa is about helping people, not necessarily curing them. Our goal is first of all to help people feel better about themselves, gain more clarity about their lives, help them prioritize and become more effective in their actions, and—perhaps most important—contact a deeper source within themselves. I was taught, "To the extent that we influence the mind, we influence the entire system, and to that extent the person is better."

There are two essential elements in this process: *Viyoga* and *Saṃyoga*. Viyoga literally means "separation." In the context of Yoga therapy, Viyoga refers to the process of separating ourselves from whatever is undesirable in our lives. As an eliminative process, it involves the purification of both mind and body. It also involves letting go of unhealthy attachments, giving up self-destructive behavior, and breaking detrimental relationships.

Saṃyoga literally means "linking together." In the context of Yoga therapy, Saṃyoga refers to the process of linking to whatever is positive and productive in our lives. It involves the development of mental qualities such as kindness, courage, patience, and compassion. It also involves establishing appropriate priorities, practicing virtues, and cultivating positive relationships.

The work of Yoga therapy can be called a *kaya kalpa*. This expression, coming from Āyurveda, is often presented as a science of immortality. In fact, kaya kalpa refers literally to the reorganization, reconstruction, and rejuvenation of our mind and body through our practice. It involves a progressive reintegration of the entire system and a creation of harmony in every aspect of our lives.

The ancient masters visualized the human system as a bird with five essential parts: a head, two wings, a body, and a tail. This bird, in turn, was visualized in five dimensions, each considered to be the "embodied soul" of the previous dimension. These dimensions are known as *mayas*—meaning "that which spreads" (to be distinguished from *māyā*, which means illusion). Each dimension, in turn, consists of five essential parts. Simplifying this complex model: The first dimension, *anna maya*, refers to our gross physical body. It includes the muscles, bones, organs, and tissues of our system. The second dimension, *prāṇa maya*, refers to the vital metabolic functions that sustain our life and health. It includes the operation of all of our physiological systems. The third dimension, *mano maya*, refers to our mental faculties of perception and cognition, and includes all the knowledge gained through our education and other external sources. The fourth dimension, *vijñāna maya*, refers to our inner and intuitive capacity to understand. It includes faith or ability to trust, values or sense of right and wrong, communication skills, state of mind, and patterns (saṃskāras) from our past that continue to influence our present attitudes and behavior. The fifth dimension, *ānanda maya*, refers to our spiritual or "heart" relationship to each moment and to life itself. It includes our longings, what pleases us, our sense of joy, our sense of fulfillment, and our focus on and union with whatever we most cherish.

Because these dimensions mutually interrelate and interpenetrate, a condition that manifests in one dimension will impact all others. For example, someone who has an accident and suffers long-term chronic low-back pain may begin to suffer from fatigue, troubled digestion, depression, and a negative attitude toward life. On the other hand, someone who suffers from low self-esteem may likewise progressively develop depression, fatigue, troubled digestion, and even joint pain.

The basic principle of Yoga cikiṭsa is that diseases are symptoms of imbalance; and, therefore, the orientation of Yoga cikiṭsa is to restore balance. According to the ancient masters, three main methodologies can be used to purify and strengthen our systems and so move toward health: *āhāra* (diet); *vihāra* (activity); and *auṣadhi* (medicine). The teaching is that the first two methods are preferable and that the third should be used as a last resort. These three methods alone can work to transform the first three dimensions of our systems—physical, vital, and mental. The ancient teachings warn us that because our past patterns are a strong force, depending upon the seriousness of our condition, healing can take time. The only way to ultimately overcome dysfunctional patterns and thereby effect deep and lasting change in our lives is if our practice penetrates to the dimension of ānanda maya, the heart.

As we will see in the section on emotional health ahead, these traditional teachings are confirmed by our present understanding of the power of emotion to influence our physiology, thoughts, and behavior. Neuroscientists are becoming progressively more convinced that the emotional brain is able to override the rational brain and that, though we tend to consciously identify with our rational brain, we connect to life most deeply through our emotions.*

If we think about the times we have been touched deeply in our hearts, it is usually in the context of some relationship. This is easily seen in the relationship between a parent and a child. Of course, this relationship has the power to transform our lives for better or for worse. And when we are affected at that level, as we will see in more detail later in this book, everything else in our system is affected.

In the fourth dimension of our being (vijñāna maya), the head of the bird represents faith. Faith is a quality of confidence and trust, without a need for external confirmations. It is a deep and intuitive knowing that calms the mind and puts the heart at rest. Faith, according to the tradition, is the "ultimate medicine" for the emotional mind.

Our natural capacity for faith is linked to our past patterns but is strengthened or weakened by our associations. Thus the ancient masters taught that the most important aspect of healing was right association (*sat sangha*). For this reason they stressed the importance of relationship—to the divine (whatever that may mean to you), to the teacher (who represents our own potential to grow), and to the spiritual community. According to the tradition, the one-on-one relationship between a teacher and a student is the first Yoga and the basis from which to develop and sustain a personal practice. Of course, for this relationship to be most effective, there must be mutual confidence, trust, and openness. Such a relationship is between hearts and not simply at the level of information exchange. Thus the masters have said that sat sangha is essential for deep healing. With that as a foundation, the other methodologies (diet, activity, and medicine) will work powerfully to restore and revitalize our health and well-being.

*Cytowic, Richard E., *The Man Who Tasted Shapes* (New York: Tarcher/Putnam, 1993), p. 462.

Our health problems may be related to congenital factors; patterns acquired in childhood; the result of an accident, an unhealthy lifestyle, chronic stress; or any combination of these or other factors. At a practical level, many methods can be applied to help us in our journey to health, including postures and their adaptations, breathing techniques and ratios, sounds and associated meanings, meditations, visualizations, rituals, and prayers, relationships (sat sangha) with others, education and study, and dietary and other lifestyle changes. All these methods work to reinforce the commitment to ourselves required to bring our lives back into balance and to create a foundation for the development of our highest potential.

Although there are many means and methods for working to restore balance in the human system, the basic orientation of any treatment is either that of reduction or purification (*langhana*) or that of tonification or building (*brahmaṇa*).

Reduction (langhana) therapy is called for when there is some kind of excess in the system that must be reduced: for example, excess weight, toxicity, hyperactivity, or anxiety. In Yoga practice, langhana techniques include exhalation, short hold after exhalation, forward bends, some twists, and headstand. Chanting, visualization, and meditation techniques can also be adapted to have a langhana effect. Langhana techniques are generally cooling (*candra*) and conserve energy. Because it is oriented toward eliminating conditions that may lead to further imbalance and disease, langhana therapy can also be preventative. In certain cases where it is necessary to increase the heat (*agni*) in the body in order to purify the system of toxins, brahmaṇa techniques are used to produce a langhana effect.

Tonification (brahmaṇa) therapy works to nourish the system. This is useful in conditions such as general weakness, low energy, specific debilities, or lack of confidence. In Yoga practice, brahmaṇa techniques include inhalation, hold after inhalation, back bends, and shoulder stand. Chanting, visualization, and meditation techniques can also be adapted to have a brahmaṇa effect. Generally, brahmaṇa techniques increase heat (agni) in the body and build energy. Because tonification is oriented toward building the system back up, it is particularly useful during convalescence. In these cases, where cooling (*candra*) techniques help to nourish the system and conserve energy, langhana techniques are used to produce a brahmaṇa effect.

These definitions are theoretical and overlapping. In practice, we often need to use both orientations and to mix a variety of methods. For example, in the sequence presented ahead for the chronic fatigue patient, we begin with a gentle brahmaṇa approach to increase her energy; however, because too much heat will deplete her energy and leave her exhausted, we end with a gentle langhana approach to lower her body heat and conserve energy.

Among individuals, there are vast differences—physically, psychologically, and spiritually. The same long-term, stressful circumstances can create a complex of symptoms—anger, high blood pressure, elevated cholesterol levels, and Temporomandibular Joint Disease (TMJ) in one person, and depression, fatigue, loss of appetite, and poor posture in another. In fact, any number of different symptoms can result from the same cause; and any number of different conditions can result in the same or similar symptoms. Depression, for example, can cause loss of appetite, sleep disorders, and fatigue. Problems with digestive, endocrine, or nervous system function can cause the same symptoms. In addition, food allergies, heavy metal toxicity, nutritional deficiencies, candida, chronic structural problems, and various forms of infections can lead to these same symptoms.

Theoretically, the Yoga tradition has practices that address any kind of condition, at any level of our system. At the same time, it should be clear that effective practice must respect the unique needs, interests, liabilities, and potentials of each individual by developing a practice that is adapted to that uniqueness. Further, every individual's condition will change over time, and thus their own practice must evolve. This kind of teaching cannot be mass-marketed. That is its gift and, at the same time, its limitation.

Anyone can benefit from a personal practice, no matter their condition. Deep work usually requires a one-on-one contact with a qualified teacher over time to establish what should be practiced, how it should be practiced, and how the practice should evolve. Finally, however, the effectiveness of a practice is not guaranteed no matter how well it is adapted to your needs, because it is your own motivation, confidence in the practice, ability to understand your condition, and ability to sustain your practice that will ultimately determine its effectiveness.

Increased self-awareness will enable you to accurately assess your condition; and the commitment to a personal practice will enable you to break unconscious and self-destructive behavioral patterns and establish new ones that will lead to positive change. Understanding the nature and functions of your body's various systems will enable you, over time, to experience directly the way they are affected by your attitudes, diet, and behavior. Through practice, you enter into a new relationship with yourself and your condition. On the one hand, you will build the energy required to break the habits and tendencies that you know to be self-destructive. On the other hand, you will be taking concrete and effective steps to reorganize your systems. The limiting factor in this approach, of course, is the necessity for personal practice. Without practice, there will be no results. But if we engage in simple practices consistently, we will be amazed at their capacity to change us deeply. Yoga therapy is an experiential process that requires *and* develops self-awareness and self-regulation as the foundation for healing.

Because of the interconnectedness of our various systems, we can initiate change in our overall condition by working through the body, the breath, and/or the mind. A process that leads to an alert and relaxed state of mind can also lead to increased control over what we normally think of as automatic functions. In the same way that the negative states of depression, anxiety, and anger—to name just a few—adversely impact our system, positive states of relaxation, joy, and love have a deeply restorative effect.

The specific methods and practices we choose will depend on our condition. As a general rule, we tend to begin all therapeutic practices by focusing on the spine and the breath. As we will see ahead, all of the fundamental systems of the body converge in the spine. And—as we have already seen—we can influence our state of mind, other aspects of our physiology, and our structure through the breath. In this process, linking the breath to the movement links the mind to the body and makes the movements conscious. As we increase our awareness of the body, we are better equipped to work with and regulate it.

Thus we begin with simple exercises of breath and movement, focusing on the spine, as a safe and effective start to our practice. We use various means to focus our attention and increase the flow of vital energy (*prāṇa*) to problem areas. As our practice develops, we will add other techniques, as appropriate, to deepen its effects and meet specific needs. The starting point for this work is variable also, and depends on the condition of each individual. We can see the graph below as an example of progression. Minus one represents someone with a very serious condition, and ten represents someone in optimal health.

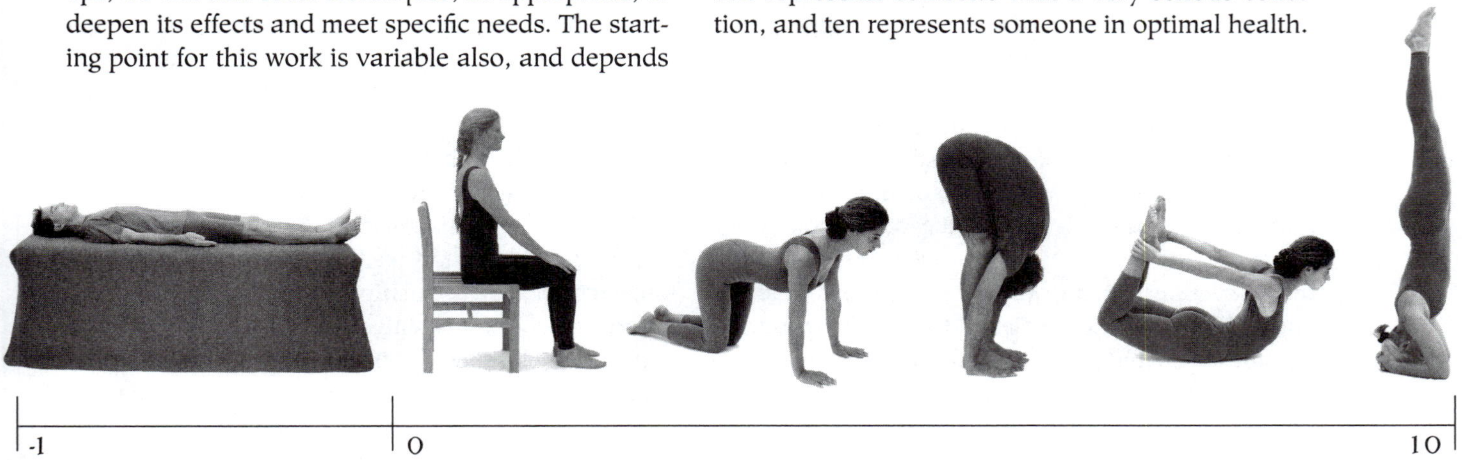

Depending upon where the person is on the graph, we start at a different point on the scale. For serious diseases, we usually begin lying on a bed or seated on a chair, and bring awareness to the breath.

No matter our starting point, the goal is to deepen our self-awareness and to integrate body, breath, and mind. As we progress in our practice, we can shift our focus away from physical and/or mental limitations toward our higher potential; away from weakness toward strength; away from pain toward well-being; away from anxiety, anger, and depression toward relaxation, contentment, and joy. We can feel better about ourselves, stabilize and elevate our moods, develop clearer perception, increase mental energy and alertness, have a greater sense of physical wellbeing, and find a sense of direction and a deeper purpose in our life.

A final note before we move on to specific methods in the following sections: unless we are able to find a competent teacher, we should consider very carefully the choices we make in developing our own practice. Our intention may be clear—improving our condition through our activity—yet some practices we believe to be positive may actually be detrimental to achieving our intended goals. The great Yoga teacher Krishnamacharya, who brought the Viniyoga tradition into this century, had a wonderful expression for this kind of practice: *aṅga bhanga sādhanā* (literally, "limb-harmful-practice"), a sādhanā that is useful for one thing but harmful in some other way.

For example, Krishnamacharya considered running, for many people, to be an aṅga bhanga sādhanā. In that context, he said, "Running is for horses!" What he meant was that though running may be good for some parts of our body (such as the respiratory and cardiovascular systems), it can also be harmful for other parts (such as the ankles, knees, and hips). I have seen people jogging along the freeway in heavy traffic at midday under the hot sun without a hat. This is a classic aṅga bhanga sādhanā: refining the system and at the same time exposing it in some destructive way.

People take up this and other aṅga bhanga sādhanā practices in the belief that they are going to get more fit. They find encouragement to continue from the fact that they suddenly feel better. In the beginning and for some time thereafter, they may *feel* better, especially if they've been sedentary, but in the long run they are also doing themselves harm.

Although we strongly suggest that you make every effort to work with a well-trained and experienced teacher, the principles and practices in this book are meant to steer you away from this sort of activity. As you increase your self-awareness, proficiency, and understanding, you will become ever more readily able to recognize aṅga bhanga sādhanā practices for what they are. Any practice, even a Yoga practice, can become an aṅga bhanga sādhanā when wrongly applied: an important part of the continuing work of personal practice, therefore, will be monitoring yourself to determine whether the practice you are engaged in is right for you.

As you will see from the case studies that follow, the technology of practice is secondary to, and emerges out of, the relationship that develops in the environment of the session between the teacher and the student. Each case must be handled individually. In my work, I develop an active relationship with each student. In order to work out an appropriate practice and make lifestyle suggestions, I find out other aspects of the student's character beyond the manifest symptoms. I repeat: because of the multiple variables between individuals suffering from the same condition, it would be inaccurate to suggest that we can prescribe a set practice for any condition.

In the sections ahead, we will present examples of Yoga cikiṭsa practices designed to work with specific chronic aches and pains, chronic diseases, and emotional health. The first section concerns common aches and pains. It contains a brief presentation of the skeletal and muscular systems to provide a foundation for understanding related problems, followed by a detailed discussion of three main aspects of these systems—neck and shoulders; upper and lower back; and sacrum, hips, and knees—and the common aches and pains that affect them. Each of these sections is followed by particular case studies and related practice sequences.

The next section concerns chronic disease. It contains a brief description of the functions of the eight main physiological systems, providing a foundation for understanding chronic related problems, and describes the various conditions of excess and deficiency that affect them. Each category is followed by a case study and related practice sequence.

The last section concerns emotional health. It contains a discussion on the brain; a discussion of the reciprocal relationship between our conceptual mind, our emotional states, and our physiology; and a discussion of the Yoga tradition's view of emotional states and how to manage them. Also included is a description of three stressful emotional states: anger and anxiety, which are presented as states of hyper arousal; and depression, which is presented as a state of hypo arousal. Case studies of hyper and hypo conditions are followed by related practice sequences.

Chapter 3

Common Aches and Pains

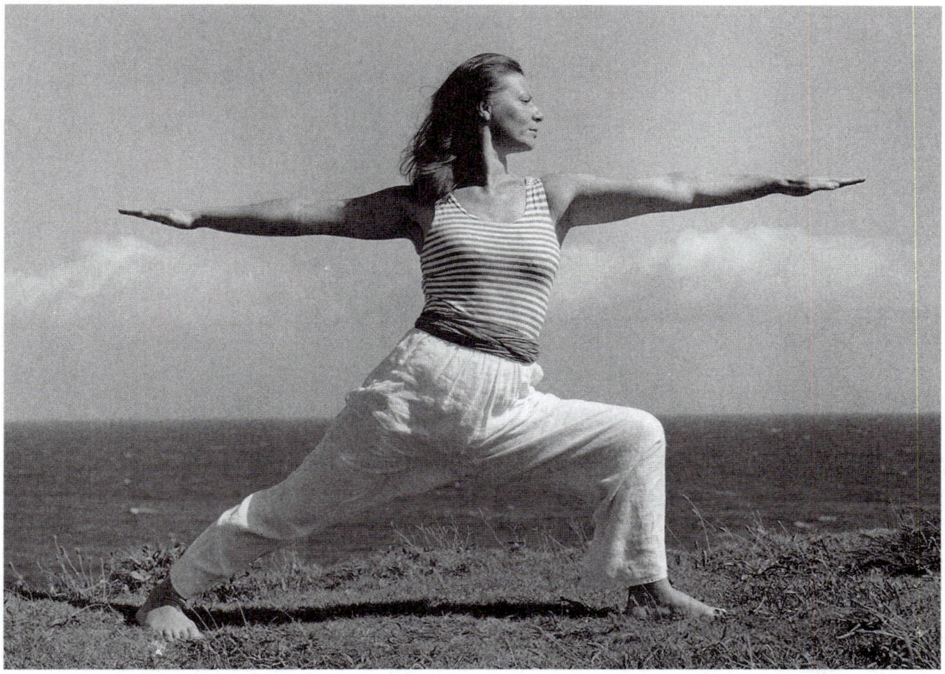

Skeletal System

The skeletal system of the human body is a complex network composed of several kinds of bones, joints, and connective tissues, each of which is a functional unit designed to serve a particular purpose. Most of the bones and joints appear in pairs, with one on the right and one on the left side of the body. The process of bone formation is called ossification, and all of the bones have a unique structure, formed to suit their special function.

The different parts of the skeleton are connected either by attachments or by joints. The attachments include membranes, muscle tendons, ligaments, and discs. The muscle tendons and ligaments are attached to the bones by collagenous fibers growing through the bone membrane and into the compact bone tissue.

Joints are points in the skeletal system where two or more bones meet (articulate) and are usually attached to each other by connective tissue, which determines the range of movement that is allowed. The immovable joint is an articulation of two bones that have been almost fused together and, as exemplified

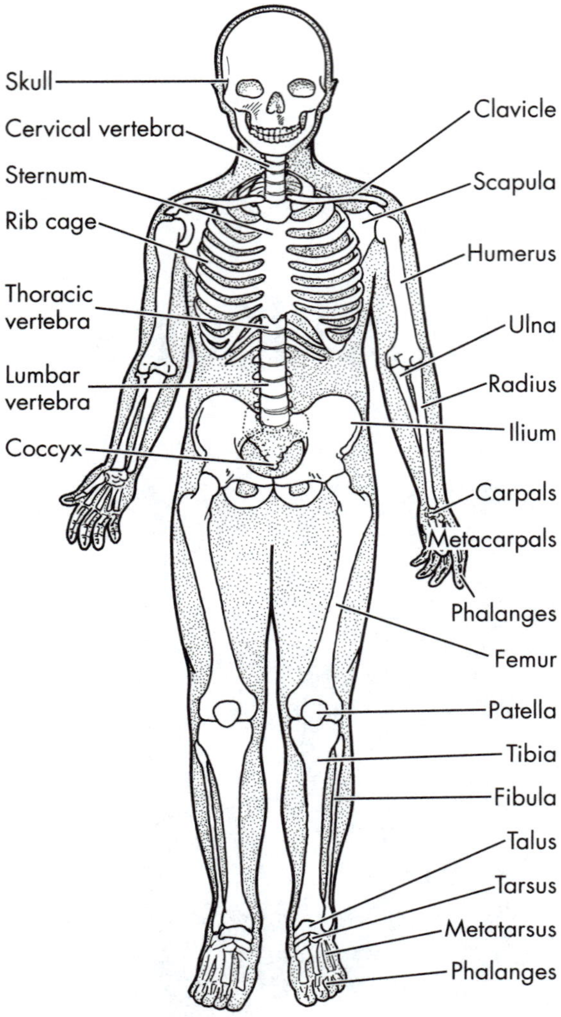

Appendicular Skeleton

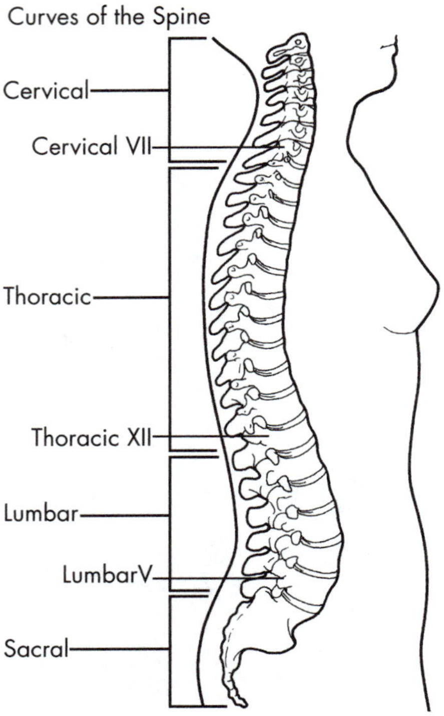

Axial Skeleton

by the bones at the juncture of the cranium, cannot be moved by muscular force. The slightly moveable joint allows a restricted range of motion due to the structure of the bones and connective tissue around it, as exemplified by the joints in the spine existing between its vertebral bodies and between the sacrum and the ilia. The freely moveable joint, known as a synovial joint, allows a relatively large range of motion. Its bones are always enclosed in a joint capsule, containing a synovial membrane, which produces a lubricating fluid and provides nutrients to its cells. Tough collagen fibers, known as ligaments, surround these synovial membranes, binding the respective bones together and limiting the range of their movement. Synovial joints vary in the movement that they allow. For example, the elbows and knees only allow movement in a single plane, while the hips and shoulders allow movement in many directions.

The skeletal system can be divided into axial and appendicular skeletons. The axial skeleton forms the vertical axis of the spine, from the tailbone (coccyx) at the bottom to the cranium at the top. The appendicular skeleton includes the shoulder girdle and attached arms and hands, and the pelvic girdle and attached legs and feet. Our discussion of the structure of the skeleton will be restricted to the spine (vertebral column) and to the pelvic and shoulder girdles that intersect it.

Axial Skeleton

The spine has four distinct segments, consisting of the cervical, the thoracic, the lumbar, and the sacral.

Each spinal segment contains a given number of vertebrae: the cervical spine has seven vertebrae; the thoracic spine has twelve, each of which is attached to one or more pair of ribs; the lumbar spine has five; and the sacrum has five, including the coccyx at its base, which consists of several small, fused vertebrae. The twelve ribs (costae) of the thoracic spine are known as the rib cage. In the front, counting from the top, the first seven pair of these ribs are attached to the breastbone (sternum). Ribs eight through ten are fused to rib seven before it attaches to the sternum, and ribs eleven and twelve are called floating ribs because they have no anterior attachment at all.

The thoracic and sacral spines, including the coccyx, support and protect the major organs of the body. These sections of the spine are formed during fetal development, although the sacrum itself only becomes fully fused sometime after puberty. The cervical and lumbar spines help position the body weight over the legs, and these sections of the spine are also not fully developed until after puberty.

The spine can be considered as a mechanism for the support and transfer of weight. In a standing position, all the weights of the body must be transferred through the spine to the pelvic girdle, down through the legs, and to the ground. The primary weights of the body are the head, the rib cage and its contents, and the pelvic basin and its contents. The upper three spinal segments balance their loads in line with the body's central axis, and the entire spine is balanced on the wedge-shaped sacrum at its base.

In the front (anterior) portion of the spine, the vertebrae are separated by a kind of hydraulic system called intervertebral discs. These discs are part of a self-contained fluid system that absorbs shock, permits some compression, and allows movement. They are made up of an outer layer of fibroelastic cartilage that encapsulates a more pulpy, highly elastic center of colloidal gel. These intervertebral discs act as shock absorbers, allowing slight movement of one vertebra on another as the gel adjusts anteriorly, posteriorly, or laterally within its semi-elastic container. There are no discs in the sacrum or coccyx.

In the posterior portion of the vertebral column, between each pair of vertebrae, a complex of bony structures protects the spinal cord and serves as the site for muscular attachments and, in the thoracic spine, for forming joints with the ribs.

The major ligaments of the spinal column are the long anterior longitudinal ligaments that run down the front of the spinal column, the ligamentum flavum, which runs between the posterior parts of the neural arches, and the posterior longitudinal ligament, which runs down the back of the vertebral bodies.

Appendicular Skeleton

The shoulder girdle consists of two paired bone segments: the right and left scapulae (shoulder blades), and the right and left clavicles (collarbones). The scapulae ride on the upper back (dorsal) portion of the rib cage; the clavicle lies above the front (ventral) portion of the rib cage. The scapula articulates with the outer part of the clavicles and with the upper arm (humerus) at a ball-and-socket joint, allowing movement in all planes. The inner part of the clavicle articulates with the sternum (breastbone) and the first pair of ribs, and is the only direct connection between the shoulder girdle and the axial skeleton. The shoulder girdle itself is composed of the shoulder blades and the muscles that position, support, and move them, and it is this shoulder girdle that guides and controls the movements of the arms.

The shoulder joint has the greatest range of motion of any joint in the body. However, because of its great mobility, it is relatively unstable and, therefore, susceptible to injury. The shoulder has several large pockets of synovial fluid (bursae) that help to reduce friction from the wide range of movement of the arms. Accordingly, excessive stress, from repetitive movement or pressure, can cause inflammation of the bursae (bursitis), resulting in restricted movement. Also, imbalances or injuries to the shoulder girdle itself can decrease the functional efficiency of the upper body, which, in turn, can influence the balance and integrity of the structure as a whole.

The sacrum is the foundation platform upon which the spinal column is balanced. It is firmly attached to the two hipbones at the sacroiliac joint. These hipbones (coxa) are formed from the fusion of three separate bones: the ilium, ischium, and pubis, which, together with the sacrum and coccyx, constitute the pelvis.

The pelvis is centrally balanced between two ball-and-socket joints, formed by the rounded heads of the two thighbones (femurs). The heads of the femurs fit into sockets (acetabulum) at the end of each of the hipbones (ilium). The femurs themselves are attached to the hipbones by their own large ligaments (iliofemoral, ischiofemoral, and pubofemoral) and, in each case, by a smaller ligament (ligamentum teres) that attaches the femur head directly to the socket (acetabulum). These structures are dense and strong, making the hip a very stable joint and capable of transferring weight from the pelvis, through the thighbones, to the knees, the lower legs, the ankles, and the feet.

The knees are very complicated joints. In fact, they are really like two separate joints: one between the upper and lower leg; the other between the kneecap (patella) and upper leg. The knee joint is stabilized by seven major ligaments, a pair of fibrocartilage pads (menisci) that cushion the articulating surfaces of the upper and lower legs, fat pads for further cushioning, and the muscle tendons of the thigh extensor muscles (quadriceps femoris). The complexity of this joint, combined with its vital role in daily activity, makes it highly susceptible to injury, including torn meniscus, strain to one of its many ligaments, and injury to the kneecap.

As we have seen, the spine consists of four distinct sections. Beginning at the pelvis and moving up the spine, the angle of each of these spinal sections determines the curvature of the spinal section immediately above it. First, there is the pelvis, which rotates back and forth on the joints described above, determining the angle of the sacrum in relation to itself and creating the plane from which the lumbar spine ascends. The lumbar spine ascends upward at an angle perpendicular to this plane, so that its own curve is necessarily determined by the angle of the sacrum to the pelvis. As the pelvis is tilted, that angle increases, causing the lumbar spine to begin at a sharper angle to horizontal and forcing it to arc through a sharper curve in order to return to the midline. Accordingly, if the pubic bone is elevated, a smaller angle is thereby created, depressing the sacrum and permitting a more erect lumbar spine. As the pelvic angle necessarily determines the degree of lumbar curvature, so also the lumbar curvature influences the thoracic curve. There is limited anterior-posterior flexion-extension mobility in the thoracic spine. Thus the thoracic spine balances as a more or less rigid moving segment at the thoracolumbar joints (see page 136); in this case maintenance of equilibrium is a structural given. Finally, the cervical spine balances the head and keeps it at the center of gravity. Thus it can be truly said that pelvic rotation is the basis for erect posture, and that when the pelvis is aligned, as it is designed to be, a stable base of support is present for diverse and powerful movements. Such alignment is one of the goals of Yoga therapy.

Besides its role of support, leverage, and protection of various organs, the skeletal system has two other essential functions: bone marrow produces our red blood cells, and it stores essential minerals (primarily calcium) and energy reserves (lipids), essential for the functioning of our bodies.

The most common problematic chronic conditions of the skeletal system are osteoporosis, osteoarthritis, and rheumatoid arthritis.

Osteoporosis is a condition characterized by a reduction of bone mass, resulting in lighter and more fragile bones, which, therefore, are more easily broken and more difficult to heal. Besides the customary hormonal treatment from health professionals, further treatment can include dietary modification to increase calcium intake and exercise programs that stress the bones and thereby stimulate bone growth.

Osteoarthritis is a degenerative condition of the articular cartilages in synovial joints. It results in subsequent degeneration of the underlying bone structure and inflammation of the joints. It is a condition that usually affects people over sixty years of age and is thought to be linked to a genetic predisposition. A very carefully considered program of Yoga therapy may be helpful to reduce pain, increase confidence, and increase range of motion.

Rheumatoid arthritis is an inflammatory condition of the synovial membranes. It results in subsequent breakdown of the articular cartilage and damage to the underlying bone structures. The cause of this condition is uncertain, although speculation ranges from bacterial or viral infection to allergy to genetic predisposition. In addition to drug therapies to reduce inflammation, regular exercise is thought to slow the process of this disease.

There are also abnormal curvatures of the spine that can be degenerative and can lead to more serious conditions. These include kyphosis, lordosis, and scoliosis. Kyphosis is an abnormal exaggeration of the thoracic spine that creates a rounded upper back. Though this condition is often congenital, it can develop as the result of poor postural habits and/or long-term activity where the body is hunched forward. Lordosis is the abnormal exaggeration of the lumbar curve that creates a hollow or swayed low back. This condition is also often congenital, but it too can be developed by poor postural habits, by wearing high heels, and even from the weight distribution that occurs during pregnancy. Scoliosis is the abnormal lateral curvature and rotation of the spine, often revealed by one hip and/or shoulder higher than the other. Severe scoliosis is congenital, but mild forms of it can be developed through chronic one-sided activities and poor postural habits.

Poor posture restricts circulation, respiration, digestion, and elimination. It can also negatively impact our confidence and self-image. However, a well-conceived program of Yoga practice can significantly improve even the most serious of such postural problems, and, in fact, all but the most progressed will usually get great benefit from a carefully designed program of Yoga therapy.

Beyond these conditions, there are other injuries to the skeletal system that are, unfortunately, quite common. Perhaps the most common are injuries to the intervertebral discs. Discs naturally degenerate with age, reducing their cushioning effect. However, if there is serious strain from an accident or a sport or work-related injury, the nucleus may break through the capsule that encloses it, resulting in a herniated or ruptured disc. These are painful and lead to severely limiting conditions that may require surgery. Therefore, people who have serious disc conditions should seek out professional care. On the other hand, many disc conditions can be effectively treated by a combination of rest and a carefully conceived program of physical or Yoga therapy.

Other problematic conditions of the skeletal system result from accidents, activity-related injuries, or chronic structural stress. Chronic structural stress may be the result of dysfunctional movement patterns. Some of these conditions include bursitis, sprains to the ligaments or tendons, and tendinitis. Bursitis is the inflammation of the bursa around the joint capsules. Tendinitis is the inflammation of the connective tissue that surrounds the tendons. All of these conditions require time and rest to heal. Two main strategies for working with these conditions are recommended: First, identifying and eliminating, as much as possible, sources of stress to the damaged area, including developing new and more functional movement patterns; second, carefully increasing the circulation to the area, bringing nutrients and eliminating the toxic buildup that interferes with healing.

After considering the muscular system in the sections ahead, we will present examples of the way in which Yoga therapy can be adapted to work with a variety of the common aches and pains.

Muscular System

All of the movements of the body, including the internal movements of the physiological processes, are dependent upon the action of muscles. There are three primary types of muscle tissue: cardiac (heart) muscle; smooth (visceral) muscle, which is located in the walls of all organs other than the heart; and

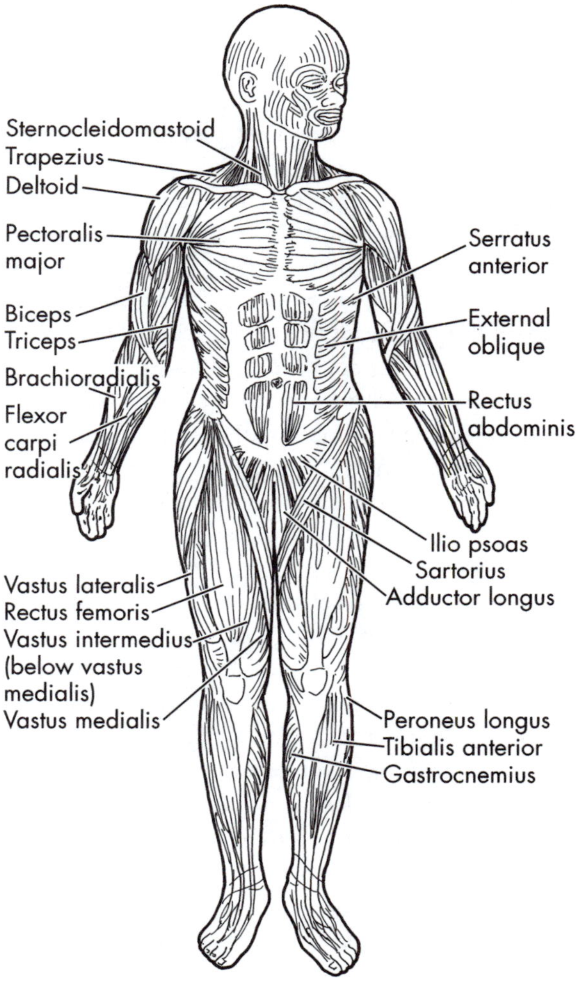

striated (skeletal) muscle. All muscle tissue shares certain characteristics: excitability, contractibility, extensibility, and elasticity. *Excitability* means that the muscle is able to receive and respond to stimuli. *Contractibility* means that the muscle changes shape as a result of stimuli, usually becoming shorter and thicker (flexion). *Extensibility* means that the muscle can be stretched beyond its normal length (extension). *Elasticity* means that the muscle easily returns to its normal length after it has been stretched. The cardiac and smooth muscles push fluids and solids through the internal channels of our bodies. The skeletal muscles, along with tendons, connective, and neural tissues, move the bones of the skeleton. Our discussion will focus on the skeletal muscles.

Three layers of connective tissue form a part of each muscle: the outer part, which surrounds the muscle and separates it from surrounding tissue and organs; the central part, which divides the muscle into individual bundles; and the inner part, which surrounds and connects the individual muscle fibers within each bundle. These three parts of the connective tissue blend together at the end of each muscle, forming the *tendons,* which attach the muscles to the bone. This connective tissue also contains the nerves and blood vessels that control and nourish the muscles.

Muscle fibers contract and actively shorten through a complex process of biochemical and neural activation. When the muscle receives a stimulus from the motor nerves, its center portion contracts, pulling on the connective tissue, which in turn pulls on the bones to which it is attached. After a muscle contracts, it returns to its normal length, either through the contraction of opposing muscles or through its own natural elasticity.

There are three types of muscular contraction: concentric, eccentric, and isometric. Concentric contraction occurs when a muscle shortens and, by so doing, moves a bone segment. Eccentric contraction occurs when a muscle lengthens against resistance. For example, when we squat, the leg extensor muscles lengthen at the same time that they contract, insuring that the force of their own movement remains less than that of the force opposing them. Isometric, or static, muscle work occurs when a muscle neither shortens nor lengthens so that, as a result of neither overcoming nor being overcome by resistance, its contraction is sustained.

A muscle has a resting tension called muscle tone. A muscle with too little muscle tone is usually weak and flaccid, while one with too much is hard and lacks elasticity. On the other hand, a healthy muscle, when at rest, is firm and yet soft. If a muscle is not stimulated through activity, it will lose muscle tone, mass, and power. Irreversible muscle atrophy can occur as a result of paralysis due to spinal injuries and various autoimmune and neurological conditions. However, because regular stimulation is needed to keep the muscles powerful and to maintain their activity (endurance), reversible muscle atrophy can also result from irregular use.

Muscle contraction requires fuel, which is supplied in the form of high-energy molecular compounds, through a complex biochemical process known as glycosis (yielding ATP, CP, and glycogen). In this process, the necessary energy reserves are produced when oxygen, glucose, and fatty acids from the bloodstream are combined and absorbed by the muscle fibers. Thus, normal muscle function is dependent upon sufficient energy reserves, which in turn are dependent upon adequate circulatory supply and normal oxygen concentrations in the blood.

There are two complex metabolic processes by which a muscle builds up and consumes its energy reserves. In moderate muscular activity, the increased energy demands on the muscles are met through a biochemical process known as *aerobic respiration.* In this process, the respiratory and cardiovascular functions increase to provide the required materials by which energy is generated. However, at peak levels of muscular exertion, the energy demand on the muscles exceeds what can be met by the respiratory and cardiovascular systems. In this case, the energy is provided by a different, and less efficient, biochemical process called *anaerobic glycosis.*

Aerobic exercise both increases muscle endurance and strengthens the respiratory and cardiovascular systems. It includes activities that provide a sustained increase in both respiratory and cardiovascular function, such as hiking and swimming. Anaerobic exercise, on the other hand, results in enlargement of the muscles. It is usually short and intensive, such as weight lifting, hiking quickly up a steep hill, or swimming at top speed in a race.

Excessive anaerobic activity depletes the muscles' energy reserves and causes the buildup of lactic acid, a by-product of anaerobic glycosis. The result is muscle fatigue and possibly cramping. After fatigue, a muscle must remove the buildup of lactic acid generated by anaerobic activity and rebuild its energy reserves. In this process, the body is aided by the circulatory system and the action of the liver, which helps to absorb the lactic acid and convert it back to glucose.

After any muscular activity or exercise, the body must also recover oxygen utilized during the activity. Thus the increased rate and depth of the breath continues for some time after the muscles are at rest. In addition, muscular activity or exercise generates heat, which increases the overall body temperature. This heat is released through perspiration, which also continues for some time after the muscles are at rest.

There are approximately seven hundred skeletal muscles, all of which begin (the origin) and/or end (the insertion) in the skeleton. These muscles are paired in an agonist-antagonist relationship to each other and, based on this relationship, form groups that, through the alternation of contraction and extension, determine movement in any part of the body. The agonist muscles are responsible for movement by contraction; the antagonist muscles relax and usually lengthen as the agonist muscles contract. In most movements, other muscles (synergists) also act to either stabilize the point of origin or to assist at the point of insertion. For example, when the arm moves on the shoulder girdle, it must be held firm by the contraction of certain muscles that are attached to it and whose coordinated action is essential for efficient movement of the body.

Following this general presentation, we will now briefly discuss the organization of the muscular system in terms of its axial and appendicular musculature.

Axial

The axial musculature includes all of the muscles of the head and neck, the muscles of the back (posterior), front (anterior), and sides (lateral) of the trunk, and the muscles of the pelvic floor. In muscles of the head and neck, we are including those responsible for facial expression, verbal communication, eating and drinking, and eye movements. Muscles of the trunk are responsible for flexion, extension, and rotation of the head, neck, and trunk. The anterior and lateral muscles of the trunk also form the muscular walls of the thoracic and abdominal cavities and include the respiratory muscles (see the medical drawing on p. 139 with names of major groups). They variously compress the abdomen, expand the thoracic cavity, and elevate or depress the ribs. The muscles of the pelvic floor compress, close, and/or lift the various openings and organs of the pelvic cavity.

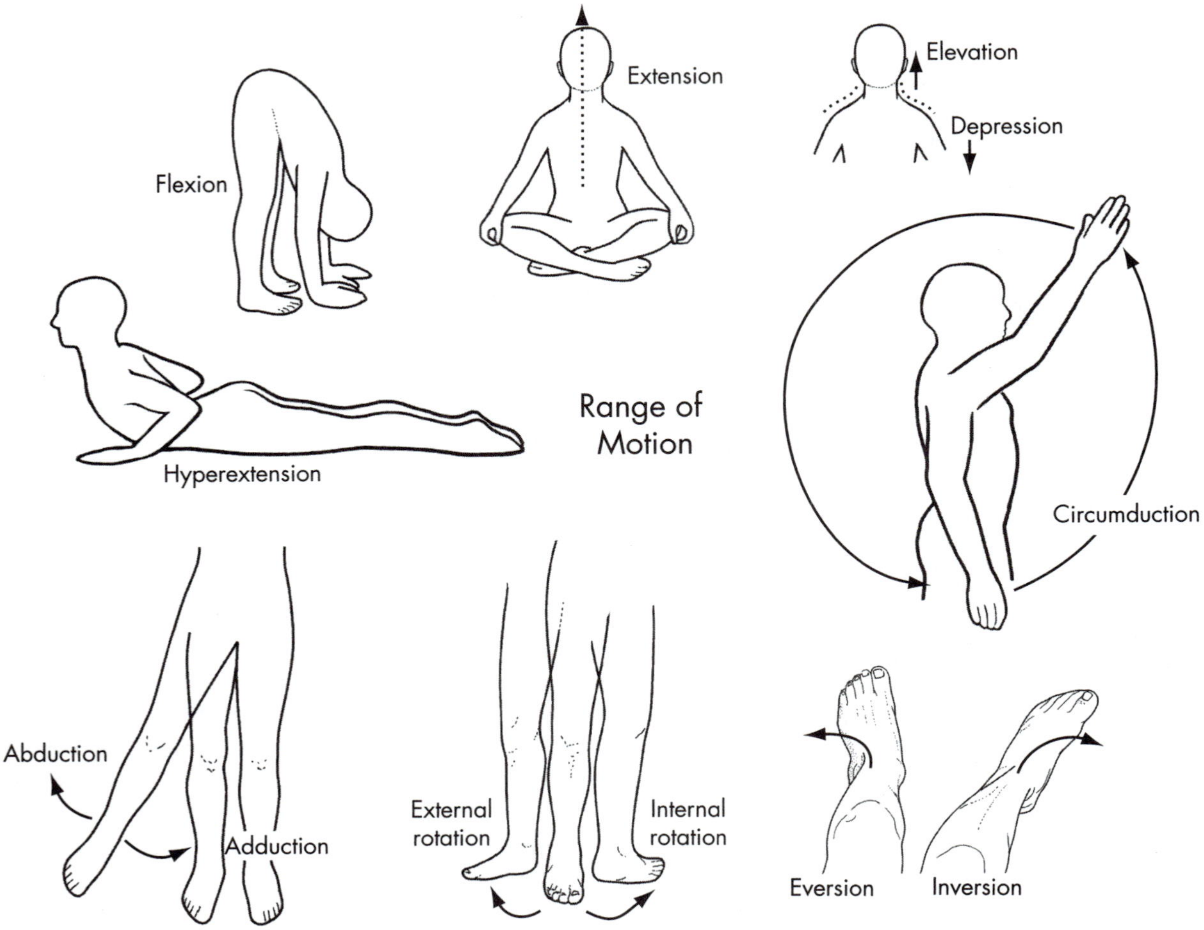

Appendicular

The appendicular musculature includes the muscles of the shoulders and arms and the muscles of the pelvic girdle and legs. Muscles of the shoulders include those muscles that elevate, depress, protract, adduct, abduct, and rotate the shoulder girdle. They also include muscles that flex the neck and rotate the head. Muscles of the shoulder likewise flex, extend, adduct, rotate, pronate, and supinate the upper arm, forearm, wrist, palm, and fingers. Muscles of the legs include those muscles that variously extend, flex, rotate, adduct, and abduct the thighs and lower legs (see the medical drawing on p. 139 with names of major groups). They also include muscles which flex the hip and the lumbar spine. Muscles of the ankles, feet, and toes (dorsi and plantar) variously flex, evert, and invert the feet and toes.

Serious conditions of the muscular system are rare. They include conditions, such as muscular dystrophies (which are congenital) and myasthenia gravis (thought to be an immunological malfunction), that result in weakness and deterioration of the muscle tissue. People with these conditions should be under direct professional care, and with that as a foundation, many will benefit from a carefully conceived program of Yoga therapy.

Accident-, sport-, or work-related injuries, such as muscle cramps and strains, are more common. These conditions respond well to rest, cold and heat therapies, liniments and oil applications, acupuncture, and massage. A more serious example of an activity-related injury is a hernia, in which a portion of an organ protrudes through an opening in a muscle. Hernias are usually the result of intense pressure in the abdominal or pelvic cavity, such as may occur from straining to lift an excessive weight. Sport or workplace injuries can often be avoided by proper training, adequate warm-up, and good equipment. In addition, proper diet will help the body generate the energy the muscles need to perform well and, therefore, avoid injury.

Beyond these conditions are the common, chronic aches and pains that we often assume to be an inevitable part of a normal life. Included in this category is the tendency of muscles, with aging, to develop increased amounts of connective tissue (fibrosis), which limits elasticity and which restricts movement and circulation. In fact, many of these common complaints can be avoided all together, or significantly improved. Sedentary people will benefit from adopting a well-planned exercise program. Active people with chronic, low-grade aches and pains would do well to reexamine their fitness program, as many well-intentioned people begin an exercise program and end up with injuries. And, in both cases, many common aches and pains can be alleviated by a regular commitment to a simple Yoga practice.

In the sections ahead, we will present examples of the way in which Yoga therapy can be adapted to improve a variety of these common aches and pains.

Neck and Shoulders

Many people suffer from chronic tension in the neck and shoulders. This may be experienced as mild to severe pain in the neck and/or shoulders, as mild to severe tension in the jaw (TMJ) and/or head, as mild to severe limitation in the mobility of the head, or as mild to severe restriction in the movement of the arms.

Before we begin to work with these conditions, it is important to find out whether there is serious damage to the cervical discs or the rotator cuff in the shoulder joints. If there is numbness or tingling sensations in the arms or hands, sharp, electric, and immobilizing pains in the neck, or sharp pains in the shoulders, it is best to seek professional diagnosis. In such conditions, Yoga therapy may assist the healing process, but the wrong practice may actually make matters worse. In working with tension, restricted movement, and chronic pain, we also want to understand the musculoskeletal condition and the neuromuscular patterns that condition our movements.

Musculoskeletal conditions of the neck and shoulders that contribute to these problems include having one shoulder higher than the other, one shoulder rotated forward, one scapula pulled in more than the other toward the spine, the head leaning to one side, the head jutting forward relative to the spine, and a flattened cervical curve. All of these structural conditions relate to corresponding muscular imbalances, chronic muscular contractions, and/or muscular weakness. Because the condition of the muscles and joints are causally related to neuromuscular mechanisms and movement patterns, there may also be joint instability and hypermobility or joint rigidity and lack of mobility.

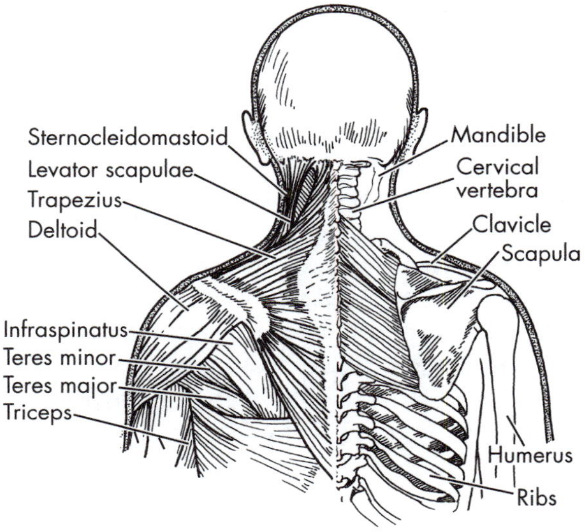

The origin of these conditions may be compensatory, habitual, or the result of stress, physical activity, or improper training. A common compensatory mechanism, for example, is excessive tension on one side of the neck and shoulders due to a congenital curvature of the spine. A very common habitual pattern is lifting the head upward as we bend forward, creating tension and compression in the back of the neck. A common stress pattern is lifting the shoulders toward the ears in reaction to tense situations. An example of a common physical activity that creates tension is talking on the phone while cradling the telephone between the shoulder and ear, and, at the same time, working with the hands. These conditions are also complicated in cases of breast-feeding moms and baby-carrying moms and dads. An example of problems due to improper training can, unfortunately, be found in many Yoga students who have been taught to pull the spine with the head when moving into backward bends and moving out of forward bends.

In conditions of chronic pain combined with restricted movement, there is always some form of muscular contraction linked to specific neuromuscular movement patterns. As the Yoga process involves learning what tools can be used to unravel such limiting mechanisms and then applying those tools, our job is to explore the mechanisms of contraction, identify them, and learn how to release them. It is also important to recognize that most conditions affecting the neck and shoulders reflect a poor functional integration of the head, neck, and shoulders and attached arms, rib cage, and upper back and, therefore, that the methodology for working these conditions involves working to adjust this functional relationship.

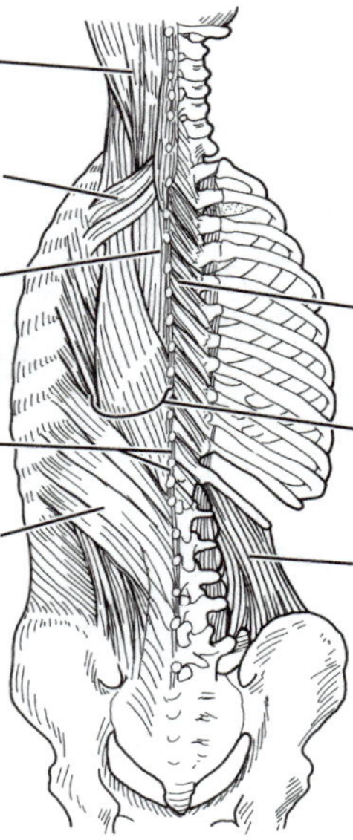

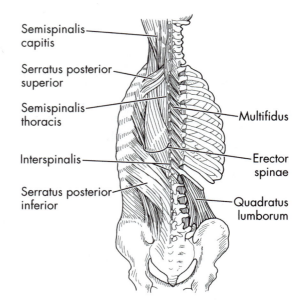

The neck connects the head to the shoulders and upper back. Muscles attach from the head, through the neck and shoulders, to the rib cage and upper back. In working the neck, one of the main principles is to work the neck by adjusting the relationship between the head and shoulders. Our normal pattern is for the head and shoulders to turn in the same direction: If we look to the right, the shoulders naturally follow to the right; If we turn our shoulders to the right, the head will follow to the right. To adjust this relationship, we can either stabilize the shoulders as we turn the head, or turn the shoulders in one way and the head in the other. As these practices are based on the principle of opposition, in both cases the effect will be to stretch the neck and shoulder muscles on the opposite side of the direction to which the head is turning. In the second case, however, the stretching effect is stronger.

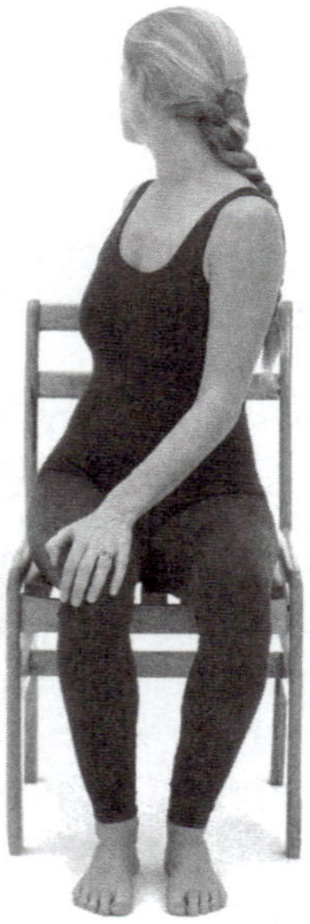

Shoulders and head turn in same direction

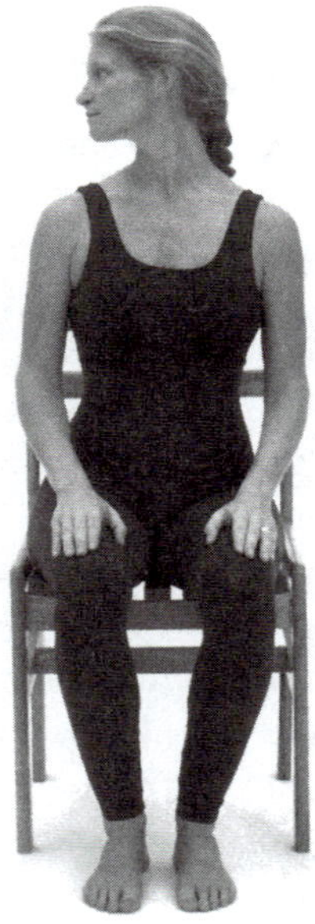

Shoulders stable head turns

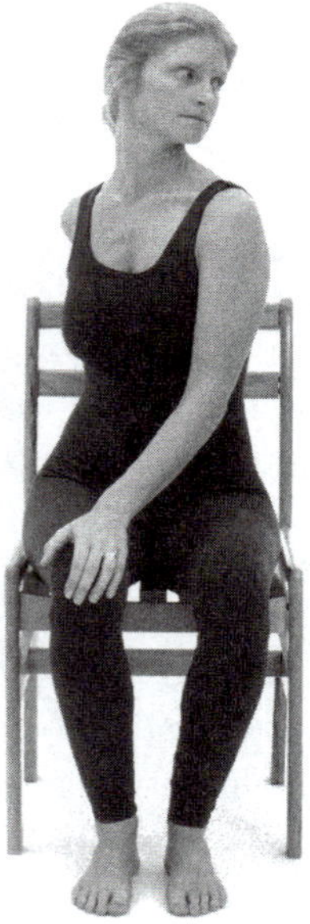

Shoulders turn one way, head the other

When the head is turned in one direction, muscles on one side of the neck are stretched while muscles on the other side are contracted. When the head is turned in the other direction, both sides of the neck are worked through alternated contraction and stretching. The effect is an increase in circulation to the muscles, both strengthening and relaxing them.

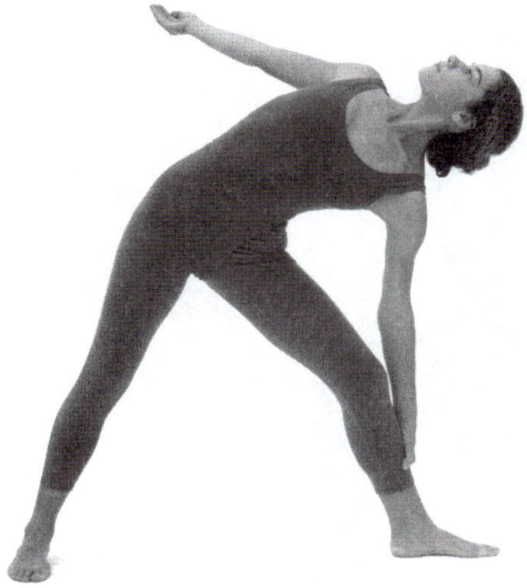

head up

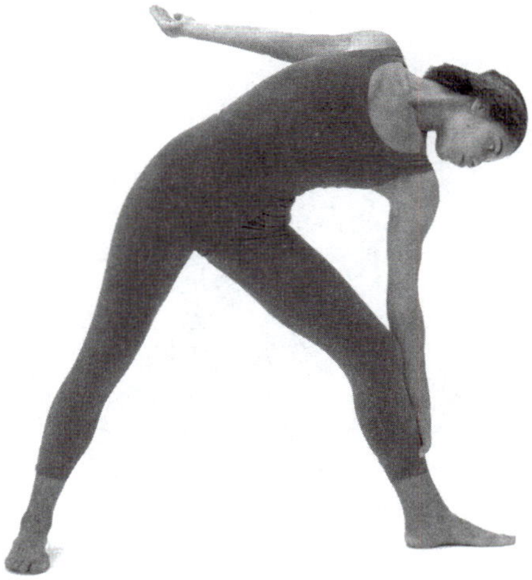

head down

Besides turning the shoulder girdle, we can also bring the shoulders forward, spreading the scapula in the back and compressing the chest in the front. Or, we can pull the shoulders back, compressing between scapula and spine and stretching the chest in the front. This results in increased circulation, strength, and relaxation for the muscles that bind the shoulder girdle through the rib cage and to the spine.

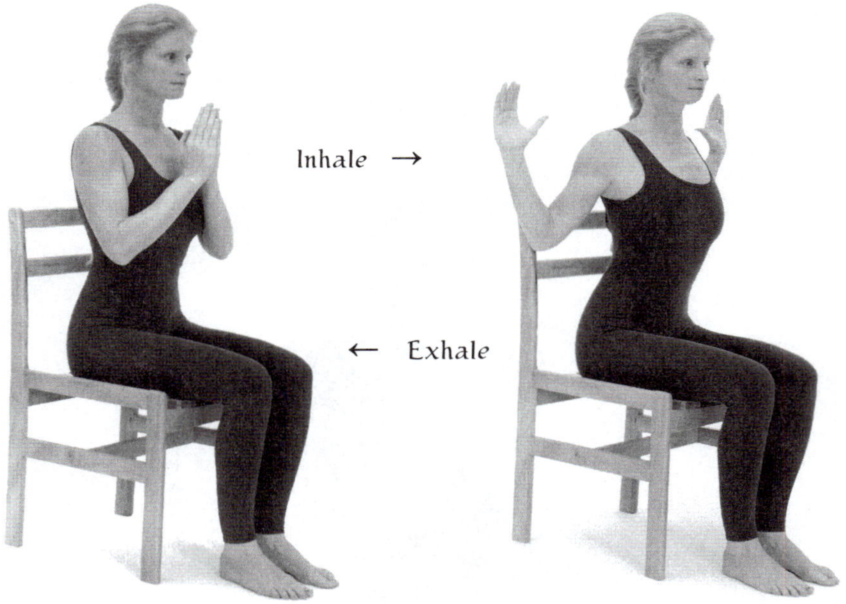

If we coordinate this process with arm movements, we can integrate a similar action with other muscles that bind the shoulders to both neck and upper back. By raising and lowering the arms alternately, we can also contract and stretch these muscles, increasing circulation and strengthening and relaxing them.

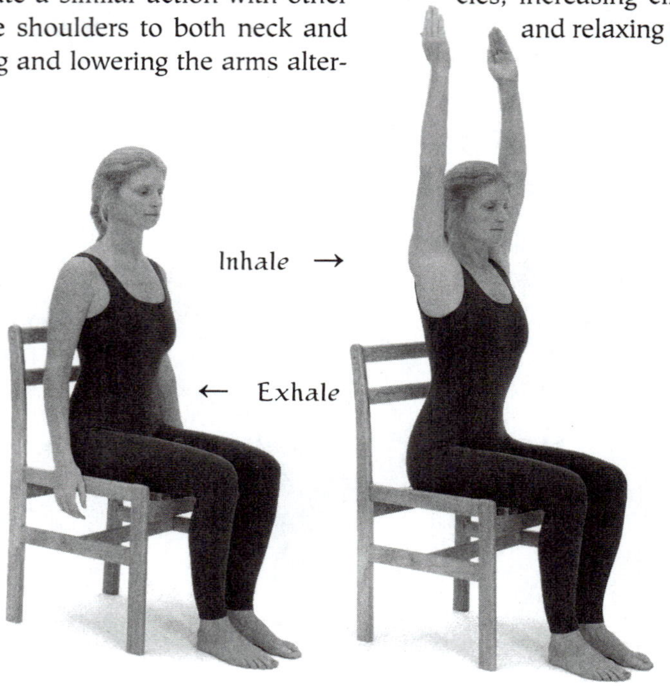

The cumulative effect of these actions is to free binding muscle contraction, restore balance between various structural parts, and establish new and more appropriate movement patterns.

In the methodology of practice, we use a combination of movement and static positions. Movement has the effect of working the paired muscles (agonist and antagonist) alternately, warming them up, increasing circulation, and bringing a more balanced development. Staying in a fixed position, on the other hand, prolongs the stretching and contraction of particular muscles, deepening the work in specific areas.

In the more advanced Yoga postures, we are able to create leverage by wrapping the arms around the legs in various ways. With any leveraged posture, we can deepen the above-mentioned effects, though there are increased risks to the joints. These risks can be mediated, however, by the proper technique, as will be discussed in the context of the practices that follow.

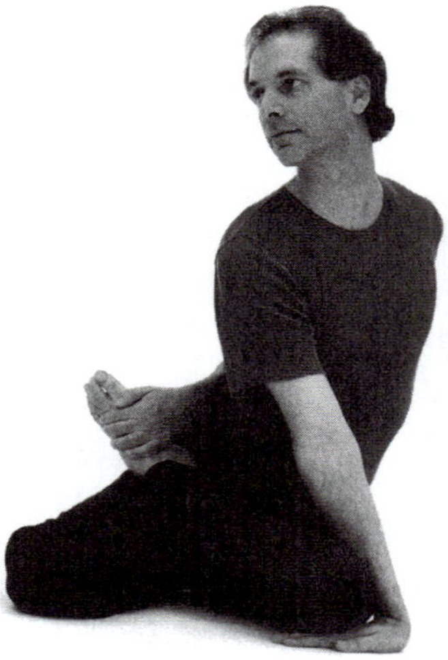

If the more serious conditions mentioned at the beginning of this section are ruled out, then much relief can be had from simple Yoga techniques. Through these techniques, we explore the imbalances in our body and find ways to improve our condition. We work with a variety of techniques, focusing around the neck, shoulder girdle, and upper back, strengthening weak muscles, releasing chronic contractions, stabilizing joints, increasing mobility and flexibility, establishing new movement patterns, and bringing integrity to the structure.

If there is pain, we find the parameters of movement where no pain exists. To this end, we first identify the general area where pain exists. Then, slowly, carefully, without any stress, we stretch and contract, beginning to increase the range of motion and also increasing circulation and avoiding irritation through the use of simple "micro" movements. When there is strong pain, we don't push into a position, making the condition worse, and we avoid positions that are locked, favoring those that allow unrestricted and easy movement. I worked with a woman once who had broken her neck. We started very simply, raising her hands partway out to the side and lowering them again, while gently turning her head. As a result of starting slowly, recognizing her limitations, and slowly increasing the parameters of her movement without going into the pain, in only a few weeks there was significant improvement.

Therefore, the first principle is simple movement. From sitting in a chair, on inhale, raise your arms out to the side and about halfway up. Then, on exhale, simultaneously turn your shoulders to the right, look to the right, lower your right arm, and bring your left hand to your right shoulder. Finally, on inhale, raise both arms out to the side and turn your head and shoulders to the middle. Repeat on the other side.

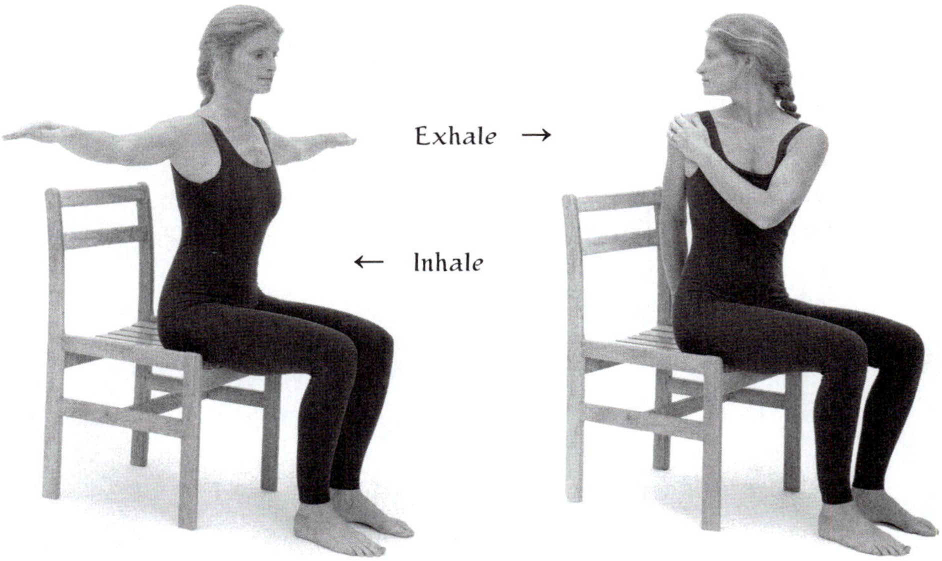

The next principle is stabilizing one part of the body and moving another part from the fixed base. From the same seated position, on inhale, put your hands on the right side of your collarbone. On exhale, turn your head slightly to the left. On the next inhale, lean your head slightly back and pull your chin up while depressing your collarbone slightly down. Stay in the stretch as you exhale, and then return to the neutral position. Can you feel the strong stretching of the muscles on the right front side of your neck? Now try this on the other side.

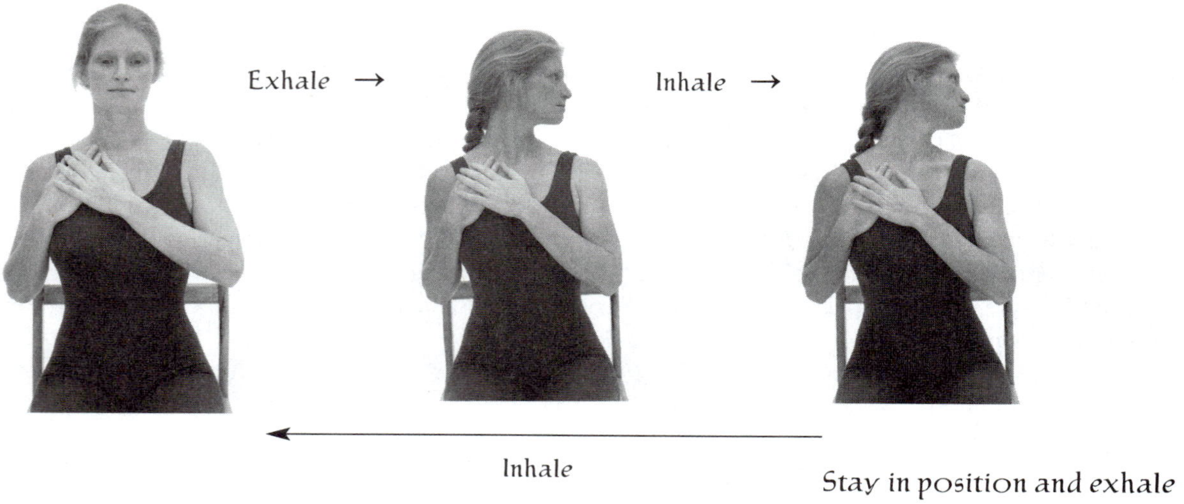

The next principle is opposition. The exercise is stronger and involves more compression on one side. Sitting on a chair with arms, place both hands on the right arm of the chair. On exhale, twist your shoulders farther to the right as you turn your head to the left. On inhale, lean your head slightly back to the left and pull your chin up. Stay in the stretch as you exhale, and then return to the neutral position on inhale. Relax and feel the right side of your neck. Then repeat these movements on the other side.

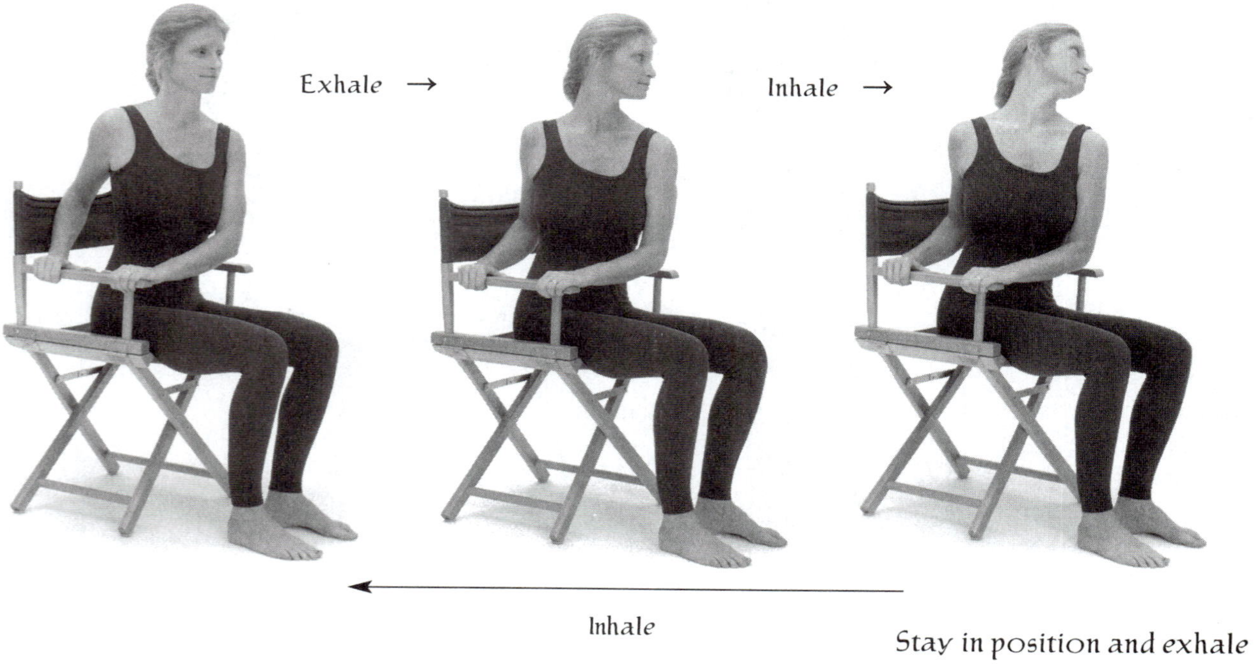

In addition to stretching and increasing circulation to the neck and shoulder area, we often need to strengthen the supporting structures of the shoulders and upper back. Another student of mine had long-term chronic pain in the neck and shoulders, with corresponding weakness in the shoulders and upper back. To deal with this situation, one of our long-term goals was to strengthen her upper back and shoulders in order to provide a more stable base for her neck. After a period of preparation we were able to introduce some external weight. From sitting in a chair, I had her raise and lower each arm separately, while holding small, half-filled plastic water bottles in each hand. After a few weeks, there was already a marked reduction of tension and an increase in strength. She no longer complained of tension or pain in her neck and was happily able to intensify her practice. In using this kind of technique, however, it is important not to pull the spine with the shoulders. Rather, we must lift the chest first, feeling the arms rising as an extension of this lift. Otherwise the techniques we use to strengthen our body may in fact increase tension and pain.

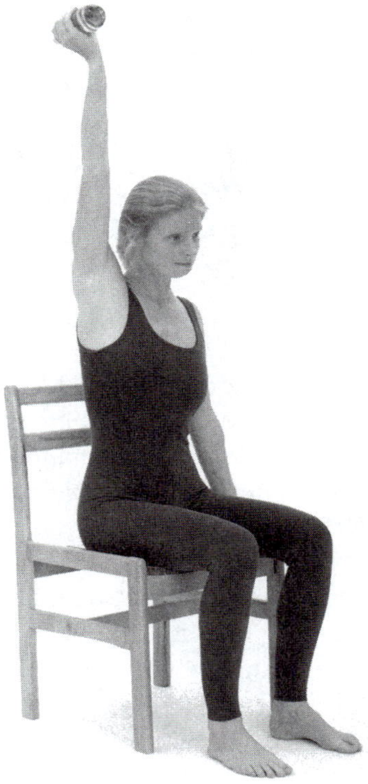

incorrect

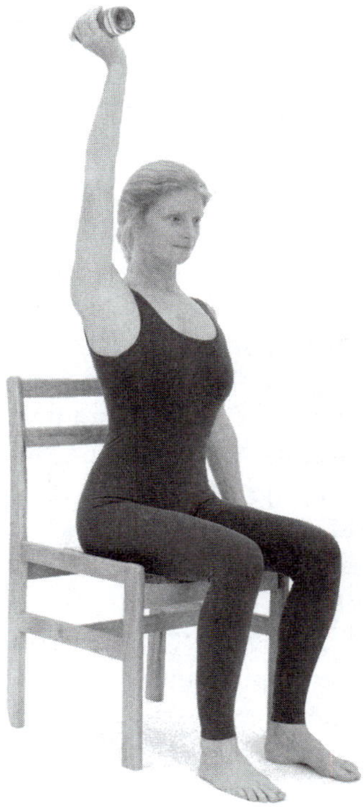

correct

These simple exercises, in which we isolated and worked the neck and shoulders, have an educational value. In a full Yoga therapy practice, however, we use movements that integrate the whole body. This is based on the recognition that what is happening in the area of the neck and shoulders is, ultimately, linked not only to the upper back and rib cage, but to the low back, sacrum, hips, and legs. Lasting improvement necessarily involves the functional integration of the entire body.

The underlying methodological orientation of the following sequences is to support this functional integration, while focusing the work in the head, neck, shoulders and arms, and in the upper back and upper part of the rib cage. They present a progression from therapeutic to developmental work specific to the neck and shoulders.

Working with the Neck and Shoulders (A Developmental Approach)

This practice was developed for F.M., a twenty-six-year-old architect. At our first session, F.M. said that she had chronic mild tension in her neck and shoulders, and recurring sharper pains between the shoulder blade and spine on her right side. She said it felt like a knife in her back.

When I asked about her work, she told me that she spent many hours each day seated or standing over a drafting table, making precise technical drawings. She told me she was right-handed. She said that her neck was constantly "going out" and that she regularly went to a chiropractor for adjustments. She said she got temporary relief, though not in the area between the scapula and spine. A friend had told her about our work, and she wanted to see if it would help.

F.M. had good coordination and supple joints. And yet her body lacked structural stability. She told me that even if she drove her car too much, her neck would bother her for days. When I asked what she was doing for exercise, she said she was not involved in any regular program. I asked her if she would be willing to do a regular Yoga practice on her own, and she said, "That's what I am here for."

My plan was to develop a practice that would strengthen and stabilize her neck. As we worked together, I found that there was a lot of tightness and congestion between the scapula and spine. I added to her practice movements that would stretch the area between the scapula and the spine, to help free her neck.

Over the next several months we met once a week and developed the following course. I asked her to go for a walk in the morning before work and to do the practice after work and before dinner. In the first few weeks, she told me that when she did Marīcyāsana she would feel popping sounds in her upper back, between the shoulder and the spine on the right side. After that, she said her shoulder felt more open and her head felt as if it was floating away from her spine.

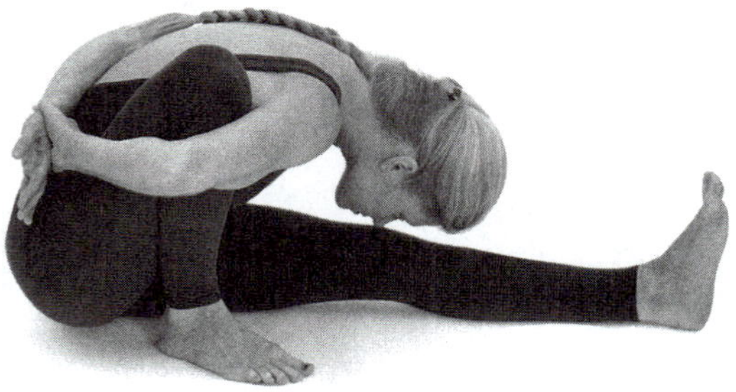

About six months after F.M. stopped her weekly sessions, she came in for a "checkup." She told me that she had been able to maintain her practice and that she felt much more stable and rarely went to the chiropractor anymore. She also told me that she joined the Sierra Club and went often on organized hikes in the mountains. She told me that she is now able to carry a pack without problems. I asked her how she manages with the four-wheel roads they have to take to get to the trailheads. She told me that now that she has her practice, she is much more confident that she can handle any tension that may arise.

A Practice for the Neck and Shoulders (Developmental)

1.
POSTURE: Vajrāsana, asymmetrical adaptation.
EMPHASIS: To gently stretch neck.
TECHNIQUE: Stand on knees with left arm over head, right arm folded behind back, and head turned to center.

On exhale: Bend forward, sweeping left arm behind back, turning head to right and resting on left side of face.

On inhale: Return to starting position.

Repeat on other side.

NUMBER: 4 times on each side, alternately.
DETAILS: *On exhale:* Keep buttocks higher than hips, and rest side of face on floor. Keep most of body weight on legs.

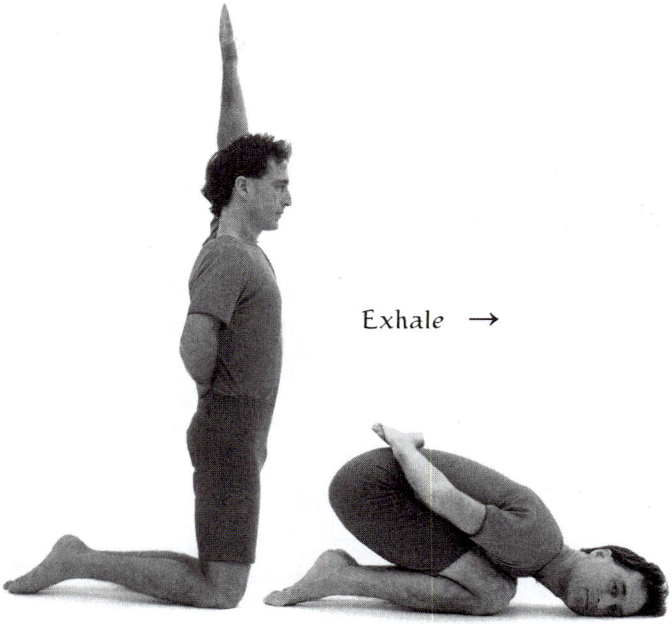
Exhale →
← Inhale

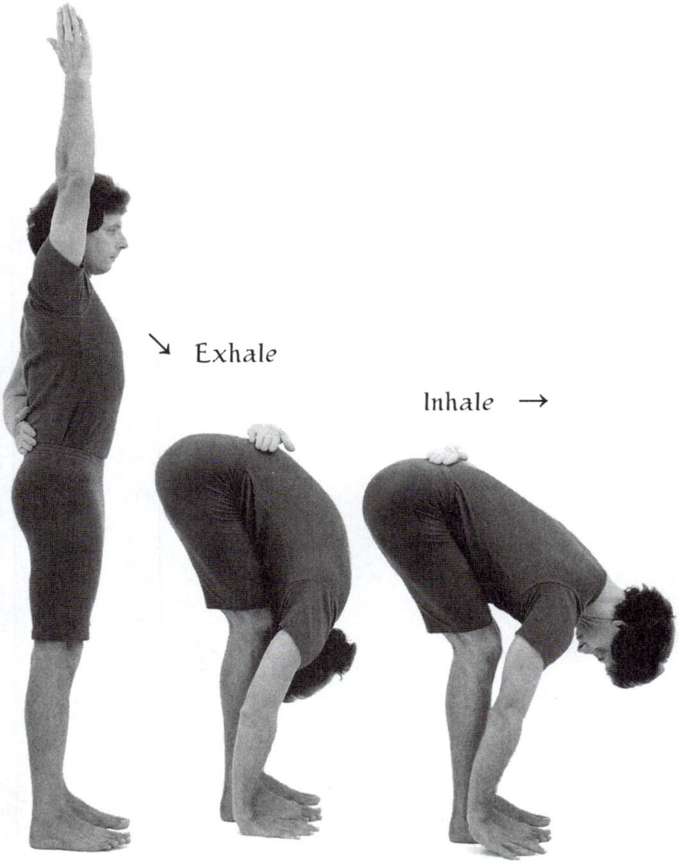
↘ Exhale
Inhale →
← Inhale
← Exhale

2.
POSTURE: Uttānāsana, asymmetrical adaptation.
EMPHASIS: To stretch back and shoulders, one side at a time.
TECHNIQUE: Stand with right arm over head, left arm folded behind back.

On exhale: Bend forward, bringing chin down, belly and chest toward thighs, and right hand to side of right foot.

On inhale: Keeping right hand by foot, lift chest and flatten upper back. Allow chin to lift slightly only toward end of inhale.

On exhale: Return to forward bend position.

On inhale: Return to starting position.

NUMBER: Repeat 4 times on each side, one side at a time.
DETAILS: *On inhale:* Lift chin slightly toward end of inhale. *On exhale:* lower chin.

3.

POSTURE: Parivṛtti Trikoṇāsana.

EMPHASIS: To stretch and strengthen neck by alternately rotating head up and down in coordination with movement of shoulder girdle and arm.

TECHNIQUE: Stand with feet spread wider than shoulders and with arms out to sides and parallel to floor.

On exhale: Bend forward and twist, bringing right hand to floor, pointing left arm upward, and twisting shoulders left. Turn head down toward right hand.

On inhale: Maintaining rotation, and with left shoulder vertically above right, bring left arm up over shoulder and forward, turning head to center and looking at left hand.

On exhale: Return to previous position with left arm pointing upward. Turn head up, looking toward left hand.

On inhale: Return to starting position.

Repeat on other side.

NUMBER: 6 times each side, alternately.

DETAILS: Keep down arm vertically below its respective shoulder, and keep weight of torso off arm. Knees can bend while moving into twist.

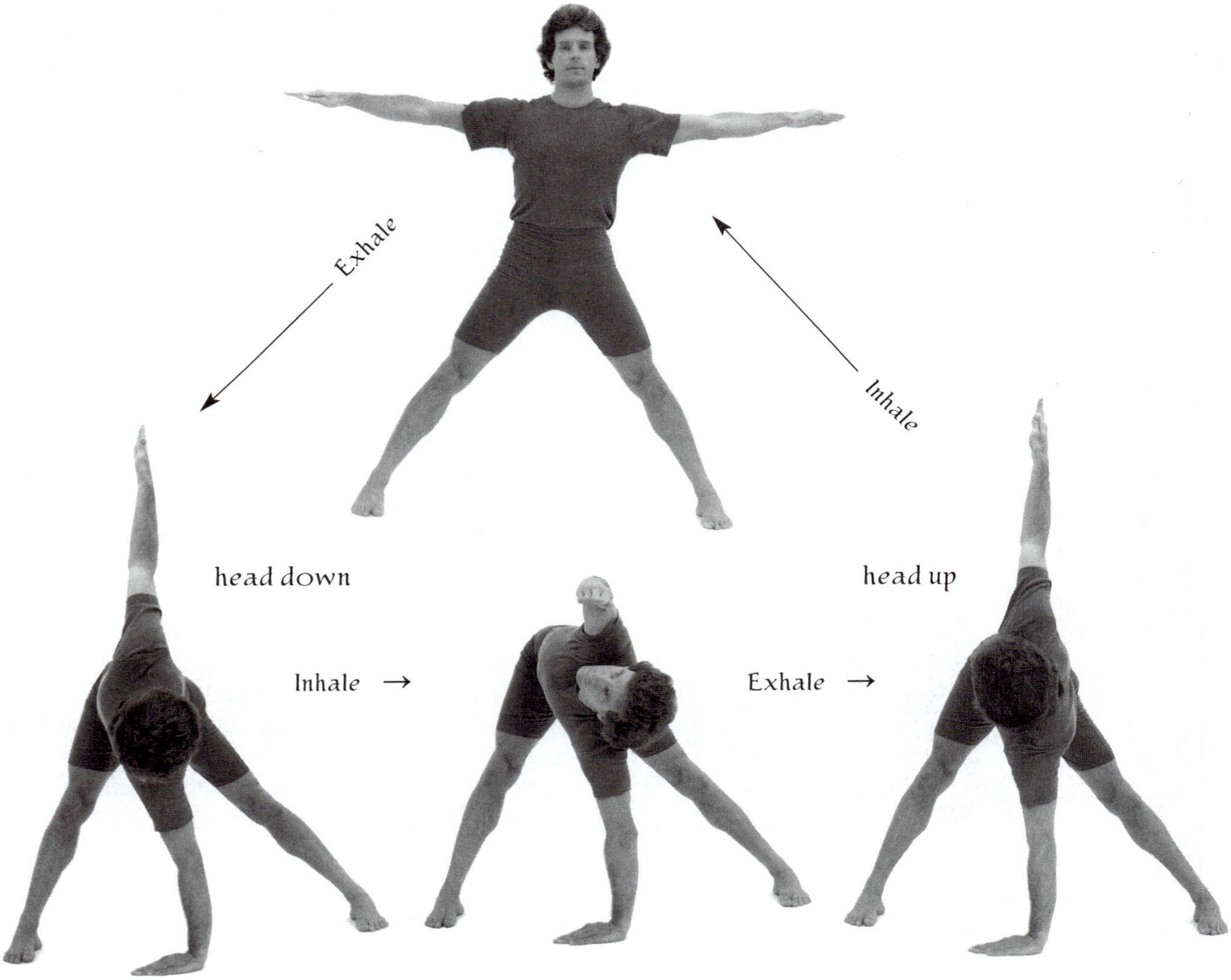

4.

POSTURE: Vajrāsana adaptation.
EMPHASIS: To gently stretch neck and to make transition from standing twist to prone back bend.
TECHNIQUE: Stand on knees with head to center and arms over head.

On exhale: Bend forward, sweeping arms behind back, turning head to right, and resting left side of face on floor.

On inhale: Return to starting position.

Repeat on other side.

NUMBER: 4 times each side, alternately.
DETAILS: *On exhale:* Keep buttocks higher than hips while resting face on floor. Keep most of body weight on legs.

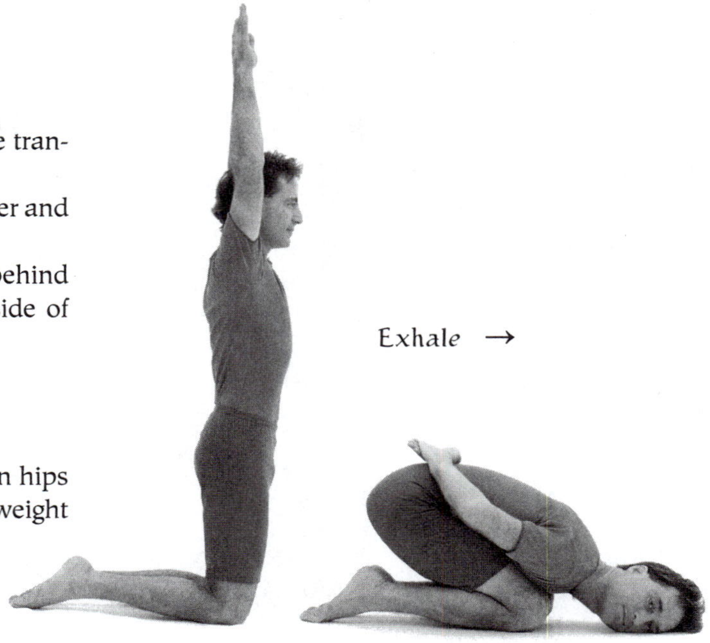

5.

POSTURE: Ardha Śalabhāsana.
EMPHASIS: To integrate movements of upper back, shoulders, and neck.
TECHNIQUE: Lie on stomach, turning head to right, crossing hands over sacrum, and turning palms up.

On inhale: Lift chest, right arm, and left leg, and turn head to center.

On exhale: Lower chest and leg while sweeping arm behind back and turning head to left. Repeat on other side.

NUMBER: 6 times each side, alternately.
DETAILS: *On inhale:* Lift chest slightly before leg, and emphasize chest height. Keep pelvis level. *On exhale:* Turn head opposite arm being lowered.

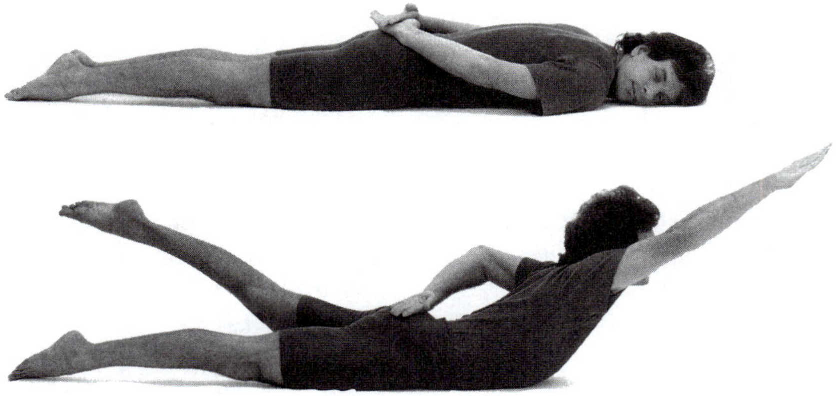

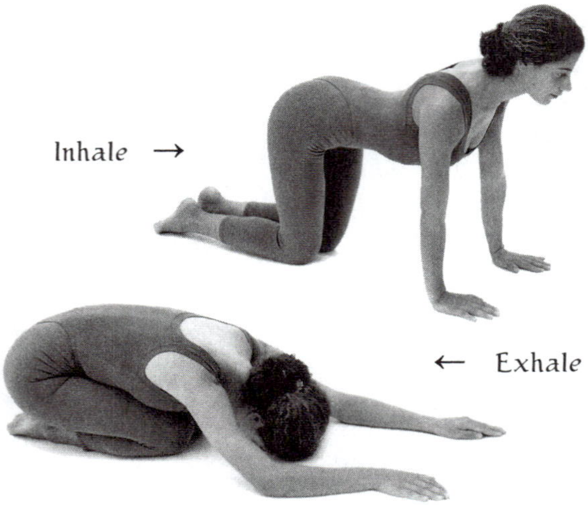

6.

POSTURE: Cakravākāsana.

EMPHASIS: To make transition from back bend to twist.

TECHNIQUE: Get down on hands and knees, with shoulders vertically above wrists, and with hips above knees.

On inhale: Lift chest up and away from belly.

On exhale: Gently contract belly, round low back, and bring chest toward thighs.

NUMBER: 8 times.

DETAILS: *On inhale:* Lead with chest, keeping chin slightly down. Avoid compressing low back; rather, feel chest expanding. *On exhale:* Round low back without collapsing chest over belly. Avoid increasing curvature of upper back. Let chest lower toward thighs sooner than hips toward heels.

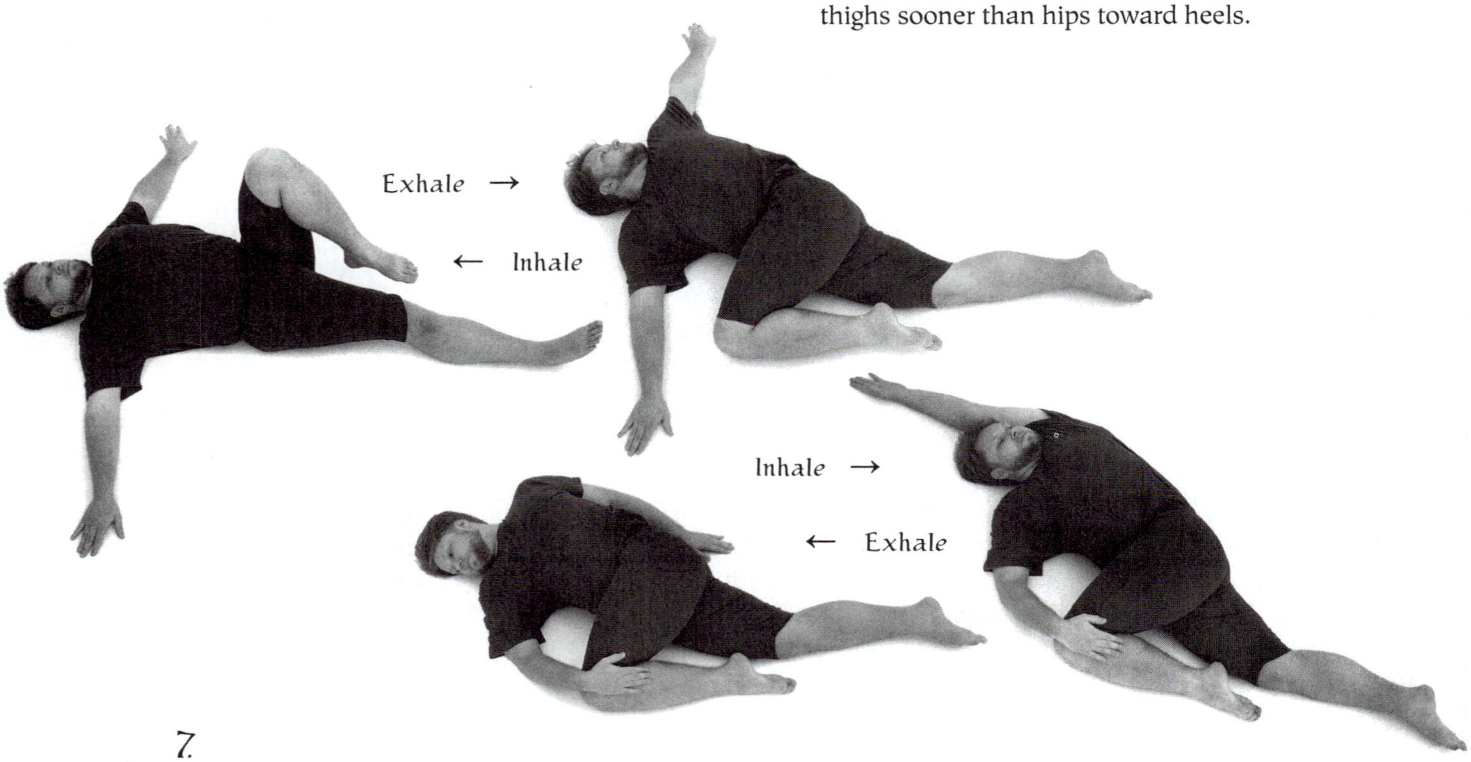

7.

POSTURE: Jaṭhara Parivṛtti.

EMPHASIS: To stretch front of shoulder and massage area between shoulder blades and spine.

TECHNIQUE: Lie flat on back, with arms out to sides and left knee pulled up toward chest.

On exhale: Twist, bringing left knee toward floor on right side of body while turning head left.

On inhale: Return to starting position.

Repeat 4 times.

On fifth repetition, stay in twist, holding knee with hand.

On inhale: Sweep left arm, palm up, wide along floor toward ear, while turning head to center.

On exhale: Lower arm back to side while turning head *right.*

Repeat 6 times.

Repeat on other side.

DETAILS: *On exhale:* While twisting right, keep angles between left arm and torso and between left knee and torso less than ninety degrees.

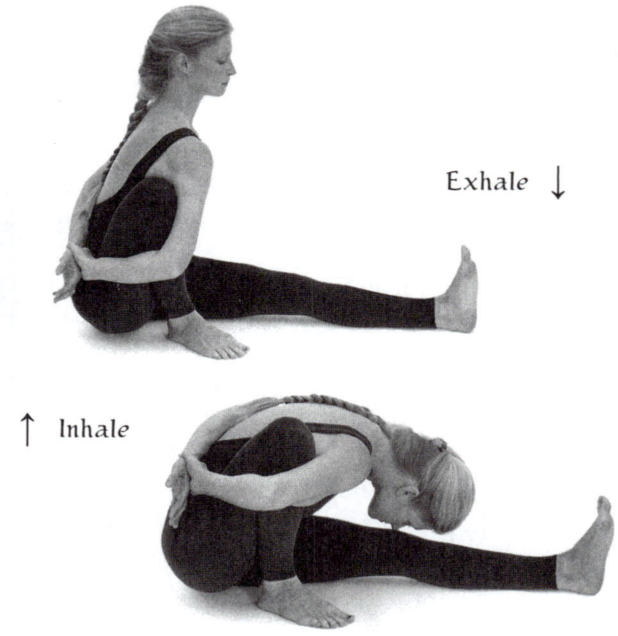

8.

Posture: Marīcyāsana.

Emphasis: To stretch muscles between shoulder blades and spine, and from shoulders to neck.

Technique: Sit with left leg extended forward, right knee bent with heel close to sit bone and knee toward chest. Wrap right arm, from inside of right thigh, around outside of right thigh and behind back. Wrap left arm behind back and grasp left wrist with right hand.

On inhale: Lift chest and flatten upper back, bringing left shoulder forward and keeping it as level with right shoulder as possible.

On exhale: Bend forward, bringing chest down toward left leg.

Repeat 6 times.

Wait, in a symmetric position, feeling quality of space in right shoulder.

Repeat on other side.

Details: Allow right sit bone to come off floor when bending forward. Allow left knee to bend on exhale.

9.

Posture: Dvipāda Pīṭham adaptation.

Emphasis: To stretch neck and upper back, spreading shoulder blades and massaging between them.

Technique: Lie on back with arms relaxed and pointing upward, fingers interlocked and palms down, knees bent, and feet on floor, slightly apart and comfortably close to buttocks.

On inhale: Press down on feet and, keeping arms relaxed, raise pelvis and lower chin until neck is gently flattened on floor.

On exhale: Return to starting position, extending arms upward, pulling shoulder blades away from spine, and feeling massage of upper back on the way down.

Number: 8 times.

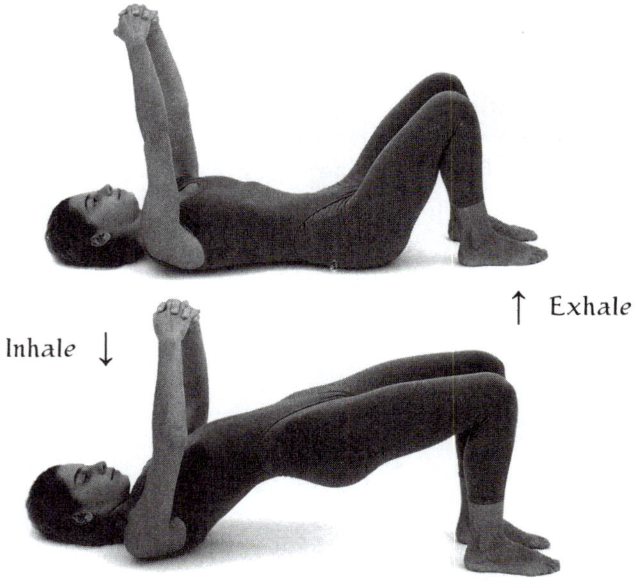

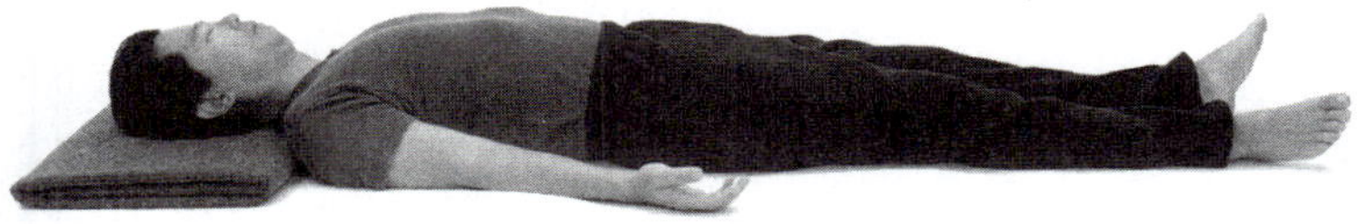

10.

Posture: Śavāsana with support.

Emphasis: To rest.

Technique: Lie flat on back with head on small pillow, arms at side, palms up, and legs slightly apart. Close eyes. Relax body fully, keeping mind relaxed and alert to sensations in body.

Duration: Minimum 3 to 5 minutes.

Working with the Neck and Shoulders (A Therapeutic Approach)

This practice was developed for G.R., a forty-three-year-old building contractor. His wife was a student at our school. He was suffering from chronic neck tension and pain, and also had recurring headaches. On the phone, he told me that his headaches had been getting worse, and that he realized that he had to do something to help himself.

In our conversations together, I learned that he had begun to back away from the heavier work of framing houses but was still involved with the finish carpentry. As we discussed his condition, he realized that the fumes from the finishes and the intense sounds and vibrations of the tools were significant contributing factors to his headaches.

As we began to work together, I could see that he had strong but very tight muscles. He could barely turn his head without displacing his shoulder girdle. G.R. was busy, and he felt that a fifteen- to twenty-minute program was all he could do. He said he would like to practice in the evening before bed.

We started with simple movements of the arms, shoulders, and head coordinated with breathing. Over the few weeks that we worked together, we evolved the following course. He told me that it not only increased the mobility of his head but that it improved his sleep.

I heard from his wife that he was very happy with the work we had done together. She told me that he had learned to reduce the tension in his neck and control his headaches through the practice.

About a year later, G.R. came back to see me. He told me that he had hurt his low back playing golf and was hoping I could help him. I told him I was surprised that he had the time to play golf, remembering how busy he had been. He told me that he had hired a foreman and was able to be off the job site more often. He had decided that he had had enough stress and strain on the job, and he said that he now spent more time working up bids and negotiating deals than cutting boards and hammering nails. He told me he much preferred using his body for sport and making a living with his mind. I asked about his neck pain and headaches, and he told me that they hadn't been a problem since the time we had worked together the previous year.

A Practice for the Neck and Shoulders (Therapeutic)

1.

POSTURE: Śavāsana adaptation.
EMPHASIS: To gently mobilize chest, upper back, and shoulders.
TECHNIQUE: Lie on back with knees bent, feet on floor, and arms down at sides.

On inhale: Raise left arm straight up over head and toward floor behind you.

On exhale: Return to starting position.

Repeat on other side.

NUMBER: 4 times on each side, alternately.
DETAILS: Move arm progressively farther toward floor behind you with each successive inhale.

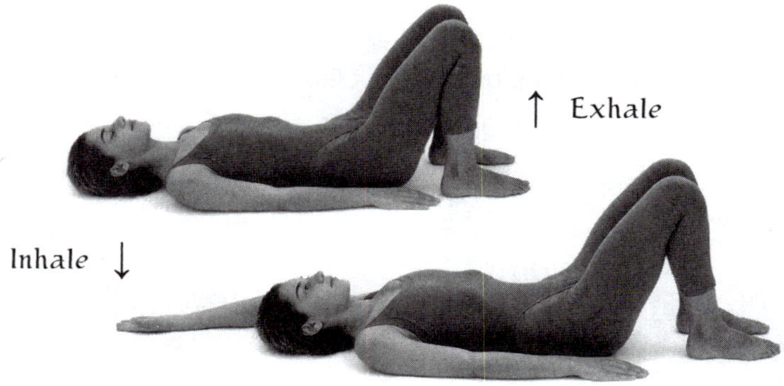

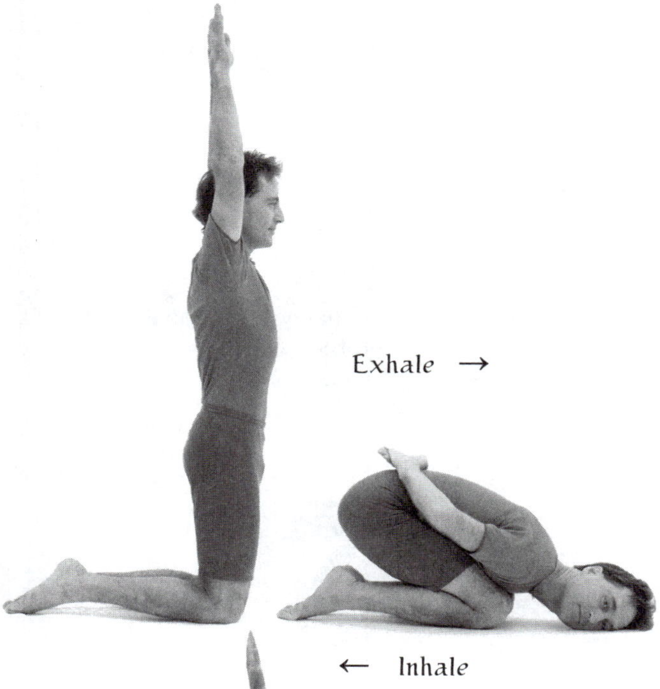

2a.

POSTURE: Vajrāsana.
EMPHASIS: To mobilize upper back and shoulders.
TECHNIQUE: Stand on knees with arms over head.

On exhale: Bend forward, sweeping arms behind back, and bring hands to sacrum, keeping palms up.

On inhale: Return to starting position.

NUMBER: 4 times on each side, alternately.
DETAILS: *On exhale:* Bring chest to thighs before bringing buttocks to heels. Rotate arms so palms are up and hands are resting on sacrum. *On inhale:* Expand chest and lift it up off of knees as arms sweep wide.

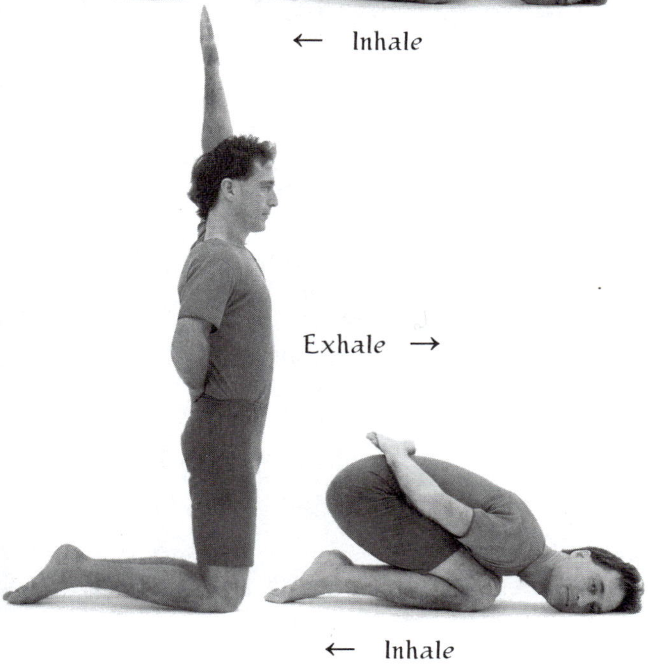

2b.

POSTURE: Vajrāsana, asymmetrical adaptation.
EMPHASIS: To gently stretch neck and to integrate neck and shoulders with arm movement.
TECHNIQUE: Stand on knees with left arm over head, right arm folded behind back, and head to center.

On exhale: Bend forward, sweeping left arm behind back, turning head to right, and resting on left side of face.

On inhale: Return to starting position.

Repeat on other side.

NUMBER: 4 times on each side, alternately.
DETAILS: *On exhale:* Keep buttocks higher than hips while resting side of face on floor. Keep most of body weight on legs.

3.

Posture: Dvipāda Pīṭham adaptation.
Emphasis: To stretch neck and shoulders, and to integrate neck and shoulders with arm movement.
Technique: Lie on back with arms down at sides, knees bent, and feet on floor, slightly apart and comfortably close to buttocks.

On inhale: Keeping chin down, press down on feet, raising pelvis and raising left arm up over head to floor behind, until neck is gently flattened on floor.

On exhale: Return to starting position, lowering left arm and turning head right.

On inhale: Move into upward position again, raising right arm and turning head center.

On exhale: Return to starting position, lowering right arm and turning head left.

Number: 4 times each side, alternately.

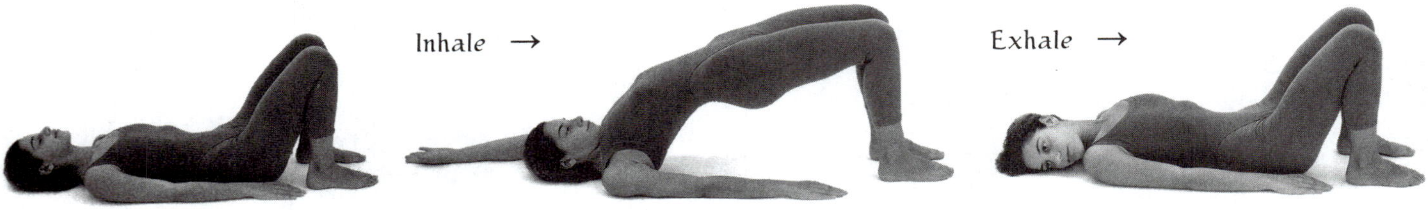

4.

Posture: Apānāsana.
Emphasis: To gently stretch low back.
Technique: Lie on back with both knees bent toward chest and feet off floor. Place each hand on its respective knee.

On exhale: Pull thighs gently but progressively toward chest.

On inhale: Return to starting position.

Number: 12 times.
Details: *On exhale:* Pull gently with arms, keeping shoulders relaxed and on floor. Press low back down into floor and drop chin slightly toward throat.

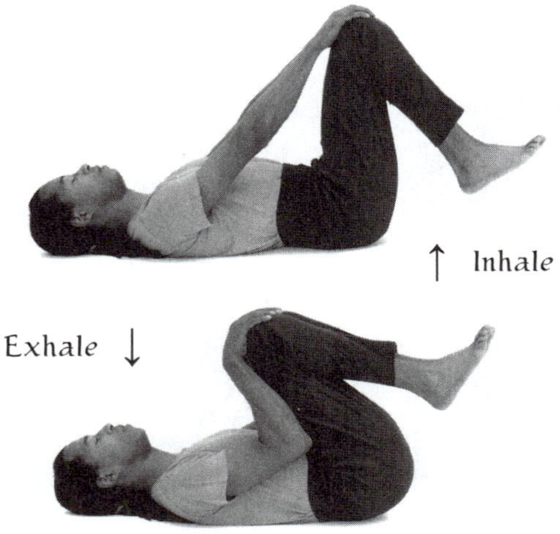

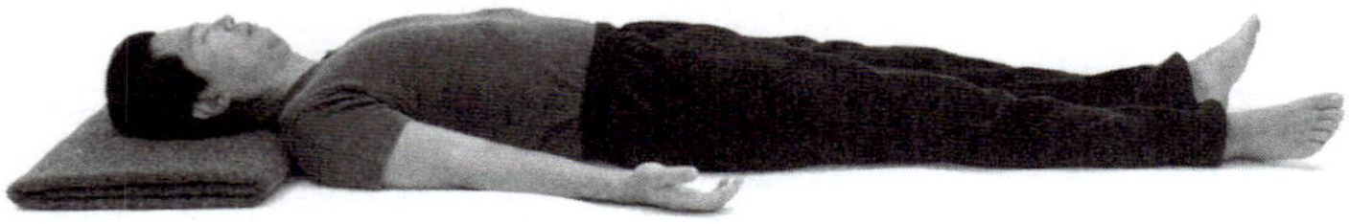

5.

Posture: Śavāsana with support.
Emphasis: To rest.
Technique: Lie flat on back with head on small pillow, arms at sides, palms up, and legs slightly apart. Close eyes. Relax body fully, keeping mind relaxed and alert to sensations in body.
Duration: Minimum 3 to 5 minutes.

Upper and Lower Back

Many people suffer from tension and pain in the back. These conditions are variable and relate to the condition of the spinal curves and their supporting musculature. They may involve mild to severe pain in the upper back (thoracic spine) and/or lower back (lumbar spine), and there may be mild to severe rigidity and restricted movement in either or both of these spinal segments.

As with neck and shoulder conditions, it is important to assess the cause of the pain. In particular, we want to find out whether there is serious damage to any of the intervertebral discs. If this is the case, there will be numbness or tingling sensations in the legs and feet, or sharp, electric, and immobilizing pains in the back. When these symptoms are present, it is best to seek professional diagnosis, because, while Yoga therapy may assist the healing process, the wrong practice may actually make matters worse.

In working with tension, restricted movement, and/or chronic pain, we need to consider the interrelated effects of three potentially contributing factors: our musculoskeletal condition; the neuromuscular patterns that condition our movements; and the biomechanical relationship that exists between the main spinal curves themselves.

General musculoskeletal conditions of the spine that may contribute to these problems include mild to severe examples of the following conditions: excessive curvature of the upper back (kyphosis), causing it to be accentuated and resulting in inward collapse of the chest, or decreased curvature of the upper back, causing it to flatten and resulting in "military spine"; excessive curvature of the lower back (lordosis), causing it to be accentuated and resulting in compression in the back part of the intervertebral discs, or decreased curvature of the lower back, causing it to flatten and resulting in compression in the front part of the intervertebral discs; and lateral displacement in the lower and/or upper parts of the back (scoliosis). All of these structural conditions relate to corresponding muscular imbalances, chronic muscular contractions, and/or muscular weakness. In addition, there may be intervertebral rigidity and corresponding movement restriction, or instability and corresponding hypermobility—all of which are causally related to habitual movement patterns.

The origin of these conditions may be congenital

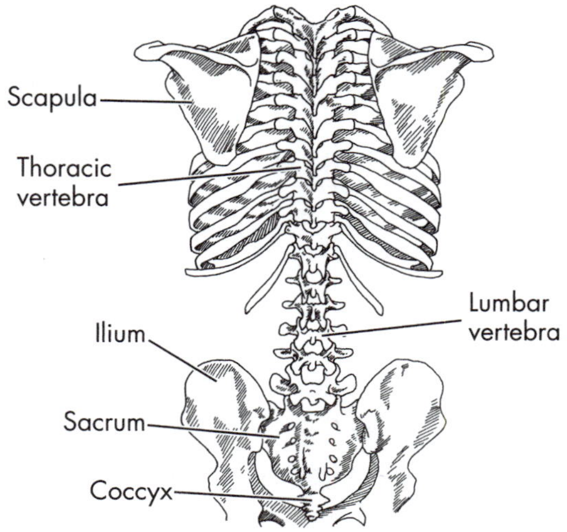

(from birth) or acquired. Individual tendencies in the spinal curves are usually established early in the growing process and may be exaggerated by repetitive activity. Excessive rounding of the thoracic curvature (kyphosis), for example, can be increased by any activity that requires long hours of bending forward, such as the work habits of an office worker, a taxi driver, or a dental hygienist. The congenital tendency to excessive curvature of the upper back can also be increased by carrying objects such as babies or groceries over long periods of time. And the congenital tendency to have a flattened upper back can likewise be increased by weight-bearing activity that requires the back muscles to contract. Curvature of the lumbar spine (lordosis) can be increased by natural developments such as pregnancy or carrying babies in the arms, and even dads may develop an increased lumbar curve by years of carrying their children. The tendency to excessive curvature of the lower back is also increased by wearing high heels or by sitting at a desk, leaning the torso forward toward a computer screen.

It is important to realize that conditions in the upper back and lower back are interconnected. If one spinal curve increases, the other usually increases to compensate. When, for example, a woman is in advanced stages of pregnancy, there is a tendency for the lumbar curve to increase and for the hips to push forward. This creates the dual condition of lumbar lordosis and sway back. In this condition, there would naturally be a tendency to fall forward. As a natural compensatory mechanism, the thoracic curve may increase, displacing some weight backward to help the body restore equilibrium.

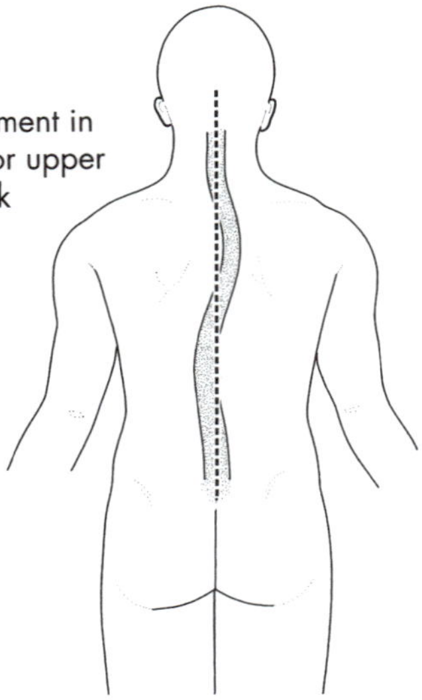

In addition to this kind of weight distribution, the supporting musculature will contract to support those body segments that are out of vertical alignment. As an example, from a standing position, and while holding a plastic water bottle in your hands, try raising your arms forward and up halfway, until they are parallel to the ground. You will notice a slight backward displacement of your shoulders, and, after a short while, you will also notice muscle tension in your shoulders and upper back. This is because both compensatory weight distribution and muscular contraction are necessary to maintain this position.

Upper Back

Let's take some time now to consider our upper backs. When the curvature of the upper back increases, the chest tends to collapse over the belly. Over time, muscles in the front of the spine tighten, and it becomes increasingly difficult to lift and expand the chest. Flattening an exaggerated curvature in the upper back involves not only strengthening the musculature that runs behind the spine, but also stretching those muscles that run in front of the spine.

Based on this musculoskeletal point of view, in āsana practice, the basic instruction given for inhalation is to simultaneously expand the chest horizontally, lift the ribs vertically, lengthen in the front of the torso, and flatten the upper back. This has the effect of strengthening the muscles in the back while stretching those in the front of the spine. Then, as the lungs deflate and there is less pressure in the thoracic cavity as a result of exhalation, we can also effectively isolate the middle and upper areas of the back and displace them forward.

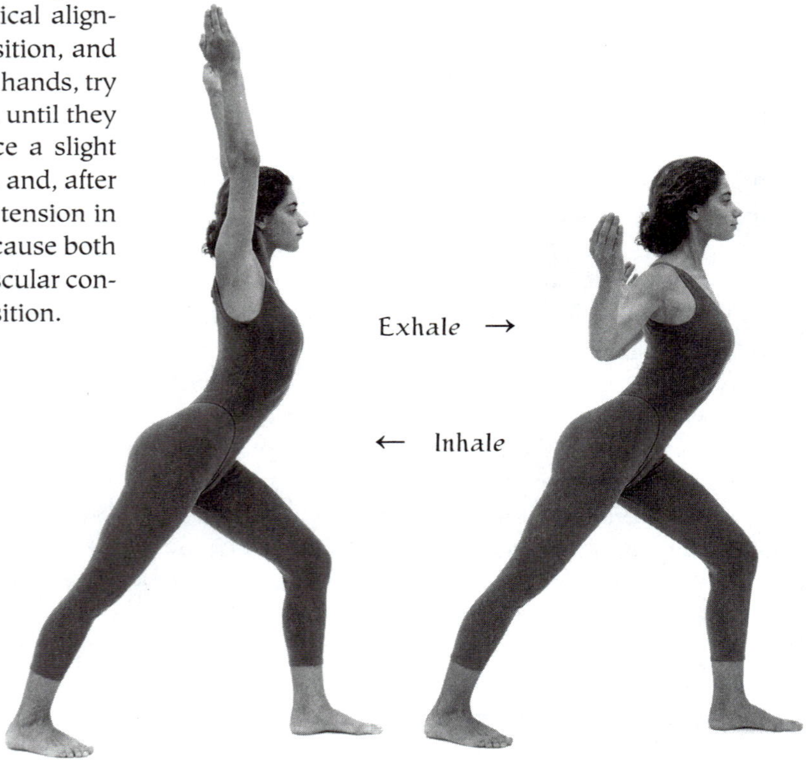

If we coordinate this process with movements of the shoulder girdle and the arms, we can deepen this effect. For example, if the shoulder blades are pulled back toward each other as the arms are opened wide, the rib cage expands and the upper back is pushed forward. As this action is repeated, muscles in the front and back of the spine are alternately stretched and contracted, increasing circulation, and strengthening and relaxing them. If the arms are also raised up over head, singly or together, we can deepen the stretching of the musculature in the front of the spine, relaxing it and allowing the chest to lift more freely. In fact, in the more advanced Yoga postures, we use the arms as levers to help expand the chest and flatten the upper back more intensely or to stretch the muscles in the front of the torso more deeply. Of course, using leverage increases risk to the joints and must be done with careful preparation.

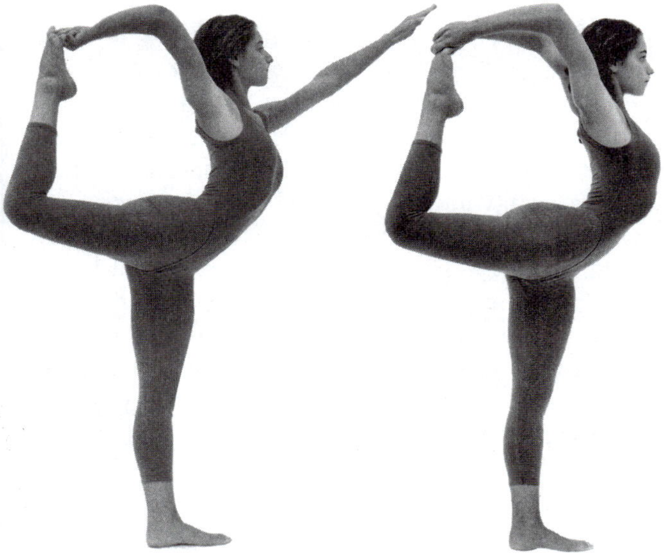

Both the lower back and the neck and shoulders can function as release valves for stress in the upper back. We must remember that in working to flatten the curve of the upper back, there is a great tendency to simply increase the curve of the lower back. And if we are successful in blocking the curve of the lower back, we must be careful not to bring too much stress to the neck and shoulders.

The first principle in working with an increased curvature of the upper back is simple movement coordinated with breathing. Sitting in a chair, move forward so that your back does not touch the back of the chair. Place the palms of your hands on the corresponding knees. On inhalation, raise one arm forward and straight up over your head. Take the arm back as far as is comfortable—behind the ear if possible—feeling the stretching on that side of the front of your torso and all the way down to the belly. On exhale, return the palm to the knee. Repeat on the same side a few times, waiting to feel the residual sensations in the front of your body. Then repeat the same procedure on the other side.

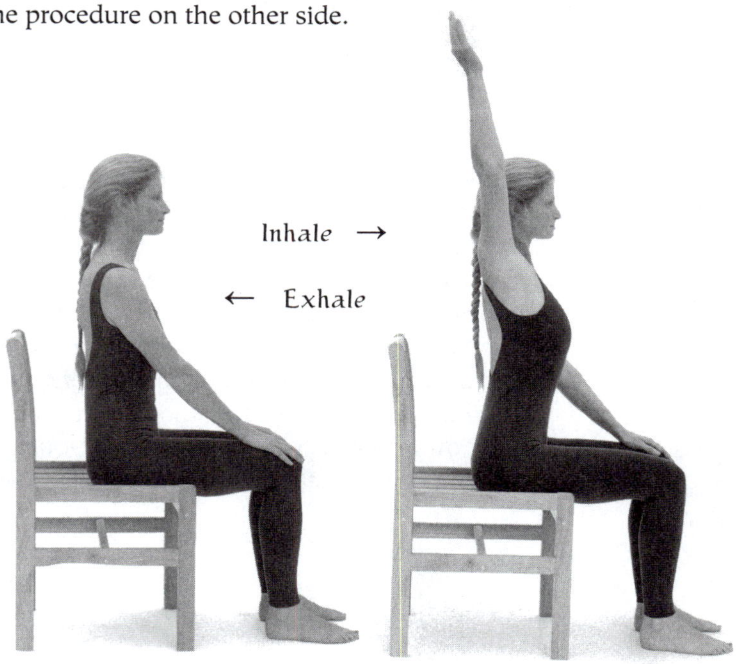

Next, place your palms together in front of your heart. On inhalation, while pulling the shoulder blades back toward each other, expand the chest horizontally and open the palms outward until they move behind your shoulders. At the same time lift the chest slightly up and away from the belly, feeling the stretching in the front of the torso. On exhale, return to the starting position with the palms together in front of your heart. Repeat several times.

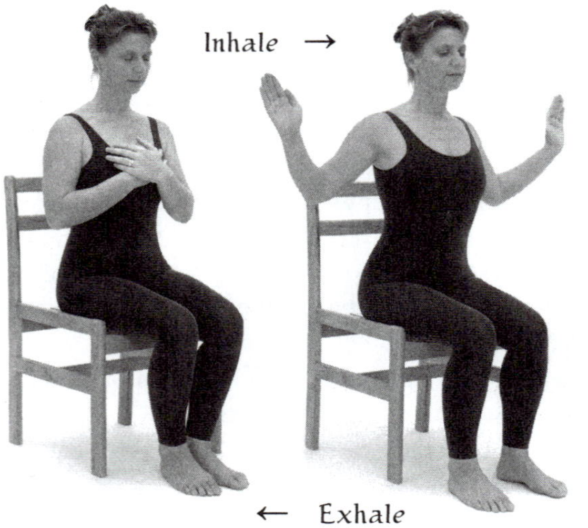
Inhale →
← Exhale

The next principle is that of using the arms as levers, and it is accomplished by using exhalation to push the mid-thoracic forward. Sitting forward on a chair, place both palms on your knees. On inhale, lift the chest upward, stretching the front of the torso, while pulling gently backward on your knees with your hands. On exhale pull a bit more strongly backward with your arms while pulling your shoulder blades toward each other and pushing your upper back forward. Repeat a few times and then relax. The arms can be used more strongly as levers when they are raised over the head or when the hands are behind the back.

In the practice that follows, you will experience examples of this action.

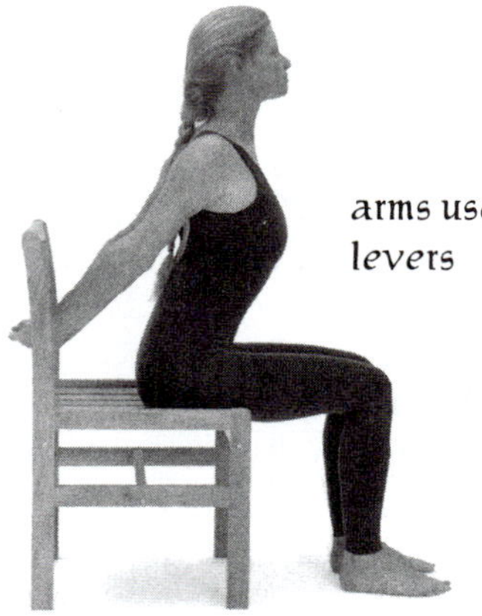
arms used as levers

These are simple exercises designed to show you the fundamental principles for working with increased thoracic curve. They are exercises that isolate the upper back and are primarily useful for their educational value. In practice, the upper back does not function in isolation but is dependent on the position of the lower back. Also, the muscles that run in the front and back of the spine connect all the way down to the pelvis. The sequence that follows is oriented toward working with conditions of increased curvature of the upper back and corresponding tension and mild pain.

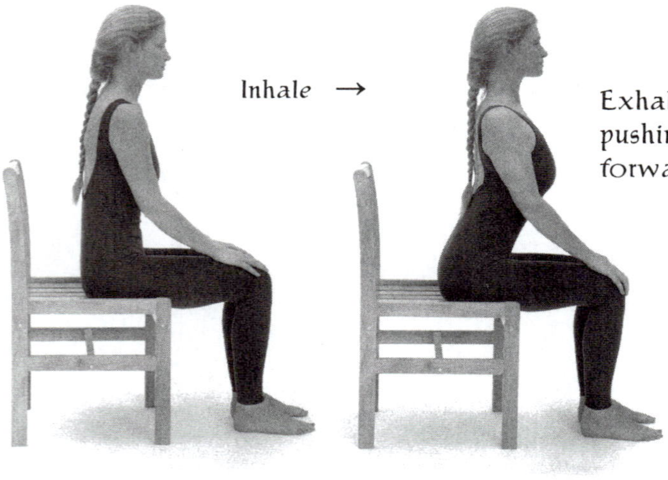
Inhale →
Exhale in position pushing upper back forward

Working with Kyphosis

This practice was developed for P.M., a thirty-four-year-old single mom. P.M. worked as a seamstress. She came because she felt that her posture was getting progressively worse. She recognized that carrying her baby and sewing were contributing factors to the problem of her posture, and she wanted to find a way to work with it.

P.M. had an exaggerated thoracic curve and a corresponding restriction in her inhalation. Over several months, we evolved the following practice. My strategy was to deepen her capacity to inhale, expand her chest and flatten her upper back, and to stretch her psoas, abdomen, and diaphragm.

Initially, P.M. resisted the practice. One day she came to me and told me she had had a dream where she angrily told me to leave her back alone! But after several weeks, she began to move through her resistance and actually enjoy the practice.

As we got to know each other, I asked her whether she had any plans for her future. Although she was a competent seamstress, it didn't satisfy her. I learned that she had completed all the course work necessary to take her teacher certification but had failed the exam several years back. She was so shocked that she had failed that she had just dropped it and returned to sewing. She told me that she could have taken the exam again but lacked confidence in herself and feared failing again. I reminded her about how she had persevered and overcome the resistance to working with her upper back, and I strongly encouraged her to prepare herself to take the exam again.

P.M. continued her practice and started coming to group classes once a week. In the following year, she passed her teacher's exam and found a job doing what she loves—teaching first grade. She tells me that she is happy with her job, feels more open in her body, and has more confidence in herself.

Upper Back: A Practice for Kyphosis

1.

Posture: Vajrāsana.
Emphasis: To warm up body, using movement to open chest and flatten upper back.
Technique: Stand on knees with arms over head.

On exhale: Bend forward, sweeping arms behind back, and bring hands to sacrum, palms up.

On inhale: Return to starting position.

Number: 8 times.
Details: *On exhale:* Bring chest to thighs before bringing buttocks to heels. Rotate arms so palms are up and hands are resting on sacrum. *On inhale:* As arms sweep wide, open chest, pull shoulder blades back, and flatten upper back.

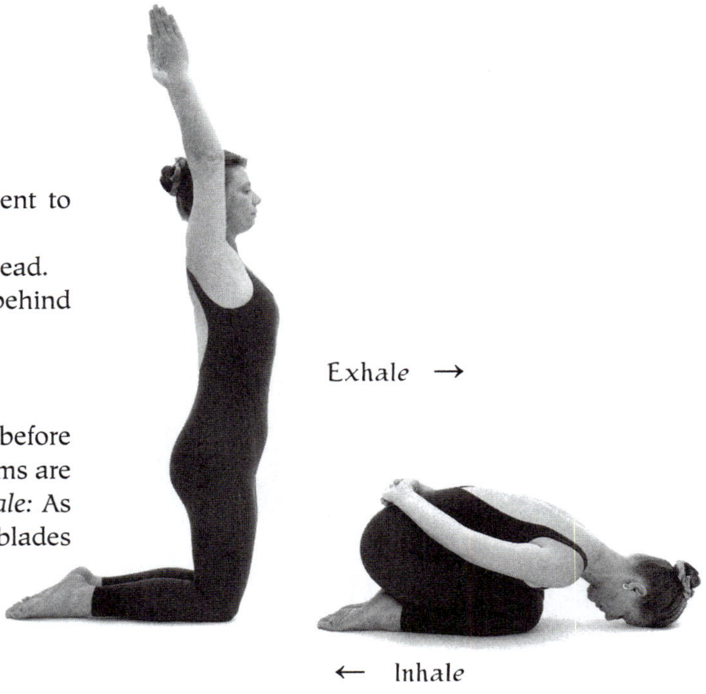

2.

POSTURE: Vīrabhadrāsana.

EMPHASIS: To strengthen muscles of back, expand chest, and flatten upper back. To introduce short hold after inhalation.

TECHNIQUE: Stand with left foot forward, feet as wide as hips, and arms at sides.

On inhale: Simultaneously bend left knee, displace chest slightly forward and hips slightly backward, bring arms out to side, with elbows slightly bent and shoulders back. After inhale hold breath 4 seconds.

On exhale: Return to starting position.

NUMBER: 6 times each side.

DETAILS: *On inhale:* Keep hands and elbows in line with shoulders. Feel opening of chest and flattening of upper back, not compression of lower back. Keep gaze forward and head level. Keep weight on back heel.

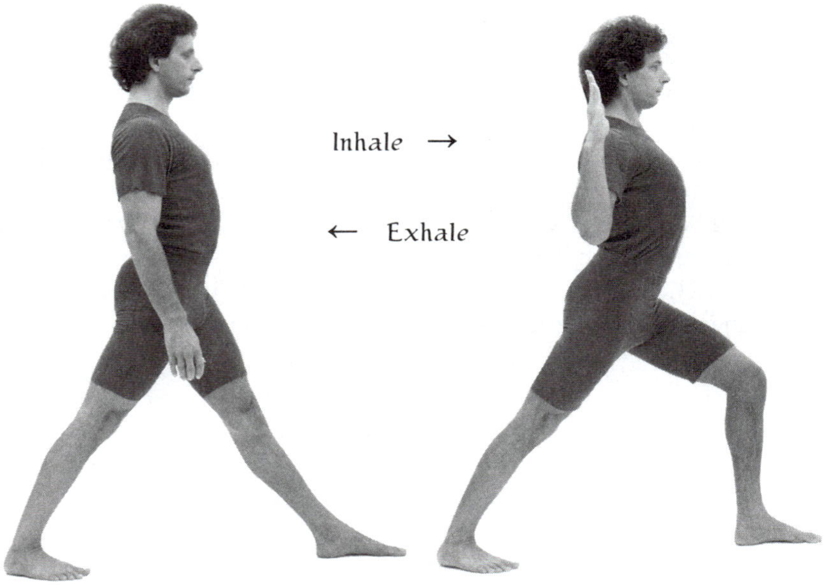

3.

POSTURE: Godhāpīṭham.

EMPHASIS: To contract musculature of upper back and flatten thoracic curve. To stretch front of torso, particularly psoas muscle.

TECHNIQUE: Kneel on left knee, with right leg extended straight behind, hands on floor on either side of left knee.

On inhale: Lift rib cage forward and up while pulling down and back with hands, pushing chest forward and flattening upper back.

On exhale: Bend elbows and lower chest to thigh.

Repeat 4 times.

Then stay up in stretch 4 breaths, each side.

DETAILS: *On inhale:* Pull down and back with hands, rather than pushing up. Drop shoulders and pull shoulder blades back. *On exhale:* While staying in posture, push mid-thoracic forward. Avoid compressing low back.

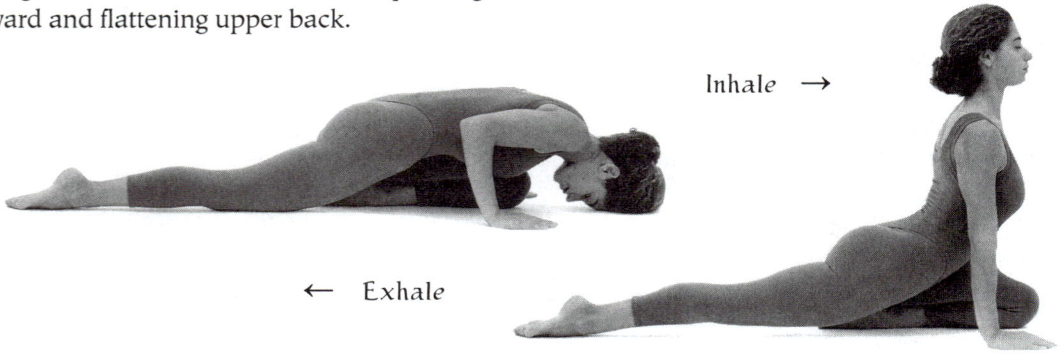

4.

POSTURE: Bhujaṅgāsana adaptation.

EMPHASIS: To gently stretch and expand rib cage. To flatten upper back with arm variation.

TECHNIQUE: Lie on belly with arms behind back, palms up and resting on sacrum, and head turned to one side.

On inhale: Lift chest, sweeping arms wide and forward, and turning head to center.

On exhale: Bend elbows and pull them back toward ribs, lifting torso higher and flattening upper back.

On inhale: Extend arms forward again.

On exhale: Return to starting position, turning head to opposite side.

NUMBER: 6 times.

DETAILS: When bending arms, keep palms and elbows at same level.

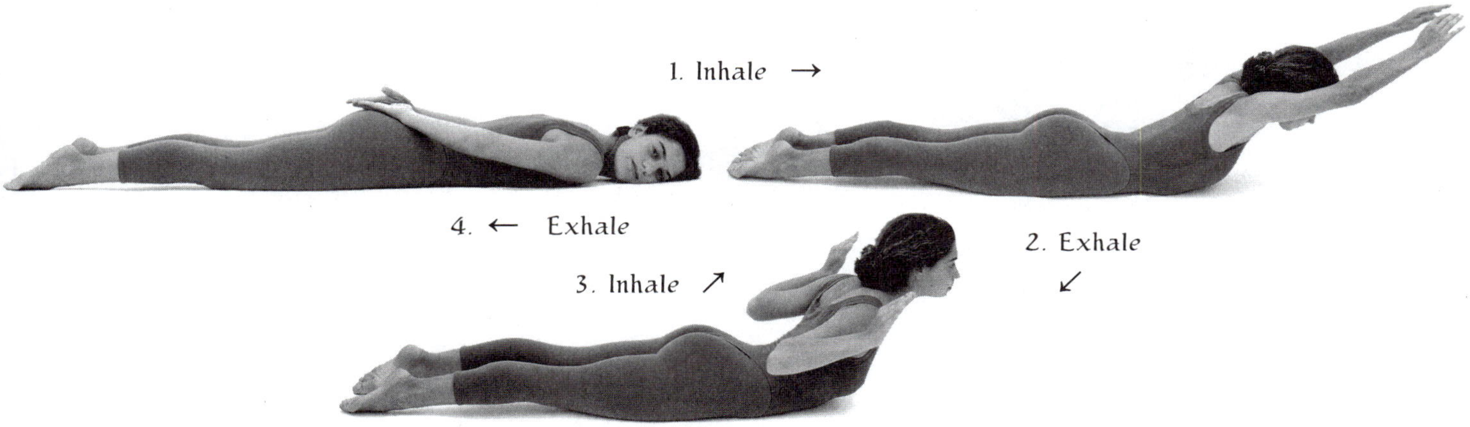

5.

POSTURE: Dhanurāsana.

EMPHASIS: To expand chest, stretch front of torso, and flatten upper back.

TECHNIQUE: Lie on stomach, resting on forehead, with knees bent and hands grasping ankles.

On inhale: Simultaneously, press feet behind you, pull shoulders back, lift chest, and lift knees off ground.

On exhale: Return to starting position.

Repeat 4 times.

Then stay in position 4 breaths.

DETAILS: While staying in position, lift chest slightly higher *on inhale*.

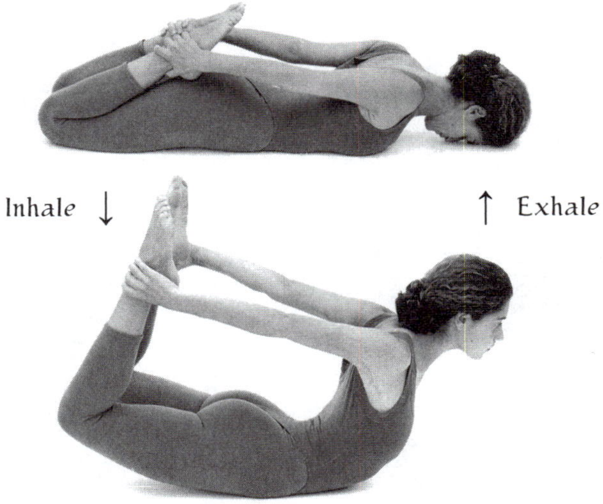

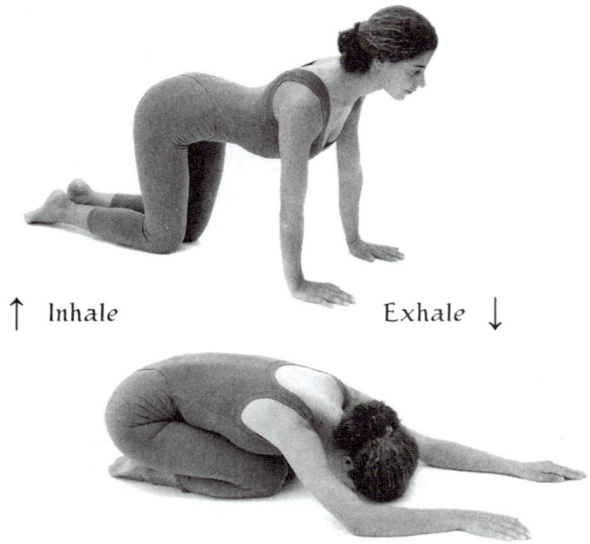

6.

Posture: Cakravākāsana.
Emphasis: To stretch and relax low back after deep back bend.
Technique: Get down on hands and knees, with shoulders vertically above wrists, and hips above knees.

On inhale: Lift chest up and away from belly.

On exhale: Gently contract belly, rounding low back and bringing chest toward thighs.

Number: 8 times.
Details: *On inhale:* Lead with chest, keeping chin slightly down. Avoid compressing low back; rather, feel chest expanding. *On exhale:* Round low back without collapsing chest over belly. Avoid increasing curvature of upper back. Let chest lower toward thighs sooner than hips toward heels.

7.

Posture: Ūrdhva Prasārita Pādāsana.
Emphasis: To extend spine and flatten it onto floor. To stretch upper back.
Technique: Lie on back with arms down at sides, legs bent, and knees in toward chest.

On inhale: Raise arms upward all the way to floor behind head and legs upward toward ceiling.

On exhale: Return to starting position.

Repeat 4 times.

Then stay in position 4 breaths, with fingers interlocked and palms out.

Details: *On inhale:* Flex feet as legs are raised upward. Keep knees slightly bent and keep angle between legs and torso less than ninety degrees. Push low back and sacrum downward. Bring chin down.

While staying in position: *On exhale,* Flex knees and elbows slightly. *On inhale:* Extend arms and legs straighter.

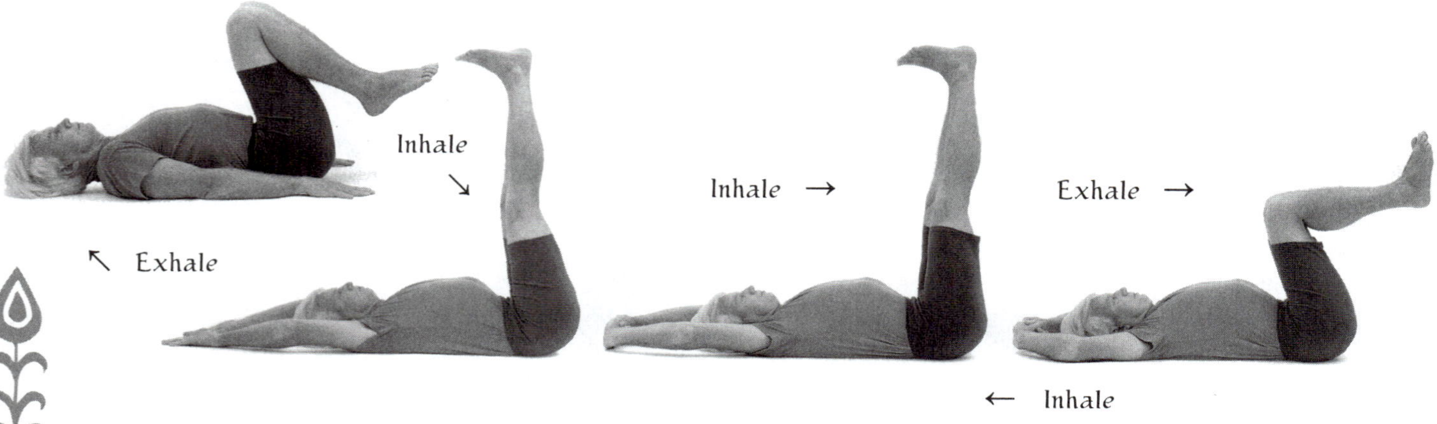

8.

POSTURE: Paścimatānāsana adaptation.
EMPHASIS: To strengthen muscles of upper back. To further flatten back with arm variation.
TECHNIQUE: Sit with legs forward, back straight, and arms raised over head.

On exhale: Bend forward, bending knees slightly, bringing chest to thighs, and palms to balls of feet.

On inhale: Leading with chest, lift arms and torso to forty-five-degree angle from legs.

On exhale: Bend elbows back toward ribs and displace upper back forward.

On inhale: Extend arms forward again.

On exhale: Bring chest and arms back to forward bend position.

On inhale: Return to starting position.
NUMBER: 6 times.
DETAILS: Same arm variation as used in numbers 2 and 4.

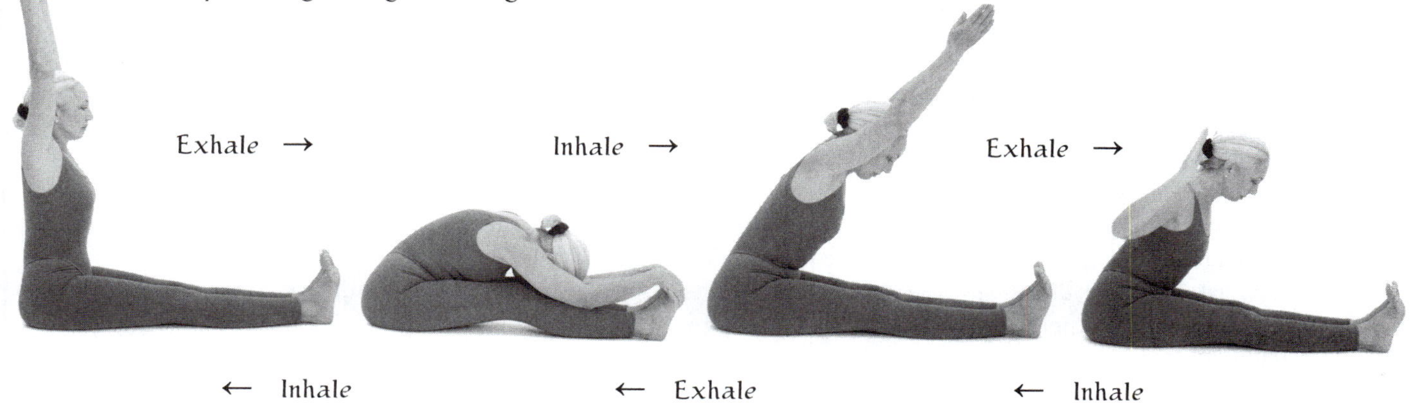
Exhale →
Inhale →
Exhale →
← Inhale
← Exhale
← Inhale

9.

POSTURE: Dvipāda Pīṭham.
EMPHASIS: To relax upper back.
TECHNIQUE: Lie on back with arms down at sides, knees bent, and feet on floor, slightly apart and comfortably close to buttocks.

On inhale: Pressing down on feet and keeping chin down, raise pelvis up until neck is gently flattened on floor and arms are overhead on floor behind.

On exhale: Return to starting position.
NUMBER: 6 times.
DETAILS: *On inhale:* Lift spine, vertebra by vertebra, from bottom up. *On exhale:* Unwind spine, coming down vertebra by vertebra.

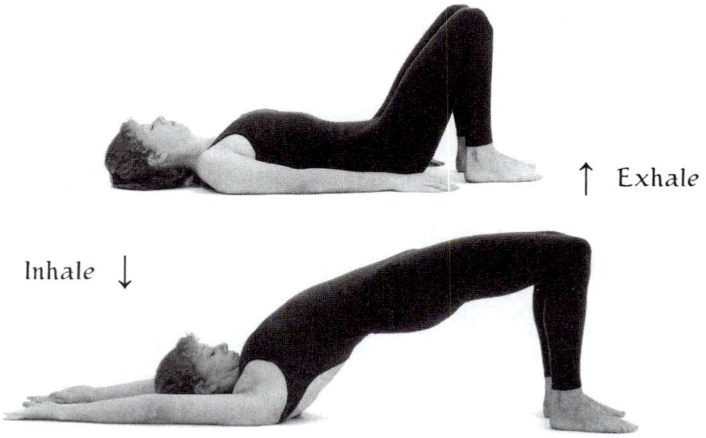
↑ Exhale
Inhale ↓

10.

POSTURE: Śavāsana with support.
EMPHASIS: To rest.
TECHNIQUE: Lie flat on back, arms at sides, palms up, and legs slightly apart. Close eyes.

Relax body fully, keeping mind relaxed and alert to sensations in body.
DURATION: Minimum 3 to 5 minutes.

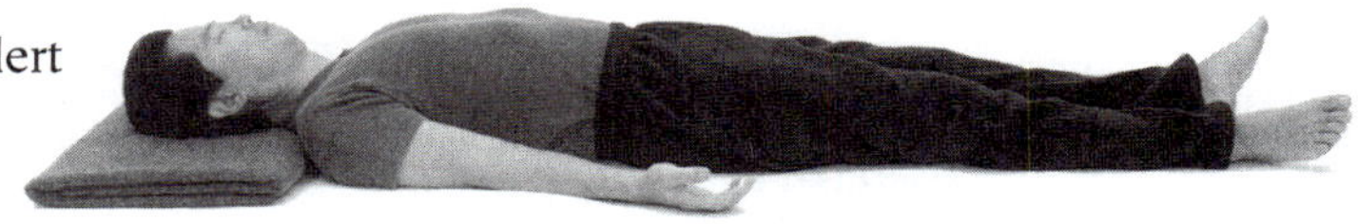

Lower Back

Now let's explore the lower back. Low back pain is perhaps the most common kind of structural pain and effects a large percentage of the population worldwide. In fact, many of the variations of this condition can be managed through simple Yoga therapeutic techniques.

It is important to understand that the curvature of the lower back (lordosis) is directly related to the angle of the pelvis. The lumbar spine rises up off its sacral base. If the pelvis is rotated forward, there will be an increased lumbar curve, sometimes referred to as a hollow back. When this occurs, there may be mild to severe compression on the back side of the lumbar's intervertebral discs. In this condition, the muscle groups running behind the lumbar spine are often chronically contracted, holding the pelvis in its forward rotation. Flattening the lumbar curve involves stretching these muscles as well as strengthening the abdominal muscles in the front of the torso. As the abdominal muscles contract from their insertion into the pubic bone, they rotate the pelvis backward, flattening the lumbar curve.

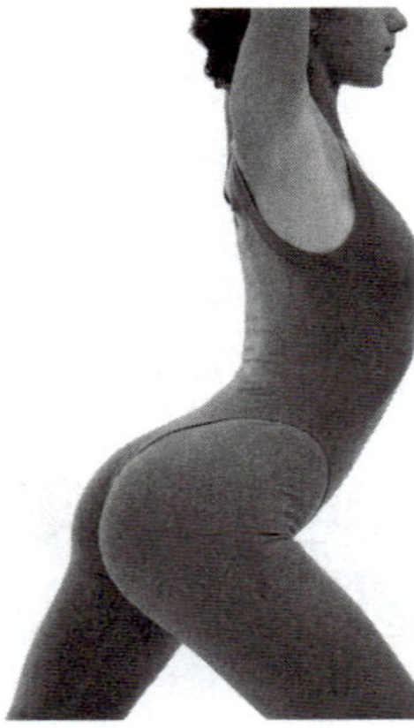

incorrect

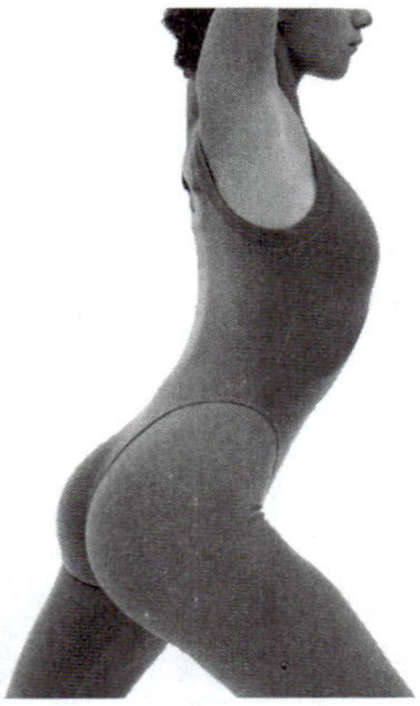

correct

Another important muscle group that relates to low back problems is the iliopsoas. These muscles run from the hips, through the pelvis, and are attached on the front of the lumbar spine. If the psoas is contracted, there may be mild to severe compression on the front side of the lumbar's intervertebral discs. If the muscles behind the spine are also contracted, then the intervertebral discs will be compressed in both the front and the back.

The condition of a contracted psoas may also be present in cases where curvature of the low back is too flattened. This condition is not as common as an increased curvature, and is most often either a congenital condition or one acquired in childhood development. This can be a serious condition, and must be managed carefully.

From the musculoskeletal point of view, the basic instruction given for exhalation in āsana practice is to contract the abdominal muscles, compressing the belly, pulling the pubic bone slightly upward, and flattening the curvature of the low back. This has the effect of stretching the muscles of the low back while strengthening the muscles of the abdomen.

Forward bending is understood as a development of this concept of exhalation and serves to deepen the stretching of the muscles of the low back. Backward bending, on the other hand, contracts the muscles of the back while stretching the muscles in the front of the spine. This alternation of contraction and stretching of the back muscles is important in healing low back pain, as it actually both strengthens and loosens those muscles, as well as stabilizes the pelvic/lumbar relationship. Backward bending can also be adapted to stretch the psoas muscles, which helps relieve intervertebral compression.

Both the upper back and the pelvis can function as release valves for the lower back. It is important to remember that, when we work to flatten the lumbar curve in forward bending, there is a tendency to increase the thoracic curve. If we keep the chest lifted and the upper back flat, we must then watch for the tendency to move from the hips, increasing stress to the lumbar/sacral junction. If the hips are loose, we have to block the forward rotation of the pelvis to assure the low back will be stretched.

The first principle for working with increased cur

vature of the low back is simple stretching movements coordinated with breathing. As an example, lie on your back with the knees bent, the hands placed on each knee, and the arms straight. As you exhale, tighten the belly below the navel, and bend the elbows, pulling the thighs toward the chest. Keep the neck and shoulders relaxed and the head on the floor. Push the low back down into the floor throughout the movement, avoiding the tendency to pull the low back up. On inhale, straighten your arms, bringing the thighs arms distance from the chest. Repeat several times. This type of simple stretching of the low back should feel good for all conditions except those involving more serious disc injuries.

The second principle is to alternate movements that gently stretch the muscles of the low back with those that gently contract them. These exercises will be part of the sequence that follows below.

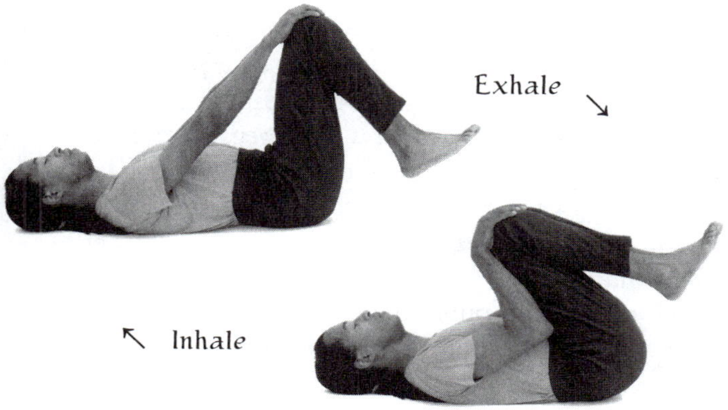

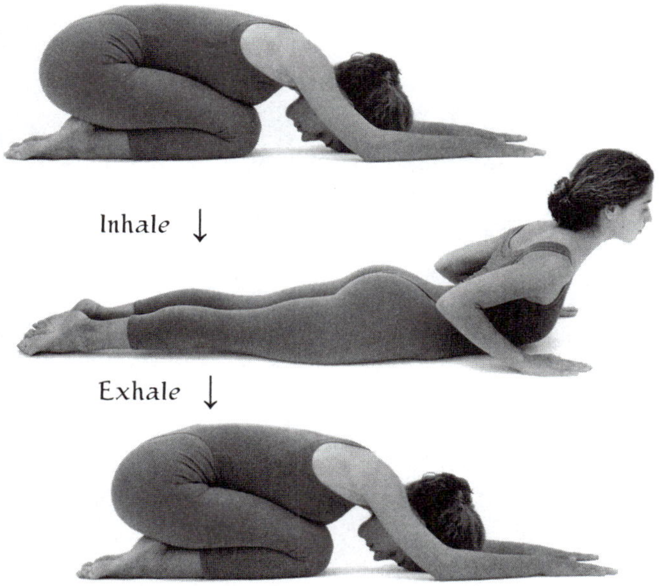

The next principle is to introduce movements that effectively stretch the psoas muscles. This usually means using asymmetrical postures, in which each side can be stretched independently. When stretching the psoas, we must be careful not to increase the compression in the low back.

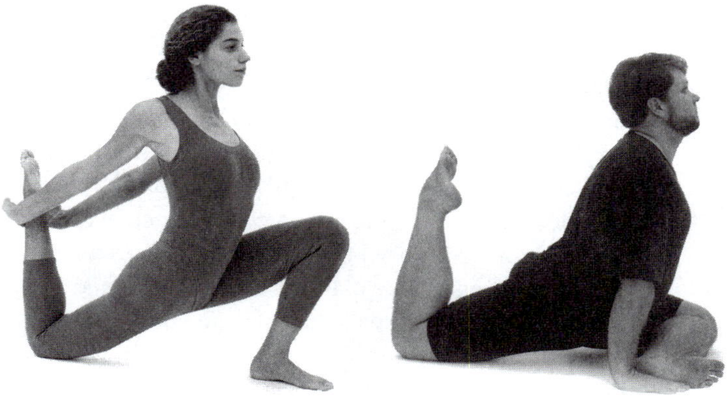

Again, the overall methodology is to begin with simple movements in which there is no pain, gradually increasing the parameters of movement and working to stretch and contract the back muscles alternately. This will increase circulation, release chronic contraction, and stabilize the area. In addition, the use of repetition will help develop new and more functional movement patterns that will carry over into daily activity.

The sequence that follows is specifically oriented to working with conditions of chronic, mild lower back pain.

Working with the Lower Back (Stretching and Strengthening)

This practice was developed for L.S., a thirty-eight-year-old successful sales representative for several major clothing lines in Hawaii. She came to see if Yoga could help her chronic low back pain.

L.S.'s work schedule was very busy. She spent a lot of time on the phone and in and out of her car, carrying boxes of samples to various stores. She also flew to the other islands regularly, with the same repetitive routine from car to store and back again.

When I asked her what else she did, she told me that she worked out regularly at the gym. I asked her if she ever slowed down. She told me she was actually afraid to stop. She told me that her husband had many creative projects that were "just about to make it" but that she had been more or less supporting them both for the past ten years. She confided that, although she loved him, she was very frustrated about the situation.

We met once a week for several months, during which time we evolved the following sequence. I observed that her hip joints were very mobile and that her low back muscles were tight and weak. My plan was to slowly stretch and strengthen her low back and stabilize the pelvic-lumbar relationship.

I had an occasion to meet L.S.'s husband, J.S., on several occasions. He was proud of his wife's success and, at the same time, ashamed that his own efforts were not bearing fruit. He told me that he felt he had to match his wife's success. His real love, he said, was playing classical guitar.

After some time, husband and wife came to meet me together. Our time was spent reflecting on different solutions to their situation. J.S. is now working with L.S. in her business and giving guitar lessons to children on the weekends. L.S. tells me that she feels her back is much stronger since she began her Yoga practice, and she rarely experiences discomfort. She told me that she never expected that finding a solution to her back problem might also lead to a solution in her marriage.

A Practice for the Lower Back

1.

POSTURE: Cakravākāsana.
EMPHASIS: To warm up body and to gently stretch lower back.
TECHNIQUE: Get down on hands and knees, with shoulders vertically above wrists and with hips above knees.

On inhale: Lift chest up and away from belly.

On exhale: Gently contract belly, rounding low back and bringing chest toward thighs.

NUMBER: 8 times.
DETAILS: *On inhale:* Lead with chest, keeping chin slightly down. Avoid compressing low back; rather, feel chest expanding. *On exhale:* Round low back without collapsing chest over belly. Avoid increasing curvature of upper back. Let chest lower toward thighs sooner than hips toward heels.

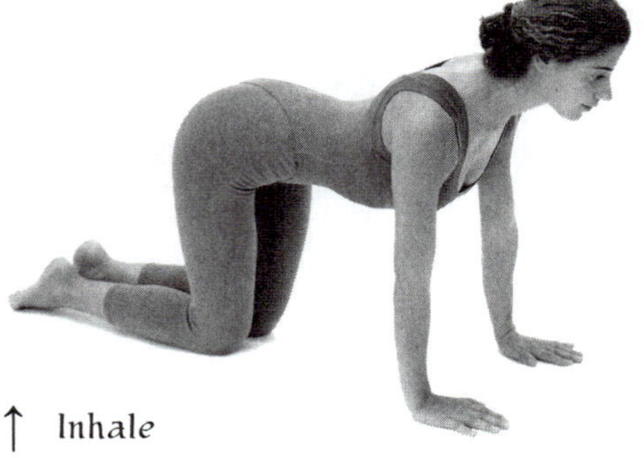

↑ Inhale

Exhale ↓

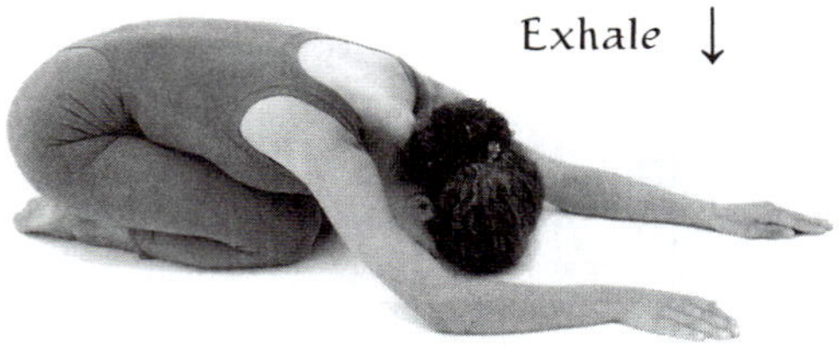

2.

POSTURE: Vajrāsana.
EMPHASIS: To further warm up body and to gently stretch back.
TECHNIQUE: Stand on knees with arms over head.

On exhale: Bend forward, sweeping arms behind back and bringing hands to sacrum, palms up.

On inhale: Return to starting position.

NUMBER: 8 times.
DETAILS: *On exhale:* Bring chest to thighs before bringing buttocks to heels. *On inhale:* Expand chest and lift it up off knees as arms sweep wide.

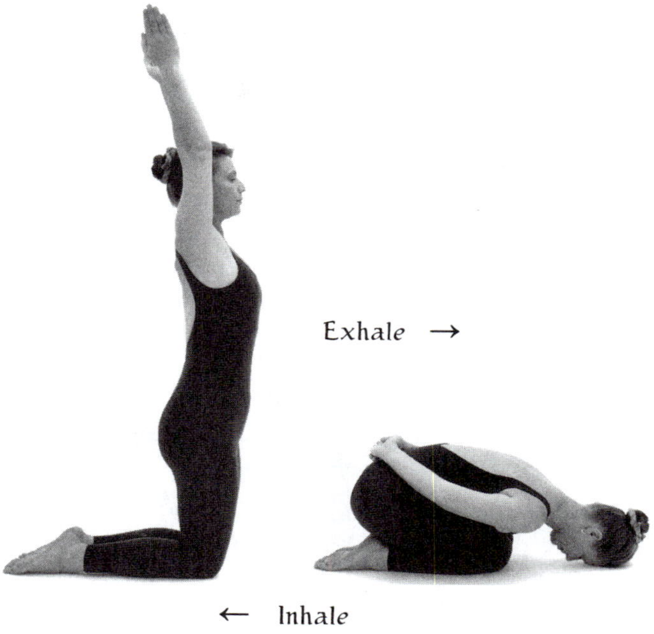
Exhale →
← Inhale

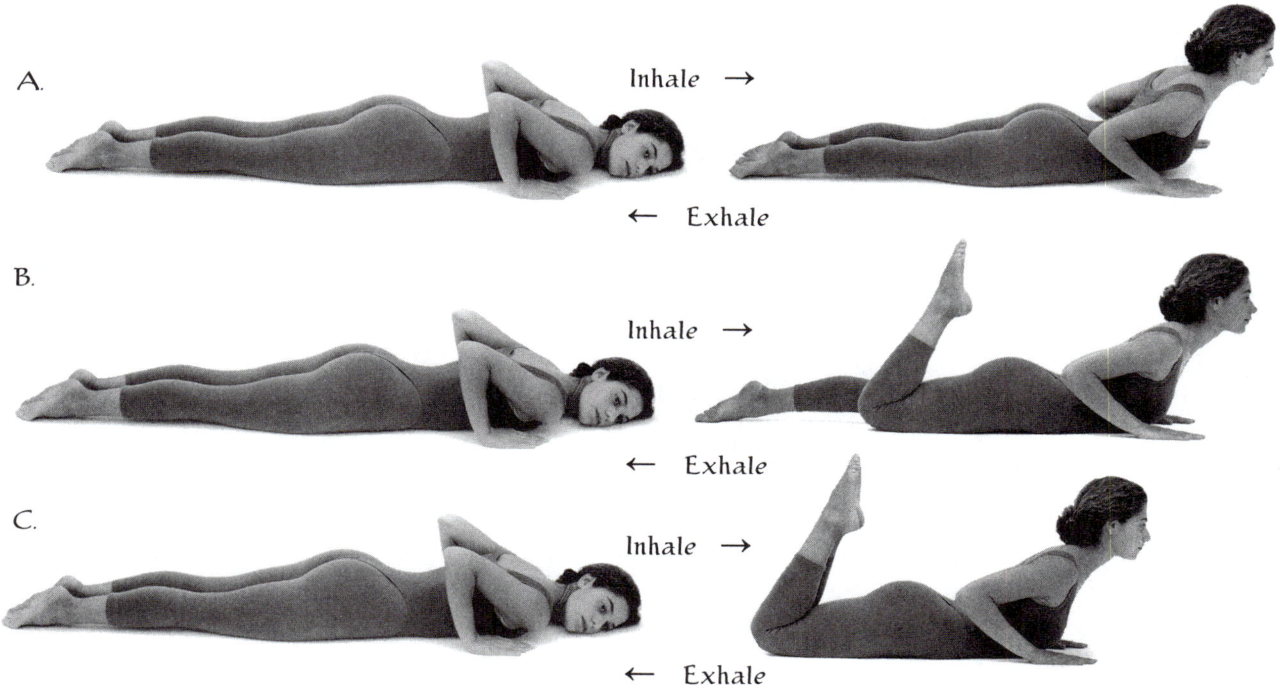
A.
Inhale →
← Exhale
B.
Inhale →
← Exhale
C.
Inhale →
← Exhale

3.

POSTURE: Bhujaṅgāsana adaptation.
EMPHASIS: To strengthen low back muscles and stabilize pelvic-lumbar relationship.
TECHNIQUE: Lie on belly, with palms on floor by chest and with head turned to one side.

A: *On inhale:* Lift chest, pulling slightly down and back with hands, turning head to center.

On exhale: Return to starting position, turning head to opposite side.

Repeat 4 times.

B: *On inhale:* As chest is lifted, bend one knee, bringing heel toward buttock.

On exhale: Return to starting position.

Repeat 2 times each side, alternately.

C: As in B, but bending both knees simultaneously.

Repeat 4 times.

DETAILS: Do not push chest higher with arms.

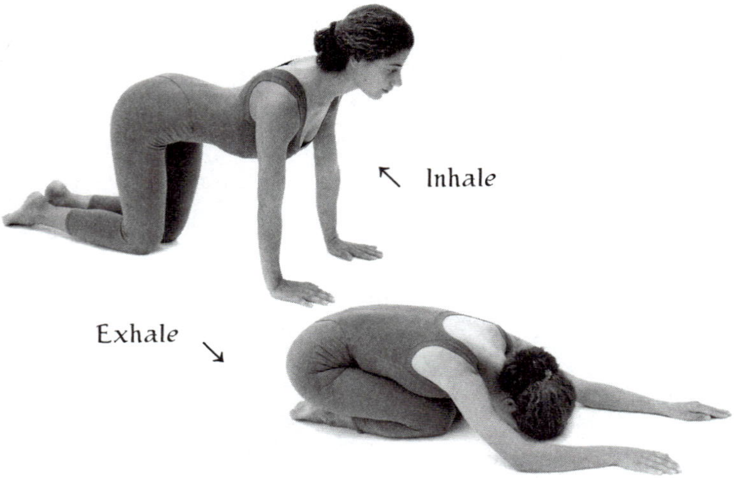

4.

Posture: Cakravākāsana.

Emphasis: To stretch and relax low back after back bend, and to make transition from prone to standing.

Technique: Get down on hands and knees, with shoulders vertically above wrists and with hips above knees.

On inhale: Lift chest up and away from belly.

On exhale: Gently contract belly, rounding low back and bringing chest toward thighs.

Number: 8 times.

Details: Move slowly, feeling gentle stretch in low back.

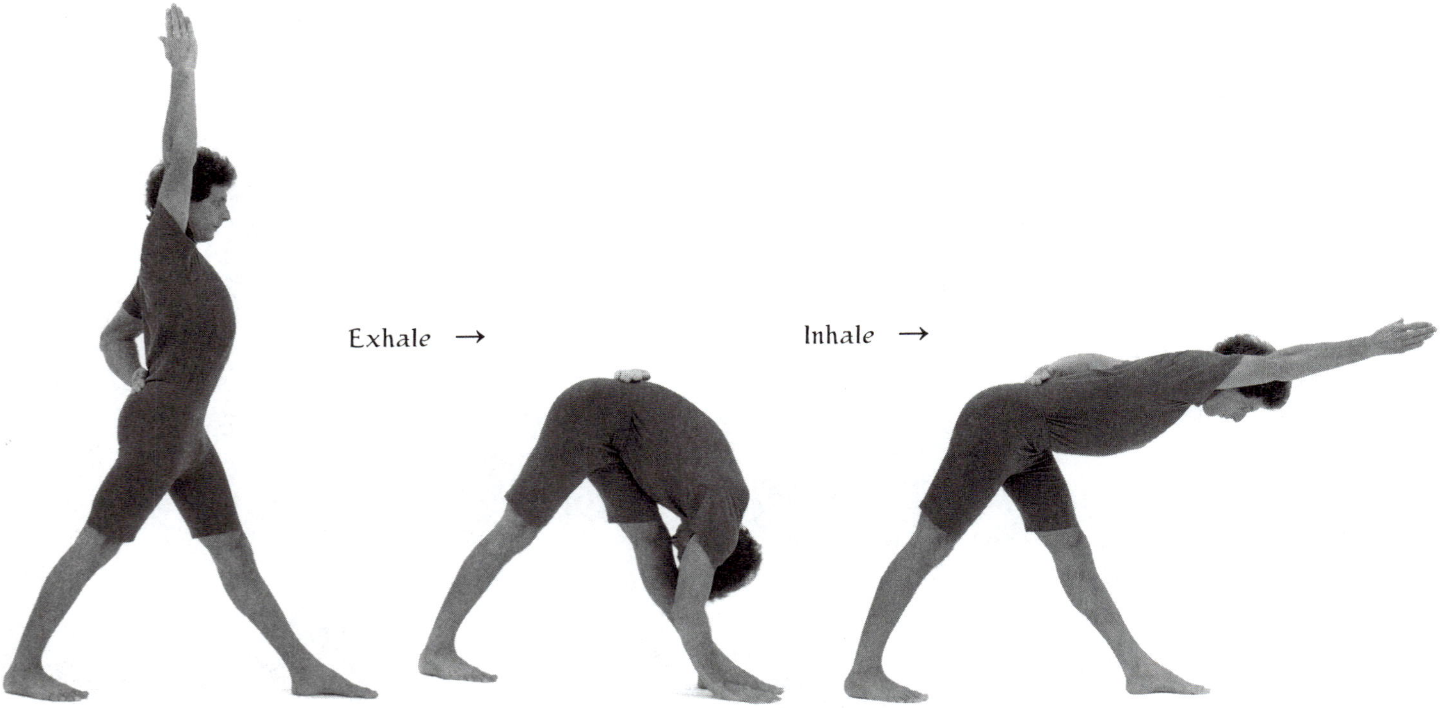

5.

Posture: Ardha Pārśvottānāsana.

Emphasis: To stretch and strengthen low back, one side at a time.

Technique: Stand with left foot forward, right foot turned slightly outward, right arm over head, and left arm folded behind back.

On exhale: Bend forward, flexing left knee, bringing chest toward left thigh and bringing right hand to left foot.

On inhale: Lift chest and arm until torso is parallel to ground.

On exhale: Return to forward bend position.

On inhale: Return to starting position.

Number: 4 times each side.

Details: Stay stable on back heel and keep shoulders level throughout movement.

6.

POSTURE: Godhāpīṭham.
EMPHASIS: To stretch front of torso, particularly psoas muscle.
TECHNIQUE: Kneel on left knee, with right leg extended straight behind, and hands on floor on either side of left knee.

On inhale: Lift rib cage forward and up, pulling down and back with hands, pushing chest forward, and flattening upper back.

On exhale: Bend elbows and lower chest to thigh.

Repeat 4 times.

Then stay up in stretch 4 breaths, each side.

DETAILS: *On inhale:* Pull down and back with hands, rather than pushing up. Drop shoulders and pull shoulder blades back. *On exhale:* While staying in posture, push mid-thoracic forward on exhale. Avoid compressing low back.

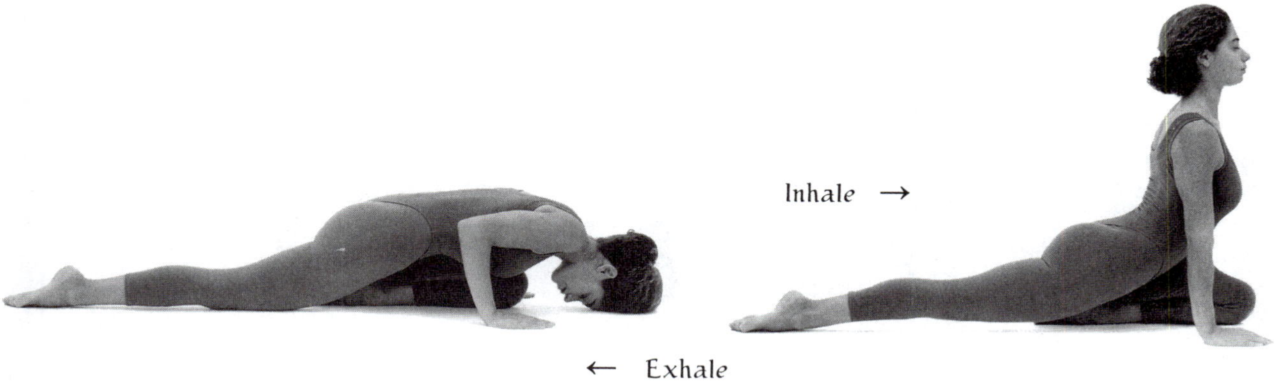

7.

POSTURE: Ardha Śalabhāsana.
EMPHASIS: To strengthen lower back.
TECHNIQUE: Lie on stomach, with head to left and palms on floor by chest.

On inhale: Lift chest and left leg, turning head to center.

On exhale: Lower chest and leg, turning head to right.

Repeat on other side.

NUMBER: 6 times each side, alternately.
DETAILS: *On inhale:* Lift chest slightly before leg and emphasize chest height. Keep pelvis level.

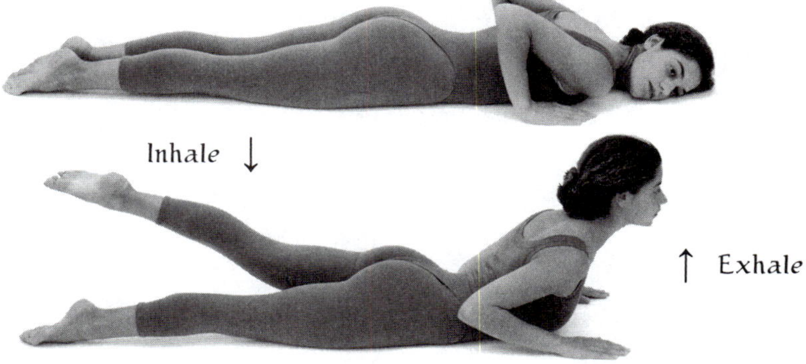

8.

Posture: Supta Eka Pādāṅguṣṭhāsana.

Emphasis: To gently stretch low back and to stretch legs, one side at a time.

Technique: Lie on back, with legs bent, left foot on floor, right foot lifted, hands holding right thigh behind right knee, and arms bent.

On inhale: Extend right leg upward, straightening arms.

On exhale: Return to starting position.

Repeat on other side.

Number: 6 times each side.

Details: *On inhale:* Flex foot as leg is raised upward. Knee can remain slightly bent. Push low back and sacrum downward. Keep chin down.

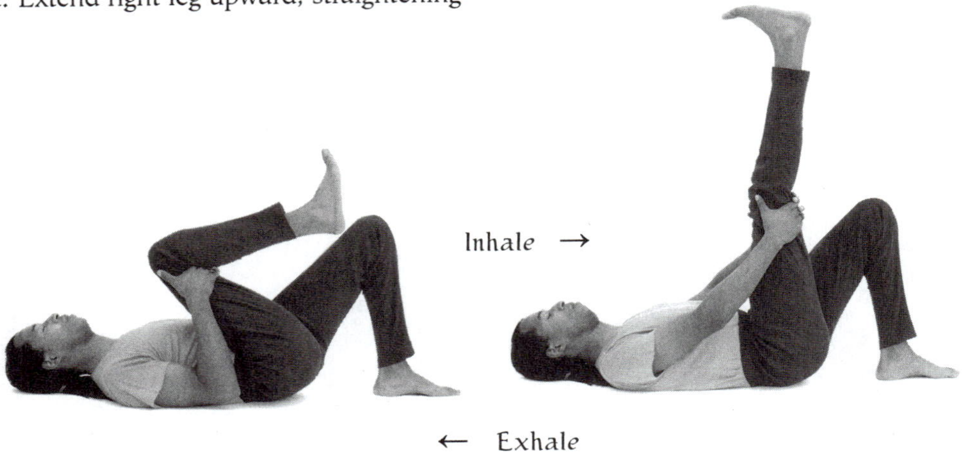

9.

Posture: Jānu Śirṣāsana.

Emphasis: To stretch lower back, one side at a time.

Technique: Sit with right leg folded in, heel to groin, left leg extended forward, right arm over head and left arm folded behind back.

On exhale: Bend forward, bringing belly and chest toward left leg and bringing right hand to left foot.

On inhale: Return to starting position.

Repeat 4 times.

Then stay down in forward bend position for 4 breaths, both arms holding left foot.

Repeat on other side.

Details: While staying in forward bend position: *On inhale:* Lift chest slightly, flattening upper back. *On exhale:* Sink from hips, bringing belly to thigh.

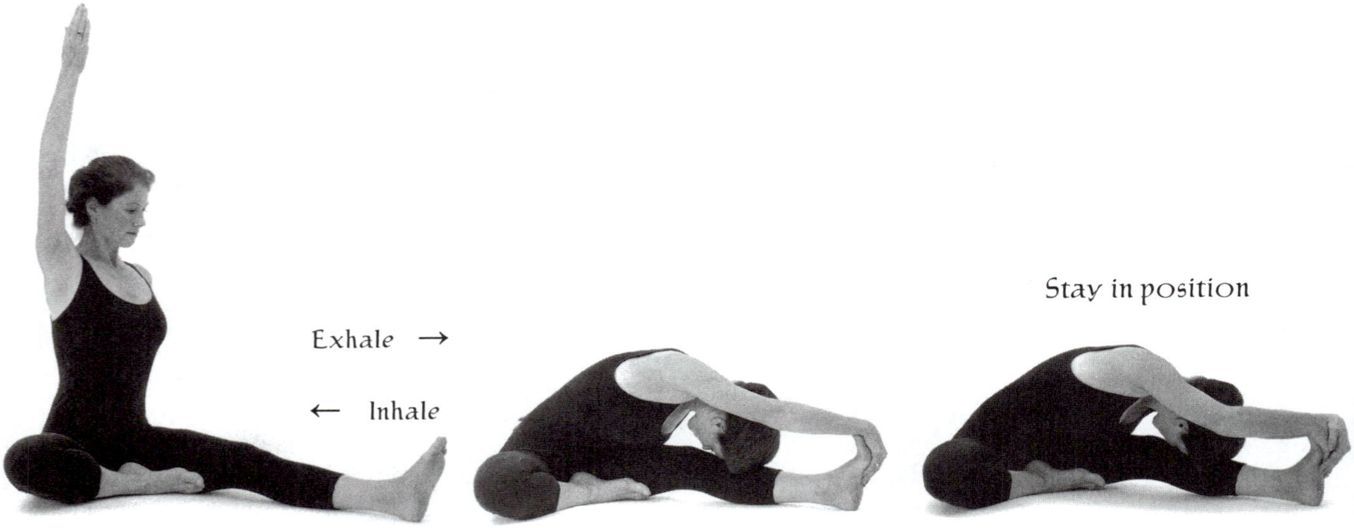

10.

POSTURE: Dvipāda Pīṭham.
EMPHASIS: To relax upper and lower back and to stretch between belly and thighs.
TECHNIQUE: Lie on back with arms down at sides, knees bent, and feet on floor, slightly apart and comfortably close to buttocks.

On inhale: Press down on feet, raising pelvis up toward ceiling, keeping chin down, until neck is gently flattened on floor, while raising arms overhead to floor behind.

On exhale: Return to starting position.

NUMBER: 6 times.
DETAILS: *On inhale:* Lift spine, vertebra by vertebra, from bottom up. *On exhale:* Unwind spine, coming down vertebra by vertebra.

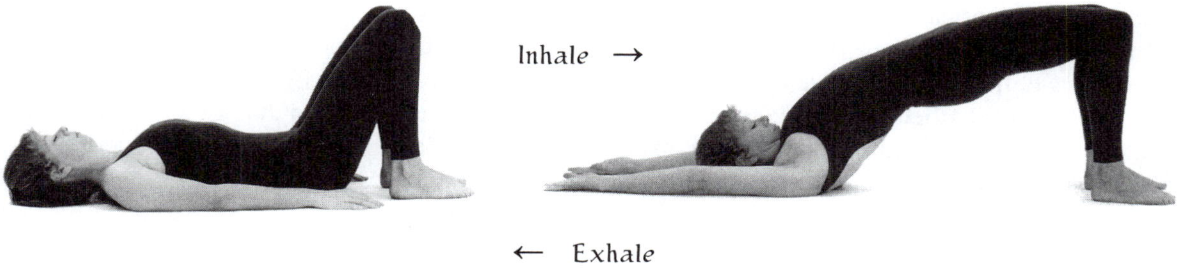

11.

POSTURE: Śavāsana.
EMPHASIS: To rest.
TECHNIQUE: Lie flat on back, with arms at sides, palms up, and legs slightly apart. Close eyes. Relax body fully, keeping mind relaxed and alert to sensations in body.
DURATION: Minimum 3 to 5 minutes.

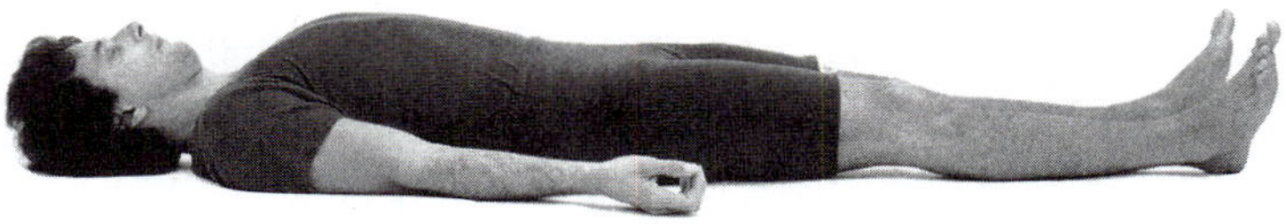

Scoliosis

Scoliosis is the lateral displacement and asymmetry in the spine. Scoliosis can be congenital or acquired. Though most of us have some degree of mild congenital scoliosis, this condition is increased by repetitive, one-sided activity. Common examples are the case of the mother who always carries her baby on one hip, or the professional tennis player, or even the professional truck driver who always wears his wallet in the same back pocket. Many children develop scoliosis from always carrying their books in one arm during the years of their primary development. Men who wear their wallets in their back pockets and who sit a lot at the office or in the car may even develop a kind of scoliosis. This is especially true if the wallet is thick with credit cards and cash! This simple habit creates a kind of stress in the spine and, over time, can even lead to serious back pain.

Congenital scoliosis is often more severe and can appear at any point along the spine. At the level of the pelvis, this condition can involve an S-like curve at the sacrum. The lumbar spine can also be severely curved. And, if there is a severe curve in the thoracic spine, the rib cage can be severely displaced. Often congenital scoliosis is a degenerative condition that, unless proper attention is given, can lead to serious problems with the back and even to organ disfunction.

There are different kinds and degrees of both congenital and acquired scoliosis. In all cases, there will be more muscular tightness on one side of the body than the other. If we look carefully at our bodies, we will see that for most of us there is some degree of imbalance between the muscles on the right and left sides of our spine. Usually one side is stronger than the other and one side has more tightness or restricted movement. Whatever the problem is, it will almost always involve the whole spine, from the sacrum through the cervical spine, as well as the pelvic and shoulder girdles. Except for the most extreme cases, these conditions respond very well to a well-conceived program of Yoga therapy. In working with them, we want to release contracted muscles and strengthen weak muscles. We want to work to bring more balance in the development of the spinal musculature. In other words: where there is hypermobility, we want to bring stability; where there is rigidity, we want to increase mobility.

The primary way of working with scoliosis is to do asymmetrical postures, so that we make each side of the body work separately and independently. If we do a symmetric posture, the looser side will absorb most of the work when stretching, and the stronger side will bear most of the work when lifting. The symmetric postures will often reinforce the imbalances, through compensation. The asymmetric postures enable us to isolate and make sure each side works. They will also bring our conscious awareness more directly to the nature of our imbalances, because of the difference in our experience when we work both sides. The more we understand this, the more we are able to adapt tools and restore or correct the imbalance.

As a general rule, we work with asymmetric postures symmetrically. That is, working both sides equally. This is important to avoid creating secondary imbalances through our work to restore balance! It may be useful to do the same number of movements on each side but make subtle shifts in the way we are moving on each side. In this way we can emphasize different things on each side while preserving balance in other areas of the body.

The following sequence offers a developmental approach to the condition of scoliosis and should be practiced when there are no conditions of acute pain.

Working with Scoliosis

This practice was developed for C.M., a sixteen-year-old student, who was brought to see me by her mother (a naturopathic physician) for help with her severe scoliosis. They first came together to group classes, to experience our work and see whether C.M. would like the practice. After some months, C.M. said she wanted to work out a program that she could do on her own.

When she was twelve, a doctor had told C.M. that her degree of scoliosis was often degenerative and that she might need surgery one day. She told me that since then she had been strongly motivated to work on her back. She had been taking regular dance classes for the past four years and was a very good dancer.

From her participation at our school, I knew that C.M. was in excellent physical condition. She was both strong and supple. She told me that she rarely experienced pain in her back. After the group class experience, C.M. told me that she realized that *Yoga was about her, not about performance.* She recognized that she could bring all of her energy and attention to work specifically on her body, and she was eager to learn more.

We took four sessions together to develop the following sequence. We worked out a general practice that emphasized asymmetric postures in order to stretch and strengthen both sides of her body independently. I asked her to pay careful attention to the differences she experienced from one side to the other in each posture that she practiced. I asked her to *let her mind link to her body through her breath* in order to feel more deeply what was happening as she practiced. I wanted her to develop as much awareness as she could about the imbalances in her body and how, through her own efforts, she could work with them.

C.M. tells me that she is very happy with her practice. She told me that since she has been practicing, she has become more aware of how she uses her body—both in dance as well as in normal daily activities. I see C.M. occasionally in group classes with her mother, who has become a regular student at our school.

A Practice for Scoliosis

1.

POSTURE: Vajrāsana.
EMPHASIS: To warm up body, gently stretching back, one side at a time.
TECHNIQUE: Stand on knees with left arm over head and right arm folded behind back.

On exhale: Bend forward, pushing left arm forward and bringing chest to thighs and hand and forehead to floor.

On inhale: Return to starting position.

NUMBER: 4 times each side, one side at a time.
DETAILS: *On exhale:* Bring chest to thighs before bringing buttocks to heels. *On inhale:* Lift chest and arm, flattening upper back upon return.

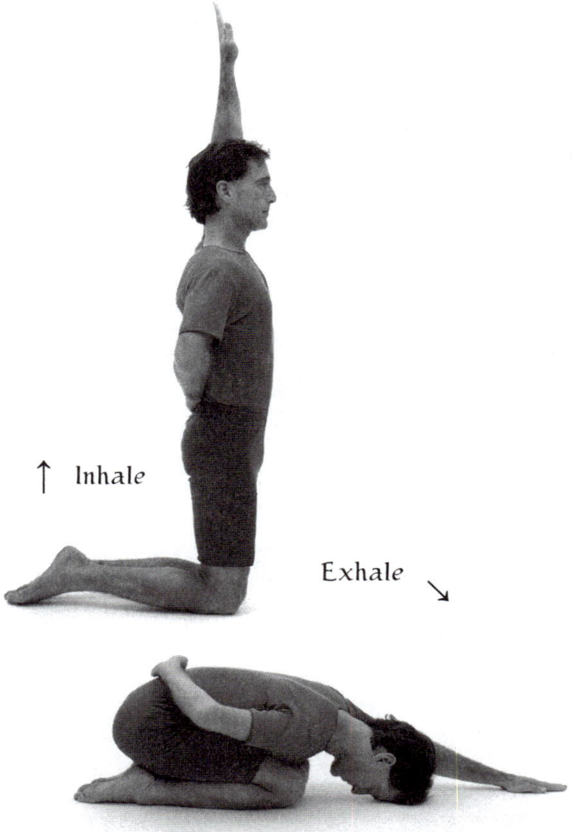

2.

POSTURE: Ardha Pārśvottānāsana.
EMPHASIS: To stretch and strengthen low back, one side at a time.
TECHNIQUE: Stand with left foot forward, right foot turned slightly outward, right arm over head, and left arm folded behind back.

On exhale: Bend forward, flexing left knee and bringing chest toward left thigh and right hand to left foot.

On inhale: Lift chest and arm until torso is parallel to ground.

On exhale: Return to forward bend position.

On inhale: Return to starting position.

NUMBER: 4 times each side.
DETAILS: Stay stable on back heel and keep shoulders level throughout movement.

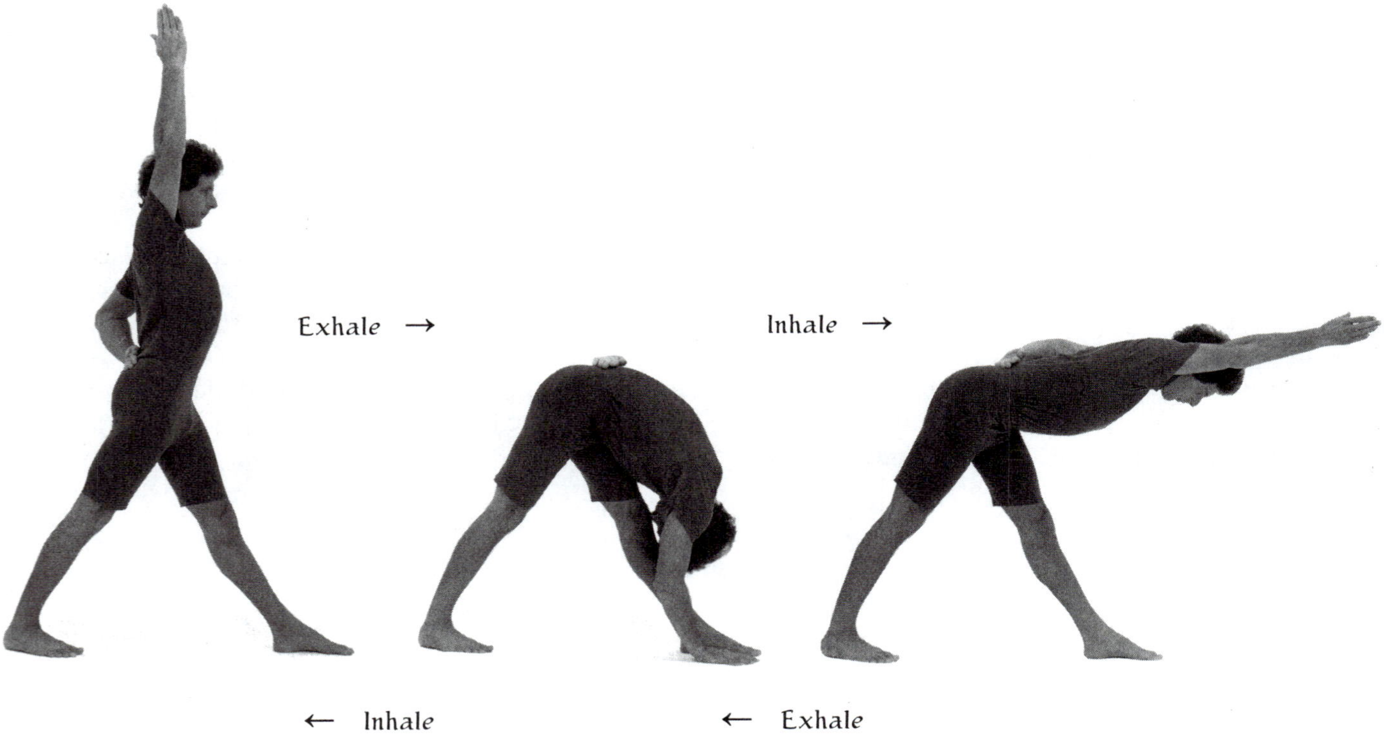

3.

Posture: Utthita Trikoṇāsana.
Emphasis: To laterally stretch torso and rib cage.
Technique:

A: Stand with feet spread wider than shoulders, left foot turned out at a ninety-degree angle to the right foot, left arm over head, and right arm straight down at waist and slightly rotated externally.

On exhale: Keeping shoulders in same plane as hips, bend laterally, lowering left shoulder and bringing left hand below left knee while turning head down toward left hand.

On inhale: Return to starting position.

Repeat.

B: With left hand down along left leg:

On inhale: Bring right arm up and forward while turning head forward toward right hand.

On exhale: Return right hand to starting position while turning head down toward left hand.

Repeat.

Number: Repeat A and B four times on each side, one side at a time.

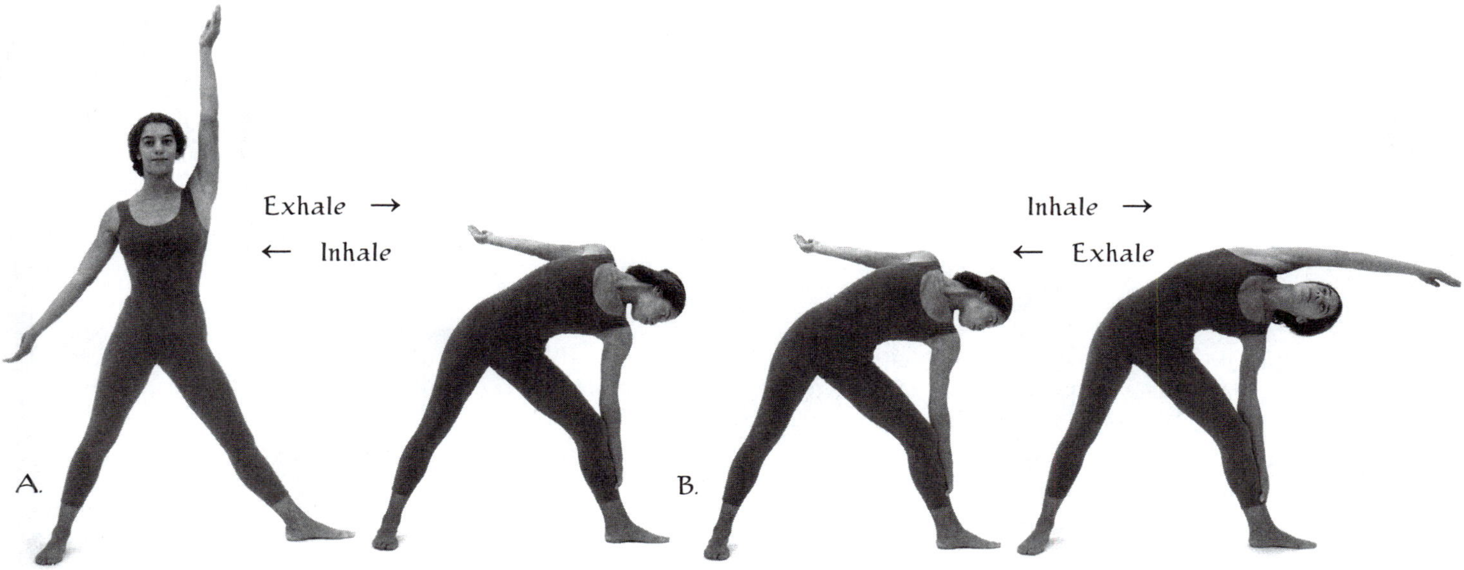

4.

Posture: Cakravākāsana adaptation.
Emphasis: To stretch low back, one side at a time.
Technique: Get down on hands and knees, with shoulders vertically above wrists, and with hips above knees. Put right knee 2 to 4 inches behind left knee.

On inhale: Lift chest up and away from belly.

On exhale: Gently contract belly, round low back, and bring chest toward thighs.

Number: 4 times each side, one side at a time.
Details: Move slowly, feeling a gentle one-sided stretch in low back and sacrum.

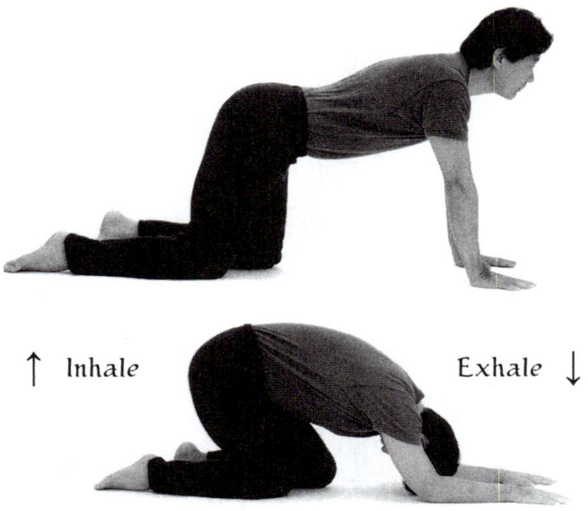

5.

POSTURE: Dvipāda Pīṭham adaptation.
EMPHASIS: To stretch neck and upper back asymmetrically.
TECHNIQUE: Lie on back with arms down at sides, knees bent, and feet on floor, slightly apart and comfortably close to buttocks.

On inhale: Keeping chin down, press down on feet, raising pelvis and raising left arm up over head to floor behind, until neck is gently flattened on floor.

On exhale: Return to starting position, leaving left arm over head.

On inhale: Move into upward position again.

On exhale: Return to starting position with arms at side.

NUMBER: 4 times each side, alternately.
DETAILS: *On inhale:* Lift spine vertebra by vertebra, from the bottom up. *On exhale:* Unwind spine, coming down vertebra by vertebra.

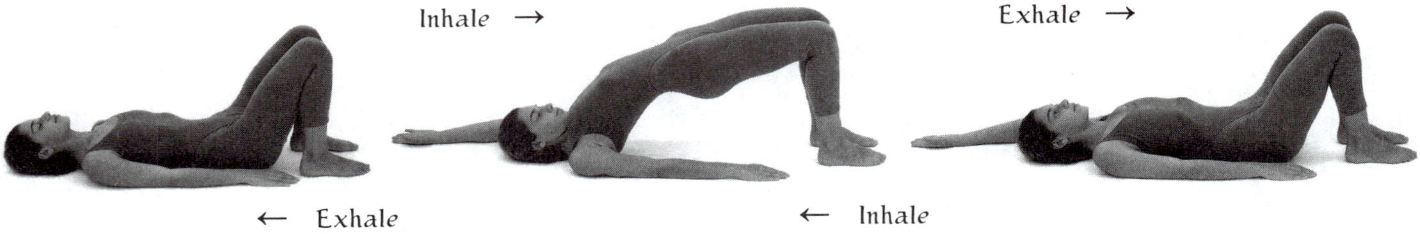

6.

POSTURE: Sarvāṅgāsana and Ekapāda Sarvāṅgāsana/Ākuñcanāsana variation.
EMPHASIS: To stretch and strengthen musculature of torso, emphasizing one side at a time.
TECHNIQUE: Lie on back.

On exhale: Raise legs and torso to shoulder stand position, placing palms on middle back for support. Keep low back slightly rounded with feet above eyes.

Stay 8 breaths.

On exhale: Lower left knee toward left shoulder.

Stay and inhale.

On exhale: Lower right leg straight toward floor behind head.

On inhale: Raise only right leg.

Repeat slowly 4 times.

Repeat on other side.

DETAILS: Move straight leg down and up slowly, keeping bent knee stable and toward chest, with heel near sit bone.

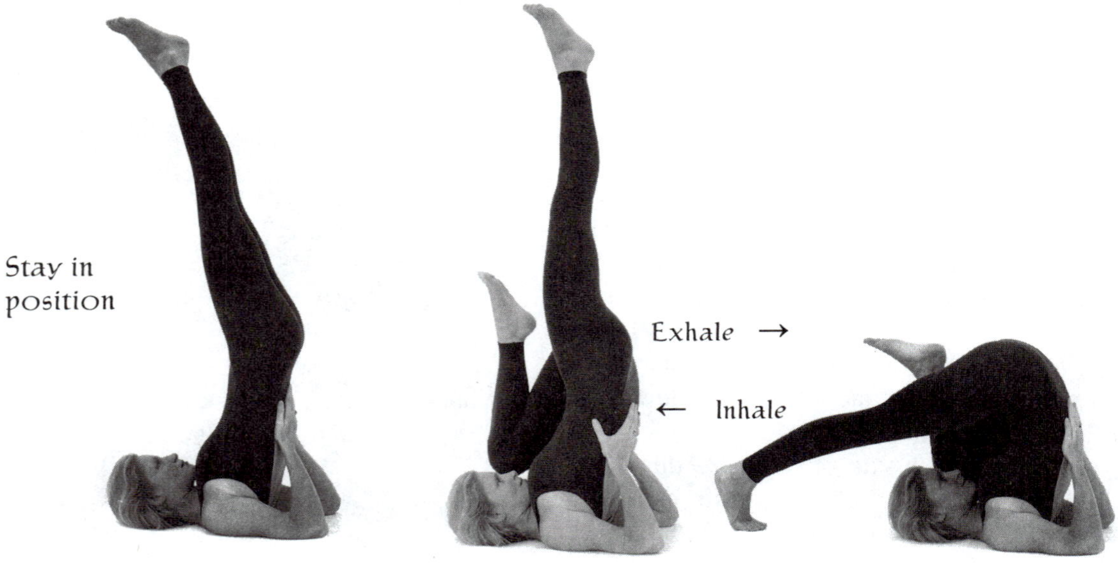

7.

POSTURE: Ardha Śalabhāsana.
EMPHASIS: To strengthen musculature of back, emphasizing one side at a time.
TECHNIQUE: Lie on stomach, with head turned to right, arms folded behind back, and palms up.

On inhale: Lift chest, right arm, and left leg, turning head to center.

On exhale: Lower chest and leg, turning head to left.

Repeat on other side.

NUMBER: 6 times each side, alternately.
DETAILS: *On inhale:* Lift chest slightly before leg, and emphasize chest height. Keep pelvis level.

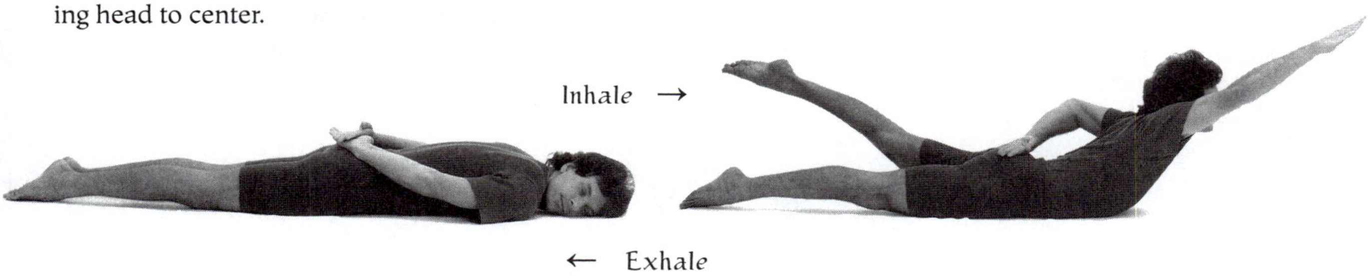

8.

POSTURE: Ūrdhva Prasārita Pādāsana, one side at a time.
EMPHASIS: To gently stretch low back and to stretch legs, emphasizing one side at a time.
TECHNIQUE: Lie on back with both knees lifted toward chest, feet off floor.

On inhale: Extend left leg upward, raising right arm up and over head to floor behind you.

On exhale: Return to starting position.

Repeat on other side.

NUMBER: 6 times each side, alternately.
DETAILS: *On inhale:* Flex foot as leg is raised upward. Knee can remain slightly bent. Low back and sacrum push downward. Chin is down.

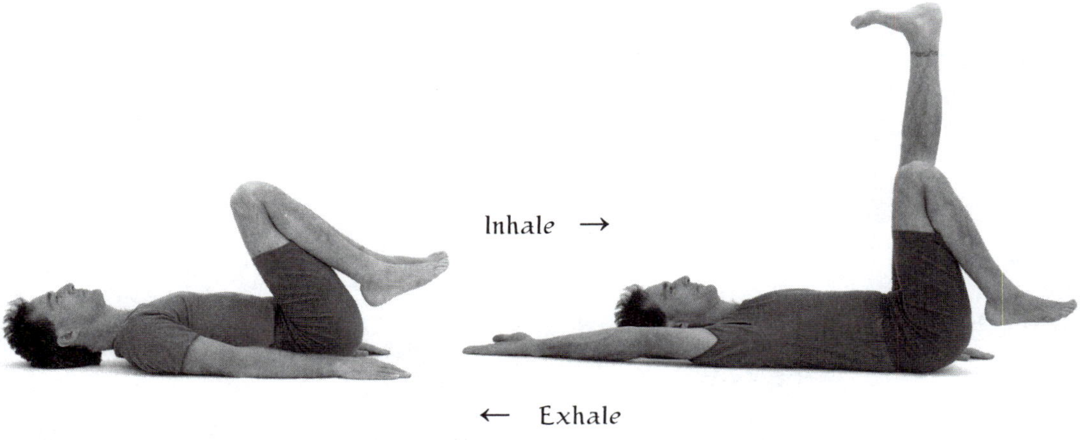

9.

POSTURE: Jaṭhara Parivṛtti.
EMPHASIS: To stretch across hips and back, one side at a time.
TECHNIQUE: Lie flat on back, with arms out to sides, and with left knee pulled up toward chest.

On exhale: Twist, bringing left knee toward floor on right side of body while turning head to left.

On inhale: Return to starting position.

Repeat 4 times.

Then stay in twist, holding left knee with right hand.

On inhale: With palm up, sweep left arm wide along floor toward ear, turning head to center.

On exhale: Lower arm back to side, turning head to left.

Repeat 6 times.

Repeat on other side.

DETAILS: *On exhale:* When twisting right, keep angles between left arm and torso and between left knee and torso less than ninety degrees.

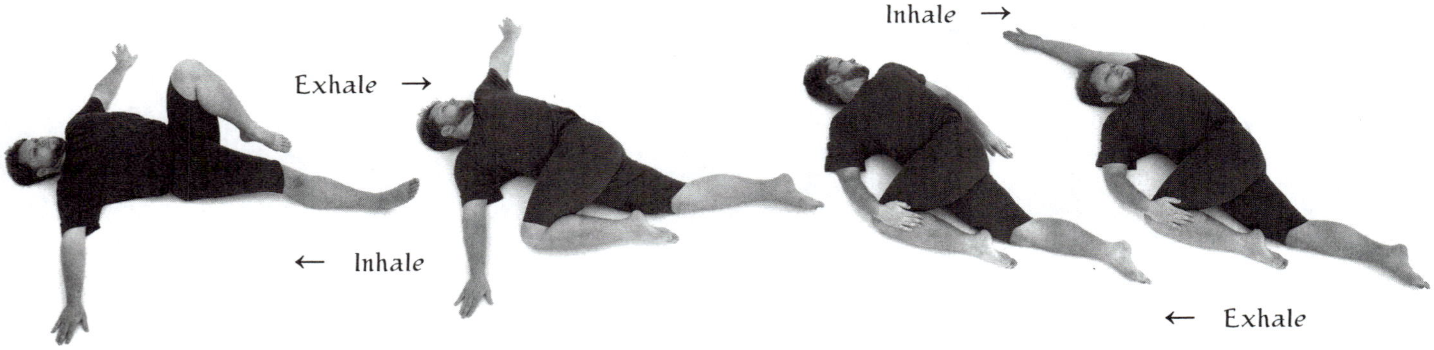
Exhale →
← Inhale
Inhale →
← Exhale

10.

POSTURE: Jānu Śirṣāsana Parivṛtti.
EMPHASIS: To deeply stretch lateral portion of torso, one side at a time.
TECHNIQUE: Sit with right leg folded in, heel to groin, left leg extended forward at an angle, left arm overhead, and right arm bent.

On exhale: Bending left knee slightly, bend laterally, bringing left hand toward left foot, keeping shoulders twisted so right shoulder is vertically above left, and turning head down toward left knee. Place right palm above right shoulder.

On inhale: Extend right arm forward, stretching right side of torso, and looking toward right hand.

On exhale: Bend right arm again, turning head down toward knee.

Repeat 4 times.

Then stay in the full stretch 4 breaths.

Repeat on other side.

DETAILS: Bend left knee enough to comfortably lower left shoulder toward knee. Keep shoulders in vertical alignment. Rotate left hand externally to grasp inside arch of left foot.

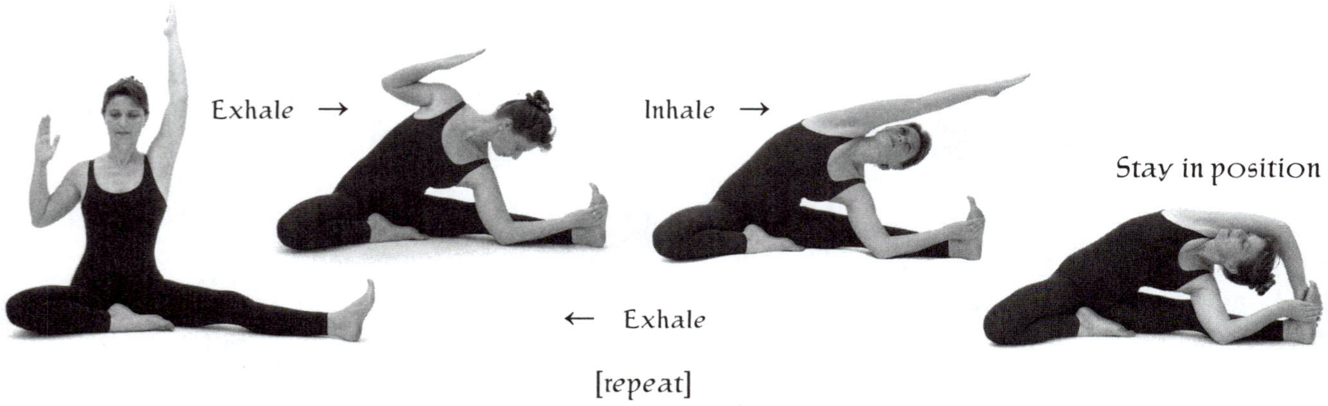
Exhale →
Inhale →
← Exhale
Stay in position
[repeat]

11.

POSTURE: Paścimatānāsana.
EMPHASIS: To relax back with gentle symmetric stretch.
TECHNIQUE: Sit with legs forward, back straight, and arms raised over head.

On exhale: Bending knees slightly, bend forward, bringing chest to thighs, and palms to balls of feet.

On inhale: Return to starting position.

Repeat 4 times.

Then stay in posture 4 breaths.

DETAILS: *On exhale:* Bend knees to facilitate stretching low back and bringing belly and chest to thighs. Move chin down toward throat. *On inhale:* Lift chest up and away from thighs, flattening upper back.

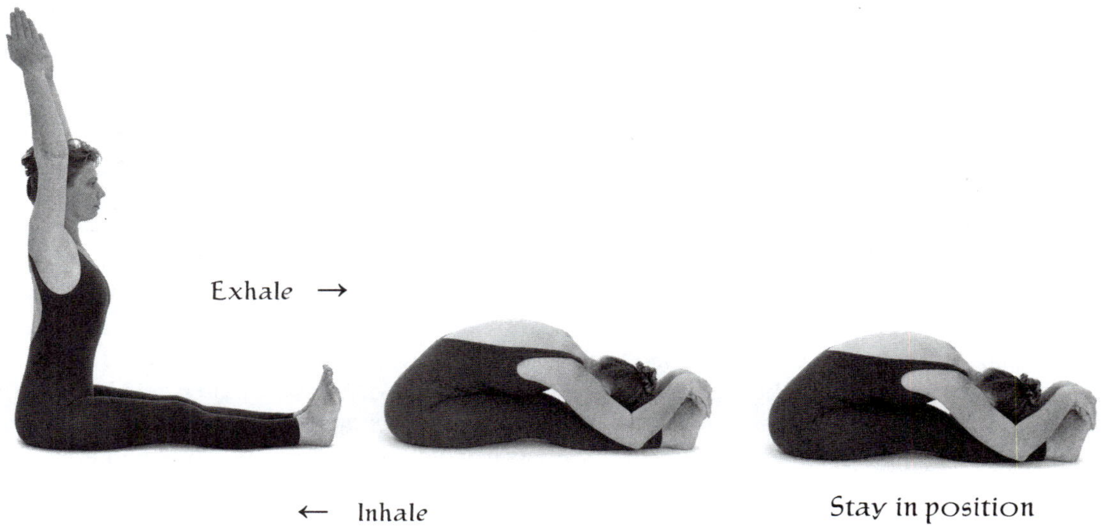

12.

POSTURE: Śavāsana.
EMPHASIS: To rest.
TECHNIQUE: Lie flat on back, with arms at sides, palms up, and legs slightly apart. Close eyes. Relax body fully, keeping mind relaxed and alert to sensations in body.
DURATION: Minimum 3 to 5 minutes.

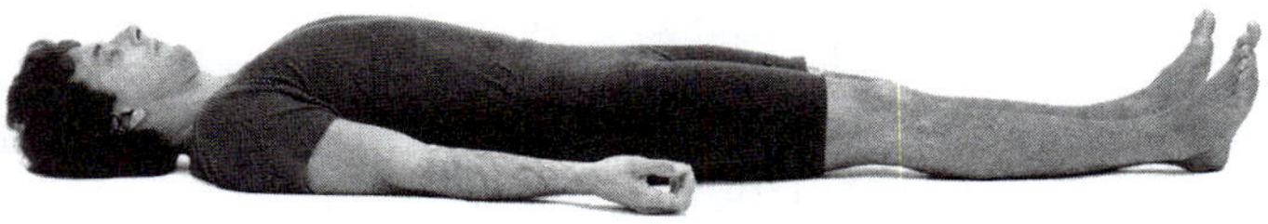

Sacrum, Hips, and Knees

Much of the low back pain that people suffer is lumbar pain, although many low back conditions also relate to the pelvis. These conditions may include mild to severe tension and pain in the sacroiliac area, the hip sockets, and the sciatic nerves. It may also include tension and pain in the groin area of the inner thighs, pain at the very top part of the front of the thighs, pain in the knees, and may involve mild to severe restriction in the movement of the legs.

Before working with these problems, it is important to assess the cause of the pain. In particular, it is important to make sure there is no serious damage to the ligaments of the sacrum, hips, and knees. We can work with sprains and strains, but if there are torn ligaments or cartilage, it is best to seek professional help. Again, in such conditions, Yoga therapy may help in the healing process, but the wrong practice may actually make matters worse.

In working with tension, restricted movement, and chronic pain, we want to understand both our musculoskeletal condition and the neuromuscular patterns that condition our movements.

The pelvis is a complex junction of the lumbosacral spine, the pelvic girdle and the attached legs. This juncture includes the various bony structures, ligamentous structures that attach the bones to each other, and muscle groups that control movements in the area. Musculoskeletal conditions that contribute to these problems include having one hip higher than the other, one hip rotated forward of the other, and/or one leg more turned in or out than the other. All of these structural conditions relate to corresponding muscular imbalances, chronic muscular contractions, and/or muscular weakness. In addition there may be joint instability and hypermobility or joint rigidity and lack of mobility. In short, conditions of the muscles and joints are causally related to neuromuscular mechanisms and movement patterns.

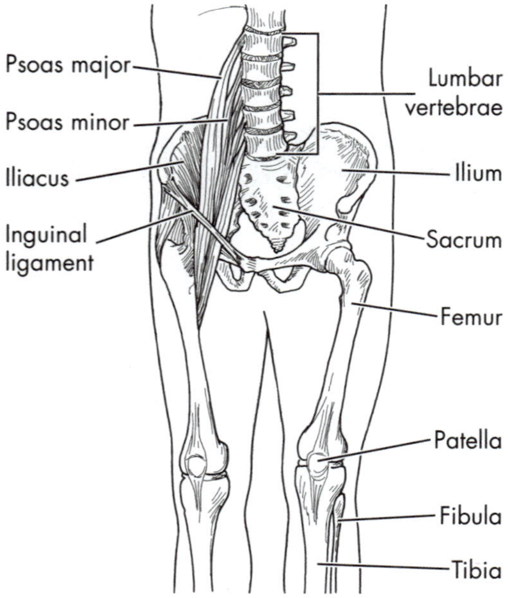

The origin of these problems may be congenital or acquired. Birth conditions can include differences in the length of the legs, lax (loose) ligaments, or shortened tendons. Acquired conditions can be the result of habitual activities due to injury or even improper training. An example of a habitual activity that creates stress in the sacrum, hips, and knees is driving a car with a standard shift. Men who wear their wallets in their back pockets often create, through this seemingly harmless habit, long-term imbalances, tension, and pain. Golfers are often troubled by sacrum pain, as are women after giving birth or, later, from always carrying the baby on one hip. Strain to the sacrum is also a common result of lifting heavy objects. Women trained in ballet at a young age also often have problems with their hips and knees. And many Yoga students have injured their sacroiliac ligaments from the stress of extreme forward bending or straining to get their legs behind their heads.

It is important to recognize that most of the conditions affecting the sacrum, hips, and knees reflect a poor functional integration between the lumbosacral spine, the pelvis, and the attached legs. The methodology for working these conditions, therefore, involves working to adjust the functional relationship between these areas.

The sacrum is a triangular-shaped wedge at the base of the spine that fits between the two sides of the pelvis. In both standing and seated positions, the weight of the spine is transferred through the sacrum to the pelvis, the sacrum acting as a bridge in weight transfer. If there is structural asymmetry in the sacrum, there will be a shear stress at the sacroiliac joints, which can result in strain and pain. From lifting increasingly heavy weight loads, for example, there is increased risk of injury, and injury to the ligaments takes time to heal.

In working with the sacrum, we want first of all to develop a balanced pelvic-lumbar rhythm. This involves both the condition of the musculature and the use of proper movement patterns. Our aim is to work to release chronically contracted muscles of both the low back and the important muscles that bind the legs, through the pelvis, to the spine (the iliopsoas group). We also want to work toward balance, strength, and flexibility on both sides of the pelvis, within each muscle group.

Many hip and knee problems are a direct result of injury or accident. Professional athletes, dancers, skiers, and Yoga practitioners, to name a few, all have increased risk to the knees. But many hip and knee problems are also the result of cumulative stress due to more subtle patterns of body use.

In working the hips and knees, the main point to consider is the tracking of the legs from the hip to the foot. Tracking refers to the way the distinct segments of the leg relate to each other, and is the result of musculoskeletal conditions and neuromuscular patterns. We can understand this phenomenon by looking at our shoes. For example, if we look at the heels of our shoes, especially shoes that we have had for a long time, we can see the way they sometimes wear evenly and sometimes are more worn on the inside or the outside edge. There are many variations of this tracking that can actually be read by looking at our shoes. The body is a weight transference mechanism within the gravitational field, body weight being transferred through the bones and joints to the earth. If there is a misalignment or imbalance, the weight is not transferred in a balanced way through the center of gravity in the joint, and the result is shear stress in the joints.

If we look further into this issue, we can notice different tracking from the ankles to the knees, and from the knees to the hips. There are people whose knees turn in, while their ankles turn out; others who have one knee that turns in more than the other; and still others who have knees that turn out. There are all kinds of tracking differences.

The origin of our tracking patterns may be in the musculature of the pelvis, the length of the bones of the legs, or even in the condition of the ankles and feet. These patterns are often linked to the way in which the femur head (greater trochanter) rotates in the hip socket (acetabulum). We can begin to understand these patterns through observation, and the bottoms of our shoes are a good place to begin. We can then try to notice how our knees turn as we walk. Of course Yoga postures, particularly standing postures, can also reveal a lot about our tracking, but, again, this requires accurate observation. For example, it is advisable to watch our knees and see how they are responding before we try to impose a rigid form on our legs.

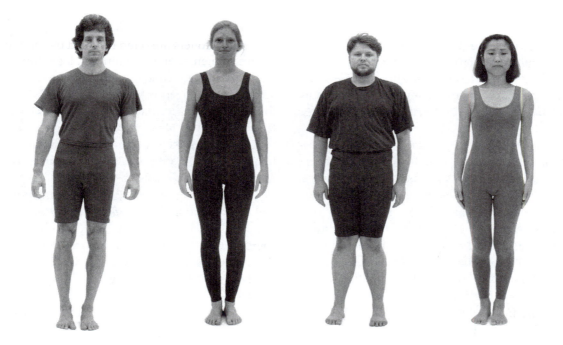

In working with any kind of a joint problem, there are three main objectives.

The first is to identify and to stop, wherever possible, activities that are causing irritation. In acute conditions, this may mean immobilizing the joint for some time. In less acute conditions, it may mean avoiding excessive weight-bearing and all forceful torquing of the joints. Or it may mean changing from a standard to an automatic car, wearing a wallet in the front pocket instead of the back, or taking a break from the golf course.

The second objective is to slowly and carefully find activities that improve the condition. This means increasing circulation to the joint, strengthening the muscles that support it, and releasing muscle spasms or chronic contractions. In Yoga therapy, this involves isolating specific muscle groups and working them gently without stress to the joints. As this presents a particular challenge for the sacrum, hip, and knee, which are all weight-bearing joints, it is most appropriate to work into these joints from supine (on the back) or prone (on the stomach) positions.

The third objective is to modify the movement patterns of the joints. For sacrum, hip, and knee problems, this means establishing a proper pelvic-lumbar rhythm and reorganizing the tracking of the legs. In Yoga therapy, this involves the repetition of carefully designed movements to re-pattern our use of the legs and hips.

In the methodology of practice, we want to introduce simple movements that increase circulation, stretch what needs to be stretched, and strengthen what needs to be strengthened. An important methodological point in working with most joint problems is to work the joint without restricting it, because, as a general rule, restricting the joint increases risk. The approach is to make the problematic area more stable and, at the same time, more flexible. This is achieved by gently contracting and stretching the muscles that support the problematic area. We then want to integrate that area with the rest of the body. This is achieved through the use of larger and more complete movements of the whole body.

The three practices that follow are designed to stabilize the sacrum, hips, and knees, and to strengthen their supporting musculature. They may be useful in certain chronic and painful conditions. They are intended to be exploratory rather than prescriptive, illustrating different tools that work the sacrum, hips, and knees. The key to this area of the body is the junction of the legs to the spine through the pelvis. Through the various postures offered in these sequences, that junction is explored from the front, back, outside, and inside of the legs and pelvis. There are many other postures that can be adapted to the sacrum, hips, and knees. And, in fact, many of these movements may not be suitable for some individuals. From these practices, we hope that you may derive ideas for working in these areas.

Working with the Sacrum

This practice was developed for R.B., a thirty-seven-year-old Yoga teacher from a city in the southwestern United States. He was visiting Hawaii on vacation, had heard about our work for years, and had come to see if I could help him with his chronic sacrum problem.

In our first session together, I asked R.B. to show me how he usually practices. I could see that R.B. was well trained in the form of the classical postures and practiced with a lot of precision and attention to details. At the same time, I could see that in his choice of postures and efforts to practice them "correctly," he was aggravating his condition. He told me that he had sensed that this was true and was frustrated with both his own practice and his teaching. He had been to see several other Yoga teachers for help, as well as other health practitioners, but was unable to find a solution.

I told him that there were two aspects to working with his condition. One was to identify what he was doing in his daily activity that was irritating his sacrum, and to modify or eliminate those activities. The other was to find out what he could do to support his healing, and add those activities to his daily routine.

On the first point, R.B. realized that *most of what he had been doing in his Yoga practice was a source of stress.* At the same time, he felt that as a teacher he had to practice. I told him there were things he could do to actually help his condition and that, once things were stabilized, he would be able to return to his regular practice. I also told him that because of this experience he would be a much better teacher.

In our discussions together, I learned that although he didn't practice while he was teaching, he regularly demonstrated the more difficult postures. I asked him to please avoid demonstrating and instead to use a student who understood the posture and was already warmed up from the practice. I also asked him to carry his wallet in his front rather than back pocket.

On the addition side, we developed the following practice over the three sessions we had together before he had to go home. The main orientation was to strengthen the muscles that surround the sacroiliac joint and increase the circulation to the sacroiliac ligament. I also suggested that he look into some nutritional supplements that would support the healing of his ligaments.

Before he left, R.B. told me that no one up till then had given him a coherent explanation about what was happening in his sacrum. He felt encouraged to have a clear direction to work with his condition. He called me several months later to say that he was feeling much better and that he was maintaining the practice I worked out for him. Since then he has continued to train with me in Hawaii and in Los Angeles. He no longer strains his sacrum in his practice, recognizing that *the form of the postures should be adapated to serve the needs of his body.* He tells me that his students really love the new, user-friendly style he now teaches.

A Practice for the Sacrum

1.

POSTURE: Cakravākāsana.
EMPHASIS: To gently mobilize low back and sacrum.
TECHNIQUE: Get down on hands and knees, with shoulders vertically above wrists and with hips above knees.

On inhale: Lift chest up and away from belly.

On exhale: Gently contract belly and round low back, bringing hips backward toward heels and bringing chest toward thighs.

NUMBER: 8 times.
DETAILS: *On inhale:* Lead with chest, keeping chin slightly down. Avoid compressing low back; rather, feel chest expanding. *On exhale:* round low back without collapsing chest over belly. Avoid increasing curvature of upper back. Go progressively lower each time, but avoid going all the way down. Let chest lower toward thighs sooner than hips toward heels.

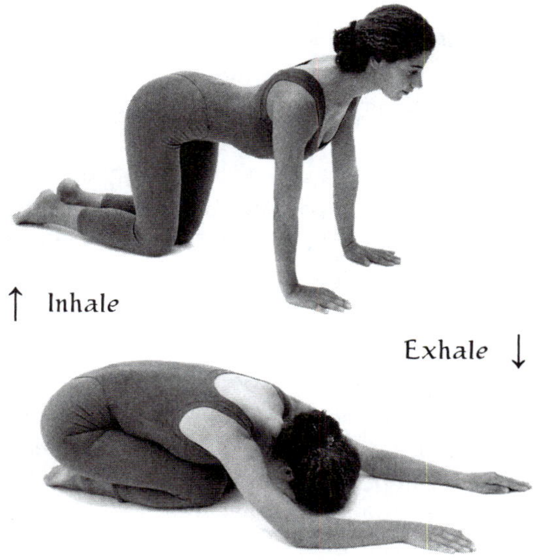

2.

POSTURE: Bhujaṅgāsana, progressively widening legs.

EMPHASIS: To strengthen large muscles of back and buttocks, strengthening musculature supporting sacroiliac joint.

TECHNIQUE: Lie on stomach, with head turned to right, palms up by chest, and legs together.

On inhale: Lift chest, turning head to center.

On exhale: Lower chest, turning head to left.

Repeat 6 times, turning head to center on inhale, and to alternate sides on successive exhales.

DETAILS: Widen legs every second repetition.

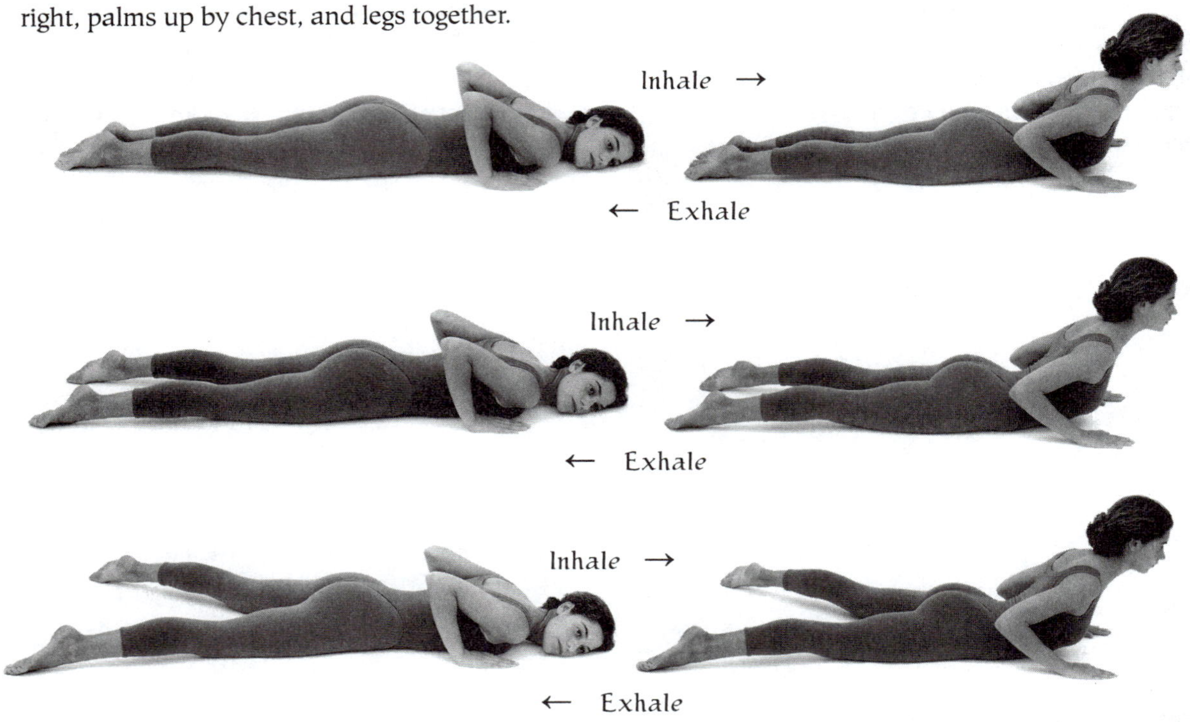

3.

POSTURE: Cakravākāsana.

EMPHASIS: To gently mobilize low back and sacrum after previous back bend.

TECHNIQUE: Get down on hands and knees, with shoulders vertically above wrists and with hips above knees.

On inhale: Lift chest up and away from belly.

On exhale: Gently contract belly and round low back, bringing hips backward toward heels and bringing chest toward thighs.

NUMBER: 8 times.

DETAILS: *On inhale:* Lead with chest, keeping chin slightly down. Avoid compressing low back; rather, feel chest expanding. *On exhale:* round low back without collapsing chest over belly. Avoid increasing curvature of upper back. Go progressively lower each time, but avoid going all the way down. Let chest lower toward thighs sooner than hips toward heels.

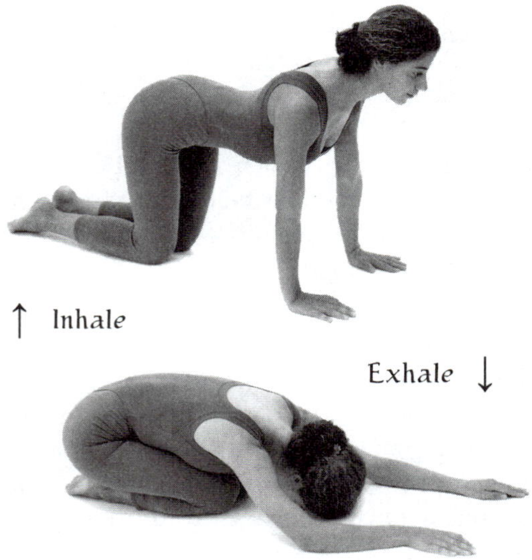

4.

POSTURE: Vimanāsana (variation of Śalabhāsana).

EMPHASIS: To strengthen large muscles of back and buttocks, strengthening musculature supporting sacroiliac joint.

TECHNIQUE: Lie on stomach, with head turned to right, palms up by chest, and legs together.

On inhale: Lift chest, turning head to center, and lift legs, opening them as wide as possible.

On exhale: Keeping chest and legs up, and keeping legs straight, bring knees together.

On inhale: Open legs wide.

On exhale: Return to starting position.

NUMBER: 6 times.

DETAILS: *On exhale:* Rotate hips inwardly to bring knees together.

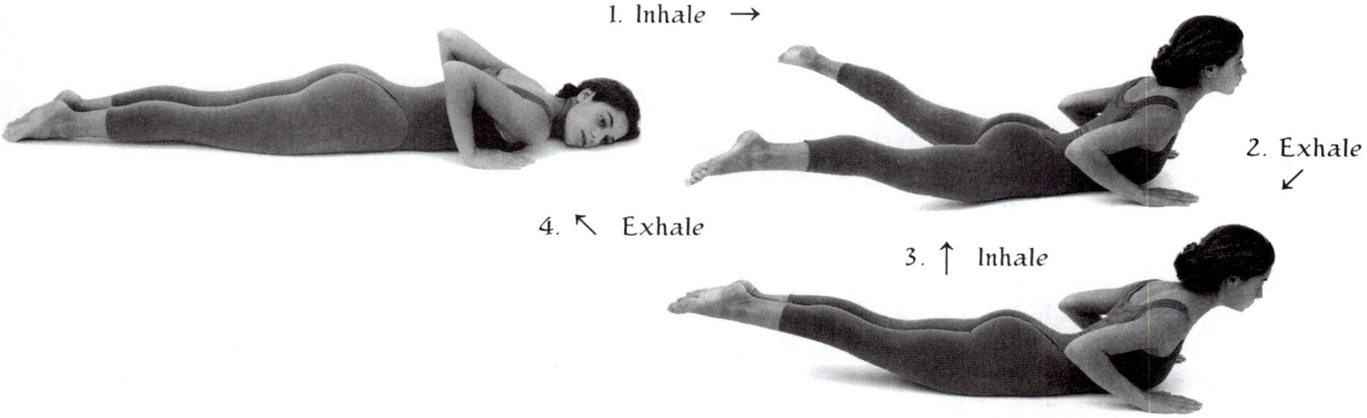
1. Inhale →
2. Exhale ↙
3. ↑ Inhale
4. ↖ Exhale

5.

POSTURE: Cakravākāsana.

EMPHASIS: To gently mobilize low back and sacrum after previous back bend.

TECHNIQUE: Get down on hands and knees, with shoulders vertically above wrists and with hips above knees.

On inhale: Lift chest up and away from belly.

On exhale: Gently contract belly and round low back, bringing hips backward toward heels and bringing chest toward thighs.

NUMBER: 8 times.

DETAILS: *On inhale:* Lead with chest, keeping chin slightly down. Avoid compressing low back; rather, feel chest expanding. *On exhale:* round low back without collapsing chest over belly. Avoid increasing curvature of upper back. Go progressively lower each time, but avoid going all the way down. Let chest lower toward thighs sooner than hips toward heels.

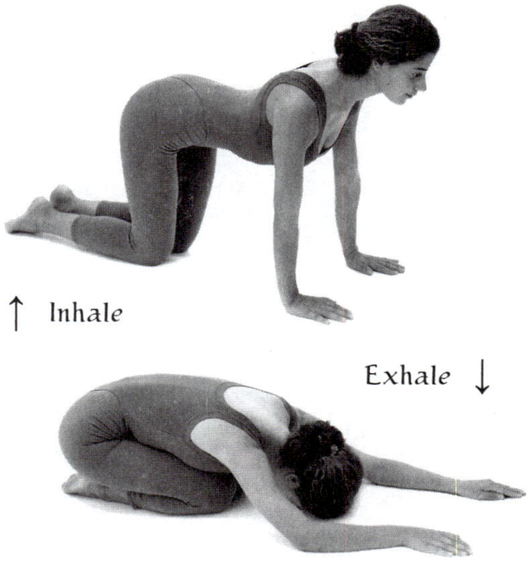
↑ Inhale
Exhale ↓

6.

POSTURE: Supta Baddha Koṇāsana.
EMPHASIS: To increase circulation to sacrum and perineal floor.
TECHNIQUE: Lie on back with knees bent and feet near buttocks. On inhale, open legs wide, bringing soles of feet together. Take up to sixty seconds to close knees together. Open legs again naturally.
NUMBER: 6 times.
DETAILS: While closing legs, keep low back flat on floor. Allow any trembling of legs that may occur.

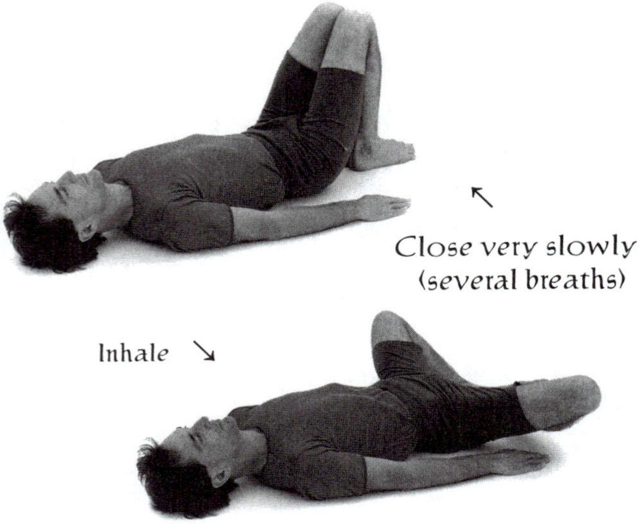

7.

POSTURE: Supported Śavāsana.
EMPHASIS: To rest.
TECHNIQUE: Lie flat on back, with arms at sides, palms up, and legs elevated and slightly apart. Close eyes. Relax body fully, keeping mind relaxed and alert to sensations in body.
DURATION: Minimum 3 to 5 minutes.
DETAILS: Place a round pillow under knees.

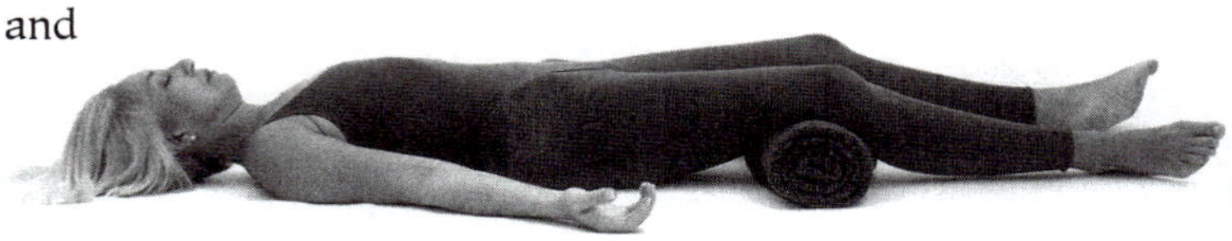

Working with the Hips

This practice was developed for E.G., a thirty-five-year-old woman who was referred to me by another student. She told me that she had gone to see a body worker who also prescribed Yoga exercises, and that she had been in serious pain ever since. The student who referred her to me had himself suffered a long history of low back pain. He told E.G. that in a few sessions with me he had learned a very simple practice that kept him pain-free. She was very hesitant about coming, but her friend convinced her she would be in good hands, and she called for an appointment.

In her first visit, I learned that she had had problems with her hips since she was a small child in Europe. She told me that she had had corrective surgery and had been in a cast for many months. She indicated that her pain was usually in the area of the hip socket and into the inner thigh. The movement of her legs at the hip was restricted. There was also some chronic pain in her low back.

E.G. told me that the body worker had given her a printed series of "hip" exercises. She practiced them for several days and had been in worse pain ever since.

E.G.'s emotions were very much on the surface, and she cried often and easily. She needed someone who would listen to her and relate to her where she was—not simply through some theoretical model. She spent a lot of time just talking about her physical and emotional condition. She confided in me that she was having a lot of difficulty in her marriage. She said her husband was very critical of her, and they argued often. She also told me that she wanted a baby, and he didn't.

My feeling was that she needed to be reassured, relaxed, and nourished. Once she was stable and out of pain, there would be time to explore her hips more deeply. I explained to her that our approach was to start slowly and work progressively toward increased strength and stability. I told her that as she began to feel better in her body, she would start to feel better about herself and might even get some more clarity about her relationship.

Her first practice consisted of only a few simple postures and some deep relaxation. She called me several days after the first session, incredulous at how much better she felt after such simple exercises. E.G. came back to see me once a week for nearly six months. In that time she was able to work progressively deeper into the region of her hips without pain, and she no longer complained about her low back.

One day she came to tell me she was going back to Europe. I asked if her husband was going with her, and she told me that they had decided to take some time apart to reassess their relationship. The following practice was evolved over the last few sessions we had together before she left. The focus was to continue stretching and strengthening the musculature of her hips.

E.G. sent me a letter from Europe a few months later. She told me that she was happy to be home with her family and that her husband was planning to come over soon. They had missed each other and were hoping to make a new start. She told me she continues to work with the practice we developed and that she is more stable and pain-free than she can remember.

A Practice for the Hips

1.

POSTURE: Dvipāda Pīṭham, progressively widening feet.
EMPHASIS: To strengthen musculature supporting hip joint.
TECHNIQUE: Lie on back with arms down at sides, knees bent, and feet on floor, slightly apart and comfortably close to buttocks.

On inhale: Keeping chin down, press down on feet, raising pelvis up toward ceiling, until neck is gently flattened on floor.

On exhale: Return to starting position.

NUMBER: 6 times.
DETAILS: Begin with feet nearly together. After 2 times, widen feet to width of hips. After 2 more times, make feet slightly wider than hips.

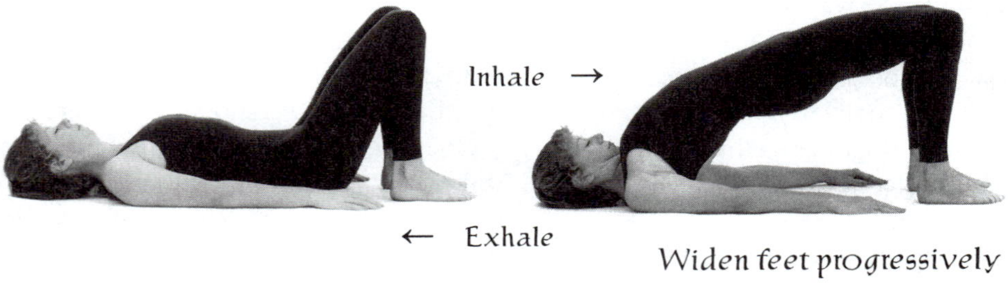

2.

POSTURE: Ekapāda Uṣṭrāsana variation.
EMPHASIS: To stretch musculature of upper and inner thigh, including iliopsoas and adductor groups.
TECHNIQUE: Stand on right knee, with knee directly below hip, and on left foot, with foot directly below left knee. Hands on left knee.

On inhale: Lift chest upward as you lunge forward, stretching front of body from right thigh to right side of abdomen.

On exhale: return to starting position.

Repeat 4 times.

Then stay in position 4 breaths.

Repeat on other side.

DETAILS: *On inhale:* While moving forward, make a slight external rotation of back leg, bringing stretch into inner thigh.

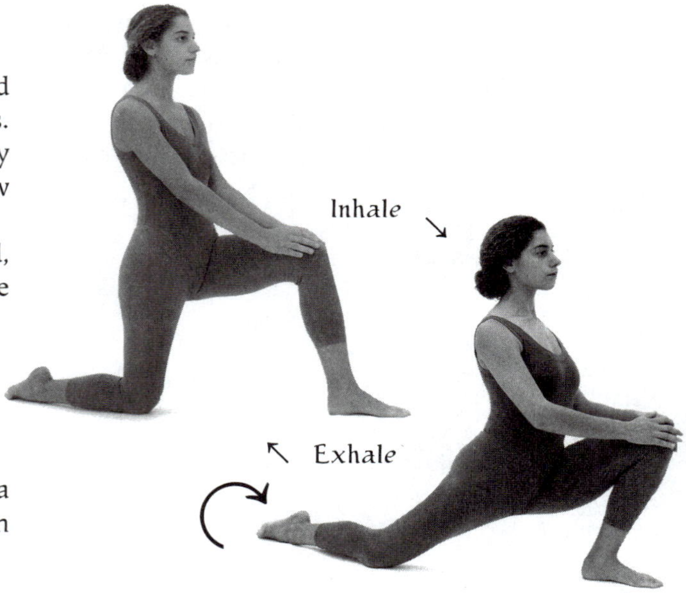

3.

Posture: Vimanāsana (variation of Śalabhāsana).
Emphasis: To strengthen large muscles of back and buttocks, strengthening hip rotator muscles.
Technique: Lie on stomach, with head turned to right, palms up by chest, and legs together.

On inhale: Lift chest, turning head to center, and lifting legs, opening them as wide as possible.

On exhale: Keeping chest and legs up, and legs straight, bring knees together.

On inhale: Open legs wide.

On exhale: Return to starting position.

Number: 6 times.
Details: *On exhale:* Rotate hips inwardly to bring knees together.

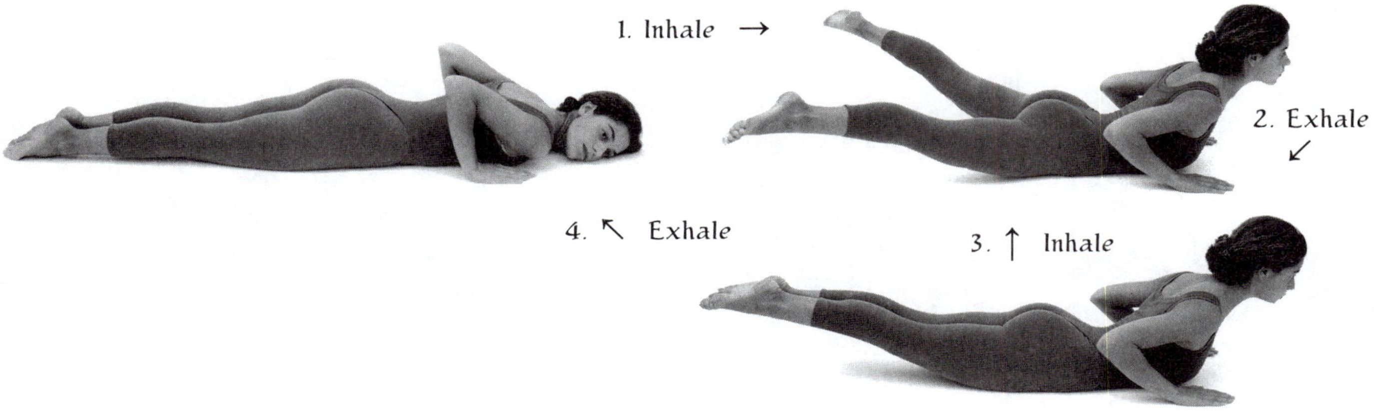
1. Inhale →
2. Exhale ↙
4. ↖ Exhale
3. ↑ Inhale

4.

Posture: Cakravākāsana.
Emphasis: To gently stretch low back after previous back bend.
Technique: Get down on hands and knees, with shoulders vertically above wrists and with hips above knees.

On inhale: Lift chest up and away from belly.

On exhale: Gently contract belly and round low back, bringing hips backward toward heels and bringing chest toward thighs.

Number: 8 times.
Details: *On inhale:* Lead with chest, keeping chin slightly down. Avoid compressing low back; rather, feel chest expanding. *On exhale:* Round low back without collapsing chest over belly. Avoid increasing curvature of upper back. Go progressively lower each time, but avoid going all the way down. Let chest lower toward thighs sooner than hips toward heels.

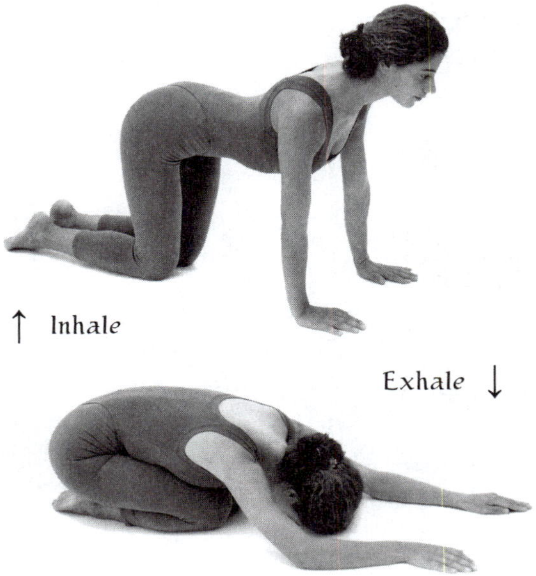
↑ Inhale
Exhale ↓

5.

POSTURE: Supta Prasārita Pādāṅguṣṭhāsana.
EMPHASIS: To stretch and contract musculature of inner thighs.
TECHNIQUE: Lie on back with knees lifted toward chest and with hands placed behind knees.

On inhale: With hands holding legs from behind knees, lift heels upward, straightening legs.

Exhale in position, placing hands on insides of knees, palms facing outward.

On inhale: Open legs wide, gently pushing legs apart with arms.

On exhale: Close legs, resisting slightly with arms.

Repeat 6 times.

Then stay with legs open 6 breaths.

DETAILS: Keep sacrum, chin, and shoulders down throughout movement. If legs are loose, hold balls of feet while staying in final position.

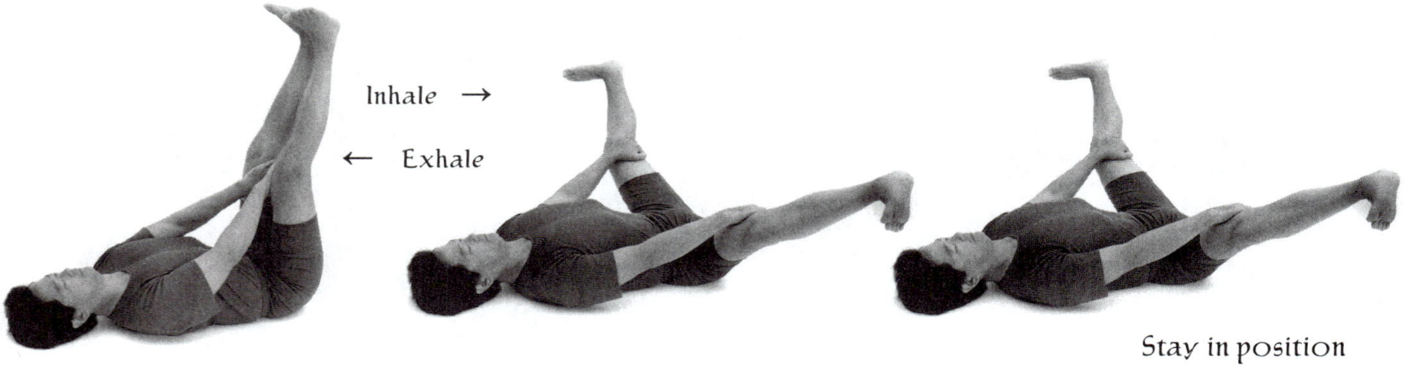

6.

POSTURE: Supta Pārśva Pādāṅguṣṭhāsana.
EMPHASIS: To stretch musculature of inner thigh.
TECHNIQUE: Lie on back with right leg lifted up toward chest, knee bent, and right hand holding right knee. Left hand on left hip.

On inhale: Push right leg right toward floor, holding left hip down with left hand.

On exhale: Return to starting position.

Repeat 4 times.

Then, from open position, hold inside of knee with right hand.

On inhale: Extend right leg straight.

On exhale: Return to starting position.

Repeat 4 times.

Then stay in extended position 4 breaths.

Repeat on other side.

DETAILS: If possible, hold extended foot with its respective hand.

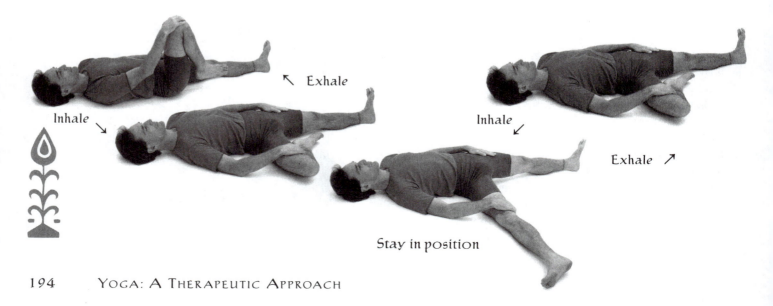

7.

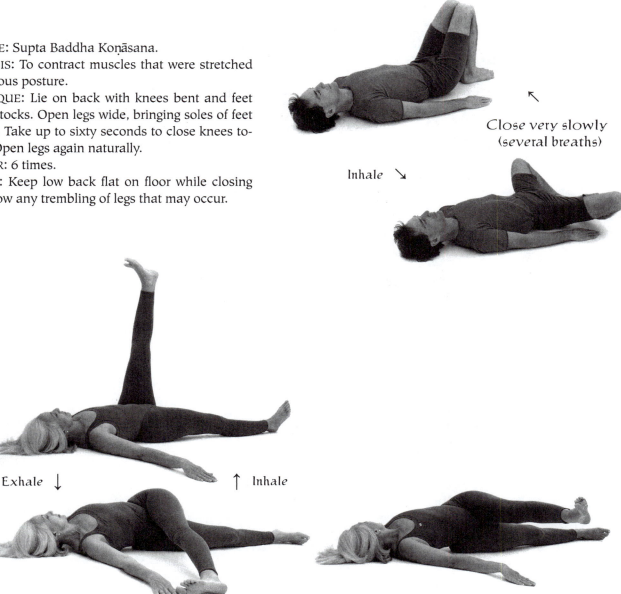

POSTURE: Supta Baddha Koṇāsana.
EMPHASIS: To contract muscles that were stretched by previous posture.
TECHNIQUE: Lie on back with knees bent and feet near buttocks. Open legs wide, bringing soles of feet together. Take up to sixty seconds to close knees together. Open legs again naturally.
NUMBER: 6 times.
DETAILS: Keep low back flat on floor while closing legs. Allow any trembling of legs that may occur.

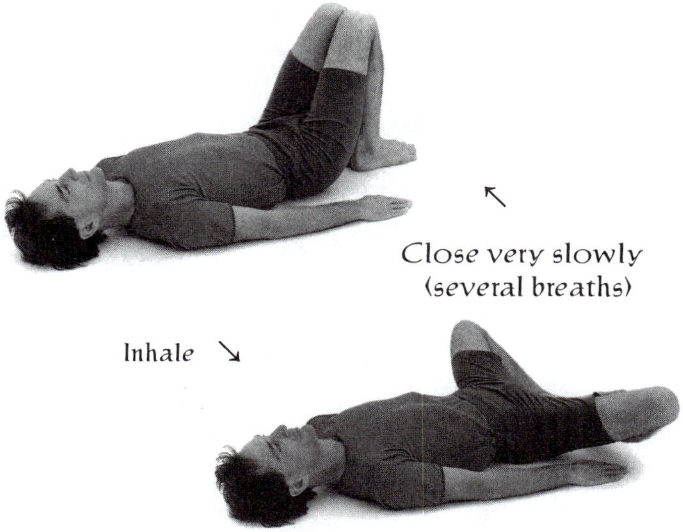

↖
Close very slowly
(several breaths)
Inhale ↘

Exhale ↓
↑ Inhale
Lift leg; stay in position

8.

POSTURE: Jaṭhara Parivṛtti adaptation.
EMPHASIS: To stretch and strengthen musculature of hip.
TECHNIQUE: Lie flat on back, with arms out to sides, and with left leg extended upward at an angle of ninety degrees to torso.

On exhale: Twist, bringing left foot to floor and toward right hand while turning head left.

On inhale: Return to starting position.

Repeat 4 times.

Then *on inhale:* from twisted position, lift left leg until parallel to ground, keeping left hip vertically above right. Hold 5 seconds.

On exhale: Return leg to floor.

Repeat 4 times.

Then lift left leg to parallel position again. Stay 4 breaths.

Repeat on other side.

DETAILS: While staying in position, explore a gentle external rotation of lifted leg, feeling work in hip abductors. Avoid straining neck.

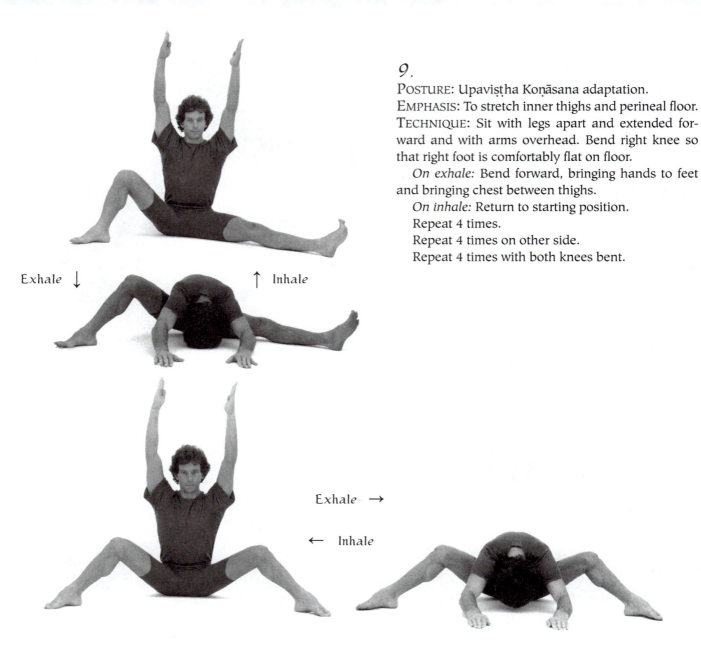

9.

POSTURE: Upaviṣṭha Koṇāsana adaptation.
EMPHASIS: To stretch inner thighs and perineal floor.
TECHNIQUE: Sit with legs apart and extended forward and with arms overhead. Bend right knee so that right foot is comfortably flat on floor.

On exhale: Bend forward, bringing hands to feet and bringing chest between thighs.

On inhale: Return to starting position.

Repeat 4 times.

Repeat 4 times on other side.

Repeat 4 times with both knees bent.

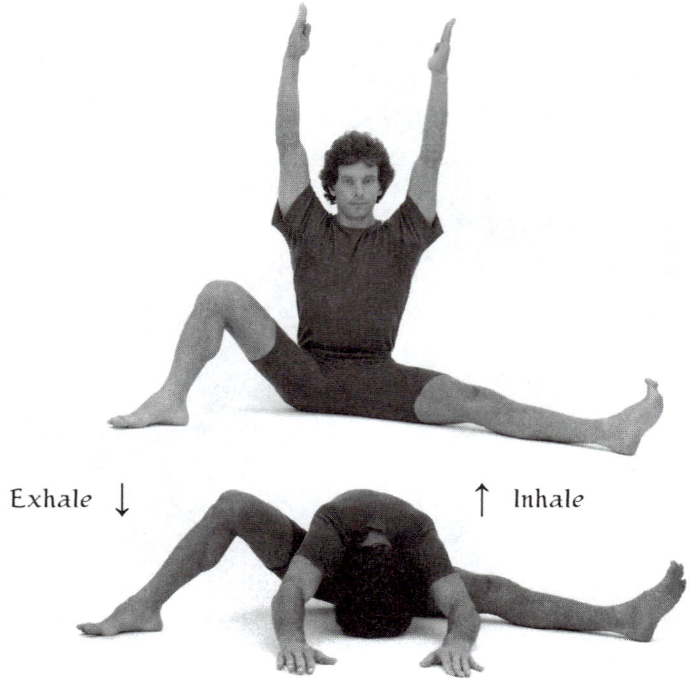

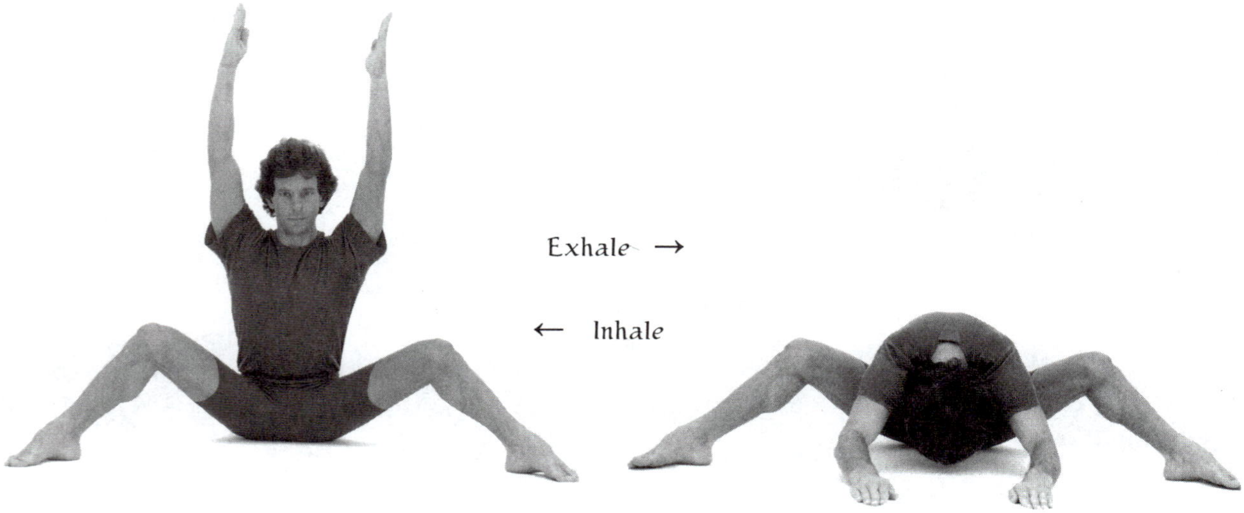

10.

POSTURE: Śavāsana.
EMPHASIS: To rest.
TECHNIQUE: Lie flat on back, with arms at sides, palms up, and legs slightly apart. Close eyes. Relax body fully, keeping mind relaxed and alert to sensations in body.
DURATION: Minimum 3 minutes.

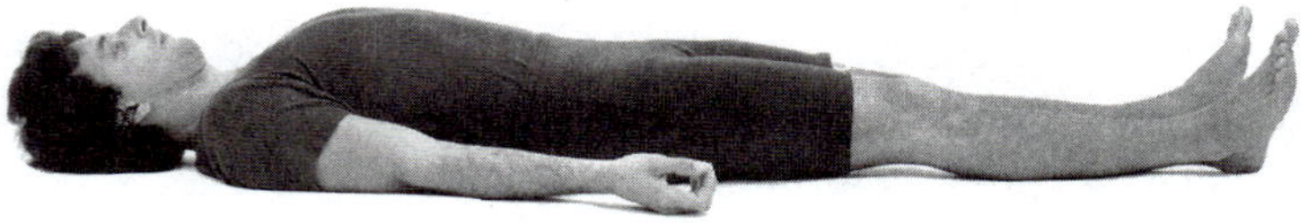

Working with the Knees

This practice was developed for P.O., a fifty-three-year-old flight attendant for a major U.S. airline. P.O. had gone on disability for a low back injury years earlier. She had come to see me, and we had worked together to get her back back into shape. Our work included techniques of breath and movement adapted to her body, as well as practical teachings from Yoga philosophy on the nature of the mind. She always told me how important those classes were for her in facing and overcoming her resistance to get off of disability. Against all expectations, she went back to work to finish out the remaining years she needed to get her early retirement benefits.

That accomplishment did a lot to boost her self-confidence and motivated her to learn more about herself. Though she had retired from the airline, she had a lot of energy and wanted to continue working. At my suggestion, she took courses at the community college in anatomy and physiology, and went on to become a licensed massage therapist in the state of Hawaii.

A few years later, P.O. came to see me complaining about recurring pains in her knees. I asked her what she had been doing, and she told me "a little massage, and a lot of gardening."

Over the next several weeks, we developed the following course designed to strengthen the musculature surrounding the knee joint. P.O. called me a few months later to report that her pain was gone and that the practice had strengthened her legs and improved her awareness of her knees. She said that, "once again," she was amazed at the effectiveness of these simple tools.

I learned a lot from P.O. She had been in A.A. for years before she came to work with me. She told me that, while A.A. had helped her pull herself out of a dysfunctional lifestyle, Yoga had helped her *to visualize her future and to take concrete steps to realize her goals.*

A Practice for the Knees

1.

Posture: Apānāsana.
Emphasis: To warm up low back without compressing knees.
Technique: Lie on back with both knees bent toward chest and with feet off floor. Place each hand behind its respective knee.

On exhale: Pull thighs gently but progressively toward chest.

On inhale: Return to starting position.

Number: 8 times.
Details: *On exhale:* Pull gently with arms, keeping shoulders down on floor and relaxed. Press low back down into floor, and drop chin slightly toward throat. Progressively lengthen exhale with each successive repetition.

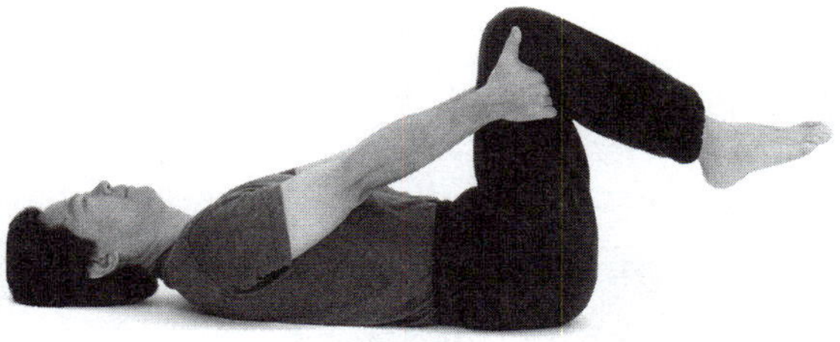

↑ Inhale

Exhale ↓

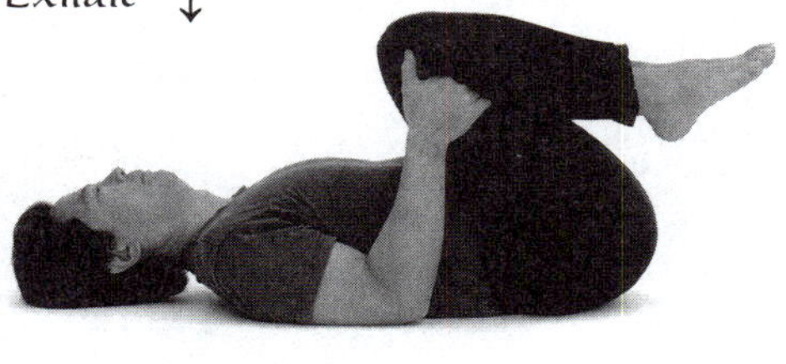

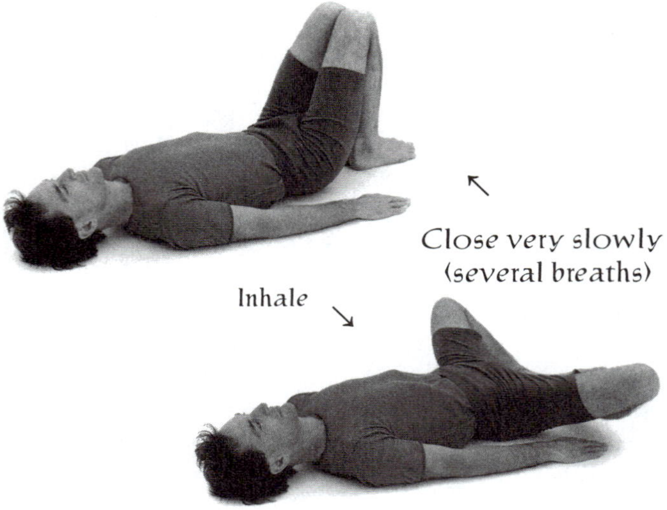

2.
POSTURE: Supta Baddha Koṇāsana.
EMPHASIS: To strengthen musculature of inner thighs.
TECHNIQUE: Lie on back with knees bent and feet near buttocks. Open legs wide, bringing soles of feet together. Take up to sixty seconds to close knees together. Open legs again naturally.
NUMBER: 6 times.
DETAILS: While closing legs, keep low back flat on floor. Allow any trembling of legs that may occur.

3.
POSTURE: Dvipāda Pīṭham.
EMPHASIS: To strengthen musculature of hips and thighs.
TECHNIQUE: Lie on back with arms down at sides, knees bent, and feet on floor, slightly apart and comfortably close to buttocks.

On inhale: Keeping chin down, press down on feet and raise pelvis up toward ceiling, until neck is gently flattened on floor.

On exhale: Return to starting position.

NUMBER: 6 times.
DETAILS: *On inhale:* Lift spine vertebra by vertebra from bottom up. *On exhale:* Unwind spine, coming down vertebra by vertebra.

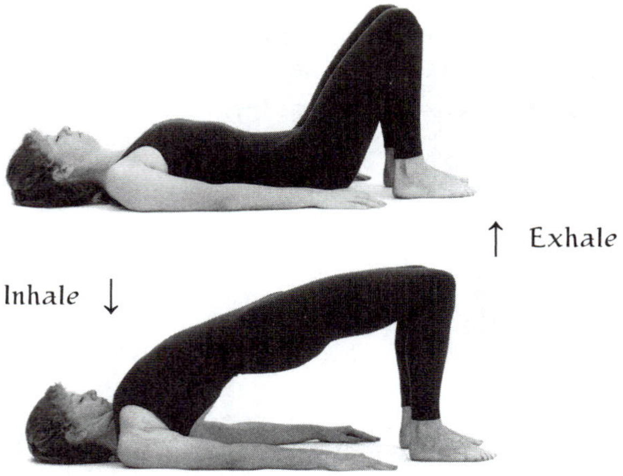

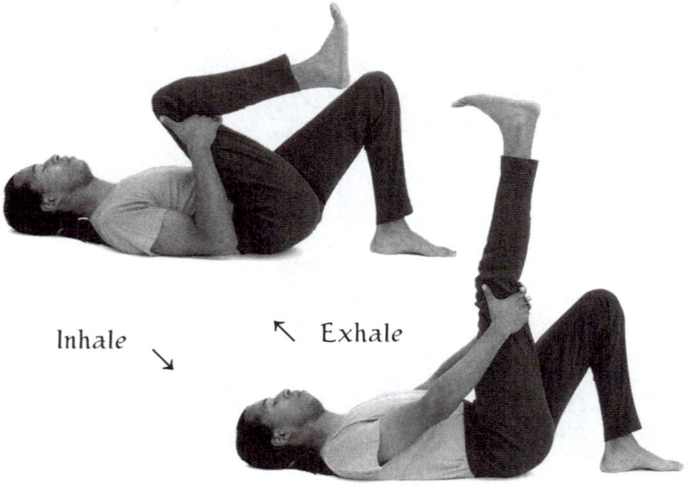

4.
POSTURE: Supta Eka Pādāṅguṣṭhāsana.
EMPHASIS: To mobilize knee joint, and to stretch and strengthen surrounding musculature.
TECHNIQUE: Lie on back, with legs bent, left foot on floor, right foot lifted, hands holding right thigh behind right knee, and arms bent.

On inhale: Extend right leg upward, straightening arms.

On exhale: Return to starting position.

NUMBER: 6 times each side.
DETAILS: *On inhale:* Flex foot as leg is raised upward. Keep knee slightly bent. Push low back and sacrum downward. Keep chin down.

5.

POSTURE: Ardha Śalabhāsana adaptation.
EMPHASIS: To strengthen the musculature of the legs, particularly at the back of the knees.
TECHNIQUE: Lie on stomach, with head turned to left and with palms on floor by chest.

On inhale: Lift chest and left leg, turning head to center.

On exhale: Stay in position.

On inhale: Slowly bend left knee, bringing heel toward buttock.

On exhale: Return to starting position, turning head to right and straigthening leg slowly.

Repeat 4 times each side, alternately.

Then stay up in position with both legs lifted and repeat 4 times.

DETAILS: Bend and straighten legs slowly.

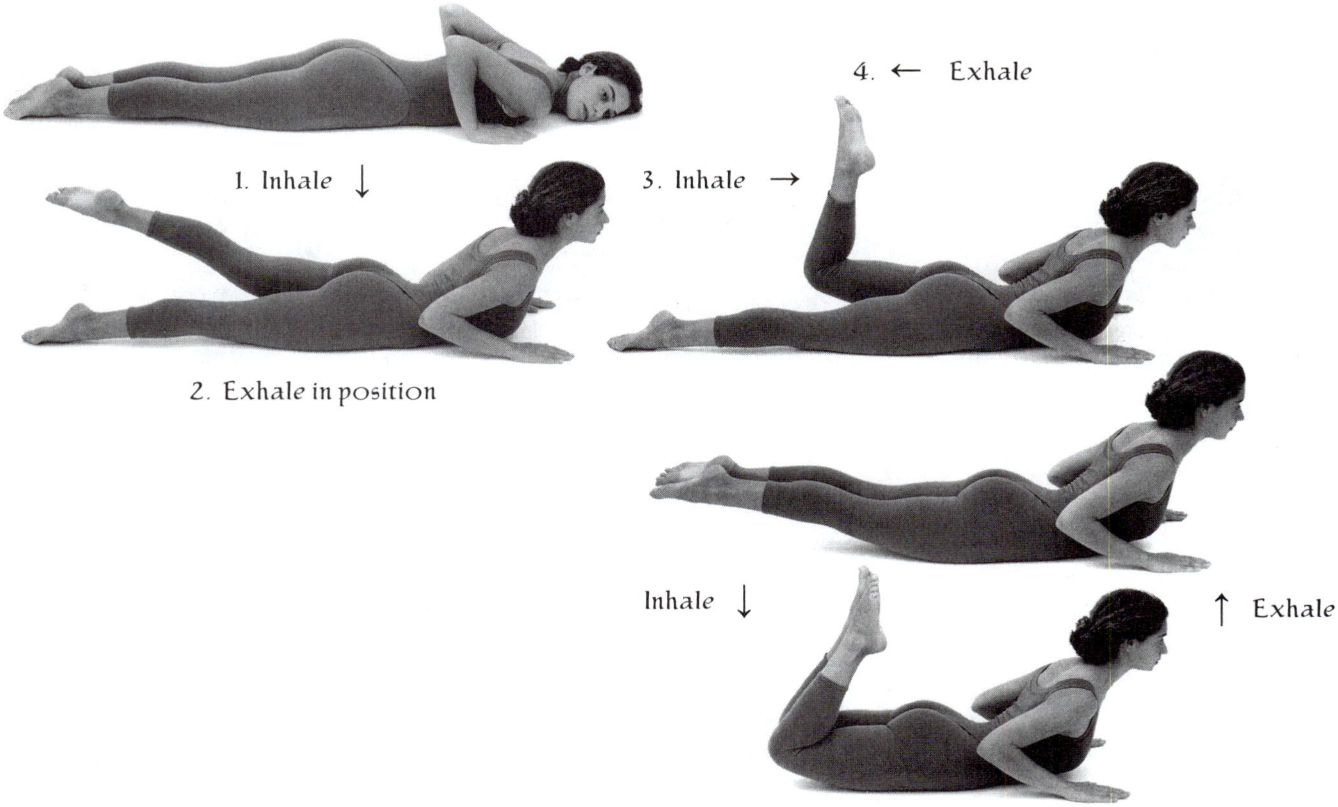
1. Inhale ↓
2. Exhale in position
3. Inhale →
4. ← Exhale
Inhale ↓
↑ Exhale

6.

POSTURE: Supta Pādāṅguṣṭhāsana.
EMPHASIS: To stretch and relax lower back. To mobilize knee joint and to stretch and strengthen surrounding musculature.
TECHNIQUE: Lie on back with legs bent, knees lifted toward chest, hands holding thighs behind knee, and arms bent.

On inhale: Extend legs upward, straightening arms.

On exhale: Return to starting position.

NUMBER: 6 times.
DETAILS: *On inhale:* Flex feet as legs are raised upward. Slightly bend knees. Push low back and sacrum downward. Keep chin down.

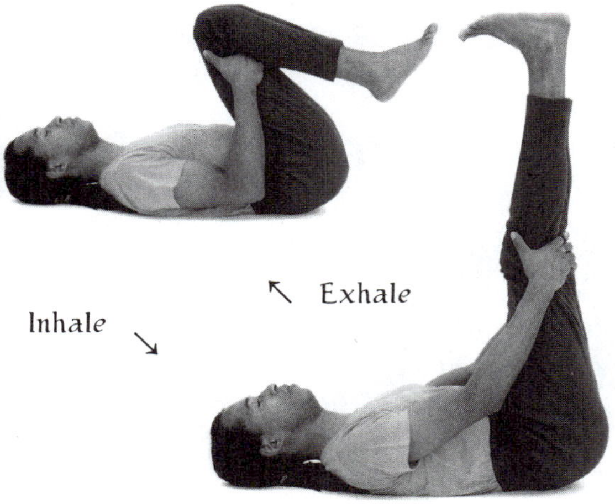
↖ Exhale
Inhale ↘

7.

POSTURE: Jaṭhara Parivṛtti.
EMPHASIS: To stretch and strengthen musculature of hip and outside of thigh.
TECHNIQUE: Lie flat on back, with arms out to sides and with left knee pulled up toward chest.

On exhale: Twist, bringing left knee toward floor on right side of body while turning head left.

On inhale: Return to starting position.

Repeat 4 times.

Then, from twisted position, lift knee up off floor several inches, keeping left hip vertically above right. Hold 5 seconds. Lower knee to floor.

Repeat 4 times.

Repeat on other side.

DETAILS: While staying in position, explore a gentle external rotation of lifted leg, feeling work in the hip abductors. Avoid straining neck.

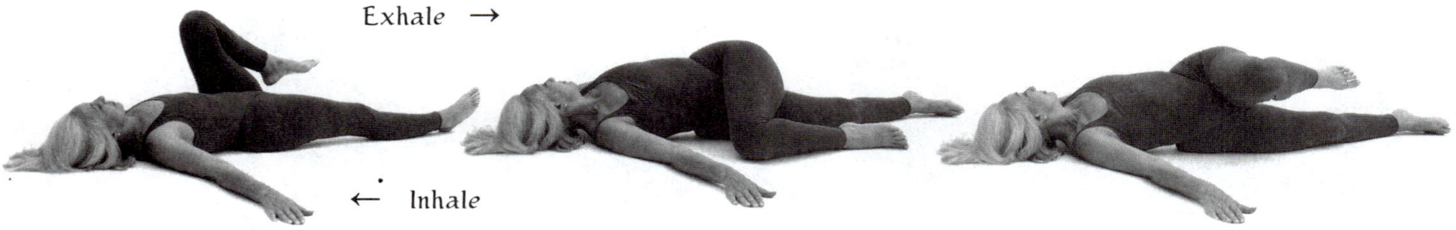

Lift knee, hold position briefly

8.

POSTURE: Apānāsana.
EMPHASIS: To gently stretch low back without compressing knees.
TECHNIQUE: Lie on back with both knees bent toward chest and with feet off floor. Place each hand behind its respective knee.

On exhale: Pull thighs gently but progressively toward chest.

On inhale: Return to starting position.

NUMBER: 8 times.
DETAILS: *On exhale:* Pull gently with arms, keeping shoulders down on floor and relaxed. Press low back down into floor, dropping chin slightly toward throat. Progressively lengthen exhale with each successive repetition.

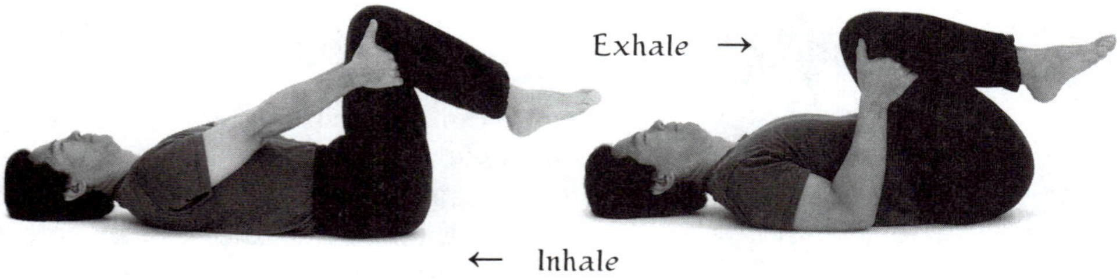

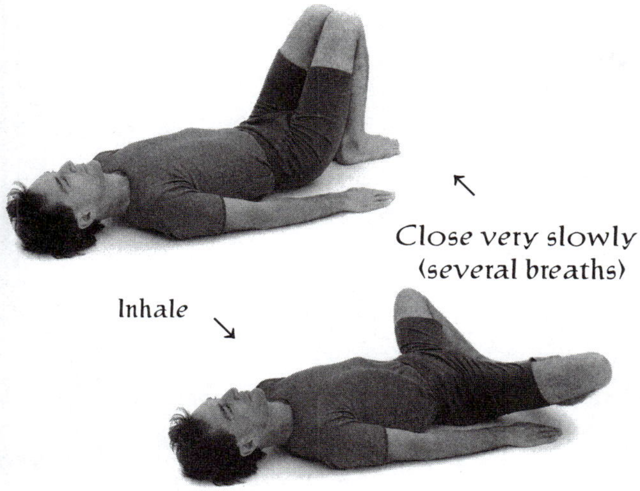

9.

POSTURE: Supta Baddha Koṇāsana.
EMPHASIS: To strengthen musculature of inner thighs.
TECHNIQUE: Lie on back with knees bent and feet near buttocks. Open legs wide, bringing soles of feet together. Take up to sixty seconds to close knees together. Open legs again naturally.
NUMBER: 6 times.
DETAILS: Keep low back flat on floor while closing legs. Allow any trembling of legs that may occur.

10.

POSTURE: Dvipāda Pīṭham.
EMPHASIS: To strengthen musculature of hips and thighs.
TECHNIQUE: Lie on back with arms down at sides, knees bent, and feet on floor, slightly apart and comfortably close to buttocks.

On inhale: Keeping chin down and press down on feet, raise pelvis up toward ceiling, until neck is gently flattened on floor

On exhale: Return to starting position.

NUMBER: 6 times.
DETAILS: *On inhale:* Lift spine vertebra by vertebra from bottom up. *On exhale:* Unwind spine, coming down vertebra by vertebra.

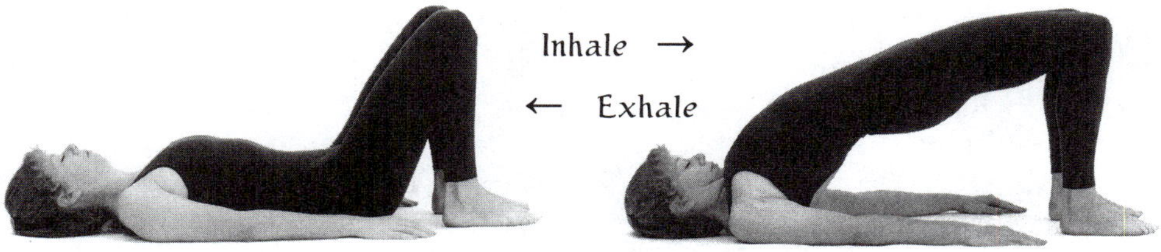

11.

POSTURE: Śavāsana with support.
EMPHASIS: To rest.
TECHNIQUE: Lie flat on back, with arms at sides, palms up, and with legs slightly apart. Close eyes. Relax body fully, keeping mind relaxed and alert to sensations in body.
DURATION: Minimum 5 minutes.

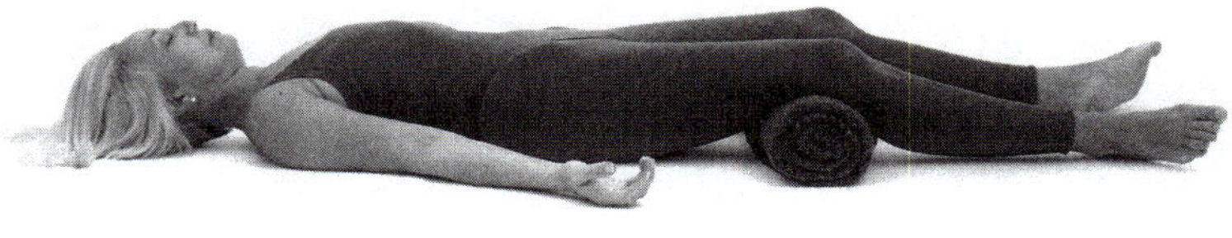

Chapter 4

Chronic Disease

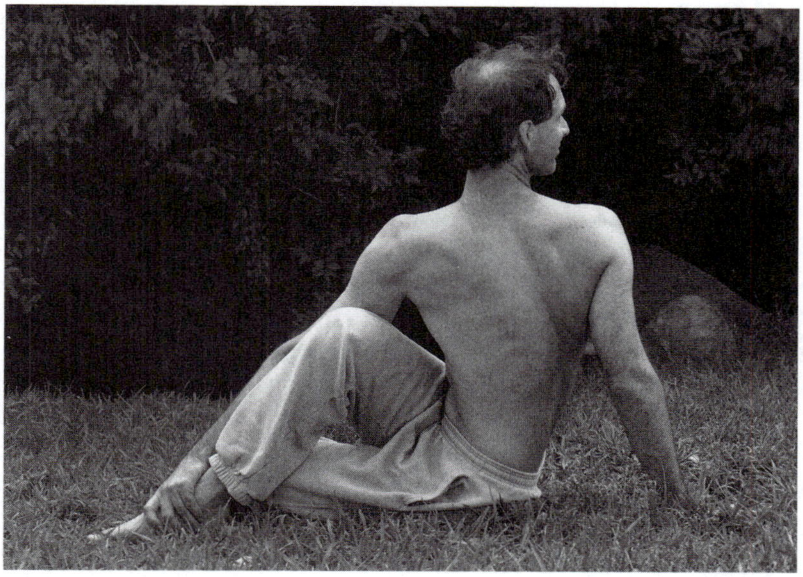

Digestion and Assimilation

In this system, food is transformed into nourishment for the cells of the body through the functions of various organs, including the mouth, teeth, tongue, salivary glands, throat, stomach, pancreas, liver, gall bladder, the small and large intestines, and the rectum. In a complex chemical process, masticated food is mixed with fluids from the organs and is broken down into nourishing elements, which are absorbed into the bloodstream and then throughout the body, and into wastes, which are eliminated.

The functional processes of the digestive system include the following:

Ingestion, in which food enters the body and begins to be processed by the actions of the jaw, teeth, and tongue, is mixed with secretions of the salivary glands, and is swallowed.

Digestion, in which food is chemically broken down into organic components through the action of acids, enzymes, and buffers secreted by the digestive tract and its accessory organs. In addition to chemical processes there are the mechanical actions of the stomach and intestines, which churn, mix, and move substances through the system.

Absorption, in which these organic elements are moved into the fluid that feeds the cells of the body.

Assimilation, in which the nutrients of the cells are utilized.

Elimination, in which the indigestible wastes from the digestive process are eliminated from the body through processes of dehydration and defecation.

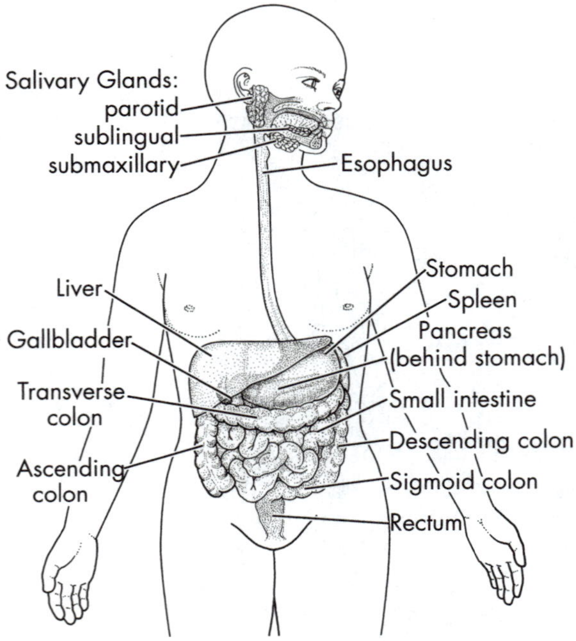

The complex process of turning food into the energy necessary to maintain life and health is regulated by the body's own natural capacity. Ideally, the body should absorb the maximum nutritional value from the food ingested and efficiently eliminate the indigestible residue. The starting point of this fundamental process is the choice of foods we put into our mouths, as well as the state of our minds and bodies when we eat. That food choice is not always determined by the true needs of the body, and we often are not eating in the optimal frame of mind or physical state.

For so many of us, what we eat is based on convention, habit, or convenience. We often eat on the run, or in the midst of other activity, regardless of our emotional state. The result is often indigestion, which compromises our ability both to absorb the maximum nutritional benefits of our food and to eliminate waste. Improper digestion further results in a weakened condition and an accumulation of toxicity, which can then become the cause of various diseases. These diseases may manifest in the digestive system itself or elsewhere. Of course, problems of the digestive system are not always caused directly by what and how we eat: the body is an integrated whole, and there can be a variety of complex causes leading to any given condition. And there are many different problems that may manifest within the digestive system itself, in one or several of the different digestive organs.

There is an ideal among the yogis that, if we were truly in touch with our bodies, we would instinctively know what foods we needed to eat every time we felt hunger, and that if we are not clear about what we should eat, it would be better not to eat at all. Furthermore, the body and mind should be in a relaxed and pleasant state, without hurry or agitation: if we are excited or upset, either physically or emotionally, we should not be eating. While eating, we should take time to really taste and savor each bite. After eating, there should be relaxed time to digest before we engage in activities that stimulate our systems.

When our digestion is strong, our body feels light and strong. We have plenty of energy. If there are no other complications, we sleep deeply and wake up feeling refreshed. Our skin color is good, our breath and body odor pleasant, and we have a high resistance to disease.

When our digestion is poor, we lack energy. Our sleep may be disturbed, so that we may feel tired even after a full night's rest. We are likely to accumulate toxins. Our complexion may be pasty, and the odor of our body and breath unpleasant. We are more susceptible to disease and more liable to experience hypersensitivity, irritability, heaviness or dullness, or other manifestations of emotional instability.

We can usually assess the condition of our digestive system by looking at our stools after defecation. This is, of course, a somewhat sensitive topic in our society. However, if we can overcome our squeamishness, much can be learned about how our body is responding to the foods we are eating and the way we are eating them. Some things to look for are whether the stool is too hard and compacted, or too loose, whether it tends to sink or float, and the intensity of its odor. The healthiest stool is well formed, almost like the shape of our intestines, floats, and doesn't have a very strong odor. This feedback is useful in deepening the process of self-reflection about what and how we eat, and how this contributes to our overall health and well-being.

When we suffer from digestive problems, we can help ourselves through the appropriate combination of lifestyle changes and Yoga practices. This may include changes in diet, taking appropriate supplements and/or medicinal remedies, as well as following the therapeutic guidance of our health practitioners. And, although we cannot solve these conditions exclusively through Yoga practice, we can be sure that a carefully constructed practice of āsanas and prāṇāyāma makes our whole system function more efficiently and in that way brings more balance into our system. Yoga therapy is not a substitute for medical attention. It is an aid to whatever else we may be doing under our own guidance or under the supervision of a professional.

Although the entire digestive system ideally functions as an integrated whole, problematic conditions can manifest in different organs. All of these conditions can be loosely grouped into two distinct categories: conditions of excess (hyper conditions) and conditions of deficiency (hypo conditions). The ancient yogis used the image of fire (*agni*) to understand the power of digestion. Following this theory, digestive disorders reflect some imbalance in this internal fire. In hyper functioning, the digestive fire is too strong; in hypo functioning, it is too weak. If the fire is either too strong or too weak, food is not properly broken down into its respective nutrients. As a consequence, the body does not receive the nourishment it needs to thrive and the undigested food becomes a source of toxicity in the body, weakening the system and creating the conditions for disease.

There is a paradox in working therapeutically with these extremes of the digestive system, because we work toward balance—in both cases—through relaxation. The well-known "fight-or-flight" response of our sympathetic nervous system actually stops the digestive process. Our organism developed such that, in cases of emergency, all available energy is redirected to the reflexes and musculature we need for survival. Thus blood is taken out of the digestive system and distributed to the muscles, heart, and brain, and the blood vessels in the digestive system contract, inhibiting digestion. This sympathetic response happens whenever we are under stress. In fact, many digestion problems come from a chronically stressed, over-amped sympathetic nervous system. Symptoms of this "sympathetic overdrive" include feeling stressed, "hyper," irritable, or rushed, along with eventual fatigue and exhaustion due to depletion of bodily reserves.

The digestive process, a parasympathetic function, works best when we are relaxed. We paradoxically calm the fight-or-flight response (sympathetic function) to stimulate the relaxation response (parasympathetic function), in order to enhance digestion.

Hyper Conditions of the Digestive System

Hyper conditions of the digestive system include the following:

Conditions of the stomach: stress-based excessive gastric acid secretion, ulcers, and heartburn (not including cases of hiatus hernia).

Conditions of the intestines: mild chronic diarrhea, Irritable Bowel Syndrome (IBS), and Inflammatory Bowel Disease (IBD).

These conditions often involve cramps, gas, burning sensations, and overall weakness. In these conditions, there is a tendency toward irritability, burning sensations, headaches, and even fevers.

Diarrhea or loose, watery stools. There can be mild but chronic to extreme, acute conditions of diarrhea. At any level, this condition indicates poor absorption of nutrients. The causes of chronic diarrhea can be poor eating habits, including poor food combinations, excessive spices, overeating, eating oily foods, and even eating too fast or in an agitated state of mind. Diarrhea can also be an infectious condition, resulting from impure food or water. This can range from a mild case to the more severe condition of dysentery.

In addition, there are more serious diseases of the intestines, grouped from the more mild irritable bowel syndromes to the more serious inflammatory bowel diseases. IBS symptoms include crampy lower abdominal discomfort and pain, gassiness, diarrhea, or constipation. The more serious IBD conditions include colitis, Crohn's disease, and diverticulosis. In working with chronic digestive problems, it is important to rule out these more serious conditions first. As with the more serious musculoskeletal problems,

Yoga therapy may help as an adjunct to professional medical treatments, but the wrong practice may actually irritate the condition.

When there is any kind of inflammatory disease resulting in diarrhea, there is often excessive heat in the body. In this case we work to reduce the heat (*langhana*) and soothe the system. We must be extremely cautious about straining the stomach through abdominal work. Thus, simple postures are most useful, such as simple forward bends with the knees bent, gently massaging the stomach, or simple twists, like Jaṭhara Parivṛtti. The lateral variation of Jaṭhara Parivṛtti is also very useful for increasing circulation without straining the system, although it must be applied cautiously. Lengthening the exhale progressively, and coordinating these simple movements with simple low-pitched sounds will further soothe the system. In acute conditions, we use even simpler techniques.

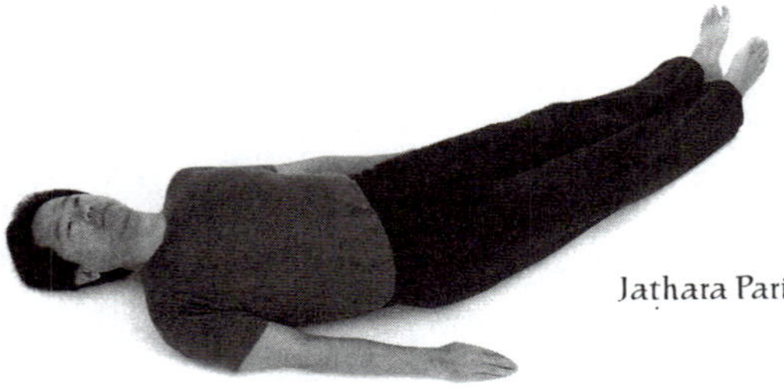

Jaṭhara Parivṛtti

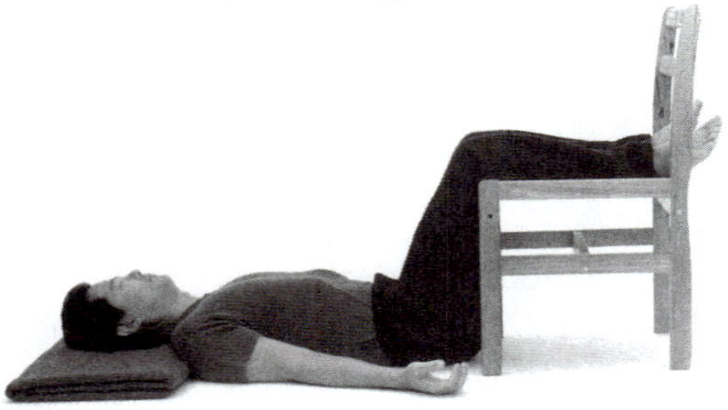

supported Apānāsana

We should avoid any strong stretching of the belly (as in deep back bends), and always exhale gently, without pulling in the belly.

The practice that follows is presented to illustrate an approach to chronic hyper conditions of the digestive system. Again, it is not prescriptive but rather indicative of an approach to these conditions.

Working with Crohn's Disease

This practice was designed for L.M., a sixty-three-year-old woman who had been diagnosed with Crohn's disease several years before. She came to see me for a general Yoga practice to support her body while she tried to work on her condition through diet, nutrition, and herbal remedies.

L.M. had a youthful energy and a very positive attitude. As I got to know her, I realized that underneath her happy countenance was an ever-present fear that she would be unable to overcome her condition and would have to have surgery—a possibility that she dreaded. Working on her condition had become the main focus of her life.

L.M. was ready and willing to develop a regular movement and breathing practice. The only structural problem that she had was an unusually deep lumbar scoliosis. I wanted to offer her a practice that would address the scoliosis, gently increase the circulation to her lower abdomen, and help her to deeply relax.

We began very simply, once a week, and over several months we evolved the following practice. She liked the practice, especially the humming, which she said helped her relax more deeply.

As we got to know each other better, we discussed the issue of surgery. I reminded her that a surgeon who specializes in her condition would have a lot of experience and that the technology was getting more and more sophisticated every year. I told her that I hoped she could open her heart to the possibility that she might have to go that route.

The day came when she told me that her doctor had scheduled the surgery. She told me that, though she was afraid, she was hopeful. The surgery was successful, and L.M. tells me she is so relieved to return to a normal life. She is still careful about her diet, but she says she no longer "obsesses" about her condition. She still does her Yoga practice and comes to work with me several times each year.

A Practice for Crohn's Disease

1.

POSTURE: Ekapāda Apanāsana.
EMPHASIS: To gently compress belly while progressively extending exhale.
TECHNIQUE: Lie on back with right knee bent toward chest, right foot off floor, left knee bent and left foot on floor. Place both hands on right knee.

On exhale: Pull right thigh gently but progressively toward chest.

On inhale: Return to starting position.

Repeat on other side.

NUMBER: 8 times each side, one side at a time.
DETAILS: *On exhale:* Pull gently with arms, keeping shoulders down on floor and relaxed. Press low back down into floor, drop chin slightly toward throat. Progressively lengthen exhale with each successive repetition.

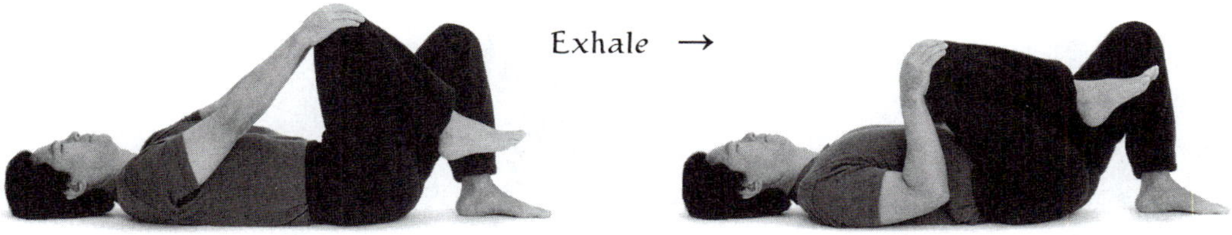

2.

POSTURE: Cakravākāsana.
EMPHASIS: To gently compress and stretch belly while working with humming sound to soothe belly.
TECHNIQUE: Get down on hands and knees, with shoulders vertically above wrists and with hips above knees.

On inhale: Lift chest up and away from belly.

Exhale with a soft, low-pitched humming sound while gently contracting belly, rounding low back, and bringing chest toward thighs.

NUMBER: 4 times with no humming; 4 times with humming.
DETAILS: *On inhale:* Avoid pulling spine with head, overarching neck. Lead with chest, keeping chin slightly down. Avoid overarching low back; rather, feel stretching in belly. *On exhale:* Round low back without collapsing chest over belly. Avoid increasing curvature of upper back. Let chest lower toward thighs sooner than hips toward heels.

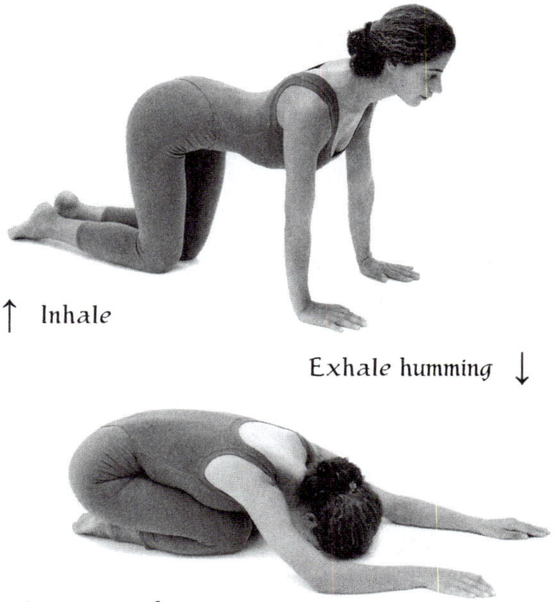

4 times no humming;
4 times with humming

3.

POSTURE: Jaṭhara Parivṛtti variation.
EMPHASIS: To gently twist and compress belly, progressively increasing number of breaths while staying in posture.
TECHNIQUE: Lie flat on back with both knees bent, thighs lifted toward chest, both feet off ground, and arms out to sides, slightly less than right angles to torso.

On exhale: Bring both knees toward floor on right side of body, twisting abdomen and simultaneously turning head left.

On inhale: Return to starting position.

NUMBER: Stay in twist 1, 2, 3, and then 4 full breaths on each side, alternating sides.
DETAILS: *On exhale:* Throughout movement, keep knees at an angle to torso that is less than ninety degrees.

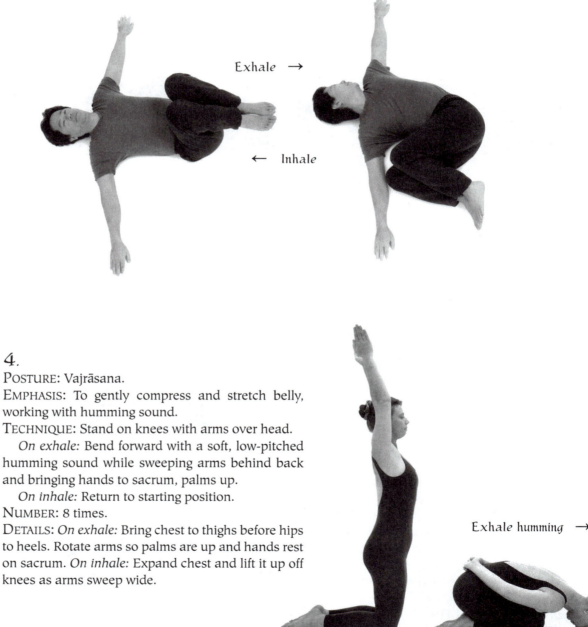

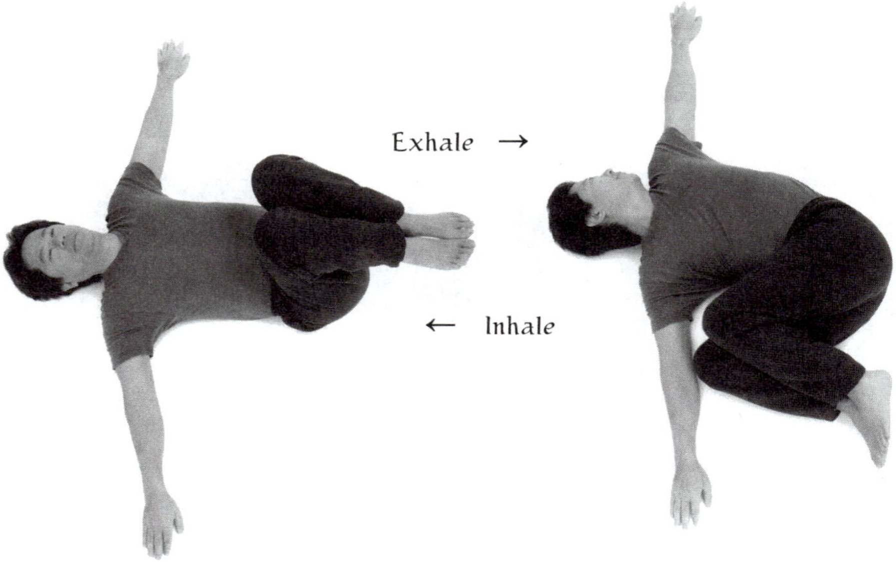

4.

POSTURE: Vajrāsana.
EMPHASIS: To gently compress and stretch belly, working with humming sound.
TECHNIQUE: Stand on knees with arms over head.

On exhale: Bend forward with a soft, low-pitched humming sound while sweeping arms behind back and bringing hands to sacrum, palms up.

On inhale: Return to starting position.

NUMBER: 8 times.
DETAILS: *On exhale:* Bring chest to thighs before hips to heels. Rotate arms so palms are up and hands rest on sacrum. *On inhale:* Expand chest and lift it up off knees as arms sweep wide.

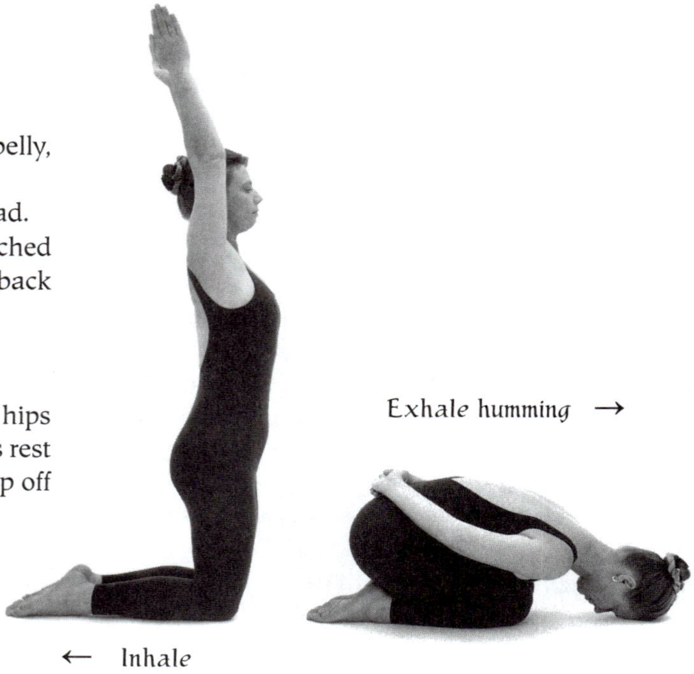

5.

POSTURE: Jaṭhara Parivṛtti variation.
EMPHASIS: To gently compress and stretch belly, using belly breathing technique.
TECHNIQUE: Lie on back with legs straight and arms flat and at a small angle from sides.

Walk both feet in small increments to left until right side of lower torso and hip are gently stretched. Raise right arm up over head.

Stay and breathe deeply, gently protruding belly *on inhale.*

Return to starting point.

Repeat on other side.

NUMBER: Stay 8 deep breaths each side.
DETAILS: Go only as far with legs as allows low back and hips to stay stable on floor. Avoid increasing arch of low back.

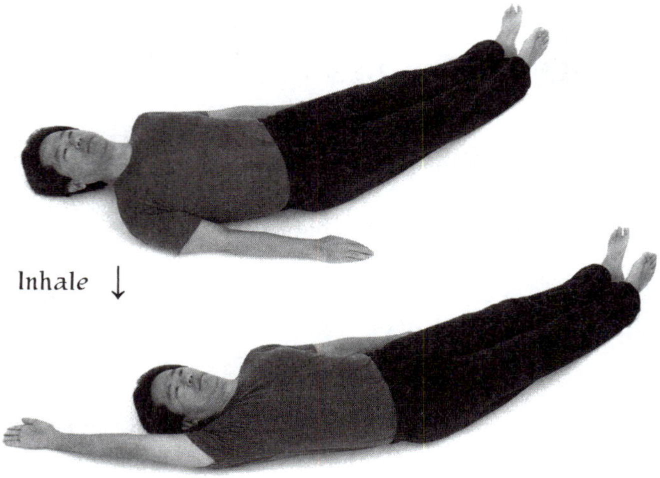

Stay in position

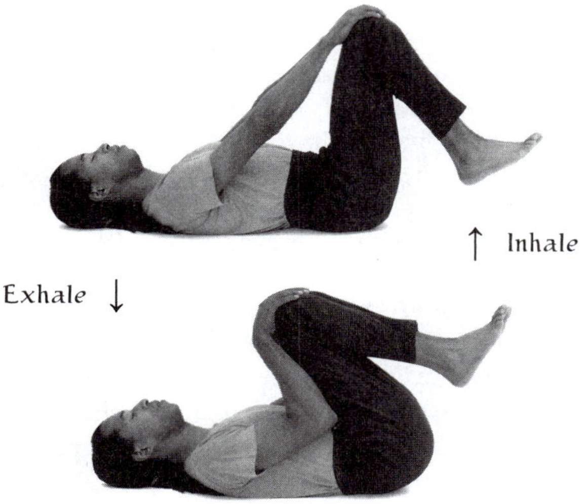

6.

POSTURE: Apānāsana.
EMPHASIS: To gently compress belly while progressively extending exhale.
TECHNIQUE: Lie on back with both knees bent toward chest and feet off floor. Place each hand on its respective knee.

On exhale: Pull thighs gently but progressively toward chest.

On inhale: Return to starting position.

NUMBER: 12 times.
DETAILS: *On exhale:* Pull gently with arms, keeping shoulders relaxed and on floor. Press low back down into floor and drop chin slightly toward throat. Progressively lengthen exhale with each successive repetition.

7.

POSTURE: Śavāsana with support.
EMPHASIS: To rest.
TECHNIQUE: Lie flat on back, with arms at sides, palms up, and legs resting comfortably on a chair. Cover closed eyes. Relax body fully, keeping mind relaxed and alert to sensations in body.
DURATION: Minimum 5 minutes.

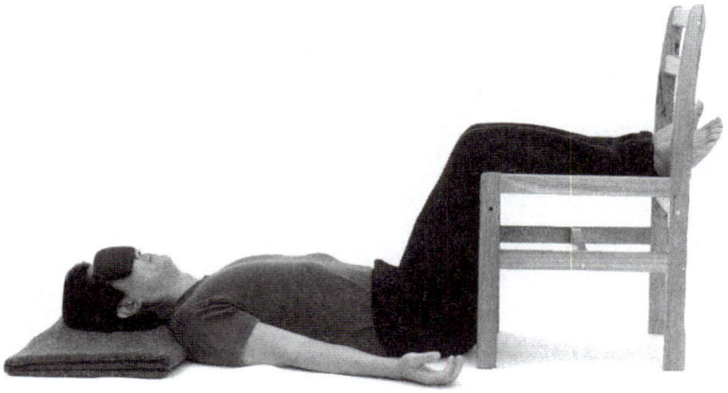

Hypo Conditions of the Digestive System

Hypo conditions of the digestive system, which involve either decreased digestive ability or decreased mobility, include the following:

> *Conditions of the stomach and small intestines:* lack of digestive enzyme, low secretion of gastric acid (hypochlorhydria—a condition that often occurs in old age).
>
> *Conditions of the large intestines:* constipation.

These conditions involve abdominal pain, gas, and indigestion (feeling bad after eating). In this condition, there is a tendency toward heaviness, lack of energy, and bloating.

Constipation involves infrequent, sluggish, and sometimes painful elimination. There may be mild to severe conditions of constipation. Chronic constipation can be caused by poor eating habits, delaying or suppressing the urge to eliminate, as well as excessive tension and anxiety. At any level, constipation indicates an inadequate elimination of wastes from the body.

Unlike hyper conditions, where we want to soothe the system, in hypo conditions we can work the abdominal area more directly in order to stimulate digestion and the movement (peristalsis) of wastes along the digestive tract. We work with a firm pulling in of the belly on exhalation, coordinated with forward bends and twists. We can even do forward bending and/or twisting postures while holding the breath out after exhalation. It is also often helpful to include some stretching of the belly through gentle backward bends. Finally, the use of segmented (krama) breathing on exhalation is also very useful for these conditions.

The practice that follows is presented to illustrate an approach to chronic hypo conditions of the digestive system. As with the previous practice, it is not prescriptive but rather indicative of an approach to these conditions.

Working with Constipation

This practice was developed for D.M., a thirty-six-year-old woman working in the commodities market. She told me she spent the better part of each day in front of a computer terminal and on the phone. She said her job was very stressful. She told me that she had been constipated for years, and although increasing the fiber intake in her diet had helped, the problem persisted. She also told me she went to the gym regularly to do low-impact aerobics.

D.M. was in good physical condition and did not suffer from chronic aches and pains. I noticed that, though she was physically toned, there was a lot of tension in her musculature—especially her jaw. I decided to develop a langhana practice for her, emphasizing exhalation, movement on hold after exhalation, forward bends, and twists. Since she regularly worked out, the main focus for this practice was to help her relax generally, and to increase circulation to and relax the lower abdomen specifically.

Over several months, we evolved the following practice. D.M. was very disciplined and was able to practice daily. She told me that often, within an hour or two after practice, she was able to have a satisfying bowel movement. I saw her again about a year after our last session together, and I asked her how she was doing. She told me that when she practices, she has no problems, but if she stops, the constipation comes back.

A Practice for Constipation

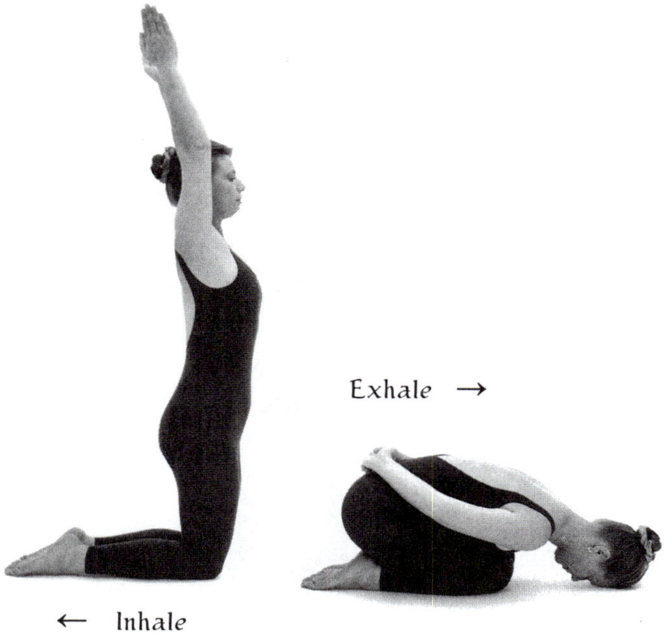
Exhale →
← Inhale

1.

POSTURE: Vajrāsana.
EMPHASIS: To compress belly and progressively extend exhale.
TECHNIQUE: Stand on knees with arms over head.

On exhale: Bend forward, sweeping arms behind back, bringing hands to sacrum with palms up.

Make each exhale progressively longer.

On inhale: Return to starting position.

NUMBER: 8 times.
DETAILS: *On exhale:* Bring chest to thighs before buttocks to heels. Rotate arms so palms are up and hands rest on sacrum. *On inhale:* Expand chest and lift it up off knees as arms sweep wide.

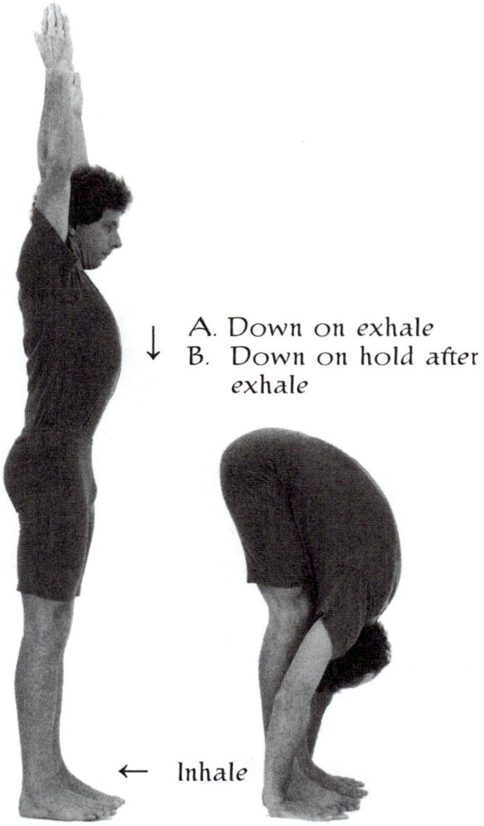
↓ A. Down on exhale
B. Down on hold after exhale
← Inhale

2.

POSTURE: Uttānāsana.
EMPHASIS: To compress belly. To introduce movement on hold after exhale.
TECHNIQUE:

A: Stand with feet slightly apart, arms over head.

On exhale: Bend forward, bending knees slightly, bringing chest to thighs, and palms to sides of feet.

On inhale: Return to starting position.

B: *Exhale* fully in starting position.

Holding breath out after exhale, bend forward, keeping belly held in.

On inhale: Return to starting point.

NUMBER: A four times. B four times.
DETAILS: *On exhale:* Bend knees to facilitate stretching of low back. Move chin down toward throat. *On inhale:* Lift chest up and away from thighs, flattening upper back. Keep knees bent until end of movement.

3.

Posture: Parivṛtti Trikoṇāsana.
Emphasis: To twist and compress belly. To achieve subtle torsion on hold after exhale.
Technique: Stand with feet spread wider than shoulders, arms out to sides and parallel to floor.

On exhale: Bend forward, bringing left hand down to floor, right arm pointing upward, twisting shoulders right. Turn head down toward left hand.

Holding breath out after exhale 4 to 6 seconds, twist slightly further.

On inhale: Return to starting position.

Repeat on other side.

Number: 6 times each side, alternately.
Details: *On exhale:* Initiate and control torsion through belly contraction. Rotate shoulder girdle until right shoulder is vertically above left. *On inhale:* Untwist torso while returning to starting position.

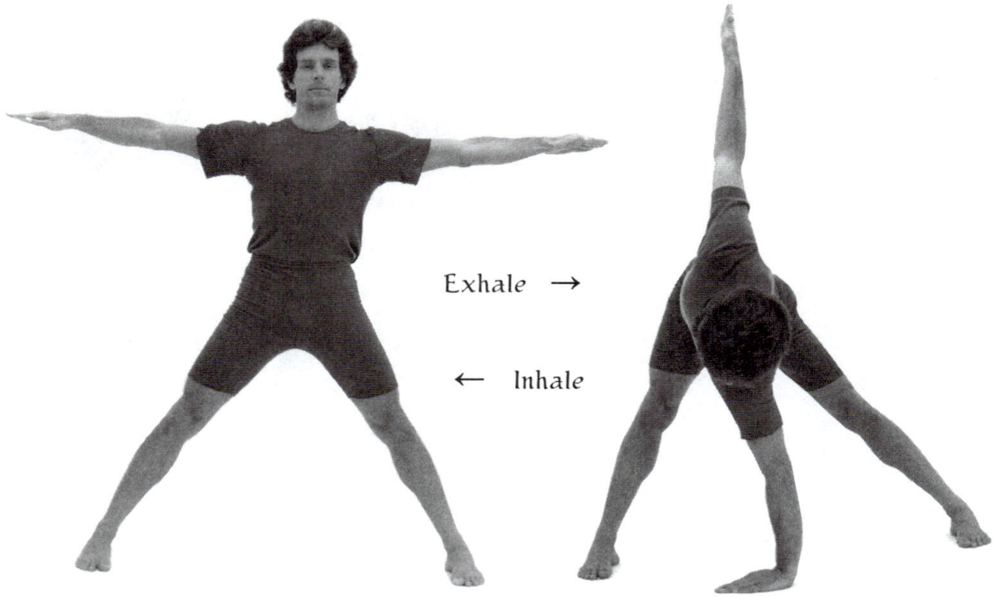

4.

Posture: Cakravākāsana.
Emphasis: To make transition from standing to supine position. To stretch rib cage on inhale and low back on exhale.
Technique: Get down on hands and knees, with shoulders vertically above wrists and with hips above knees.

On inhale: Lift chest up and away from belly.

On exhale: Gently contract belly, round low back, and bring chest toward thighs.

Number: 8 times.
Details: *On inhale:* Lead with chest, keeping chin slightly down. Avoid compressing low back; rather, feel chest expanding. *On exhale:* Round low back without collapsing chest over belly. Avoid increasing curvature of upper back. Let chest lower toward thighs sooner than hips toward heels.

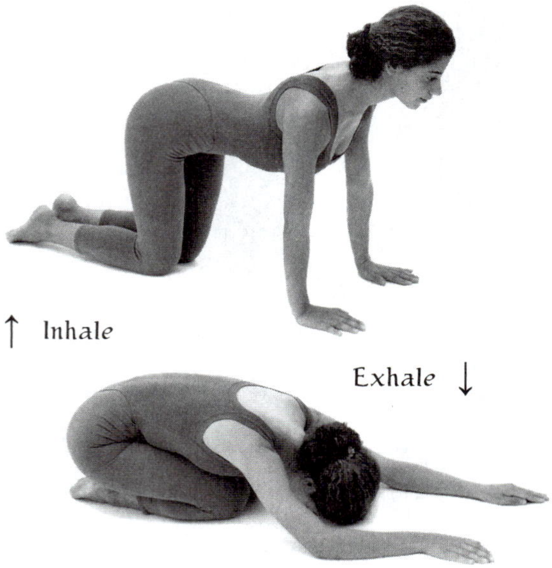

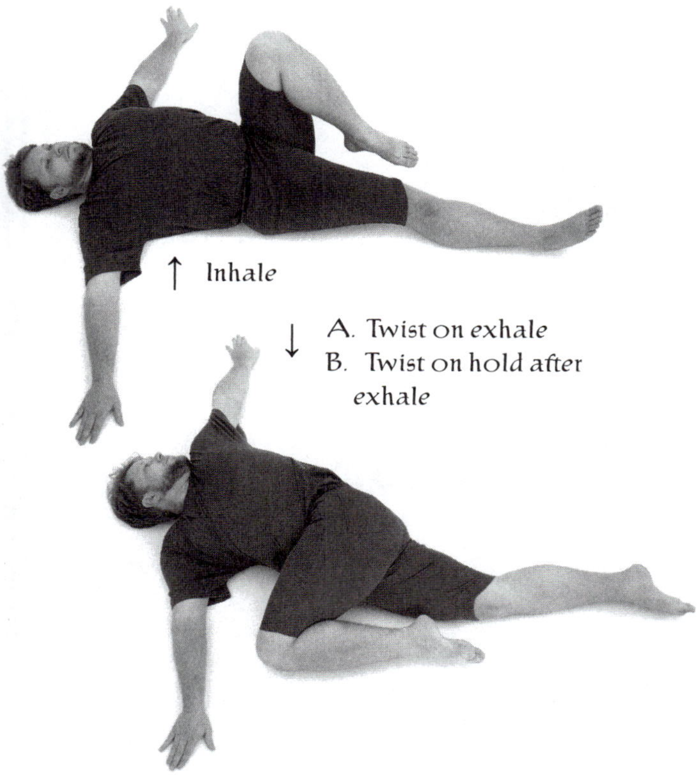
↑ Inhale
↓ A. Twist on exhale
B. Twist on hold after exhale

5.

POSTURE: Jaṭhara Parivṛtti.
EMPHASIS: To twist and compress belly. To move on hold after exhale.
TECHNIQUE: Lie flat on back, with arms out to sides and with left knee pulled up toward chest.

A: *On exhale:* Twist, bringing left knee toward floor on right side of body while turning head to left.

On inhale: Return to starting position.

Repeat 4 times.

B: *Exhale* fully in starting position. Holding breath out after exhale, twist again to right, holding belly in.

On inhale: Return to starting position.

Repeat 4 times.

Repeat on other side.

DETAILS: *On exhale:* When twisting right, keep angles between left arm and torso and between left knee and torso less than ninety degrees.

6.

POSTURE: Ūrdhva Prasārita Pādāsana.
EMPHASIS: To stimulate lower abdomen, extend spine and flatten it onto floor, and stretch legs.
TECHNIQUE: Lie on back with arms down at sides, legs bent, and knees in toward chest.

On inhale: Raise arms upward all the way to floor behind head, and legs upward toward ceiling.

On exhale: Return to starting position.

Repeat 4 times.

DETAILS: *On inhale:* Flex feet as legs are raised upward. Slightly bend knees, keeping angle between legs and torso less than ninety degrees. Push low back and sacrum downward. Bring chin down.

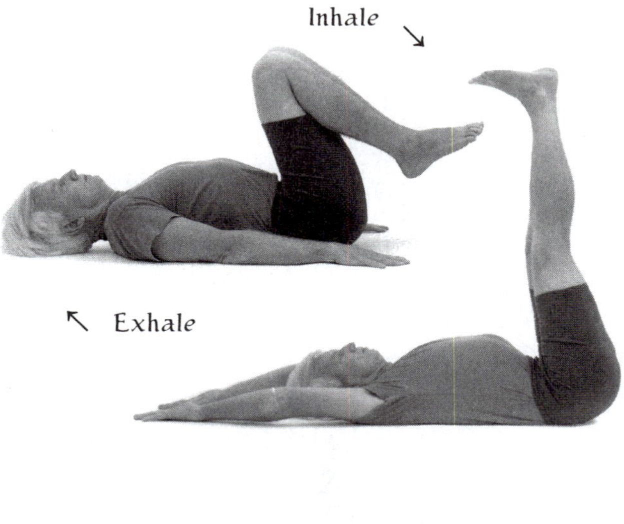
Inhale ↘
↖ Exhale

7.

POSTURE: Paścimatānāsana.
EMPHASIS: To compress belly and stretch back.
To move on hold after exhale.
TECHNIQUE:

A: Sit with legs forward, back straight, and arms raised over head.

On exhale: Bending knees slightly, bend forward, bringing chest to thighs, and palms to balls of feet.

On inhale: Return to starting position.

B: *Exhale* fully in starting position.

While holding after exhale, bend forward, keeping belly held in.

On inhale: Return to starting point.

NUMBER: A four times; B four times.
DETAILS: *On exhale:* Bend knees to facilitate stretching low back and bring belly and chest to thighs. Move chin down toward throat. Feel like diaphragm moves up while holding after exhale. *On inhale:* Lift chest up and away from thighs, flattening upper back.

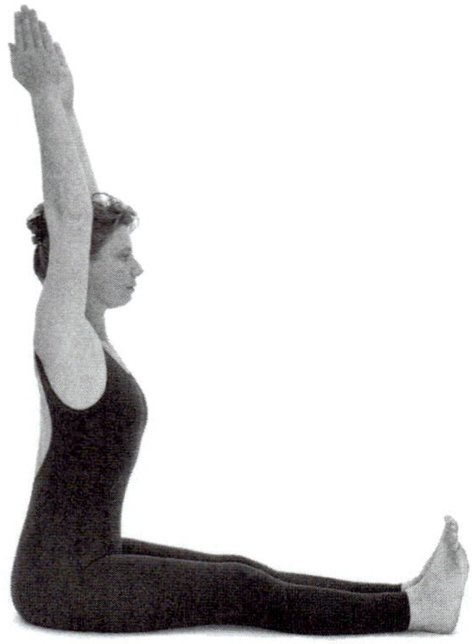

↑ Inhale

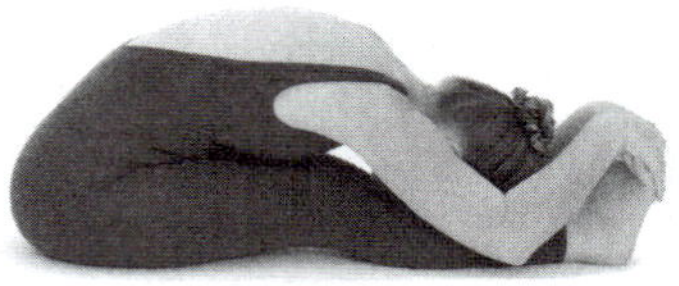

↓ A. Forward bend on exhale
B. Forward bend on hold after exhale

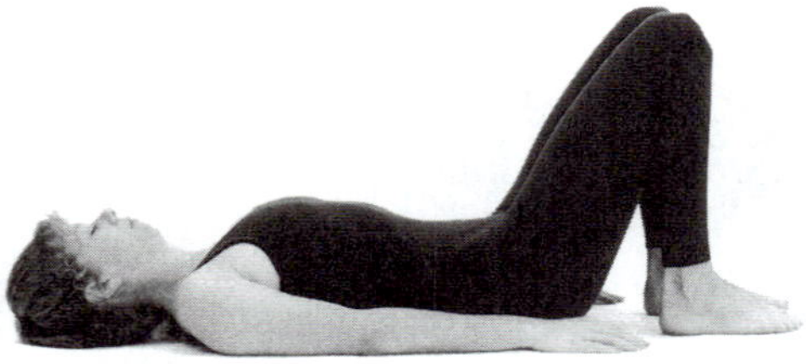

↑ Exhale

Inhale ↓

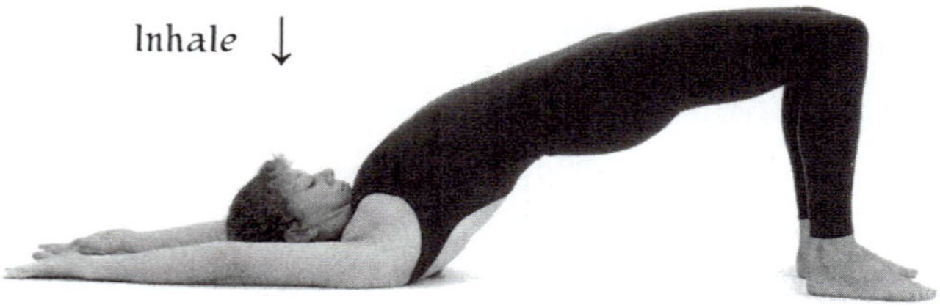

8.

POSTURE: Dvipāda Pīṭham.
EMPHASIS: To relax back and stretch belly.
TECHNIQUE: Lie on back with arms down at sides, knees bent, and feet on floor, slightly apart and comfortably close to buttocks.

On inhale: Pressing down on feet and keeping chin down, raise pelvis until neck is gently flattened on floor, while raising arms up overhead to floor behind.

On exhale: Return to starting position.

NUMBER: 6 times.
DETAILS: *On inhale:* Lift spine, vertebra by vertebra, from bottom up. *On exhale:* Unwind spine, coming down vertebra by vertebra.

9.

POSTURE: Śavāsana with support.
EMPHASIS: To rest.
TECHNIQUE: Lie flat on back, with arms at sides, palms up, legs slightly apart, with a support under the knees. Close eyes. Relax body fully, keeping mind relaxed and alert to sensations in body.
DURATION: Minimum 5 minutes.

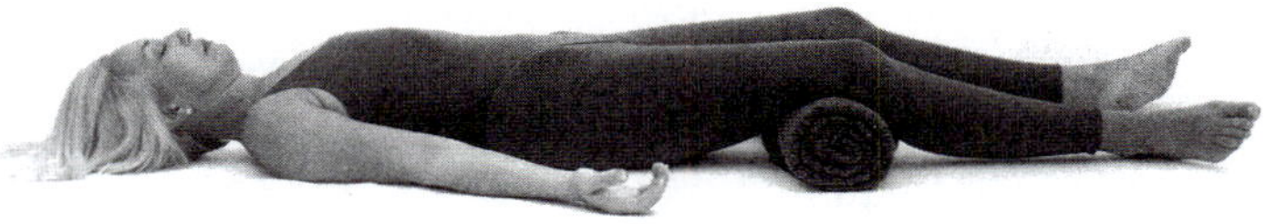

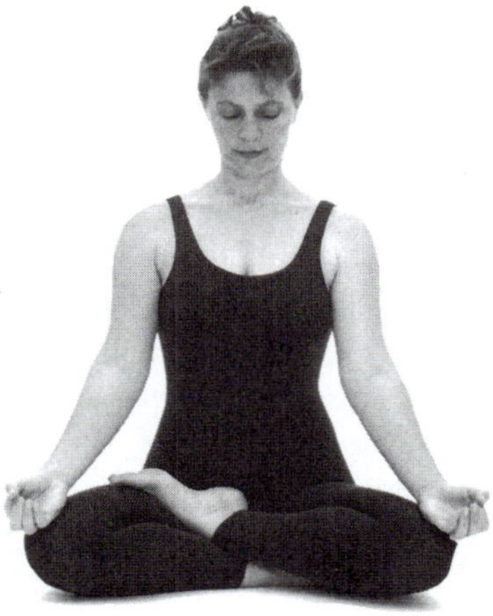

10.

POSTURE: Prāṇāyāma-Viloma Krama.
EMPHASIS: To stimulate and compress belly through segmented exhale.
TECHNIQUE:

Inhale deeply and fully.
Exhale ½ of breath in 4 to 6 seconds.
Pause in middle of exhale for 4 to 6 seconds.
Exhale remainder of breath in 4 to 6 seconds.
Hold breath out 4 to 6 seconds.
Inhale deeply.
Repeat.

NUMBER: 8 times.
DETAILS: Control first segment of exhale from pubic bone to navel. Control last segment of exhale from navel to solar plexus.

Respiratory System

Respiration is essential for the life and function of every cell in our bodies. Cells utilize oxygen and produce carbon dioxide, and it is through respiration that the cells obtain the one and eliminate the other. The respiratory system consists of the nose, nasal cavities, sinuses, pharynx, larynx (voice box), trachea (wind pipe), and the lungs—including the air passages (bronchi), the air sacs (alveoli), and the surrounding membranes (pleura). The upper part of the respiratory tract serves to filter, warm, and humidify incoming air. The lower part provides surfaces through which the vital exchange of gasses occurs.

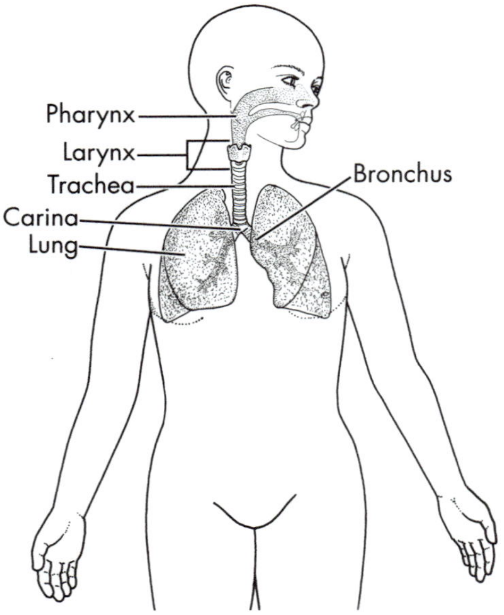

There are actually three levels of the respiratory process:

Ventilation refers to the twofold, mechanical process of inhalation and exhalation.

Delivery refers to the vital exchange (by diffusion) and transport (via circulation) of gasses between the lung surfaces and the bloodstream, between the bloodstream and the fluids surrounding the cells, and between those fluids and the cells themselves.

Utilization refers to the use of oxygen by the cells for metabolic processes, primarily the production of energy. It is through this cellular metabolism that the cells generate, store, and use energy to support and maintain bodily function.

This threefold process of respiration nourishes and purifies the blood, and thereby the entire body. The cardiovascular system provides the link between these three processes. Through inhalation, oxygen in the air passes through the lungs, into the bloodstream, and then to every cell of the body. Through exhalation, waste material (carbon dioxide) is returned from the cells, via the bloodstream, to the lungs, and is exhaled out of the body.

In addition to their vital respiratory function, the pleural membranes protect the delicate lung surfaces from changes in temperature, dehydration, and the presence of pathogens. The larynx, which includes the vocal chords, enables us to generate vocal sounds. The nose filters the air, preventing airborne particles, insects, et cetera, from entering the deeper nasal cavity and from there into the lungs.

In normal activity, the cellular demand for oxygen is met by automatic, reflexive breathing. In this process, the inhalation phase, which is active, lasts for approximately two seconds, and the exhalation, which is passive, lasts for approximately three seconds. The normal rate of respiration for an adult is between twelve and eighteen cycles per minute.

When we are exercising or otherwise stressing the system, there is significantly greater demand for oxygen, and our respiratory rate increases accordingly. When this occurs, there is a homeostatic integration of the respiratory rhythm and the cardiovascular response, so that the increased respiratory rate and the cardiac circulation are coordinated. In fact, we measure the quality of our aerobic workouts by this increase, usually measured by the increased heart rate.

It is interesting to notice that these increases in respiratory and cardiac rates occur both when we are very physically active and when we are strongly stimulated emotionally. When we are physically active, the muscles function as auxiliary pumps for the heart, assisting circulation. In this case, there is an overall developmental conditioning of the body. If, on the other hand, we are chronically emotionally stressed without being physically active, the respiratory and cardiac rates have to increase to meet the increased oxygen demand without the support of the musculature. In this case, the systems of the body are taxed in an unhealthy way.

There is an old notion among the yogis that we are all born with a certain number of breaths in this life.

The goal of the yogis was to slow down the natural respiratory rate and to develop the capacity to engage in increasingly demanding muscular activities with progressively deeper and slower breaths. This represents a somewhat different view of aerobic conditioning than the one current today, though both are oriented to the efficient oxygenation of the entire system and the development of cardiovascular fitness and stamina. Public recognition of the importance of aerobic exercise for maintaining optimal health is on the rise. Yet many people have not been able to integrate this important practice into their lives.

Usually, we are so caught up in the momentum of our activities that we are unaware of our breathing patterns. It is common for people to say, when reflecting on their breath, "I don't breathe." Of course, we are all always breathing in some fashion, but the normal patterns of breathing are usually shallow, restricted, and punctuated with holding patterns. The ancient Yoga authority Patañjali declared that these normal, disturbed, irregular habits of breathing are themselves symptoms of deep imbalances in our system. They can either indicate the presence of various mental afflictions, physical diseases, or be contributing factors to lowering our immunity and increasing our susceptibility to such diseases. When our breathing patterns are weak, we may have low energy and find ourselves easily fatigued and more emotionally stressed. When, on the other hand, our breathing patterns are deep and strong, we have increased endurance, stamina, and a sense of well-being.

In addition to developing poor breathing habits, many of us live and work in relatively toxic environments, where the need for the purification that occurs through good aerobic activity is even greater. In addition, habits like smoking tax the respiratory system and increase toxicity in the body. In fact, lung cancer is on the rise worldwide, and the vast majority of lung cancers have been directly linked to cigarette smoking. Smoking makes the air we take into our lungs dryer and contaminates it with particles that have been shown to be carcinogenic.

There are many different factors that, in combination, reduce the efficiency of the respiratory system. When this vital function is impaired, the rest of our system is negatively impacted and there are various problematic conditions that may manifest within the respiratory system itself.

Structurally, breathing is inhibited due to weak respiratory muscles, rigid and inelastic structures of the chest, and poor lung capacity. The result is often poor ventilation and oxygenation. This condition is often present when there is a sunken or shallow chest. Symptoms include weakness, low breath endurance, and fast or shallow breathing.

Infectious conditions, directly linked to a weakened immune response, that attack the respiratory system include common colds, coughs and flus, or, at a more serious level, bronchitis, pneumonia, and tuberculosis. Symptoms of these conditions range from runny nose or sore throat to accumulation of mucus and phlegm, fevers, difficulty in breathing, cough, wheezing, weakness, and chest pain.

Many allergic conditions, also linked to a defect in the immune system, attack the respiratory system. Common allergies such as allergic rhinitis or hay fever produce similar symptoms, including sneezing, wheezing, accumulation of mucus and phlegm, feeling of tightness in the chest, and difficulty in breathing. Bronchial asthma, which is less common but still widespread, is a more serious form of allergic reaction. Asthma sufferers have episodes of mild to severe breathlessness and wheezing. These episodes, commonly referred to as asthma attacks, are characterized by narrowing of the air passages and difficulty in exhalation. These attacks are usually recurring and are variable in severity. Although acute asthma can indeed be life threatening, there is no actual damage to the lung tissue.

More serious, long-term conditions, which result in actual physical damage to the respiratory tract, are chronic bronchitis and emphysema. Chronic bronchitis is the long-term inflammation of the bronchial passages. Symptoms of this condition include restricted breathing and a chronic cough that produces a thick, greenish-yellow mucus. Emphysema is a disease in which the air sacs (alveoli) are destroyed, inhibiting the vital gas exchange with the bloodstream. Symptoms of this condition include laborious breathing, gasping sounds with each breath, and debilitating weakness.

The common denominator of these conditions is the obstruction of the air flow either into or out of the lungs, or the inability of the lungs to efficiently exchange gases into and out of the bloodstream. In addition, there are the shared symptoms described above.

Breathing is perhaps the single most important activity we do to maintain our lives. When our capacity to breathe is obstructed, it is a very frightening experience. In all acute conditions, it is important to be under the guidance of medical professionals. Even in the case of chronic asthma, sufferers should receive the benefit of modern medical care. In acute asthma attacks, the use of bronchodilator drugs can be lifesaving.

The causative factors of these respiratory conditions are complex. They are clearly influenced by hereditary tendencies, improper diet, poor digestion, smoking, excessive physical exertion, lack of adequate physical exercise, poor posture, exposure to weather extremes, air pollution, infections, tension, and emotional stress.

According to the Yoga tradition, these conditions are often linked to the digestive system. With improper digestion, mucus and phlegm are produced in the stomach and accumulated in the lungs. A careful assessment of our diet, as well as other lifestyle adjustments, are essential ingredients to any program of self-improvement.

In addition to these lifestyle adjustments, and in coordination with appropriate medical care, a carefully constructed Yoga therapy program will strengthen our systems and even help people with chronic conditions to become more independent of medications.

Allergies that attack the respiratory system may be considered a kind of hypervigilance of the immune system. An asthma attack is a bronchial spasm in response to an irritation. In this case, even though the bronchial spasm is parasympathetic, the direction of practice is first to soothe and then to strengthen the system, giving particular attention to developing the capacity for exhalation.

Cases where the breathing is structurally restricted, on the other hand, may be considered hypo or deficient conditions. Here the direction of practice is to mobilize the rib cage, and particular attention is given to developing the capacity for inhalation.

In the respiratory system, however, this division of diseases and symptoms into excessive (hyper) and deficient (hypo) is not a perfect fit. Many people suffering from asthma have restricted chest mobility and would equally benefit from developing their capacity to inhale. And those with restricted chests will likewise benefit from strengthening their exhale. Therefore, the best approach for any specific condition must be developed in the context of individual body type, structural capacity, and breathing habits.

In fact, everybody will benefit from the development of their breathing capacity. The core ideas in Yoga therapy for working with respiratory conditions are relaxation, developing the breath capacity, and, in particular, achieving greater control of the diaphragm. In certain conditions, it may be more appropriate to emphasize strengthening exhalation, and in other conditions, inhalation. As we have seen, in Yoga breath training, we develop the capacity to expand the chest and abdomen on inhalation and to pull the belly in on exhalation. There are different techniques that may be applied in different situations, and we learn through training to utilize the most appropriate method for each situation.

In the sequences that follow, we will offer practices designed to increase confidence, strengthen the body, increase the capacity for inhalation and exhalation, increase circulation to all the organs, move the body fluids, and facilitate digestion and elimination.

Developing Exhalation

In the case of the asthmatic, for example, the normal breathing pattern is often reversed, with the belly coming in on inhalation and going out on exhalation. The first step in working with these conditions is breathing reeducation. We begin by training in "abdominal" breathing, where the abdomen goes out on inhalation and is pulled in on exhalation. This is developed with the help of simple positions and movements.

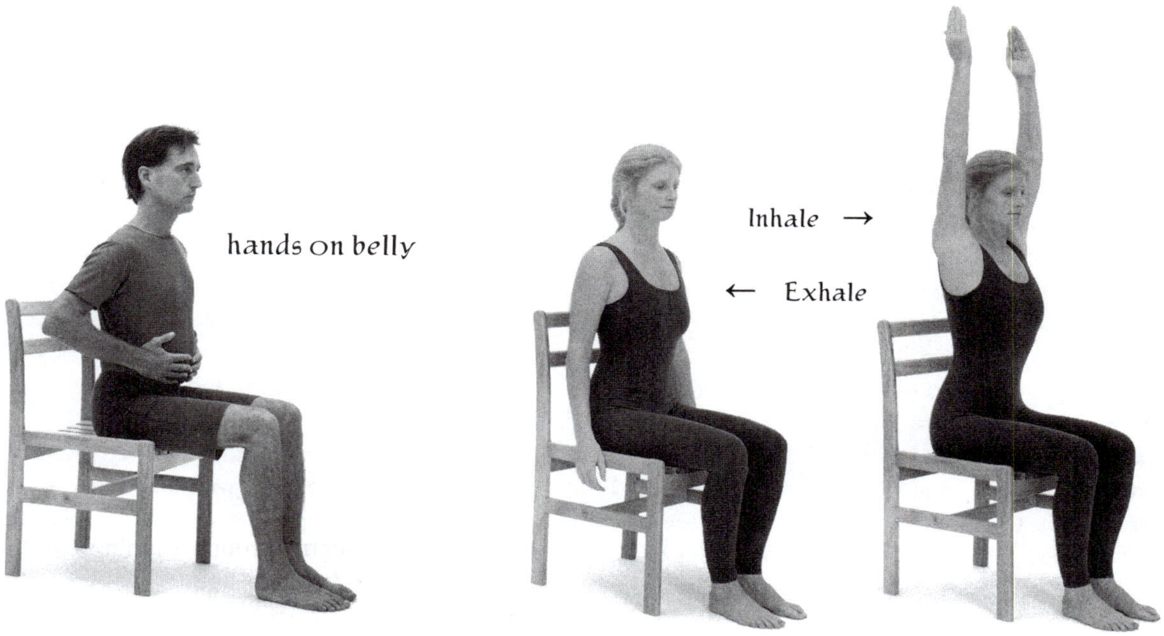

The next step is increasing the ability to deepen and control exhalation. As we have seen, exhalation is considered a technique of relaxation. This is achieved through the use of simple postures that facilitate exhalation and help the diaphragm move fully upward.

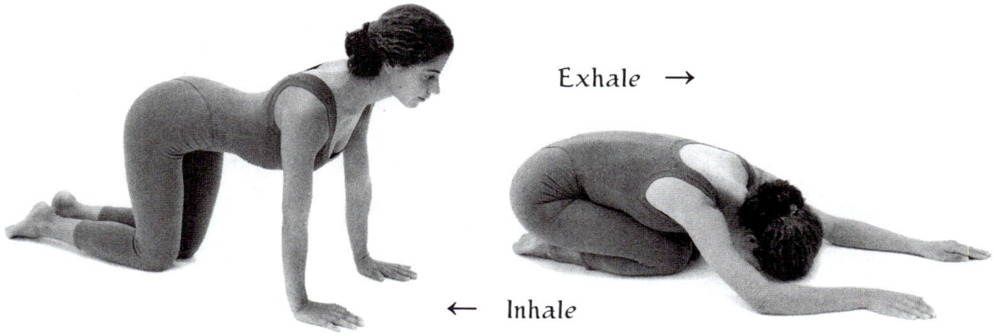

As breath control increases, we can introduce stronger positions that place a greater demand on breathing capacity. We then will begin holding the breath after exhalation.

Fear and anxiety are strong factors in any restricted breathing, and they must be respected. Progress in this direction is gradual and should proceed without forcing the system. The following sequence is illustrative of an approach to working with asthma.

Working with Asthma

The sequence that follows was developed for C.D., a forty-three-year-old woman who, when she first came to study with me, was a personnel manager for a regional telephone company. She had been suffering from asthma for many years and also complained of chronic pain in her shoulders.

C.D. had taken some group classes at our school while she was on vacation with her family. She liked our gentle approach and was hopeful for some improvement in her long-standing condition. I had the opportunity to work with her on and off over many years, both at our school and in various other cities where I teach. Her dedication to the study and practice of Yoga was clear, and, in time, she completed an extensive training program with me. She eventually left her job and is now a full-time Yoga teacher. Through her experience of learning to manage her own asthma, she has become a great resource for others suffering with the same condition.

C.D.'s faith in Yoga gave her the discipline to practice regularly for many years. When we first started working, she had a lot of fear about both her asthma and her shoulder. I noticed that the movement of her rib cage was severely restricted and that her whole upper body was weak. Any attempt to expand her chest on inhale created breathing spasms, and she was also unable to come forward in Cakravākāsana without breathing spasms.

We began with very simple movements to mobilize her chest and upper back without any emphasis on inhalation. Our next step together was to emphasize exhalation in simple forward bends. As her confidence grew, we then added inhalation techniques coordinated with arm movements. My next aim was to help her increase the mobility in her upper back and to release tension in her neck.

Over time she let me know which āsanas felt the best to her, and the following sequence emerged as the foundation for her daily practice. Over the years I noticed that she never failed to have a plastic water bottle with her. As her fear about her shoulders lessened, I suggested that she keep two of them with her while she practiced. I asked her to hold one in each hand while she did her forward bends, both seated and standing. Over time she put progressively more water in them. After her practice, I asked her to drink some of the water. She liked this idea very much. Though her asthma is still with her, she is able to manage it much better now and has much more confidence in herself. She is able to do a deep-breathing practice without spasm on most days. She tells me she feels much stronger, and her shoulder pain is, for the most part, a memory.

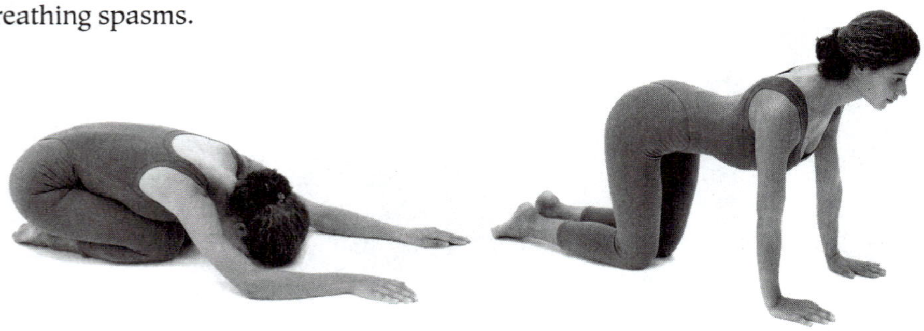

A Practice for Asthma

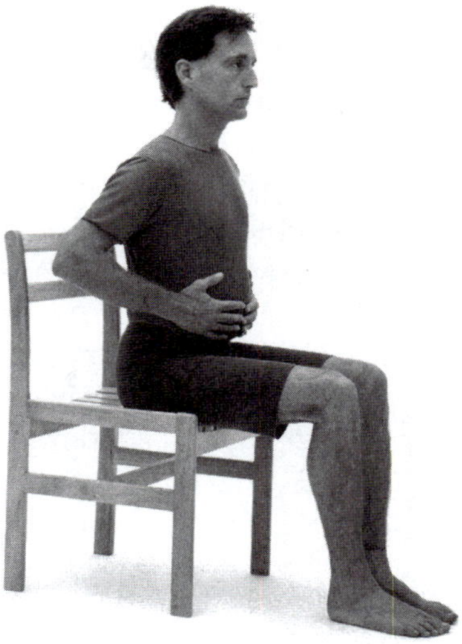

1.

POSTURE: Seated breathing.
EMPHASIS: To train abdominal breathing.
TECHNIQUE: Sit forward on a chair with spine erect and hands placed on abdomen.
On exhale: Gently pull belly in toward spine.
On inhale: Gently release belly and let it come out.
NUMBER: 12 times.
DETAILS: Make both inhale and exhale long and smooth.

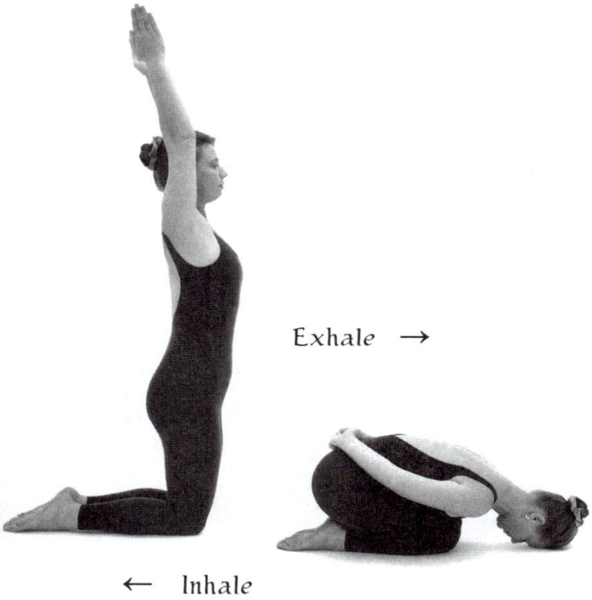

2.

POSTURE: Vajrāsana.
EMPHASIS: To compress belly. To gently mobilize rib cage. To introduce lengthening of exhalation.
TECHNIQUE: Stand on knees with arms over head.
On exhale: Bend forward, sweeping arms behind back, bringing hands to sacrum with palms up.
On inhale: Return to starting position.
NUMBER: 8 times.
DETAILS: *On exhale:* Make exhalation progressively longer with each repetition. Bring chest to thighs before buttocks to heels. Rotate arms so palms are up and hands rest on sacrum. *On inhale:* Expand chest and lift it up off knees as arms sweep wide.

3.

POSTURE: Uttānāsana.
EMPHASIS: To strengthen arms, shoulders, and upper back (holding water bottles). To compress belly and continue lengthening exhalation.
TECHNIQUE: Stand with feet slightly apart, arms over head.
On exhale: Bend forward, bending knees slightly, bringing chest to thighs and bottles to sides of feet.
On inhale: Return to starting position.
NUMBER: 8 times.
DETAILS: *On exhale:* Make exhalation progressively longer with each repetition. Bend knees to facilitate stretching of low back. Move chin down toward throat. *On inhale:* Lift chest up and away from thighs, flattening upper back. Keep knees bent until end of movement.

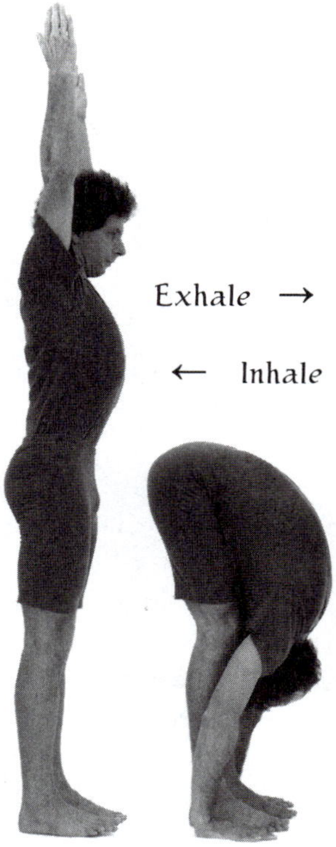

4.

Posture: Utthita Trikoṇāsana.

Emphasis: To stretch and mobilize rib cage.

Technique: Stand with feet spread wider than shoulders, left foot turned out at ninety-degree angle to right foot, left arm over head, and right arm out to the side with palm up.

On exhale: Bend laterally, bringing left hand below left knee, while twisting shoulders right. Turn head down toward left hand.

On inhale: Raise right arm up and forward, turning head to follow hand.

On exhale: Return right arm out to the side, turning head down to left foot.

On inhale: Return to starting position.

Number: 6 times each side.

Details: *On exhale:* Pull pubic bone slightly up to avoid increased lumbar curve. Bend left knee slightly. Keep shoulders in same plane as hips. *On inhale:* Stretch intercostal muscles fully on up side.

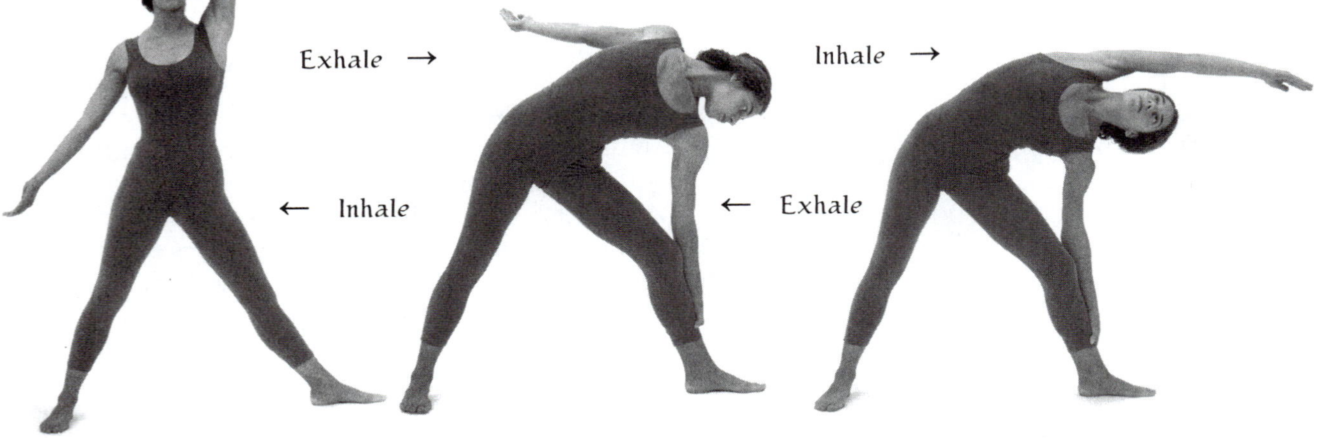

5.

Posture: Cakravākāsana.

Emphasis: To gently compress and stretch belly. To introduce humming on exhale. To transition from standing lateral bend to seated twist.

Technique: Get down on hands and knees, with shoulders vertically above wrists and with hips above knees.

On inhale: Lift chest up and away from belly.

On exhale: Gently contract belly, round low back, and bring chest toward thighs while making a gentle, low-pitched humming sound.

Number: 8 times.

Details: *On inhale:* Lead with chest, keeping chin slightly down. Avoid compressing low back; rather, feel chest expanding. *On exhale:* Round low back without collapsing chest over belly. Avoid increasing curvature of upper back. Let chest lower toward thighs sooner than hips toward heels.

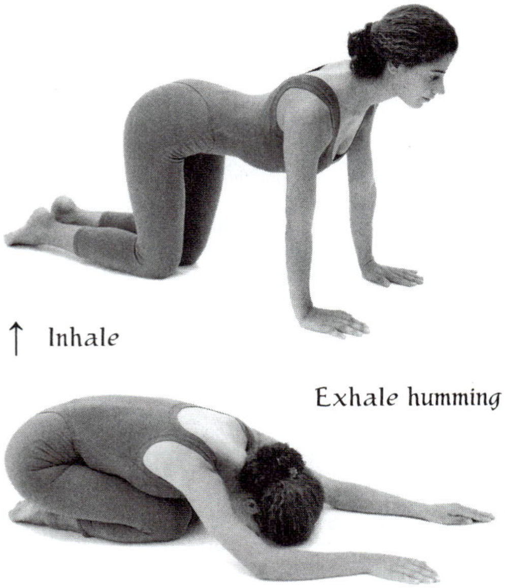

6.

POSTURE: Ardha Matsyendrāsana.

EMPHASIS: To fully exhale by deeply twisting belly and moving diaphragm upward. To introduce hold after exhale.

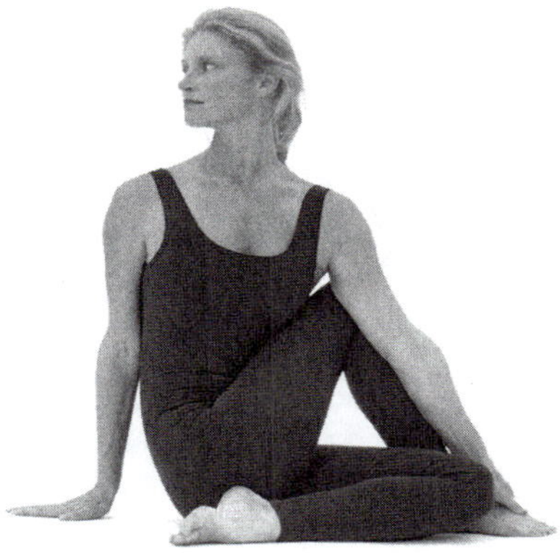

TECHNIQUE: Sit with left leg folded on floor, left foot by right hip, right knee straight up, right foot crossing over on outside of left knee, right arm behind back with palm down on floor by sacrum, left arm across outside of right thigh, and left hand on right foot.

On inhale: Extend spine upward.

On exhale: Twist torso and look over right shoulder.

Hold breath 4 to 6 seconds after exhale.

NUMBER: 8 breaths each side.

DETAILS: *On exhale:* Control torsion from deep in belly, using arm leverage only to augment twist. *On inhale:* Subtly untwist body to facilitate extension of spine.

7.

POSTURE: Paścimatānāsana.

EMPHASIS: To strengthen arms, shoulders, and upper back (holding water bottles). To compress belly and stretch and strengthen back. To deepen hold after exhale.

TECHNIQUE: Sit with legs forward, back straight, and arms raised over head.

On exhale: Bending knees slightly, bend forward, bringing chest to thighs, and bottles to feet.

Hold after exhale 4 to 6 seconds.

On inhale: Return to starting position.

NUMBER: 8 times.

DETAILS: *On exhale:* Bend knees to facilitate stretching low back and bring belly and chest to thighs. Move chin down toward throat. Feel like diaphragm moves up while holding after exhale. *On inhale:* Lift chest up and away from thighs, flattening upper back.

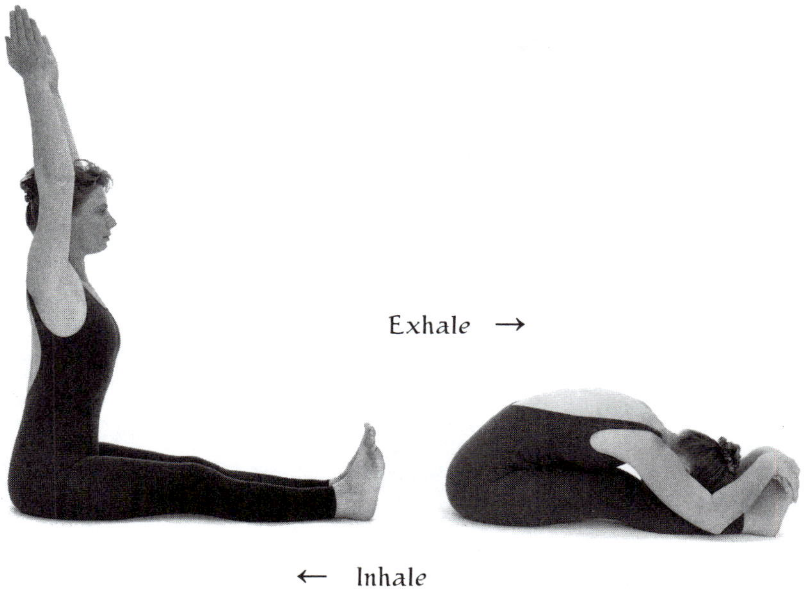

8.

POSTURE: Śavāsana.
EMPHASIS: To rest.
TECHNIQUE: Lie flat on back, with arms at sides, palms up, and legs slightly apart. Close eyes. Relax body fully, keeping mind relaxed and alert to sensations in body.
DURATION: Minimum 5 minutes.

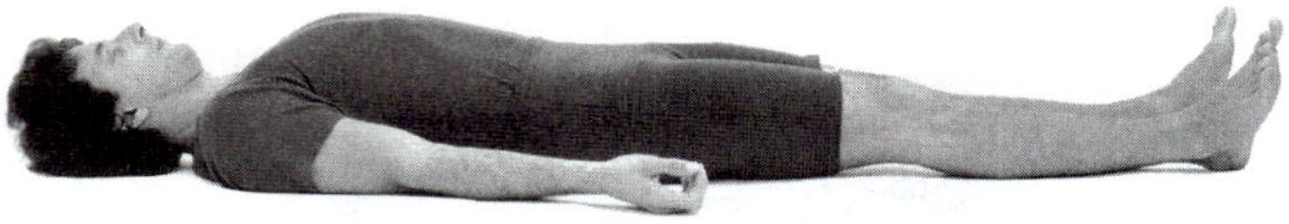

9.

POSTURE: Prāṇāyāma—Viloma Krama, three-stage exhale.
EMPHASIS: To stimulate and compress belly through segmented exhale.
TECHNIQUE:

Inhale deeply and fully.
Exhale 1/3 of breath in 3 seconds.
Pause 3 seconds.
Exhale another 1/3 of breath in 3 seconds.
Pause 3 seconds.
Complete *exhale* in 3 seconds.
Inhale deeply and repeat.

NUMBER: 8 times.
DETAILS: Contract abdomen from pubic bone to solar plexus in 3 stages. Skip the 3-second pause after the third stage of exhale.

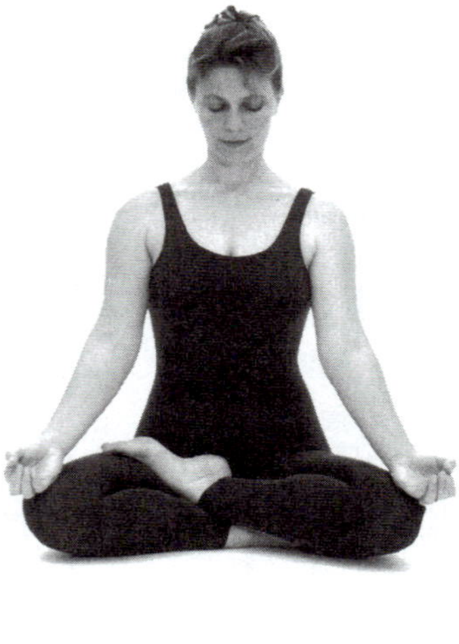

Developing Inhalation

In the case of restricted chest mobility, for example, practice is designed to progressively expand the structures of the rib cage, strengthen the respiratory muscles, and deepen the capacity for inhalation. The first step is to improve expansion of the chest on inhalation. This is facilitated by the use of simple arm movements, coordinated with breathing.

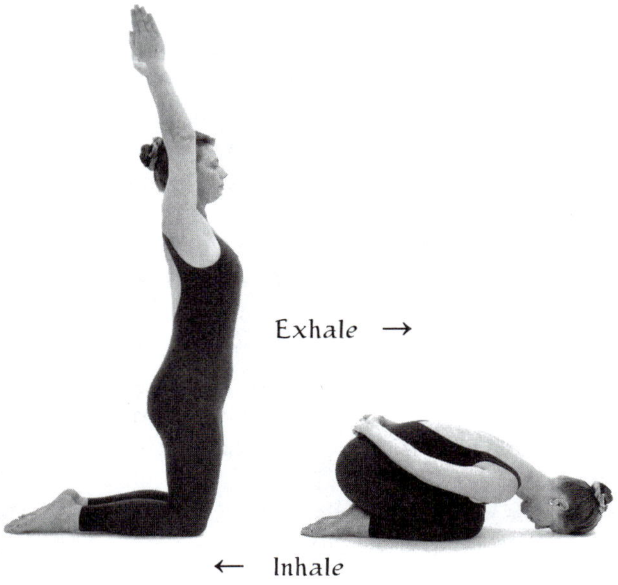
Exhale →
← Inhale

The next step is increasing the ability to deepen and control the inhalation. This is achieved through the use of simple postures that facilitate inhalation and help the chest expand even more fully.

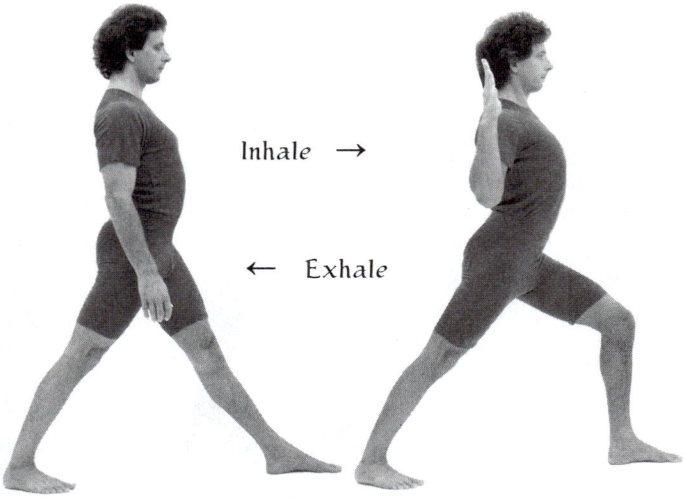
Inhale →
← Exhale

As breath control increases, we can introduce stronger positions that place a greater demand on breathing capacity. Then we will introduce holding the breath after inhalation.

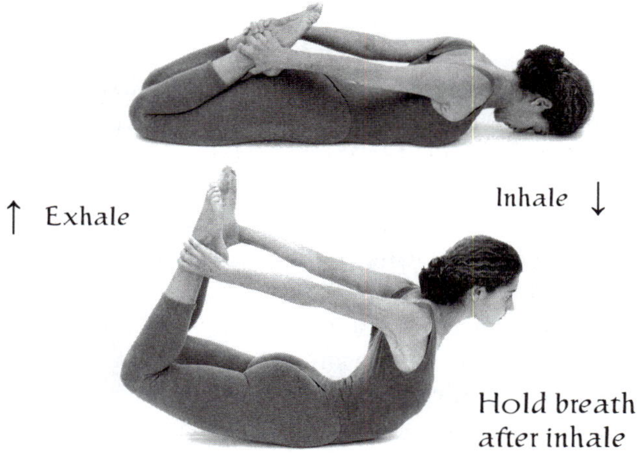
↑ Exhale
Inhale ↓
Hold breath after inhale

Working with Inhalation

This sequence was developed for G.T., the nineteen-year-old nephew of one of my students from Italy. He came to me on the advice of his aunt, who had been studying with us for some time. She was concerned that he was drifting without any direction and thought that maybe Yoga would help. G.T. came with an open and sincere attitude, though he was both uncertain and confused about his future. He had been to the United States when he was twelve, spoke some English, and liked the idea of learning some more.

Initially I asked him about how he was feeling and what he would like to do with me. His main physical concern seemed to be the narrowness of his chest, and he wondered if he could do something to help expand and develop it. He didn't talk to me about any other concerns. My impression was of a sweet and rather timid young man.

As we began working together, I discovered that he had some difficulties at school and had left before graduating. His main interest seemed to be art, and he was quite talented as a graphic artist. He had held odd jobs for the past year or two since he left school. He was not involved in any sport or physical activity.

As we were in Italy that year for about three months, I was able to follow his progress until I felt he could understand and practice the brahmaṇa sequence below on his own. It took us the full three months, working once a week, to reach this point. The emphasis of our work was postures that place a demand on the larger muscles of his body and postures that expand the chest. At the same time I wanted to keep the practice relatively short and uncomplicated, since I knew I wouldn't be able to check in with him regularly.

I somehow felt that he needed more physical and mental stimulation and hoped he would be able to find some direction. The area in Italy that he is from is hilly and full of villas, churches, and chapels. He told me about some of the special hidden places he knew of and, with my hopes for him in mind, I asked him to take me to one. Instead of driving up the steep hill to the parking lot, I suggested we walk. It was interesting for me to notice how winded he was and, at the same time, how excited to arrive at this hidden spot. I asked him if there were others around, and he said many. Since he obviously enjoyed these special places and recognized the need for more exercise, I suggested that he go on small excursions once a week, hiking up to the various sites.

G.T. enjoyed both the Yoga practice and the excursions and was able to keep them up for quite some time after I left Italy. I was happy to hear that he went back and finished school. As of this writing, G.T. is twenty-two years old and is studying art history and painting at a university in Italy.

A Practice for Inhalation

1.

POSTURE: Prāṇāyāma—Anuloma Krama, two stages.
EMPHASIS: To expand chest and deepen inhalation capacity.
TECHNIQUE:

Exhale deeply and fully.
Inhale 1/2 of breath in 4 to 5 seconds.
Pause 4 to 5 seconds.
Inhale remainder of breath in 4 to 5 seconds.
Pause 4 to 5 seconds.
Exhale slowly and fully.
Repeat.

NUMBER: 8 times.
DETAILS: *On inhale:* Expand chest from pit of throat to sternum. Then expand abdomen from solar plexus to pubic bone.

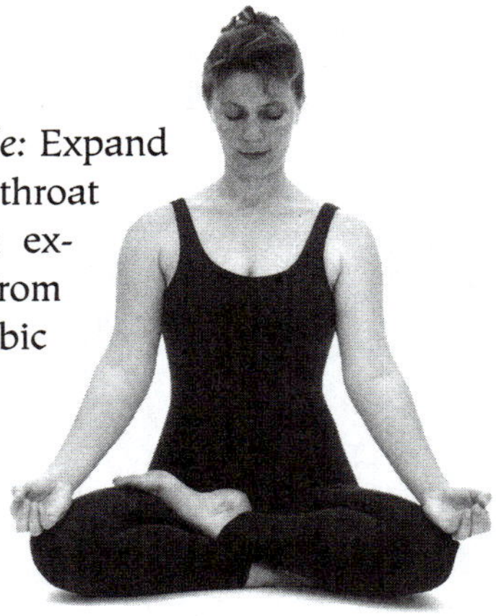

2.

Posture: Vajrāsana/Cakravākāsana Viṅyāsa.
Emphasis: To warm up body. To introduce lengthening of inhale.
Technique: Stand on knees with arms over head.

On exhale: Bend forward, bringing arms to floor in front of you.

On inhale: Lift chest up and away from belly, coming forward onto hands.

On exhale: Tighten belly, round low back, and bring chest toward thighs.

On inhale: Return to starting position.

Number: 8 times.
Details: *On inhale:* Make inhalation progressively longer with each repetition. Bring chest to thighs before hips to heels. Avoid pulling spine with head, overarching neck. Lead with chest, keeping chin slightly down. Avoid overarching low back; rather, feel stretching in belly. *On exhale:* Round low back without collapsing chest over belly. Avoid increasing curvature of upper back. Let chest lower toward thighs sooner than hips toward heels.

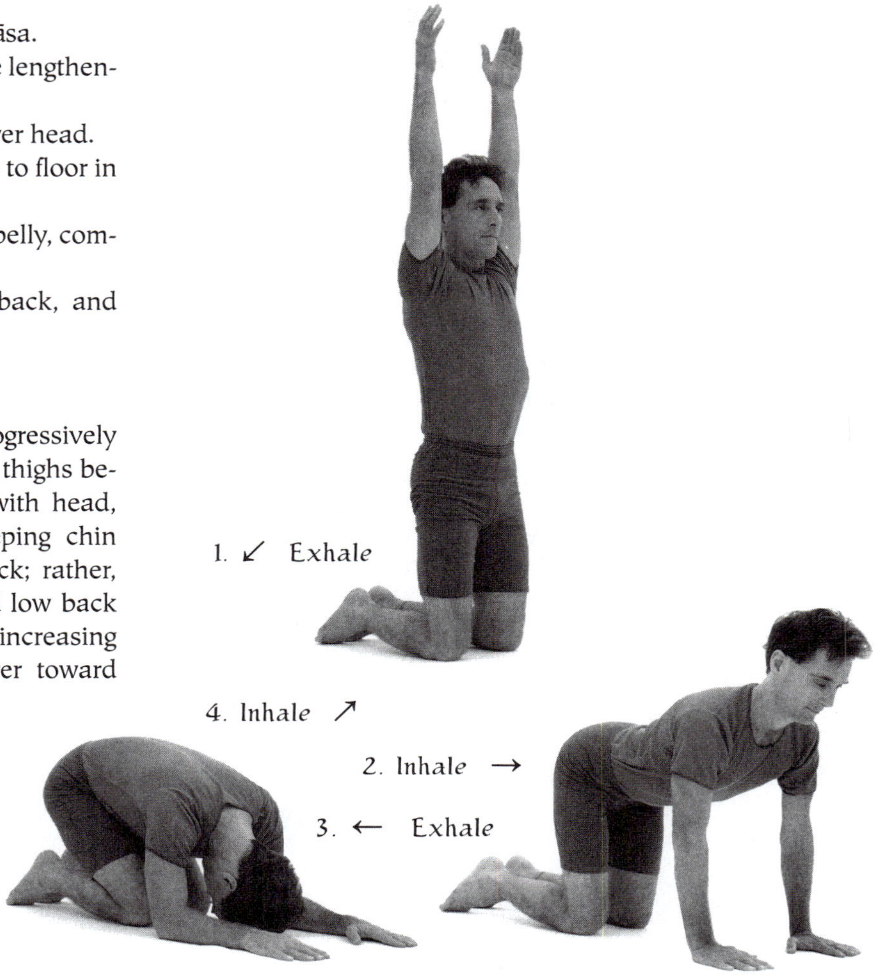
1. ↙ Exhale
4. Inhale ↗
2. Inhale →
3. ← Exhale

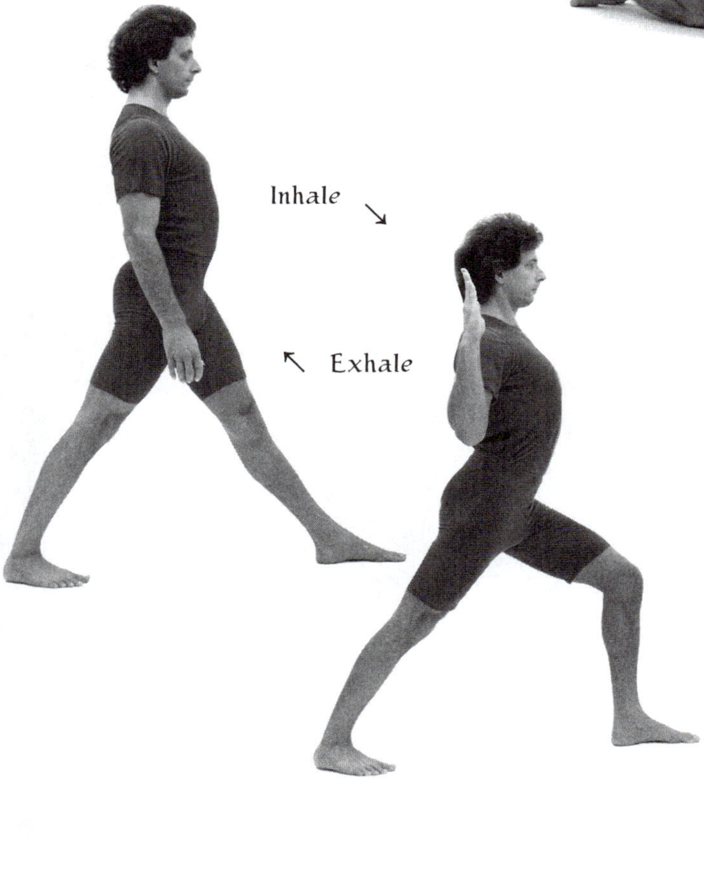
Inhale ↘
↖ Exhale

3.

Posture: Vīrabhadrāsana.
Emphasis: To strengthen muscles of back and legs. To expand chest and flatten upper back. To increase hold after inhalation.
Technique: Stand with left foot forward, feet as wide as hips, and arms at sides.

On inhale: Simultaneously bend left knee, displace chest slightly forward and hips slightly backward, bringing arms out to sides and shoulders back.

After inhale: Hold breath 2, 4, and 6 seconds, 2 times each, progressively.

On exhale: Return to starting position.

Number: 6 times each side.
Details: *On inhale:* Keep hands and elbows in line with shoulders. Feel opening of chest and flattening of upper back, not compression in low back. Keep head forward. Stay firm on back heel.

4.

POSTURE: Ardha Utkaṭāsana.
EMPHASIS: To increase inhalation while increasing demand on musculature. To strengthen legs and upper back.
TECHNIQUE: Stand with feet slightly apart and arms over head.

On exhale: Bend forward, bending knees, until thighs are parallel to ground and hips are at knee level, bringing chest to thighs and palms to sides of feet.

On inhale: Return to starting position.

Repeat, increasing inhalation by 1 or 2 seconds after every 2 repetitions.
NUMBER: 8 times.
DETAILS: *On exhale:* Push heels firmly and reach arms forward. *On inhale:* Lift chest, flattening upper back without exaggerating lumbar curve. Then straighten legs.

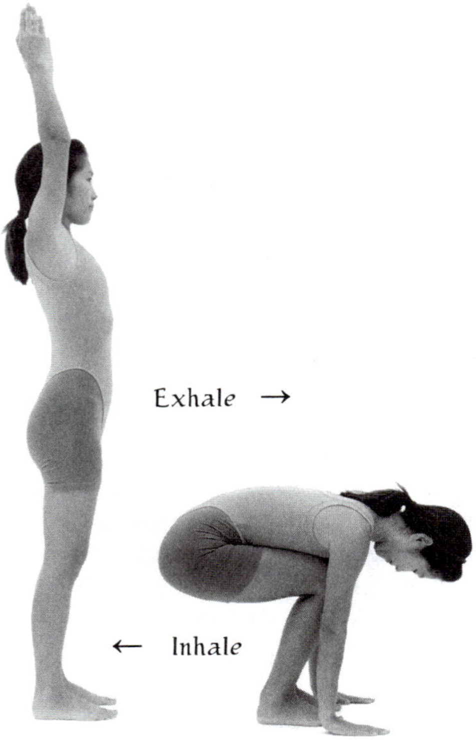

5.

POSTURE: Dhanurāsana.
EMPHASIS: To stretch and expand chest. To strengthen back and legs. To deepen inhale.
TECHNIQUE: Lie on stomach, resting on forehead, with knees bent and hands grasping ankles.

On inhale: Simultaneously press feet behind you, pull shoulders back, lift chest, and lift knees off ground.

On exhale: Return to starting position.

Increase hold from 2 to 4 to 6 seconds after inhale every second breath.
NUMBER: 6 times.
DETAILS: *On inhale:* Lift head forward, pulling ears away from shoulders. Do not collapse head backward. Keep knees from opening wider than hips.

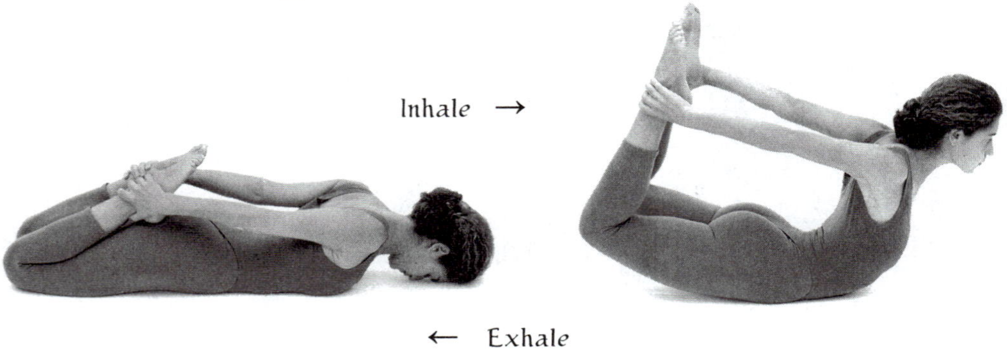

6.

POSTURE: Ūrdhva Prasārita Pādāsana.
EMPHASIS: To extend spine and flatten it onto floor. To stretch legs.
TECHNIQUE: Lie on back with arms down at sides, legs bent, and knees in toward chest.

On inhale: Raise arms upward all the way to floor behind head and legs upward toward ceiling.

Stay and stretch 2 full breaths.

On exhale: Return to starting position.

NUMBER: 4 times.

DETAILS: *On inhale:* Flex feet as legs are raised upward. Slightly bend knees, keeping angle between legs and torso less than ninety degrees. Push low back and sacrum downward. Bring chin down. While staying in position: *On exhale,* flex knees and elbows slightly; *on inhale,* extend arms and legs straighter.

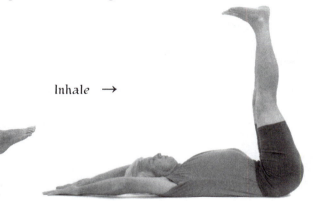

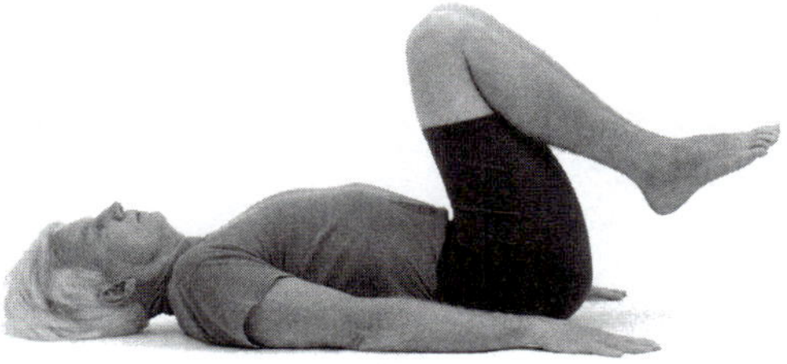

Inhale →

← Exhale

7.

POSTURE: Mahāmudrā / Jānu Śirṣāsana.
EMPHASIS: To develop both inhalation and exhalation capacity. To introduce breathing ratio. To strengthen respiratory and spinal musculature.
TECHNIQUE: Sit with right leg folded in, heel to groin, left leg extended forward, and holding left leg between ankle and knee with both hands.

On inhale: Extend spine upward, expanding chest, flattening upper back, and lengthening in front of torso.

Hold after inhale.

On exhale: Maintain posture while pulling belly firmly in.

Hold after exhale.

Remain in extended position 8 breaths. Then sink belly and chest to thigh.

Stay in forward-bended position 4 breaths.

Repeat on other side.

NUMBER: 8 breaths with spine extended; 4 breaths in forward bend, each side.
DETAILS: Ratio: begin with 6-second inhale, 3-second hold, 6-second exhale; 3-second hold. Increase to 8-second inhale, 4-second hold, 8-second exhale, 4-second hold. Bend extended leg so as to focus on spine.

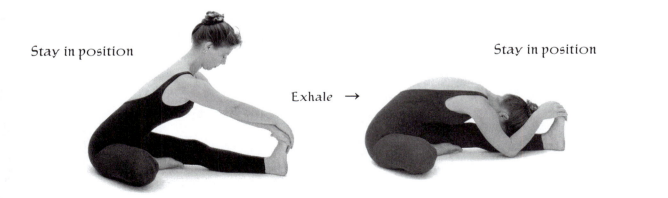

Stay in position

Exhale →

Stay in position

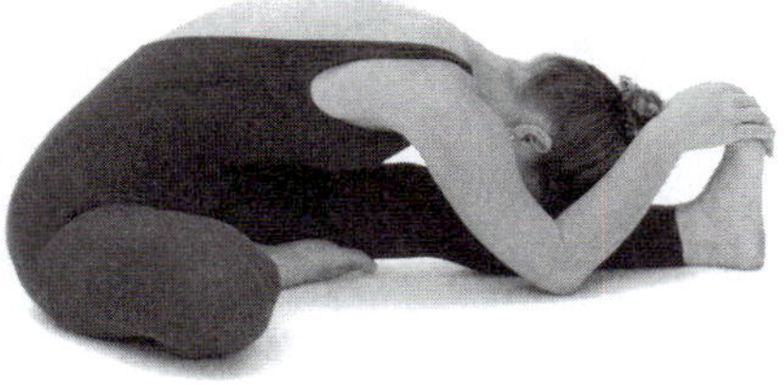

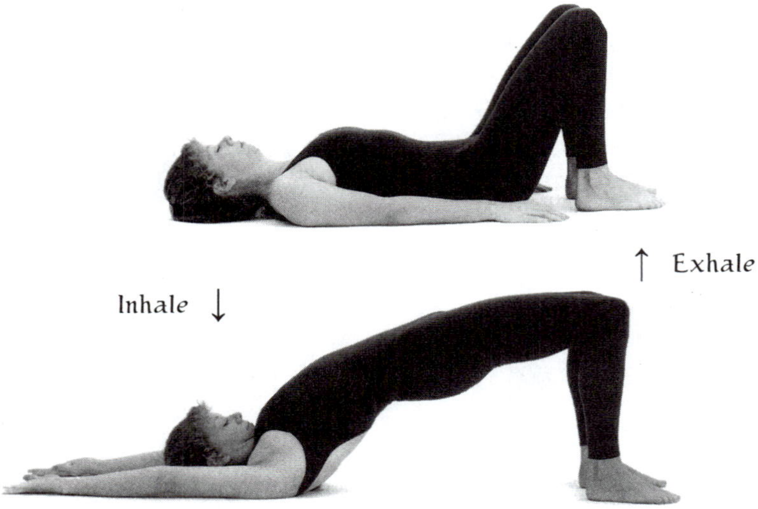

8.

POSTURE: Dvipāda Pīṭham.
EMPHASIS: To relax back and stretch belly.
TECHNIQUE: Lie on back with arms down at sides, knees bent, and feet on floor, slightly apart and comfortably close to buttocks.

On inhale: Pressing down on feet and keeping chin down, raise pelvis up toward ceiling, until neck is gently flattened on floor, while raising arms overhead to floor behind.

On exhale: Return to starting position.
NUMBER: 6 times.
DETAILS: *On inhale:* Lift spine, vertebra by vertebra, from bottom up. *On exhale:* Unwind spine, coming down vertebra by vertebra.

9.

POSTURE: Śavāsana.
EMPHASIS: To rest.
TECHNIQUE: Lie flat on back, with arms at sides, palms up, and legs slightly apart. Close eyes. Relax body fully, keeping mind relaxed and alert to sensations in body.
DURATION: Minimum 3 to 5 minutes.

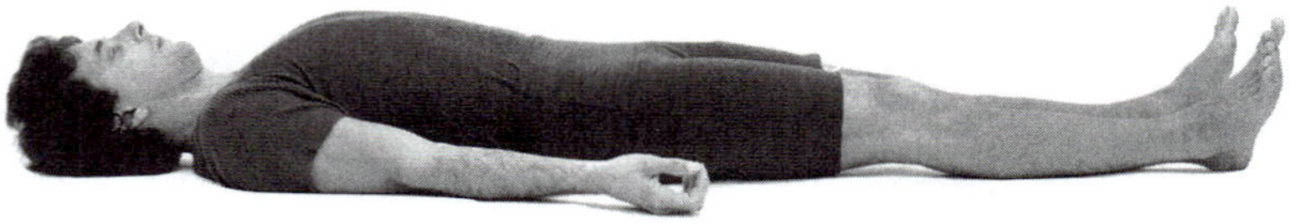

Cardiovascular System

Our cardiovascular system is essential to the life and function of our bodies. Through the bloodstream, nourishment from the digestive system, oxygen from the respiratory system, and hormones from the endocrine system are carried to every cell. Also through the bloodstream, wastes and toxins are collected from the cells and moved toward the body's main organs of elimination, including the lungs, skin, kidneys, and intestines. In this work, the cardiovascular system is aided by the lymphatic system, whose fluids aid in both absorption of nourishment from the blood and elimination of wastes from the cells.

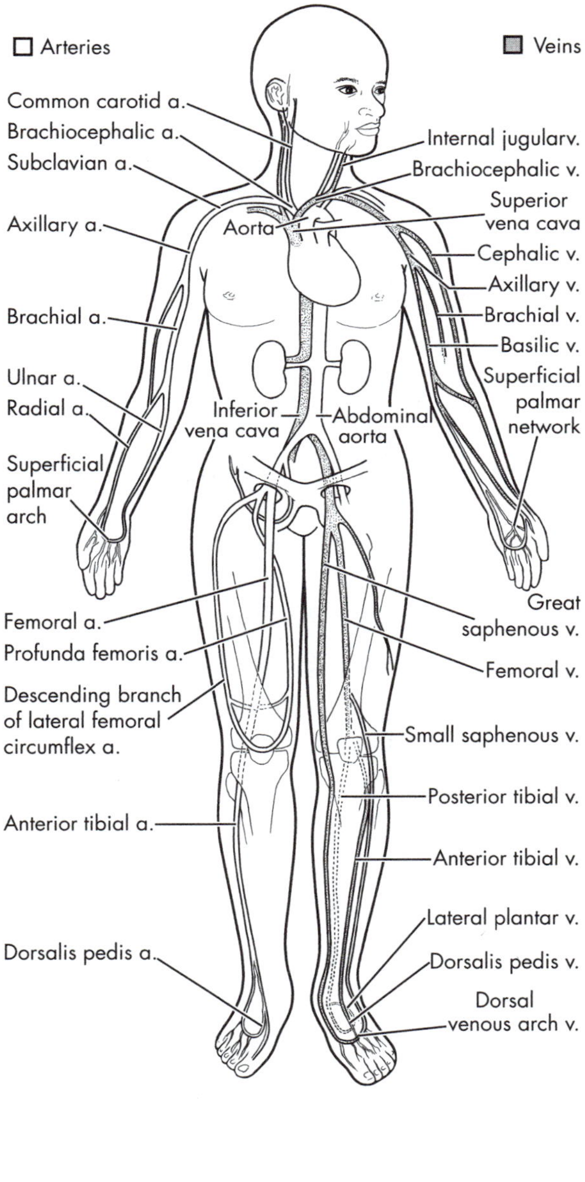

The cardiovascular system includes the heart, which pumps the blood, the circulating blood itself, and the arteries, veins, and capillaries through which the blood travels. In addition, the heart is encased in a membrane called the pericardium.

The functions of blood are varied and essential to the maintenance of life. In addition to transporting and distributing oxygen and nutrients to the cells and transporting wastes from the cells, blood delivers hormones and enzymes to specific tissues. Through buffers, it also neutralizes acids generated by muscular activity, protects from blood loss by its clotting mechanism, defends against foreign substances through its white blood cells and antibodies, and helps regulate body temperature by appropriate redistribution of heat.

The circulatory system includes a pulmonary circuit, which transports blood to and from the lungs, and a systemic circuit, which transports blood to and from the rest of the body. Arteries carry blood from the heart, veins carry blood to the heart, and capillaries carry blood between the arteries and veins. The chemical and gaseous exchanges that nourish and cleanse the cells taking place across their microscopic walls is a process called diffusion.

The central organ of the cardiovascular system is the heart, a four-chambered pump whose primary role is that of developing the pressure necessary to move a volume of blood through the system at an appropriate speed. The heart is not a continuous pump but works in cycles of contraction (systole) and relaxation (diastole), generating a pressure system that, along with a series of valves, assures that the blood flows in the desired direction.

In a simplified way the process is as follows: Purified, oxygenated blood leaves the lower left chamber (left ventricle) of the heart and travels through the body via the arteries and capillaries, delivering to the cells the materials they need to live and develop. On its journey, the bloodstream also collects wastes, including carbon dioxide, and returns, via the veins, to the heart, entering its upper right chamber (right atrium). From here it is pumped through the lower right chamber (right ventricle) of the heart into the lungs where it is oxygenated and purified of carbon dioxide and other gaseous wastes. And, finally, the blood is pumped back to the upper left chamber (left atrium), of the heart, then into the lower left chamber (left ventricle) and out again through the arteries into the body. This cycle continues from shortly after conception until the moment we die.

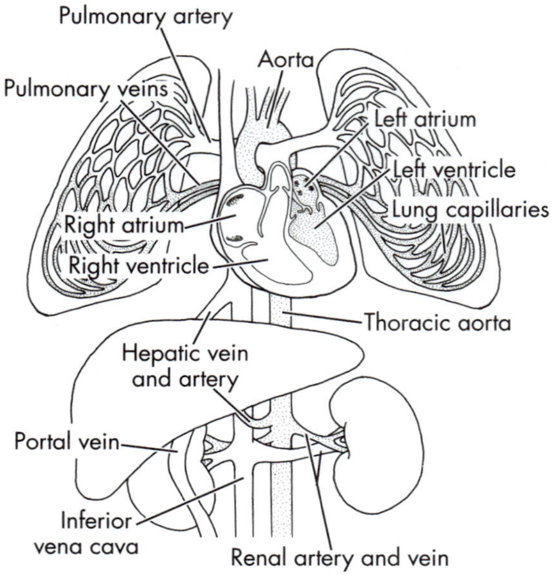

Through volume of blood, integrated actions of the heart pump, and changes in the diameters of the blood vessels (vasodilation and vasoconstriction), the cardiovascular system regulates and maintains the body's entire supply of blood. Because pressure in the system is determined by strength and rate of blood flow, volume of blood in the system, and resistance of the blood vessels, under normal circumstances an increase in heart rate will increase blood flow to the capillaries. The balance between pressure and resistance, which determines our blood pressure, is regulated by both neural (ANS) and hormonal control, which work automatically to regulate our blood flow, ensuring that our cellular need for oxygen and nutrients is met.

However, we also directly influence this complicated system through our thoughts, emotional states, and habitual activities. For instance, just think of how your body responds to emotional stimulation and how thoughts and emotions influence your heart beat. This is because strong emotions like desire, anger, anxiety, and fear speed up the heart and increase blood pressure. This is also why without an increase in physical activity, which engages the muscles to assist the blood flow, excessive cardiovascular response can in time weaken the system.

Our diet influences the volume of fluid in our system. If we have too much salt, for example, we tend to retain fluid (edema), which by increasing the volume of fluid in our body can also raise our blood pressure. If, on the other hand, we are protein deficient, we tend to lose blood volume, which lowers our blood pressure.

Exercise increases the heart rate and, during the period of exercise, tends to raise the blood pressure. If we exercise moderately, resistance in the blood vessels drops (vasodilation), the cells get more oxygen and nutrients, and wastes are more efficiently removed. The end result is a lower resting blood pressure. However, if we exercise excessively, we can actually strain and ultimately weaken our systems. At a certain point our exercise results in fatigue, stress, and, potentially, in strain and injury. In fact, according to the yogis, chronically reaching this point of fatigue by overtraining is one of the causes of disease. It is important to exercise on a regular basis, but we must beware of becoming compulsive and, in the long run, turning our health-oriented program into a stress-producing one!

Conditions that affect the circulatory system are generally grouped under the heading of heart disease. These conditions can be grouped as genetic defects, coronary heart disease, cardiomyopathy, and anemia. Genetic defects include conditions such as irregular heartbeat (cardiac arrhythmia) and heart murmurs. Coronary heart disease involves damage or malfunction of the heart that is caused by the narrowing or blockage of the coronary arteries (arteriosclerosis). Cardiomyopathy refers to diseases of the heart muscle itself such as inflammation of the heart muscle, or enlarged heart. Anemia is a condition of low concentration of oxygen-rich hemoglobin in the blood.

Causes of these conditions can include genetic predisposition, diseases (such as hypertension and diabetes mellitus), infection (myocarditis), elevated blood cholesterol, improper diet and poor digestion, being overweight, poisoning through self-destructive unhealthy habits (such as excessive smoking, drinking, or use of other drugs), tightness of the chest, excessive physical exertion, insufficient physical activity, and chronic emotional stress (including anxiety, anger, and depression).

Symptoms and *consequences* of these conditions can include rapid heartbeat (tachycardia), chest pain (angina), high blood pressure (hypertension), low blood pressure (hypotension), and finally heart attack (myocardial infarction). Serious heart conditions require the direct care and guidance of a qualified medical practitioner.

When we have heart conditions, we can really help ourselves through the appropriate combination of lifestyle changes and appropriate Yoga practices. We should take time to reflect on our diets, consider giving up smoking or other substance abuses, and regularly take time to relax. If we are overweight, it is important to begin to face this circumstance and work to bring it under control because the heart works overtime when we are chronically overweight. If our lifestyle is sedentary, we can begin a cardiovascular exercise program although, in order to avoid further stress, we should be careful to build up into it gradually.

Although we cannot resolve our heart conditions exclusively through Yoga practice, a well-conceived program of Yoga therapy can be beneficial for restoring and maintaining the balanced functioning of the cardiovascular system.

Hypertension

Hypertension—the technical term for chronically high blood pressure—is a widespread and serious condition, which, if left untreated, can lead to heart attack, stroke, accelerate the development of arteriosclerosis, and even lead to kidney failure. At present, there are effective means to control dangerously high blood pressure through medication. With this control, those who suffer from this condition can begin the process of lifestyle adjustment that can eventually reduce their dependency on medication.

Blood pressure refers to pressure within the arteries during the two phases of the heart cycle. In a blood pressure reading the first number refers to pressure in the arteries when the heart is contracting (systolic) and the second to pressure remaining in the arteries between contractions while the heart is resting (diastolic).

Although both measurements are important, it is the lower number (diastolic) that is the more important indication of hypertension. In fact, many people with high blood pressure don't even know it unless it is so high that headaches and perhaps chest pains result. Usually we discover high blood pressure when we go to see a doctor or check our own blood pressure at a local mall. In fact, after the mid-thirties, it is a good practice to have your blood pressure checked regularly and, if your diastolic pressure is consistently over ninety, to consult with your physician.

The main orientation for working with hypertension through Yoga therapy is to take a calming and conserving (langhana) approach. We should establish a regular, gentle practice including simple movements coordinated with breathing, adequate rest, simple prāṇāyāma, palming the eyes, guided relaxation and visualization, and peaceful meditations. I have worked with many people suffering from hypertension. Some have been overweight, and some have been thin. Some have had increased curvature of their upper backs and some have had excessively straight upper backs. Therefore, as high blood pressure is not generally limited to a specific type of person, in working with this condition structural and constitutional needs must be recognized and respected. Accordingly, the following sequence is designed to illustrate universal principles in working with hypertension and further individualization of the practice should be done respecting such needs.

With regards to breathing, we recommend that you avoid the following, at least initially: straining to increase the length of inhale or exhale, prolonging retention of the breath after exhale or inhale, forcing the chest to expand on inhale, and pulling the stomach in strongly on exhale. With regards to postures, we also recommend that you avoid the following, at least initially: strong standing postures, inverted postures, and moving from standing immediately to supine positions.

Working with Hypertension

This particular sequence was developed for D.M., a forty-five-year-old caretaker of the gardens of a large estate, who came to see me for help with his hypertension. He was referred to me by a physician who believed that D.M. would benefit from our work. I saw D.M. two times per week for two weeks, and then once a week over the next several months. This sequence evolved out of our work together over the first month. When we began our work together, D.M. told me that he was on medication and that he was curious to see what Yoga could do for him. Although he was physically active in his profession, he told me that he was not involved in any regular exercise program. He complained of chronic low back tension and discomfort.

We began our work together with very simple arm movements and breathing exercises, done seated in a chair. He was surprised to discover how tight his back was and how shallow his breathing.

As we got to know each other, he began to share with me more about his life. He had been living for about three years with a woman who had a daughter from a previous marriage. It seems that he and the daughter, who was just going through puberty, were not getting along. This was creating problems between him and his girlfriend, and the tension was high in the house. I could see he was both frustrated and angry and was developing resentment toward the daughter. I asked him about his work, and he told me that he spent a lot of time running a lawn mower and a Weed Eater™. Both machines have intense vibration and high-pitched sounds.

As he became more comfortable with the exercises, I added progressive lengthening of exhalation to his practice, and later some low-pitched humming sounds to help him to relax. I also introduced some postures to help strengthen and loosen his back. I strongly suggested that he avoid running the machines when he was angry and that he use ear protection to dull the sound.

In subsequent months, he told me that he had hired someone to work with him and run his machines. He also told me that he and his girlfriend and her daughter had begun family counseling. Things were much better between him and the daughter, and he and his girlfriend were planning to get married.

When I asked him about his back, he told me that he had forgotten about his back problems. He was happy to report that his doctor had reduced his medication. He was feeling much better about himself and his prospects for the future.

A Practice for Hypertension

1.

POSTURE: Arm movements in chair.
EMPHASIS: To gently mobilize rib cage while deepening inhale and exhale.
TECHNIQUE:

A: Sit on a chair or bench with back straight and hands on knees.

On inhale: Raise one arm forward and up over head.

On exhale: Return to starting position.

Repeat on other side.

B: *On inhale:* sweep both arms out to sides and up over head.

On exhale: Return to starting position.

NUMBER: A four times each side, alternately. Rest. Then B six times.
DETAILS: *On inhale:* Lift chest up and away from belly and lift chin slightly.

A.

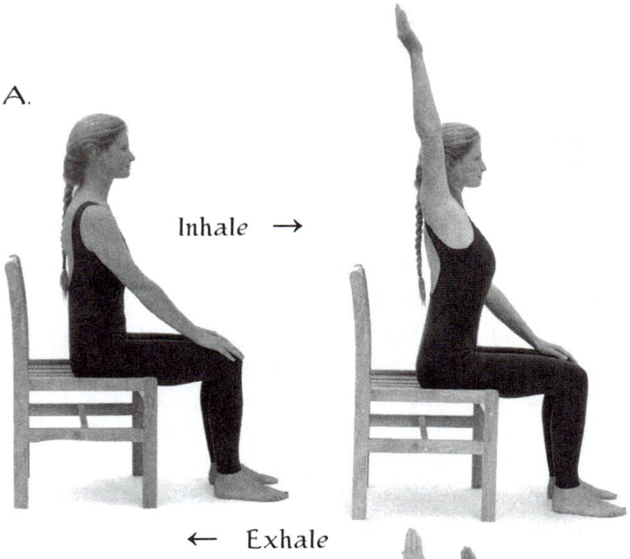

B.

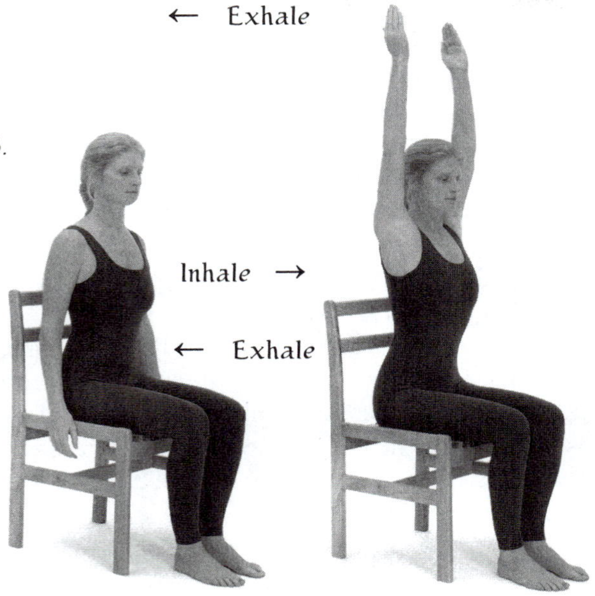

2.

POSTURE: Uttānāsana.
EMPHASIS: To extend length of exhale.
TECHNIQUE: Stand with feet slightly apart facing a chair.

On inhale: Raise arms forward and up over head.

On exhale: Bend forward, bending knees slightly, bringing chest to thighs, and palms to chair.

On inhale: Return to previous position with arms over head.

On exhale: Return to starting position.

NUMBER: 6 times.
DETAILS: *On inhale:* Lift chest up and away from thighs, flattening upper back. Keep knees bent until end of movement.

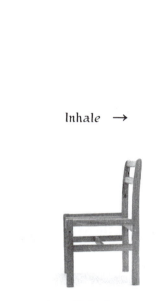

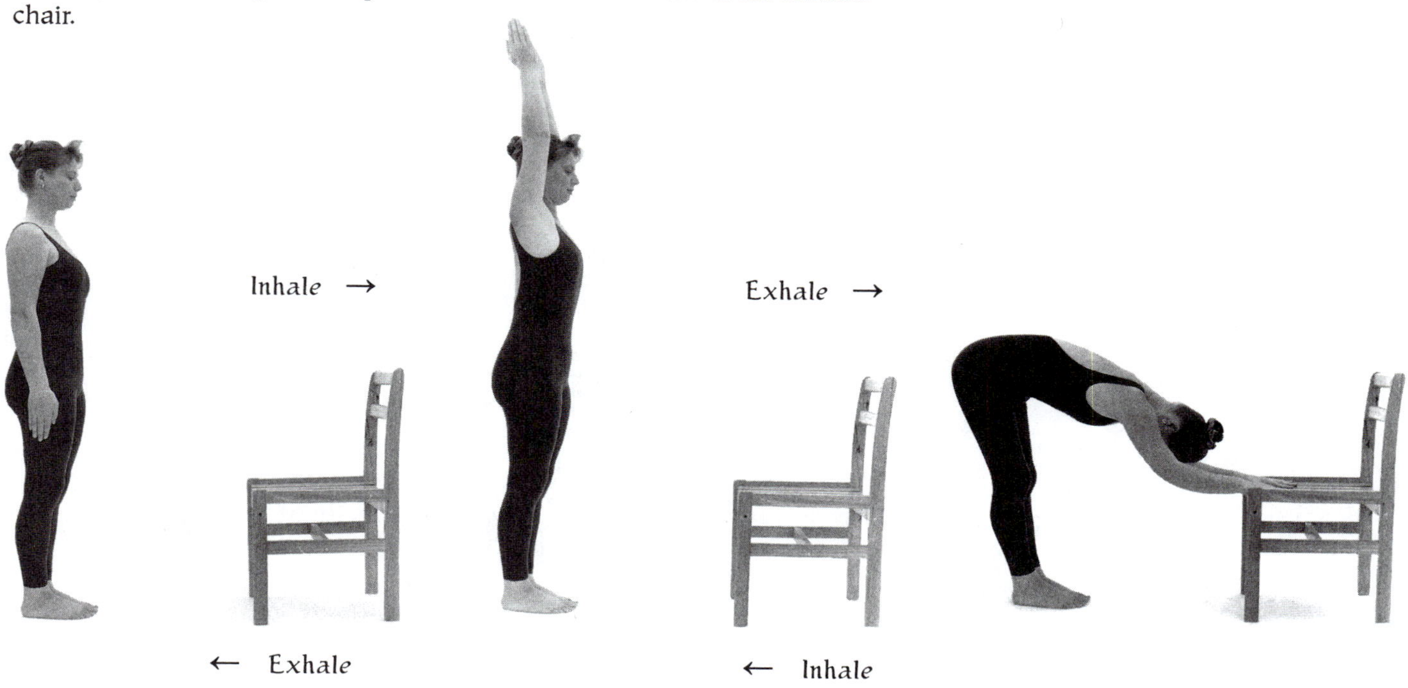

3.

POSTURE: Sitting on chair.
EMPHASIS: To relax using sound and deep breathing.
TECHNIQUE:

Inhale deeply.

Long *exhale,* using a soft, low-pitched humming sound on every other exhalation.

NUMBER: 16 breaths.

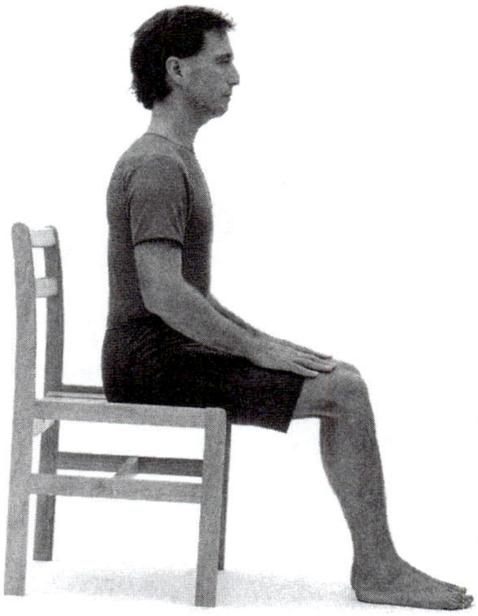

4.

POSTURE: Cakravākāsana.
EMPHASIS: To stretch rib cage on inhale. To gently compress and stretch belly on exhale.
TECHNIQUE: Get down on hands and knees, with shoulders vertically above wrists and with hips above knees.

On inhale: Lift chest up and away from belly.

On exhale: Gently contract belly, round low back, and bring chest toward thighs.

NUMBER: 8 times.
DETAILS: *On inhale:* Lead with chest, keeping chin slightly down. Avoid compressing low back; rather, feel chest expanding. *On exhale:* Round low back without collapsing chest over belly. Avoid increasing curvature of upper back. Let chest lower toward thighs sooner than hips toward heels.

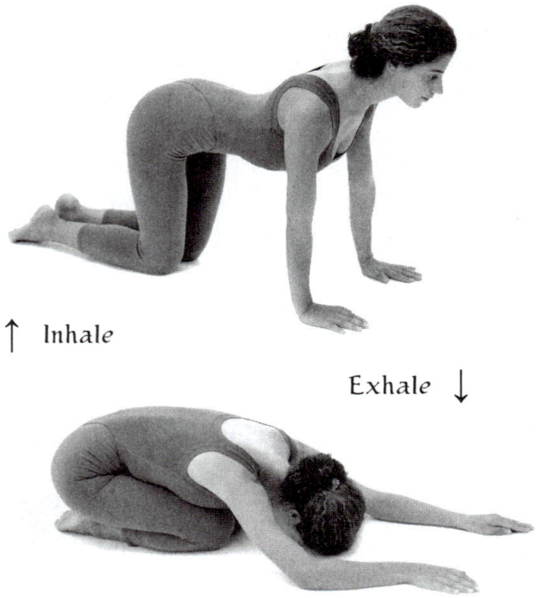

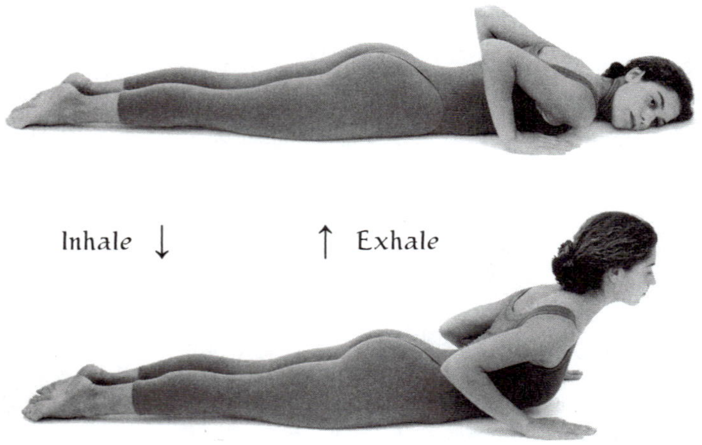

5.

POSTURE: Bhujaṅgāsana.
EMPHASIS: To gently stretch and expand rib cage, deepening inhalation.
TECHNIQUE: Lie on belly with palms by chest, head turned to one side.

On inhale: Lift chest, turning head to center.

On exhale: Lower chest to floor, turning head to opposite side.

NUMBER: 6 times.
DETAILS: *On inhale:* Use back to lift chest; don't push with arms.

6.

POSTURE: Apānāsana.
EMPHASIS: To gently compress belly while progressively extending exhale.
TECHNIQUE: Lie on back with both knees bent toward chest and feet off floor. Place each hand on its respective knee.

On exhale: Pull thighs gently but progressively toward chest.

On inhale: Return to starting position.

NUMBER: 12 times.
DETAILS: *On exhale:* Pull gently with arms, keeping shoulders relaxed and on floor. Press low back down into floor and drop chin slightly toward throat. Progressively lengthen exhale with each successive repetition.

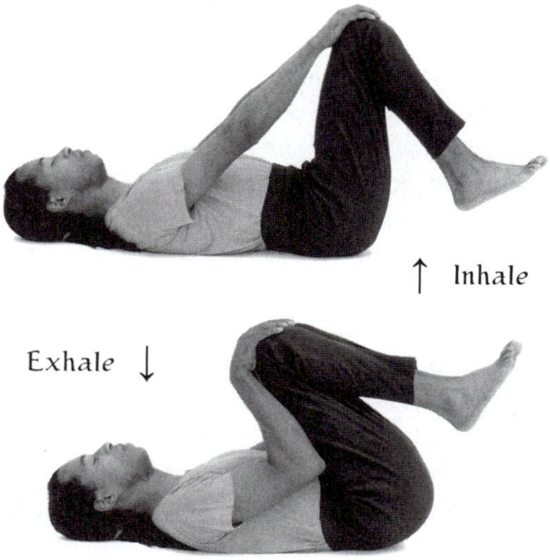

7.

POSTURE: Śavāsana with support.
EMPHASIS: To rest.
TECHNIQUE: Lie flat on back, with arms at sides, palms up, and legs slightly apart. Close eyes. Relax body fully, keeping mind relaxed and alert to sensations in body.
DURATION: Minimum 3 to 5 minutes.

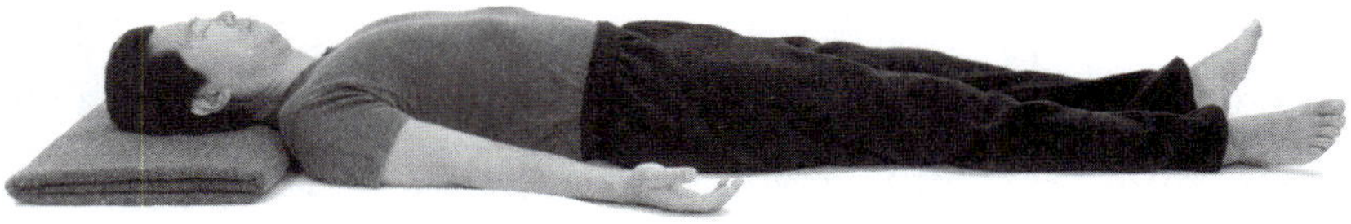

Hypotension

Hypotension is generally not considered to be as serious as hypertension, yet many people suffer from it; and serious low blood pressure can result in oxygen and nutrient deprivation in the peripheral systems. Because low blood pressure is often related to overall weakness in the system and specifically weakness of the digestive fire, it is often accompanied by lack of energy, poor circulation, coldness in the extremities, weakness of the heart muscle, and a tendency toward dizziness. Once I was in India working with a woman who had finished her practice and was resting on the floor when someone knocked on the door. She got up to a standing position suddenly, and the next thing I knew she had passed out on the floor. So, a general principle for working with hypotension is gradual transitions, particularly from a lying to a standing position. For the same reason, standing postures with the head below the waist often result in dizziness.

As with hypertension, in cases of hypotension the same principle of respecting structural differences applies. I have worked with heavyset and thin people with low blood pressure. For some, shoulder stand presents too much risk to their necks and upper back; for others shoulder stand is a wonderful posture. Therefore we recommend twisting, backward bending, shoulder stand, and some holding of the breath after inhalation, and the following sequence is illustrative of our approach and how each practice can be adapted, respecting the principles given earlier in this book, to your own unique structural needs.

Working with Hypotension

This particular sequence was developed for D.O., a thirty-eight-year-old woman who came to me without any particular complaints. She began by coming to group classes sporadically over several years. She would appear for a while and then disappear again. D.O.'s body was very flexible, and she was easily able to practice many āsanas. She always wanted to do the shoulder stand and if I didn't include it in the sequence, I would invariably find her doing it on her own at the end of the class.

After one period of absence, she came to me after class and expressed interest in seeing me privately. D.O. told me that her main interest was in spiritual matters, but that she was coming to Yoga only to help maintain her body and support her health. She told me that she was living off of a small inheritance, which kept her at a minimalist lifestyle, but that she didn't have to work. She was very much the "loner," though she went to church regularly, and I never knew her to have a boyfriend.

As we began working together privately, I noticed that although she was interested and willing to work her body, she had great resistance to working with her breath. When I commented on that, she said that focusing on her breath made her dizzy. She told me she often felt dizzy when getting out of bed in the morning. She also said that she often felt weak and without energy reserves. I asked her about her diet, and she told me that she was practically a "fruitarian."

Since she had worked with me in group classes on and off for several years, she was very familiar with our approach to āsana practice. Over several months, we evolved the following course, which I asked her to practice in the afternoon. I suggested that she go for a brisk walk in the morning, preferably with some hills to climb. I also asked to her to eat some oatmeal in the morning before her walk. At one point, I encouraged her to find some kind of work or social service to engage more actively in the community.

D.O. still shows up at group classes sporadically, but assures me she is practicing on her own. She told me that she now enjoys the small breathing exercises I gave her and no longer gets dizzy when she practices. She also happily told me that although she still wasn't working, she had begun to go to church gatherings and had met a man, and that they had recently moved in together.

A Practice for Hypotension

1.

POSTURE: Dvipāda Pīṭham.

EMPHASIS: To warm up body by engaging large muscles of thighs and buttocks.

TECHNIQUE: Lie on back with arms down at sides, knees bent, and feet on floor, slightly apart and comfortably close to buttocks.

On inhale: Pressing down on feet and keeping chin down, raise pelvis until neck is gently flattened on floor, while raising arms overhead to floor behind.

On exhale: Return to starting position.

NUMBER: 6 times.

DETAILS: *On inhale:* Lift spine, vertebra by vertebra, from bottom up. *On exhale:* Unwind spine, coming down vertebra by vertebra.

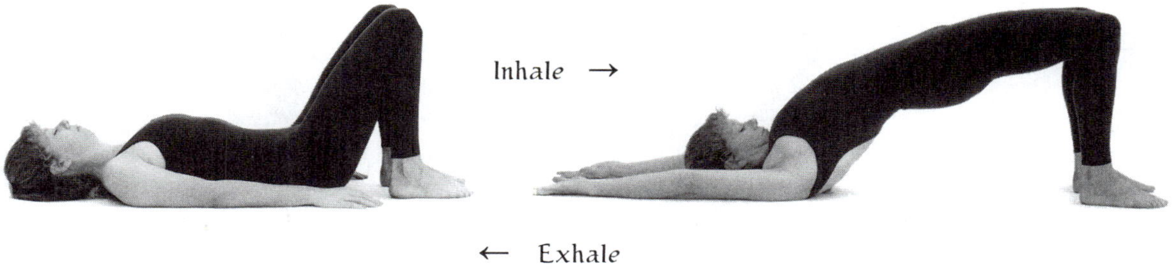

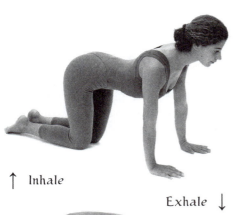

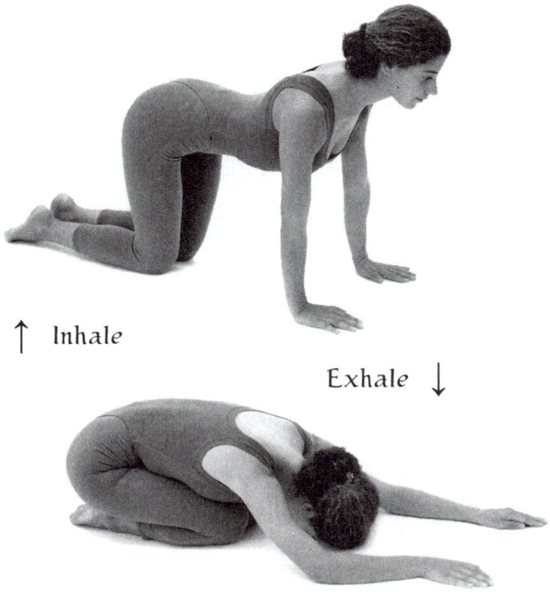

2.

POSTURE: Cakravākāsana.

EMPHASIS: To make transition from supine to standing position. To stretch rib cage on inhale and low back on exhale.

TECHNIQUE: Get down on hands and knees, with shoulders vertically above wrists and with hips above knees.

On inhale: Lift chest up and away from belly.

On exhale: Gently contract belly, round low back, and bring chest toward thighs.

NUMBER: 8 times.

DETAILS: *On inhale:* Lead with chest, keeping chin slightly down. Avoid compressing low back; rather, feel chest expanding. *On exhale:* Round low back without collapsing chest over belly. Avoid increasing curvature of upper back. Let chest lower toward thighs sooner than hips toward heels.

3.

POSTURE: Vīrabhadrāsana.
EMPHASIS: To strengthen muscles of back and legs, expand chest, and flatten upper back. To introduce short hold after inhalation.
TECHNIQUE: Stand with left foot forward, feet as wide as hips, and arms at sides.

On inhale: Simultaneously bend left knee, displace chest slightly forward and hips slightly backward, bring arms out to side, with elbows slightly bent and shoulders back.

Hold breath after inhale 4 seconds.

On exhale: Return to starting position.

NUMBER: 6 times each side.
DETAILS: *On inhale:* Keep hands and elbows in line with shoulders. Feel opening of chest and flattening of upper back, not compression of lower back. Keep head forward and weight on back heel.

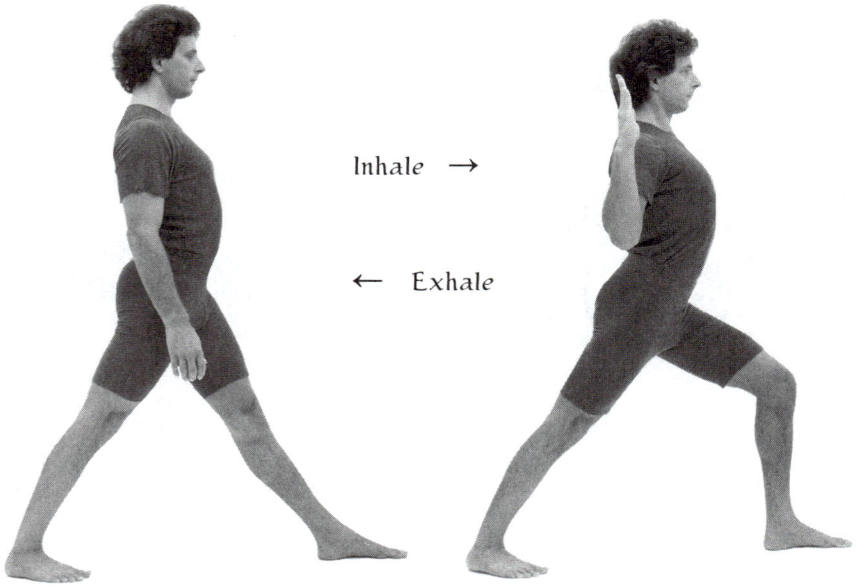

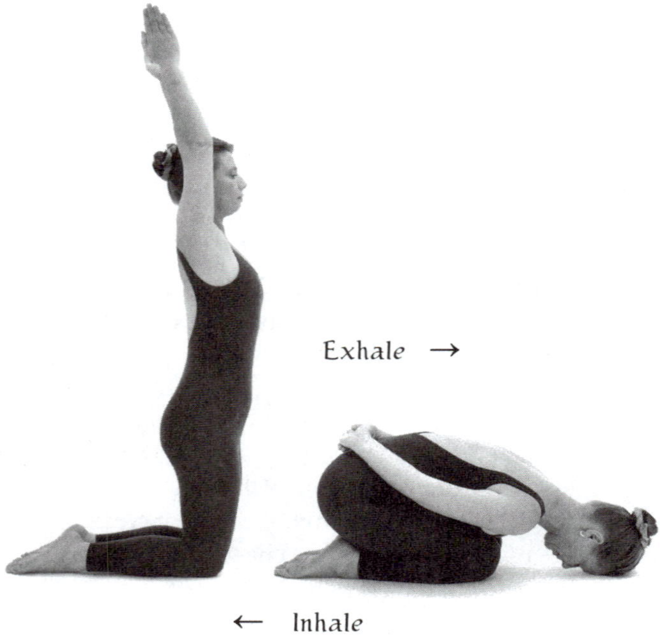

4.

POSTURE: Vajrāsana.
EMPHASIS: To make transition from standing to supine position. To stretch low back.
TECHNIQUE: Stand on knees with arms over head.

On exhale: Bend forward, sweeping arms behind back and bringing hands to sacrum, keeping palms up.

On inhale: Return to starting position.

NUMBER: 8 times.
DETAILS: *On exhale:* Bring chest to thighs before bringing buttocks to heels. Rotate arms so palms are up and hands are resting on sacrum. *On inhale:* Expand chest and lift it up off of knees as arms sweep wide.

5.

POSTURE: Dvipāda Pīṭham.
EMPHASIS: To prepare upper back and neck for shoulder stand. To engage large muscles of hips and thighs.
TECHNIQUE: Lie on back with arms down at sides, knees bent, and feet on floor, slightly apart and comfortably close to buttocks.

On inhale: Pressing down on feet and keeping chin down, raise pelvis until neck is gently flattened on floor, while raising arms overhead to floor behind.

On exhale: Return to starting position.

NUMBER: 6 times.
DETAILS: *On inhale:* Lift spine, vertebra by vertebra, from bottom up. *On exhale:* Unwind spine, coming down vertebra by vertebra.

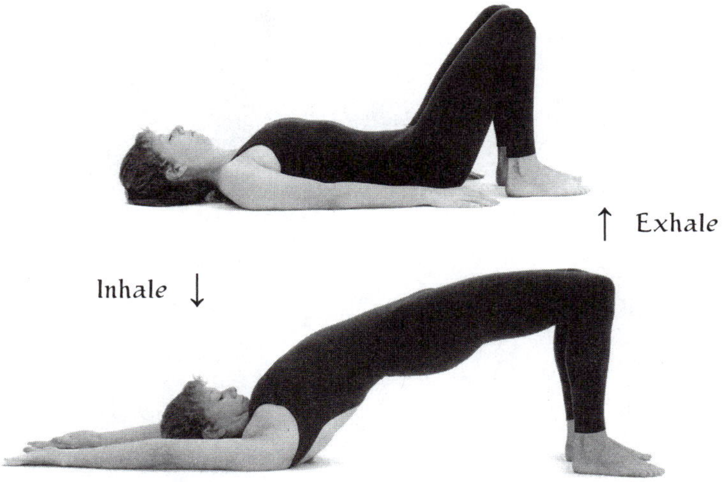

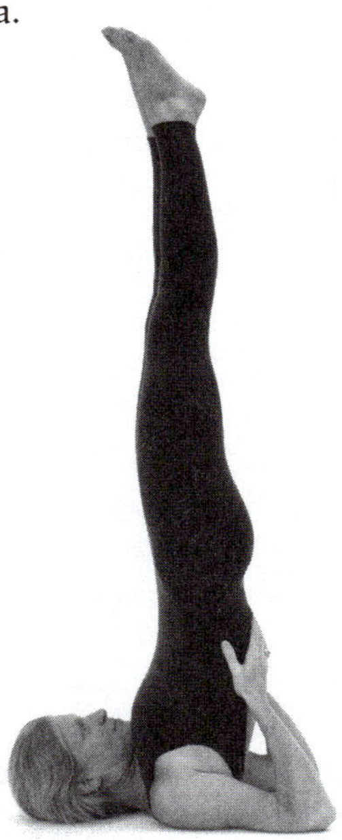

6.

POSTURE: Sarvāṅgāsana.
EMPHASIS: To invert, increasing pressure on thoracic cavity and deepening inhale and exhale.
TECHNIQUE: Lie on back.

On exhale: Flip legs up over head, lifting buttocks and lower to middle back off floor, and placing palms on middle back.

On inhale: Raise legs upward.

Stay and breathe deeply.

NUMBER: 18 breaths.
DETAILS: Place hips vertically above elbows rather than shoulders, and feet slightly beyond head.

7.

POSTURE: Ardha Śalabhāsana.
EMPHASIS: To arch upper back and neck while mobilizing arms, as a counterpose to shoulder stand.
TECHNIQUE: Lie on stomach, with head turned to right, hands crossed over sacrum, and palms up.

On inhale: Lift chest, right arm, and left leg, turning head to center.

On exhale: Lower chest and leg, while sweeping arm behind back and turning head to left.

Repeat on other side.

NUMBER: 6 times each side, alternately.
DETAILS: *On inhale:* Lift chest slightly before leg, and emphasize chest height. Keep pelvis level. *On exhale:* Turn head opposite arm being lowered.

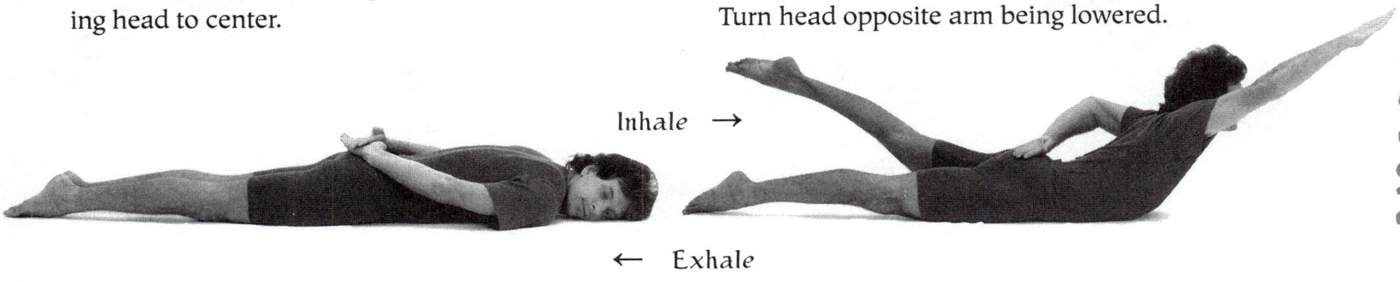

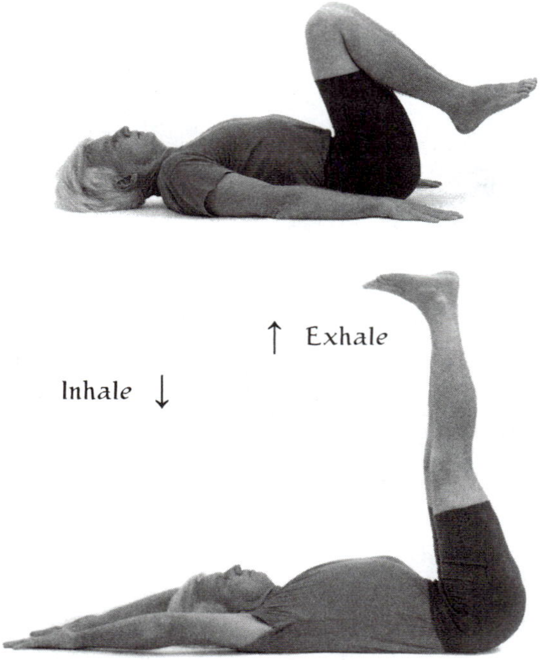

8.

Posture: Ūrdhva Prasārita Pādāsana.
Emphasis: To extend spine and flatten it onto floor. To stretch legs.
Technique: Lie on back with arms down at sides, legs bent, and knees in toward chest.

On inhale: Raise arms upward all the way to floor behind head, and legs upward toward ceiling.

Stay in stretch 2 full breaths.

On exhale: Return to starting position.

Number: 4 times.

Then stay in position 4 breaths, with fingers interlocked and palms out.

Details: *On inhale:* Flex feet as legs are raised upward. Slightly bend knees, keeping angle between legs and torso less than ninety degrees. Push low back and sacrum downward. Bring chin down. While staying in position: *On exhale,* flex knees and elbows slightly; *on inhale,* extend arms and legs straighter.

9.

Posture: Jaṭhara Parivṛtti.
Emphasis: To twist and compress belly and stretch hips.
Technique: Lie flat on back, with arms out to sides, and with left leg extended upward at an angle of ninety degrees to torso.

On exhale: Twist, bringing left foot toward right hand, while turning head left.

On inhale: Return to starting position.

Repeat 4 times.

Then stay in twist, holding left foot with right hand, 6 breaths.

Repeat on other side.

Details: *On exhale:* While twisting right, keep angles between left arm and torso and between left leg and torso less than ninety degrees. Knee may bend.

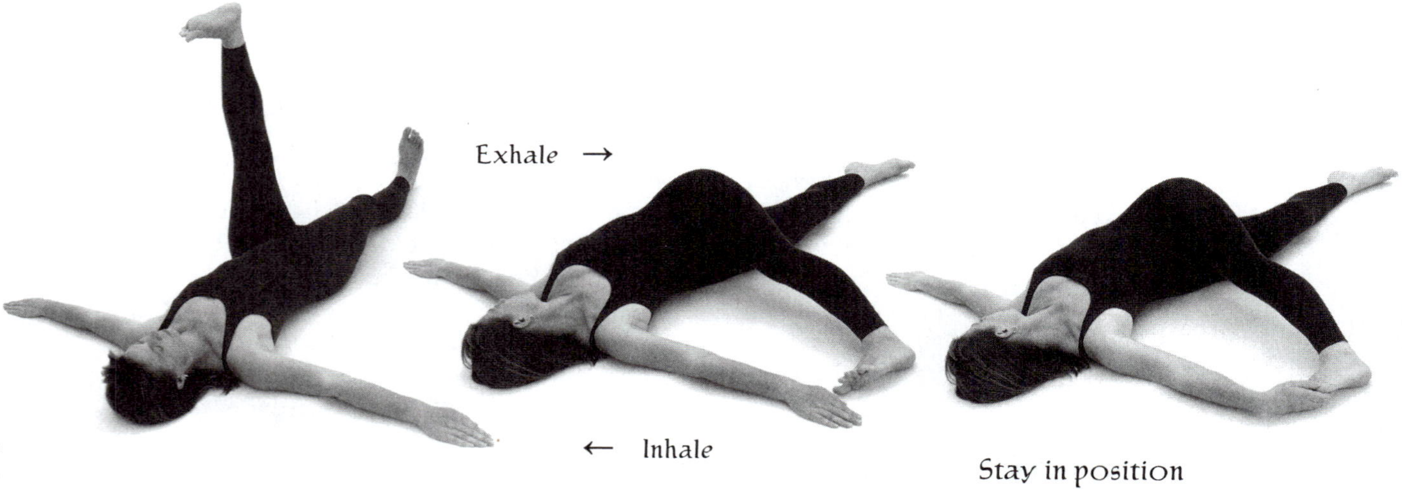

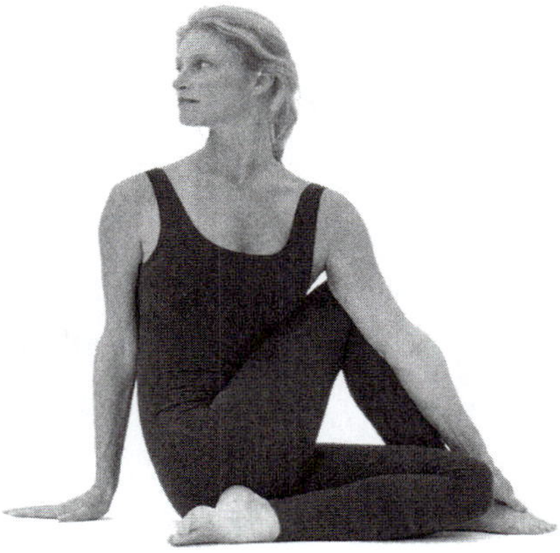

10.

POSTURE: Ardha Matsyendrāsana.
EMPHASIS: To deeply twist belly and fully exhale, emphasizing upward movement of diaphragm.
TECHNIQUE: Sit with left leg bent, left foot by right hip, and right knee straight up, right foot crossing over on outside of left knee, right arm behind back with palm down on floor by sacrum, and left arm across outside of right thigh, left hand on right foot.

On inhale: Extend spine upward.

On exhale: Twist torso and look over right shoulder.

NUMBER: 8 breaths each side.
DETAILS: *On exhale:* control torsion from deep in belly, using arm leverage only to augment twist. *On inhale:* subtly untwist body to facilitate extension of spine.

11.

POSTURE: Paścimatānāsana.
EMPHASIS: To compress belly and to stretch and strengthen back. To introduce short hold after exhale.
TECHNIQUE: Sit with legs forward, back straight, and arms raised over head.

On exhale: Bending knees slightly, bend forward, bringing chest to thighs, and palms to balls of feet.

Hold after exhale 4 to 6 seconds.

On inhale: Return to starting position.

Then stay in forward bend position 4 breaths.
DETAILS: *On exhale:* Bend knees to facilitate stretching low back and bring belly and chest to thighs. Move chin down toward throat. Feel like diaphragm moves up while holding after exhale. *On inhale:* Lift chest up and away from thighs, flattening upper back.

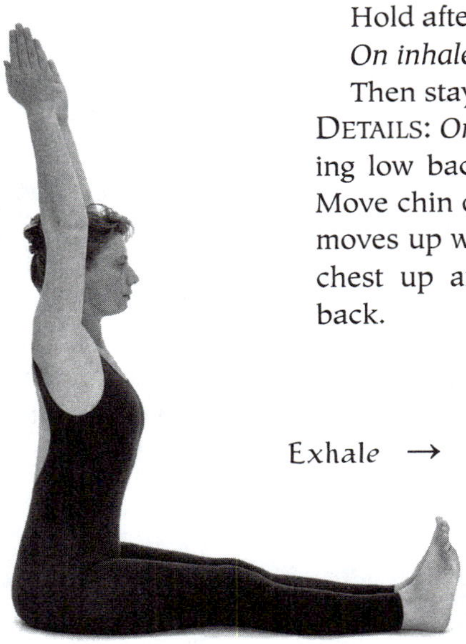

Exhale →

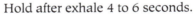

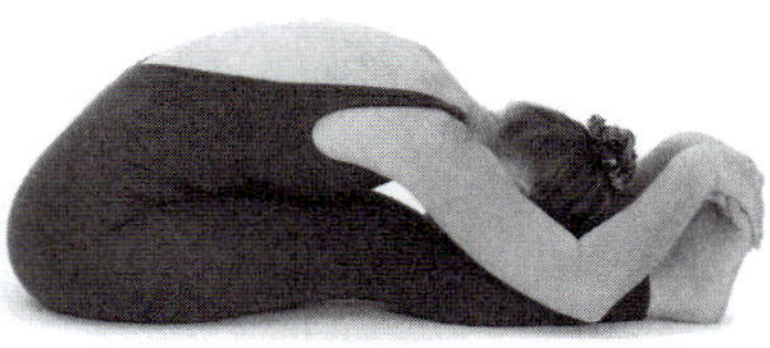

← Inhale

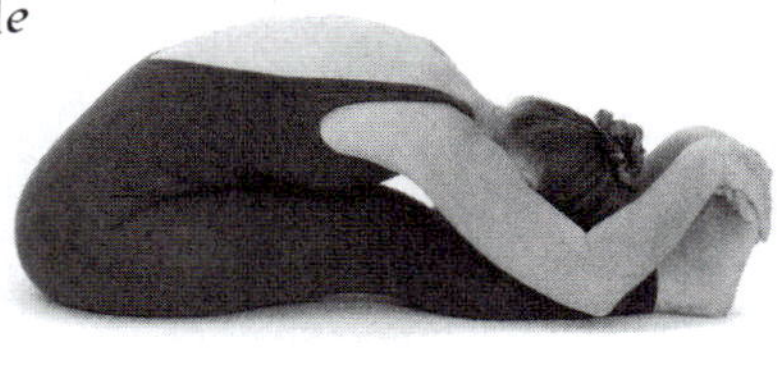

Stay in position

12.

POSTURE: Śavāsana with support.
EMPHASIS: To rest.
TECHNIQUE: Lie flat on back, with arms at sides, palms up, and legs slightly apart. Close eyes. Relax body fully, keeping mind relaxed and alert to sensations in body.
DURATION: Minimum 3 to 5 minutes.

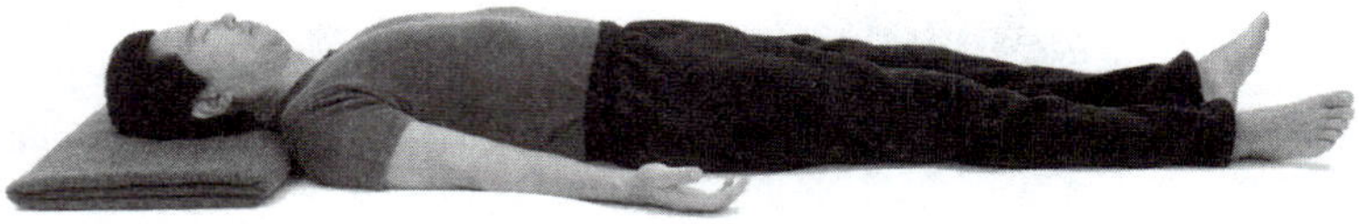

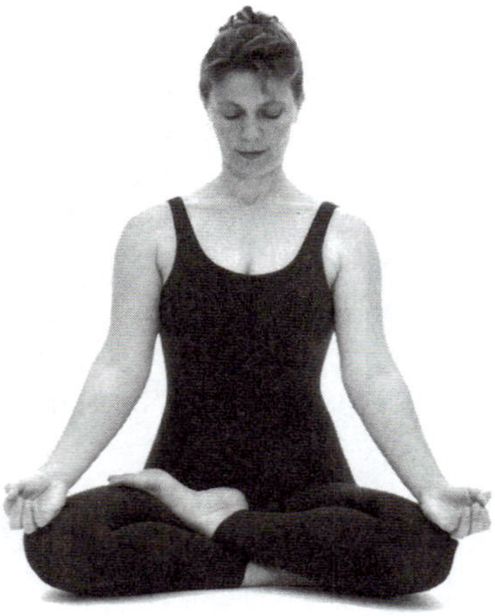

13.

POSTURE: Prāṇāyāma—Anuloma Krama, two stages.
EMPHASIS: To increase capacity to inhale and hold after inhale.
TECHNIQUE:

Exhale deeply and fully.
Inhale 1/2 of breath in 4 seconds.
Pause for 4 seconds.
Inhale other 1/2 of breath in 4 seconds.
Pause 4 seconds.
Exhale fully.
Repeat.

NUMBER: 8 times.
DETAILS: *On inhale:* Expand chest from pit of throat to solar plexus on first stage; from solar plexus to navel on second stage. Keep area from navel to pubic bone gently contracted throughout breathing exercise.

The Lymphatic System and Immunity

The lymphatic system plays an essential role in maintaining the body's health in a world of potential accidents, climatic changes, infections, parasites, and pollution. The primary function of this system is the production, maintenance, and distribution of special cells (lymphocytes), which are essential for the defense of the body against invading organisms such as bacteria, viruses, abnormal cells, and toxins. In addition, the lymphatic system helps in the delivery of nutrients and removal of wastes from the bloodstream, and in the maintenance of normal blood volume.

This system includes the lymphatic fluid, the network of vessels through which it flows, and the lymphatic organs and specialized defense cells that these organs produce.

The fluids of our circulatory and lymphatic systems are interrelated. Through a filtration process, fluid from the capillaries moves into the extracellular (interstitial) fluid surrounding most of the body's cells. As this fluid enters the lymphatic vessels, lymph is formed. The lymphatic vessels, together with smaller lymphatic capillaries, are spread throughout the body and extend into most of the body's tissue. From the lymphatic capillaries, lymph flows into larger vessels and, through a series of ducts, returns to the circulatory system.

Lymph nodes (commonly called lymph glands) are also found throughout the body, their role being to monitor and purify the contents of the lymph fluid as it moves toward the circulatory system. When we have an injury or infection, our lymph glands swell, indicating the presence and response of an increased number of defense cells.

The spleen is located between the stomach, the left kidney, and the diaphragm muscle. Because the spleen contains large amounts of both lymphatic tissue and red blood cells, the contents of the blood are monitored and purified as they pass through the spleen.

The body's vital defense cells (lymphocytes) are produced, differentiated, and stored in the lymph nodes, spleen, thymus, and bone marrow. These vital defenders of body immunity move throughout the entire system, destroying or deactivating invading organisms, abnormal cells, and toxins. T cells, which mature in the thymus, attack both our own and foreign cells that have become infected by viruses. B cells, which are produced in the bone marrow, secrete antibodies that chemically attack foreign substances (pathogens) that can cause disease. In coordination with this immediate response, the body produces specific T- and B-type "memory cells," which recognize particular pathogens and prepare the body for a more powerful and rapid defense upon future exposure to them. In addition to lymphocytes, there are other white blood cells (such as phagocytes) that contribute to the body's defense.

There are two main levels of our immune response: innate immunity and naturally acquired immunity. Innate immunity is present at birth and can be exemplified by the body's response to a scrape that becomes infected and whose innate immune re-

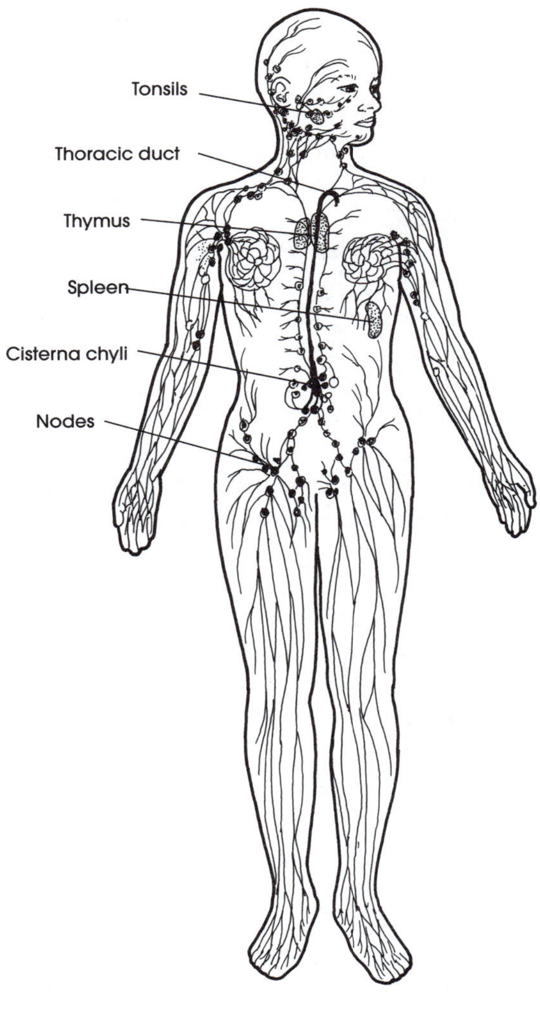

sponse is indicated through the presence of pus. Naturally acquired immunity appears following the body's exposure and subsequent response to a particular pathogen. This immunity begins to develop after birth and is continually developed as we grow and encounter new pathogens. In addition to naturally acquired immunity, there is also active immunization in which the body's response to particular pathogens is intentionally stimulated by the administration of vaccines.

The immune system and immune response are very complex and there are a large variety of conditions that result from disorders in immune function. These disorders are grouped as allergies, autoimmune disorders, and immunodeficiency diseases.

The most common and least dangerous class of immune disorders are mild allergies. In these conditions, the body reacts in a hypersensitive way to the presence of some substance that enters the body through skin, air, or food. The excessive response causes unpleasant allergic reactions, common examples being hay fever, asthma, and skin rashes.

Autoimmune disorders are often more serious. In these conditions, the immune system mistakenly attacks normal body cells and tissues. Examples of this disorder are rheumatoid arthritis, fibromyalgia, and Chronic Fatigue Syndrome (CFS). Symptoms of these conditions include muscle aches, joint pain, stiffness, multiple tender "trigger" points (fibromyalgia), general weakness, headaches, swollen lymph nodes (CFS), chronic low-grade fevers (CFS), lack of energy, difficulty sleeping, short-term memory loss, and massive fatigue.

Immunodeficiency diseases are the most serious and are characterized by the suppression of immune function. When immune function is suppressed, pathogens that are normally harmless can become life-threatening. AIDS is the best-known and most lethal of these conditions. Chronic fatigue syndrome, thought to be caused by a viral infection, can also be considered an immunodeficiency condition. Less serious is the recognized immune system depression that results from chronic stress, and because chronic stress results in less resistance to illness, people suffering from this condition are sick with abnormal frequency. Also, as the immune response is gradually depressed with age, elderly people are more susceptible to viruses and have a much higher incidence of cancer.

According to Yoga theory, the appropriate practice will increase our resistance to illness and disease. A strong digestion, deep respiratory capacity, a healthy cardiovascular system, and a balanced endocrine system all encourage the healthy functioning of the lymphatic system and immune response.

As with the other systems we have seen, we need to develop a slightly different strategy for the different classes of immune disfunction.

The general strategy for dealing with *allergic* conditions is to first build energy (brahmaṇa), stimulating the body's ability to deal with the symptoms, and then calm the system (langhana). In general, relaxation promotes wellness and restores homeostatic balance. If on the other hand there is the presence of infection or heavy toxicity, we would start with a langhana course to facilitate elimination, and then use brahmaṇa to strengthen the system.

Obviously, there are many different conditions that fall into this category, and they affect people with vastly different structural characteristics. The following practice, then, is illustrative of the general approach, and further individualization is recommended.

Working with Allergies

This practice was developed for N.P., a thirty-seven-year-old man who came to Yoga for help with his asthma and allergies. He told me that he couldn't keep a job because, sooner or later, he would be unable to handle the work environment. He would inevitably develop a reaction to someone smoking or wearing a strong perfume; or the air-conditioning would get to him, or the paint on the walls, or the dust in the carpet.

N.P. was a tall, thin man with a pasty complexion and excessive sweating of his hands and feet. He had a high level of anxiety and was at the same time highly irritable. He had spent a lot of time and money with various health practitioners and at self-help educational seminars. He knew a lot about his various allergies, as well as how to regulate his personal environment and diet. He had moved from apartment to apartment, looking for a place where he could find some relief. When he came to me, he had established a "safe zone" at his home, but, of course, he couldn't control the outside world and so was very frustrated. He asked me by phone if we had cats around the office, and to please be sure there were no flowers, or incense or candles burning in my office when he came to see me. He obviously had some preconceptions about what he might find in a Yoga school!

I asked him about his level of physical activity. His response was defensive, justifying his lack of physical exercise with the excuse of his multiple sensitivities. I suggested that if he could strengthen and increase the flexibility of his body, he would feel better about himself and his condition might improve. I assured him that we would proceed gradually, without force, and that the exercises would actually help him to relax. He agreed to try.

When we began to work together, I saw that his body was rigid and his breathing capacity limited. Over the half year that we worked together, we evolved the following sequence to generally strengthen his body, increase his flexibility, and deepen his breathing capacity. Over time, he became more relaxed with exercise and began to enjoy the practice.

My goal with N.P. was to increase his self-confidence. I also felt that regular practice would increase his digestive fire, support his immune response, and reduce his hypersensitivity.

After about six months of working together once a week, N.P. stopped coming to see me. About one year later he came back with this news: He had created his own business that he was running out of his home, and he was feeling very positive about its possibilities. He had created a niche in the tourist industry, packaging flights, accommodations, car rentals, and special activities for people looking to create an alternative vacation in Hawaii. N.P. looked well. His complexion had improved, and when I shook his hand I noticed that it wasn't sweaty. He proudly reported that he had continued his Yoga practice, and also that he had been going to the beach every morning for a long walk and a swim.

A Practice for Allergies

1.

POSTURE: Vajrāsana.
EMPHASIS: To warm up the body. To mobilize the rib cage to support respiration. To stretch low back.
TECHNIQUE: Stand on knees with arms over head.

On exhale: Bend forward, sweeping arms behind back and bringing hands to sacrum, keeping palms up.

On inhale: Return to starting position.

NUMBER: 8 times.
DETAILS: *On exhale:* Bring chest to thighs before bringing buttocks to heels. Rotate arms so palms are up and hands are resting on sacrum. *On inhale:* Expand chest and lift it up off knees as arms sweep wide.

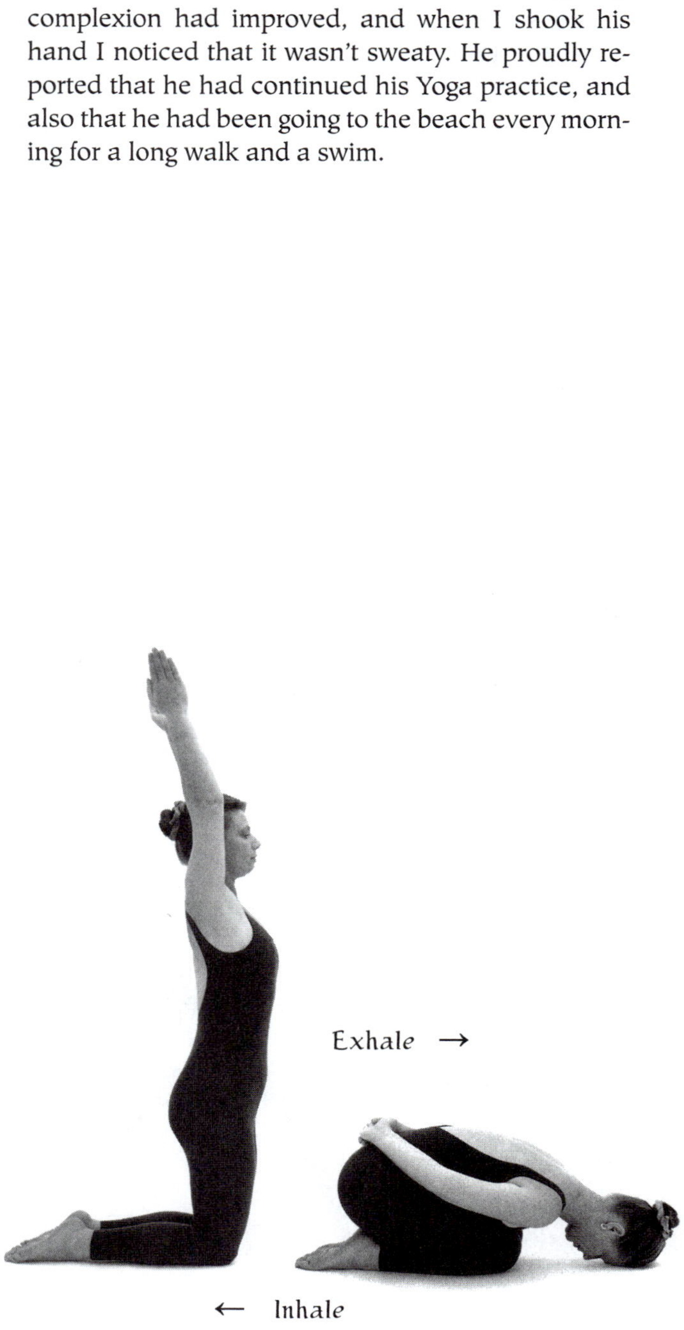

2.

Position: Ardha Pārśvottānāsana.
Emphasis: To asymmetrically stretch and strengthen back and legs.
Technique: Stand with left foot forward, right foot turned out a bit less than forty-five degrees, left arm folded behind back, and right arm raised over head.

On exhale: Bend forward, bringing belly and chest toward left thigh and right hand toward left foot.

On inhale: Return to starting position.

Repeat on other side.

Number: 8 times each side, one side at a time.
Details: *On exhale:* Keep back heel firmly down on floor. Bend front knee slightly. *On inhale:* Lift chest first, letting arms and head follow.

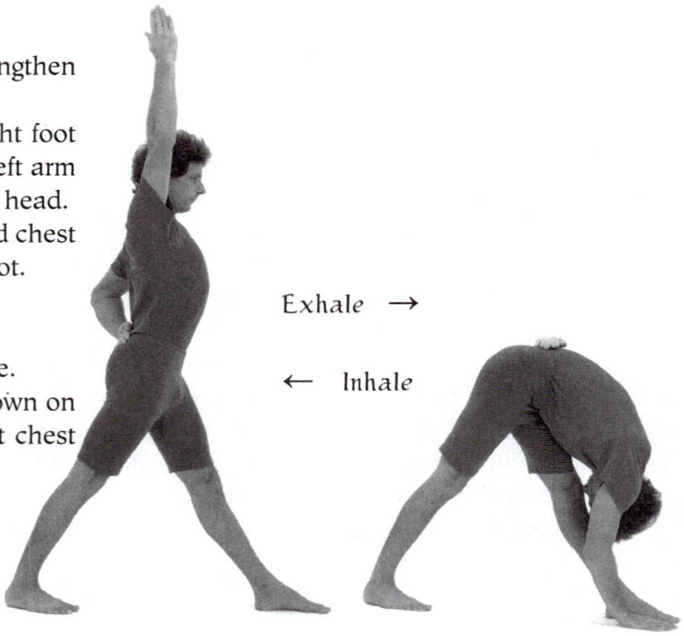

3.

Posture: Utthita Trikoṇāsana.
Emphasis: To laterally stretch torso and mobilize rib cage.
Technique:

A: Stand with feet spread wider than shoulders, left foot turned out at ninety-degree angle to right foot, left arm over head, right arm straight down at waist and slightly rotated externally, and head to center.

On exhale: Keeping shoulders in same plane as hips, bend laterally, lowering left shoulder and bringing left hand below left knee while turning head down toward left hand.

On inhale: Return to starting position.

Repeat.

B: With left hand down along left leg:

On inhale: Bring right arm up and forward while turning head forward toward right hand.

On exhale: Return right hand to starting position while turning head down toward left hand.

Repeat.

Number: Repeat A, then B four times, then repeat on other side.

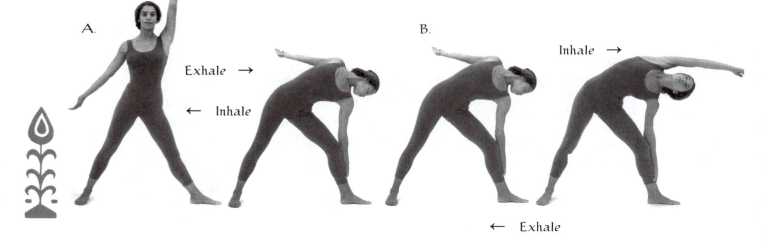

4.

POSTURE: Cakravākāsana.

EMPHASIS: To stretch and balance low back after lateral posture. To transition from standing lateral bend to prone back bend.

TECHNIQUE: Get down on hands and knees, with shoulders vertically above wrists and with hips above knees.

On inhale: Lift chest up and away from belly.

On exhale: Gently contract belly, round low back, and bring chest toward thighs.

NUMBER: 8 times.

DETAILS: *On inhale:* Lead with chest, keeping chin slightly down. Avoid compressing low back; rather, feel chest expanding. *On exhale:* Round low back without collapsing chest over belly. Avoid increasing curvature of upper back. Let chest lower toward thighs sooner than hips toward heels.

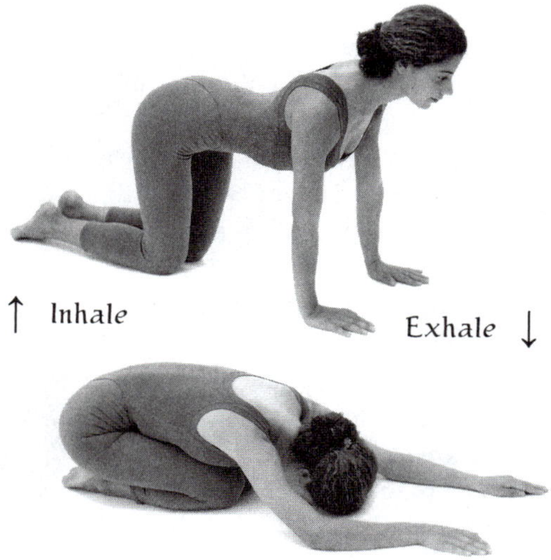

5.

POSTURE: Ardha Śalabhāsana.

EMPHASIS: To arch upper back and neck while mobilizing arms.

TECHNIQUE: Lie on stomach, with head turned right, hands crossed over sacrum, and palms up.

On inhale: Lift chest, right arm, and left leg, turning head to center.

On exhale: Lower chest and leg, while sweeping arm behind back and turning head to left.

Repeat on other side.

NUMBER: 6 times each side, alternately.

DETAILS: *On inhale:* Lift chest slightly before leg, and emphasize chest height. Keep pelvis level. *On exhale:* Turn head opposite arm being lowered.

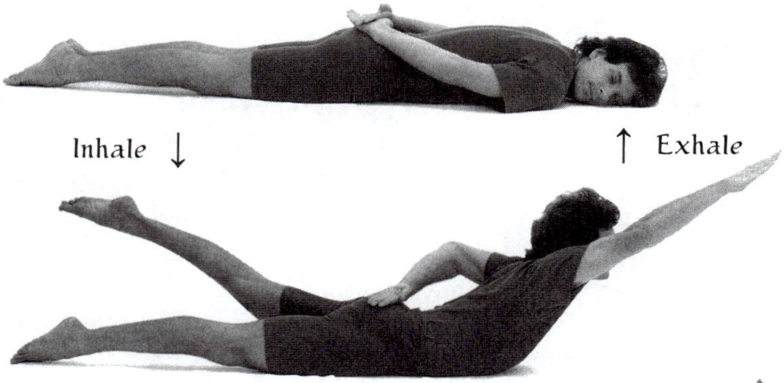

6.

POSTURE: Ūrdhva Prasārita Pādāsana, one side at a time.

EMPHASIS: To extend spine and flatten it onto floor. To stretch legs and back. To sharpen mental focus through asymmetrical adaptation.

TECHNIQUE: Lie on back with arms down at sides, legs bent, and knees in toward chest.

On inhale: Raise right arm up and over head, and raise left leg upward.

On exhale: Return to starting position.

Repeat on other side.

NUMBER: 4 times each side, alternately.

DETAILS: *On inhale:* Flex foot as leg is raised upward. Slightly bend knee, keeping angle between leg and torso less than ninety degrees. Push low back and sacrum downward. Bring chin down.

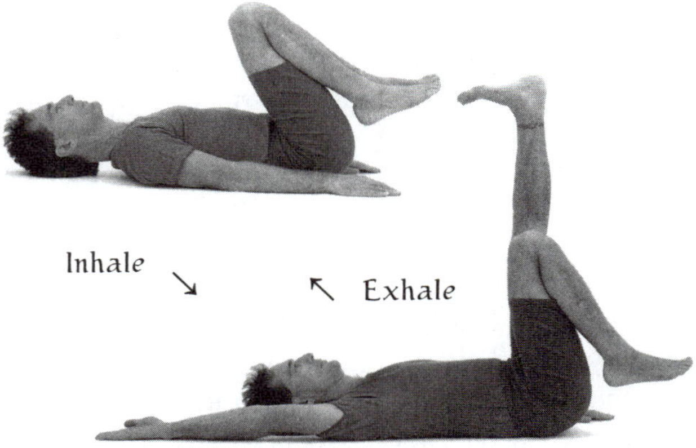

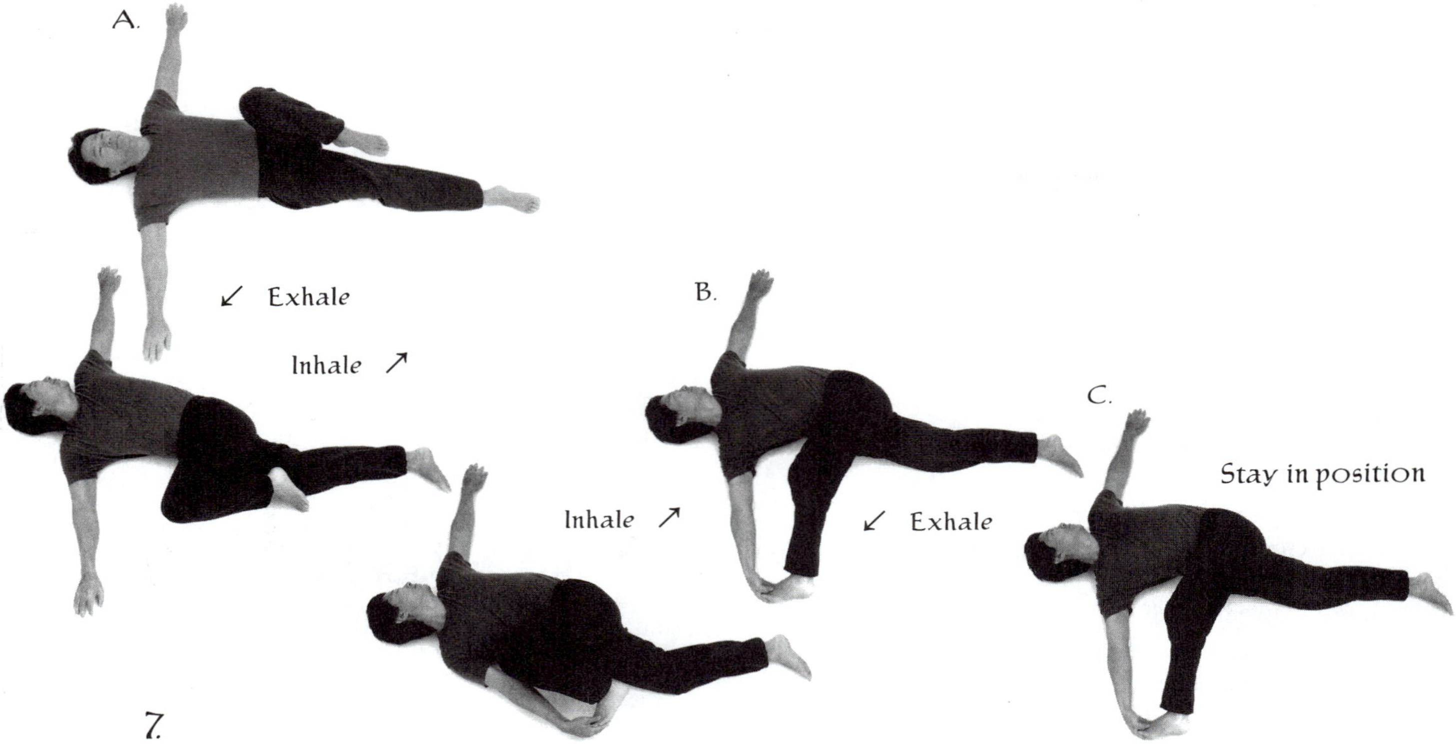

7.

POSTURE: Jaṭhara Parivṛtti.

EMPHASIS: To twist and compress belly. To facilitate exhalation.

TECHNIQUE:

A. Lie flat on back, with arms out to sides and with left knee pulled up toward chest.

On exhale: Twist, bringing left knee toward floor on right side of body while turning head to left.

On inhale: Return to starting position.

Repeat 4 times.

B. Then stay in twist, holding left foot with right hand.

On inhale: Extend leg.

On exhale: Bend leg.

Repeat 4 times.

C. Then stay in full twist 4 breaths.

Repeat on other side.

DETAILS: B: *On inhale,* straighten leg from hip, using hand to guide foot.

8.

POSTURE: Mahāmudrā/Jānu Śirṣāsana.
EMPHASIS: To develop both inhalation and exhalation capacity. To introduce breathing ratio. To strengthen respiratory and spinal musculature.
TECHNIQUE: Sit with right leg folded in, heel to groin, left leg extended forward, and holding left foot with both hands.

On inhale: Extend spine upward, expanding chest, flattening upper back, and lengthening in front of torso.

Hold after inhale.

On exhale: Maintain posture while pulling belly firmly in.

Hold after exhale.

Remain in extended position 8 breaths. Then sink belly and chest to thigh.

Stay in forward-bended position 4 breaths.

Repeat on other side.

NUMBER: 8 breaths with spine extended; 4 breaths in forward bend, each side.
DETAILS: Ratio: begin with 6-second inhale, 3-second hold, 6-second exhale, 3-second hold. Increase to 8-second inhale, 4-second hold, 8-second exhale, 4-second hold. Bend extended leg so as to focus on spine.

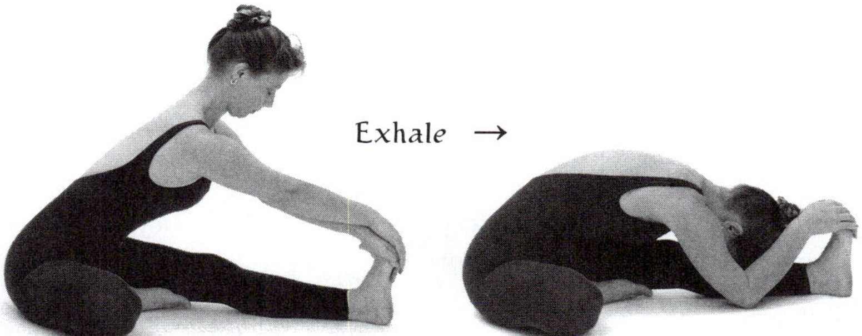

9.

POSTURE: Paścimatānāsana.
EMPHASIS: To compress belly and to stretch and strengthen back.
TECHNIQUE: Sit with legs forward, back straight, and arms raised over head.

On exhale: Bend forward, bending knees slightly, bringing chest to thighs, and palms to balls of feet.

On inhale: Holding feet, lift chest upward, flattening upper back.

On exhale: Bend forward again.

Repeat.

NUMBER: 6 times.
DETAILS: *On exhale:* Bend knees to facilitate stretching of low back, and bring belly and chest to thighs. Move chin down toward throat. *On inhale:* Lift chest up and away from thighs, flattening upper back.

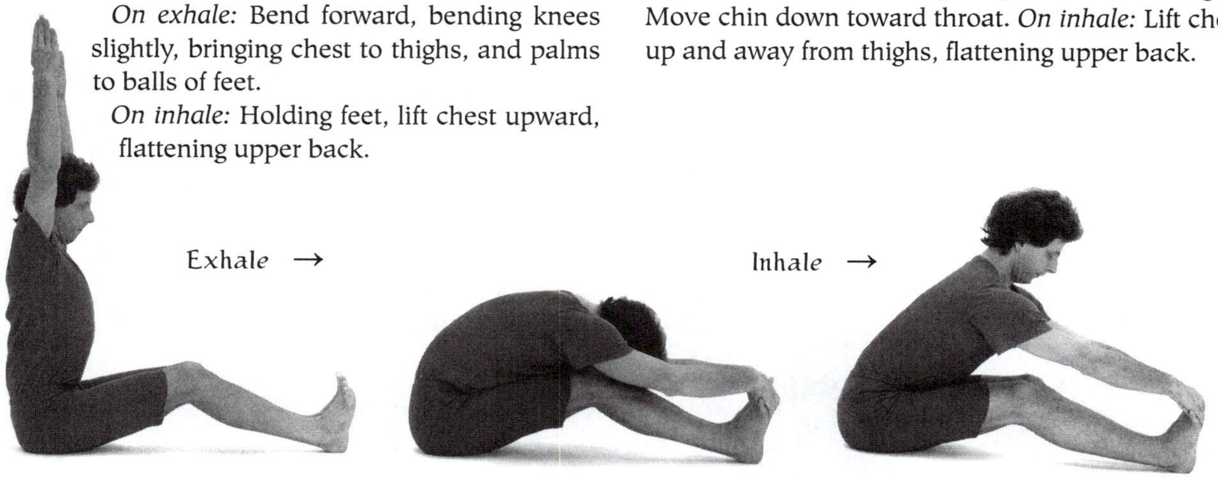

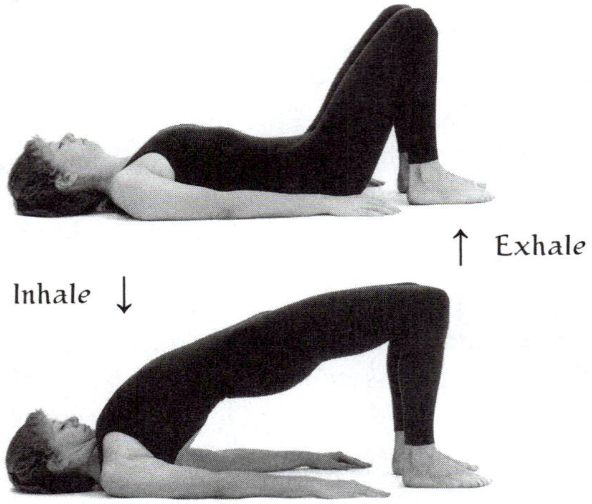

10.
POSTURE: Dvipāda Pīṭham.
EMPHASIS: To relax back and stretch belly.
TECHNIQUE: Lie on back with arms down at sides, knees bent, and feet on floor, slightly apart and comfortably close to buttocks.

On inhale: Pressing down on feet and keeping chin down, raise pelvis up toward ceiling, until neck is gently flattened on floor.

On exhale: Return to starting position.

NUMBER: 6 times.
DETAILS: *On inhale:* Lift spine, vertebra by vertebra, from bottom up. *On exhale:* Unwind spine, coming down vertebra by vertebra.

11.
POSTURE: Śavāsana with support.
EMPHASIS: To rest.
TECHNIQUE: Lie flat on back, with arms at sides, palms up, and legs slightly apart. Close eyes. Relax body fully, keeping mind relaxed and alert to sensations in body.
DURATION: Minimum 3 to 5 minutes.

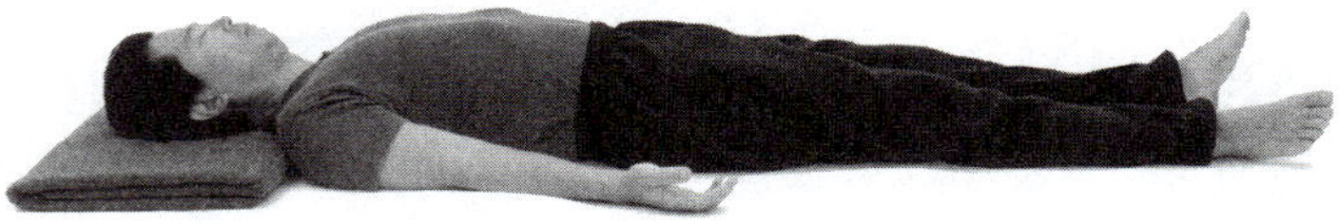

12.
POSTURE: Seated Breathing.
EMPHASIS: To increase control of inhale and exhale. To relax mind and body.
TECHNIQUE: Inhale fully; pause briefly; exhale fully; pause briefly.
NUMBER: 18 breaths.
DETAILS: Gradually lengthen inhale and exhale to comfortable maximum, sustain for a few breaths, then gradually reduce length of inhale and exhale, returning to starting point.

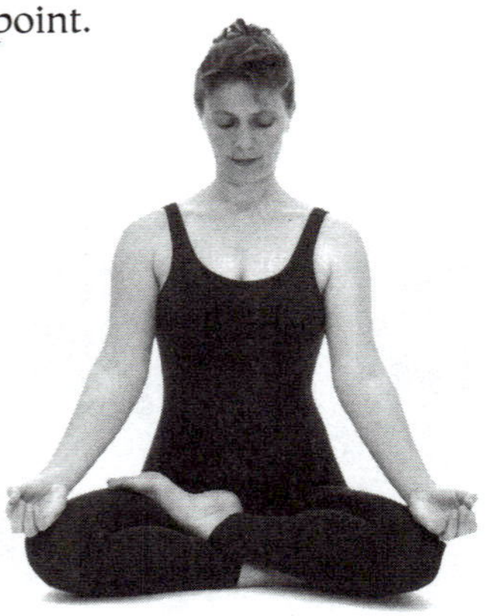

The challenge for people suffering from autoimmune and immunodeficiency disorders, such as CFS, is that their condition is often aggravated by exercise. In such cases, the strategy is to begin very simply (langhana) and to gradually build their energy (brahmaṇa). Practices must be gentle, with rest between postures and time to feel the increased flow of energy throughout the body. Individuals suffering from these conditions usually have muscular pain and weakness, so the practices must be carefully constructed to support them without aggravating this condition. The practice that follows is necessarily illustrative of these principles although, again, further individualization is essential.

Working with Chronic Fatigue Syndrome

This practice was developed for L.B., a fifty-three-year-old woman suffering from chronic fatigue syndrome. Her husband, who was a minister, had been coming to our school for group classes for several years. L.B. worked as a teacher in the local public school system.

L.B. had been suffering with her condition for many years, and she appreciated the benefits of exercise. However, whenever she got started on a program, she would inevitably suffer a setback in her condition. She had heard about our school from her husband and had finally decided to give Yoga a try.

She told me that she had very low energy, getting out of bed every morning was a struggle, that she was easily fatigued, and had occasional bouts of low-grade fever. Though she suffered from general muscular weakness, she did not seem to have the chronic muscular pains characteristic of many CFS cases.

We organized to meet once a week for several months. I had her begin very gently, seated in a chair, with simple movements coordinated with breathing. Later I asked her to do short holding of the breath after inhale. For the first month, her practice began with simple movements on a chair, then standing for one posture, and then resting in a chair again. She was encouraged by our gentle approach and continued coming to see me.

After some time, it became evident that she wanted to talk more about her personal life. I learned that she was under a lot of stress at the local high school where she taught. She was genuinely interested in education and told me that, for the most part, the students were only there because they had to be. She told me that she felt that they respected neither the learning process nor her.

After several months, she confided in me that there was not much spark left between her and her husband, and that they never did things together anymore. Then she told me that she had several "hard" drinks after dinner every evening.

As we worked together she opened up more and more. I reminded her of the picture she had painted of herself: a woman unhappy with her work and unhappy in her marriage, who did little or no exercise, and who drank. She clearly needed to make a change. I encouraged her to reflect on what she loved to do and to visualize a rewarding life. I thought that if she could get a new direction, she would be able to tap a deep source of energy inside her that would help her make a shift. I also asked her if she would be willing to make a commitment to go for a short walk and then sit and talk with her husband after dinner *before* she started to drink. I knew he would be pleased.

At a certain point, I asked her if she would be interested in using some sound in her practice. I told her that sound techniques produce vibrations that would gently stimulate the energy in her body. She was happy to try and was very pleased with the results. She told me that after using the technique, she felt nourished and revitalized. I asked her to use the time at the end of her practice, when she was feeling well, to reflect on her future and then listen to her heart.

After some time, she came to tell me she was leaving the island. She had applied and been accepted in a doctoral program in education and was excited about the future. Her husband stayed behind for several months. Then one day he came to tell me he was joining his wife. As he left, he told me that his wife had asked him to thank me for helping her to find the courage to change.

A Practice for Chronic Fatigue Syndrome

1.

POSTURE: Forward bending in a chair.
EMPHASIS: To gently mobilize rib cage while deepening inhale. To stretch back while deepening exhale.
TECHNIQUE: Sit on a chair or bench with back straight and hands on knees.
On inhale: Raise arms out to sides.
On exhale: Bend forward, bringing hands to feet.
On inhale: Return to previous position.
On exhale: Return to starting position.
NUMBER: 8 times.
DETAILS: *On inhale:* Lift chest up and away from belly, bringing palms to shoulder level with elbows bent and slightly lifted. *On exhale:* Bring hands to knees and slide them down legs toward feet.

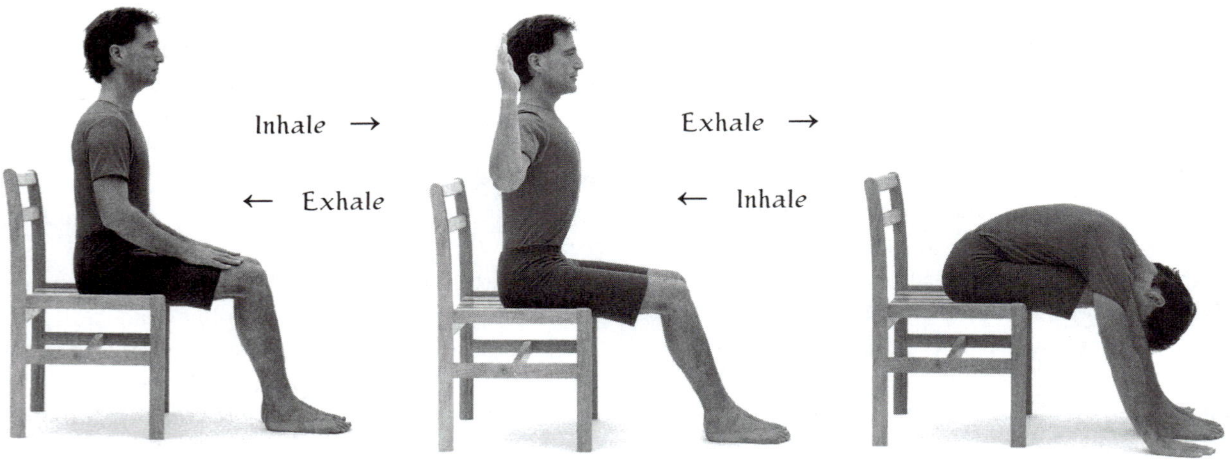

2.

POSTURE: Vīrabhadrāsana.
EMPHASIS: To build energy, strengthen muscles of back, expand chest, flatten upper back, and strengthen leg muscles. To increase hold after inhalation.
TECHNIQUE: Stand with left foot forward, feet as wide as hips, and arms at sides.
On inhale: Simultaneously bend left knee, displace chest slightly forward and hips slightly backward, and bring arms out to sides and shoulders back. Hold breath 2, 3, and 4 seconds, 2 times each in a progressive fashion.
On exhale: Return to starting position.
NUMBER: 6 times each side.
DETAILS: *On inhale:* Keep hands and elbows in line with shoulders. Feel opening of chest and flattening of upper back, not compression in low back. Keep head forward. Keep firm on back heel.

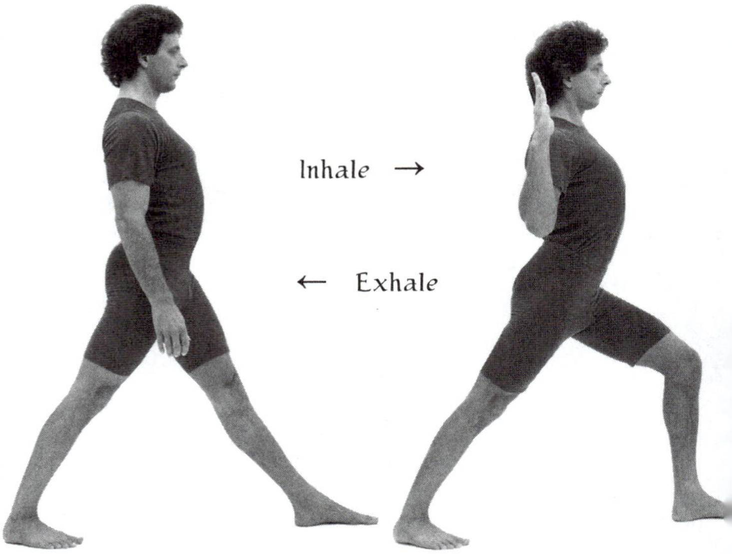

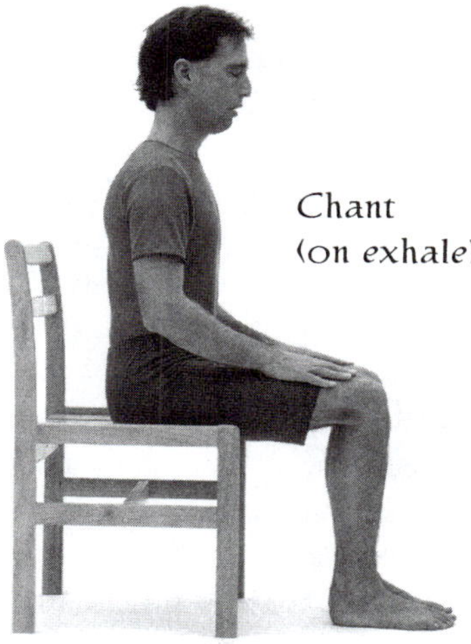

3.

Posture: Rest on chair and use of sound technique.
Emphasis: To rest and build energy through sound and pitch.
Technique: After a short rest, to deepen inhale and exhale.

On exhale: Chant **OM**. Pause briefly.
Inhale.
Repeat 3 times at low pitch.
Rest briefly.
Repeat 3 times at a middle pitch.
Rest briefly.
Repeat 3 times at a higher pitch.
Rest briefly.

Details: Chant: The "**O**" sound should last about 3 seconds, the "**M**" sound about 1 second. Both low and high pitches should be comfortable; not too low or too high.

4.

Posture: Cakravākāsana.
Emphasis: To stretch rib cage on inhale. To gently compress and stretch belly on exhale.
Technique: Get down on hands and knees, with shoulders vertically above wrists and with hips above knees.

On inhale: Lift chest up and away from belly.

On exhale: Move hips back and down toward heels, lowering chest toward thighs.

Number: 8 times.
Details: *On inhale:* Lead with chest, keeping chin slightly down. Avoid compressing low back; rather, feel chest expanding. *On exhale:* Let chest lower toward thighs sooner than hips toward heels.

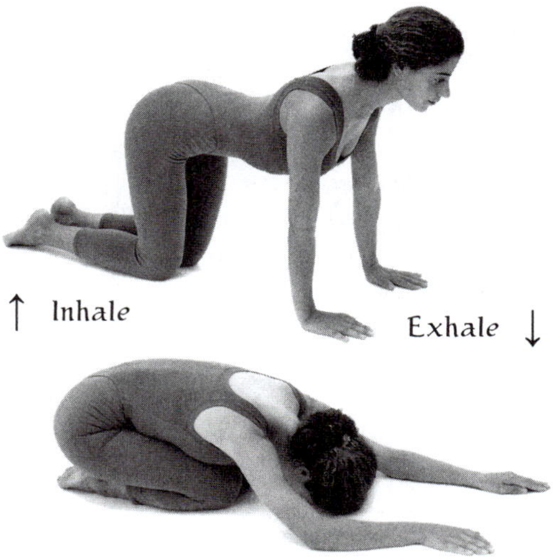

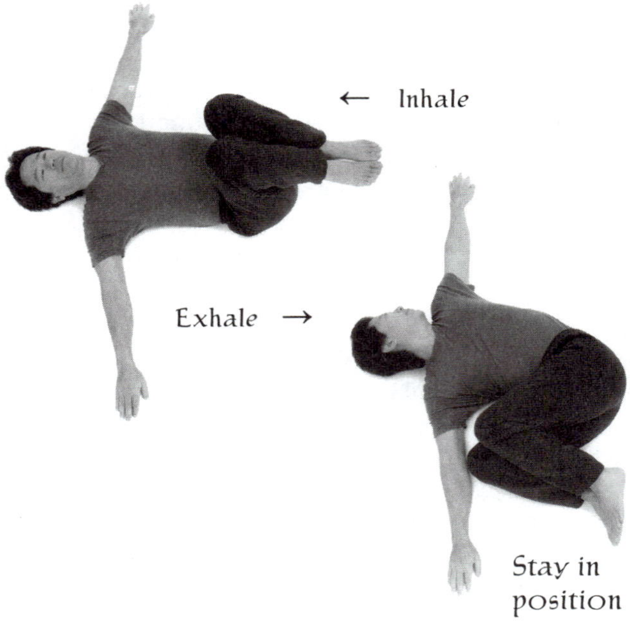

5.

POSTURE: Jaṭhara Parivṛtti variation.
EMPHASIS: To gently twist and compress belly, progressively increasing number of breaths in posture.
TECHNIQUE: Lie on back with both knees bent, thighs lifted toward chest, and both feet off ground. Arms out to sides, slightly less than right angles to torso.

On exhale: Bring both knees toward floor on right side of body, twisting abdomen and simultaneously turning head left.

On inhale: Return to starting position.

Stay in twist 1, 2, 3, and then 4 full breaths on each side, alternating sides.
DETAILS: *On exhale:* Throughout movement, keep knees at an angle to torso that is less than ninety degrees.

6.

POSTURE: Apānāsana.
EMPHASIS: To gently compress belly while progressively extending exhale.
TECHNIQUE: Lie on back with both knees bent toward chest and feet off floor. Place each hand on its respective knee.

On exhale: Pull thighs gently but progressively toward chest.

On inhale: Return to starting position.
NUMBER: 12 times.
DETAILS: *On exhale:* Pull gently with arms, keeping shoulders relaxed and on floor. Press low back down into floor and drop chin slightly toward throat. Progressively lengthen exhale with each successive repetition.

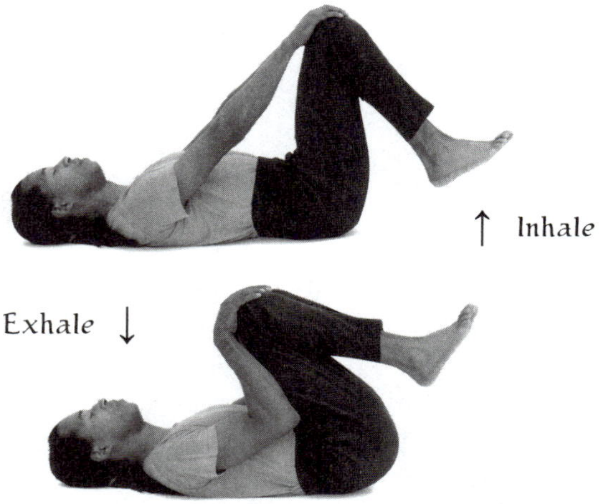

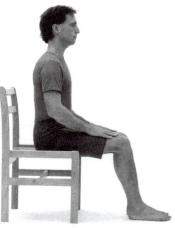

7.

POSTURE: Rest and feel vitalized, while sitting in chair.
EMPHASIS: To relax, feel nourished and alive, while sitting up.
TECHNIQUE: Sit in a comfortable chair, without slumping.
NUMBER: About 5 minutes.

Endocrine System

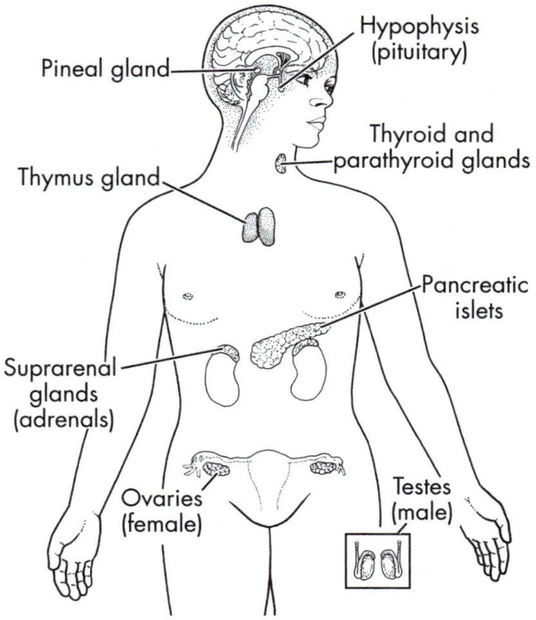

The endocrine system, along with the nervous system, monitors and regulates all the body's activity. The nervous system influences bodily function through neurotransmitters that travel on a complex system of nerve tissue that laces throughout the entire body. The endocrine system influences the function of the body by releasing chemicals, known as hormones, into the bloodstream. Hormones are complex chemical structures that, by modifying the activities of particular cells that respond to them, eventually modify the body's tissues and organs as well. In this way, they also adjust metabolic operations in response to changes in the availability of nutrients and to the body's demand for energy. In addition, they direct bodily activities such as growth, maturation, sexual development, pregnancy, and response to stress. In short, they regulate the entire metabolic process of the body.

Accordingly, the endocrine system and its function is complex and mysterious and although we understand the function of most of the hormones produced by the endocrine glands, there are still some whose function has yet to be discovered. A brief discussion of what we do know of this important system follows.

There are seven major endocrine glands in the human body, located, from the head downward, in this order: pineal, pituitary, thyroid and parathyroid (actually separate glands located together), thymus, pancreas, adrenals, and gonads. Each gland produces particular hormones, which have specific roles in the growth, development, and functioning of the body. In addition to these seven major glands, the heart, kidneys, liver, and digestive tract also produce essential hormones. And they all work, in coordination with the neural control of the nervous system, to help maintain homeostasis in the body.

The role of the pineal gland is little understood. Melatonin, a hormone released by the pineal gland, influences the body's physiological rhythms, which are linked to the day/night cycle. The production of this hormone is decreased by exposure to sunlight. People who are too often indoors or who live in locations where the winter months are dark and gray often suffer from depression, low energy, and lack of ability to concentrate (Seasonal Affective Disorder, SAD). Whether or not this is the direct result of increased melatonin production is not yet clear, but it is clear that these symptoms result from inadequate sunlight and that full-spectrum lights, which are strong enough to decrease melatonin production, are helpful in such cases.

Melatonin production is at its highest between 8:00 P.M. and 4:00 A.M. People who work late into the night under artificial lights, or who travel regularly across time zones (and suffer jet lag) often manifest symptoms similar to those suffering from SAD syndrome. Whether or not this is the direct result of decreased melatonin production is also not yet clear. Melatonin supplements that claim to help such people are also available.

The pituitary gland is the master controller of all the other glands because it releases hormones that target and regulate their functions and influence all their metabolic processes. It can be anatomically divided into two parts: the anterior and posterior. Hormones released by the anterior and posterior pituitary stimulate the thyroid (TSH) and adrenal (ACTH) glands, regulate the gonads (gonadotropins), and stimulate the mammary glands and uterus through pregnancy, birth, and lactation (prolactin and oxytocin). In addition, because the anterior pituitary releases the hormone responsible for stimulating growth (growth hormone), it may also be considered a growth gland. In addition, the posterior pituitary releases a hormone (ADH) that prevents water loss and thereby elevates blood volume and pressure.

The thyroid is both a growth and an energy gland. By producing hormones (such as thyroxine) that target most of the cells in the body, the thyroid increases our ability to utilize energy (glucose) and oxygen. By increasing metabolic rate, these hormones also increase our body temperature, enabling us to adapt to cold weather. Also, by producing hormones that target the bones, kidneys, and intestines the thyroid (releasing calcitonin) and parathyroid (releasing parathormone) together regulate the calcium concentrations in our body fluids, thereby directly influencing the growth and development of our skeletal system.

The thymus is the immune gland. It releases hormones (thymosin) that target important body defense cells, causing lymphocytes to become T cells, which are an essential part of the body's defense against viruses and infections. The thymus thereby influences the strength of our immune system. The thymus gland also releases other hormones whose functions are as yet unknown.

The adrenals are primarily energy glands. They release hormones that affect a variety of metabolic and regulatory functions in nearly all of the body's cells. The adrenal glands can be divided anatomically and functionally into two parts: the adrenal cortex and the adrenal medulla. By releasing glucocorticoid hormones into muscles, fatty tissue, and liver cells, the adrenal cortex regulates our ability to store and utilize energy (glucose). By releasing mineralcorticoid hormones into kidney cells, it also influences the sodium concentration in our urine. The adrenal medulla is essentially a part of the sympathetic nervous system. It secretes epinephrine and norepinephrine, in response to stimulation by sympathetic nerves, which increase cardiac activity and blood pressure, resulting in the familiar "adrenaline rush" that is part of the body's fight-or-flight response to perceived danger or extreme emotional stimulation.

The pancreas can be said to have two distinct functions: exocrine and endocrine. In its exocrine function, the pancreas secretes digestive enzymes that break down carbohydrates (carbohydrases), fats (lipase), and proteins (proteinase and peptidases). It also secretes sodium bicarbonates, which neutralize stomach acid. In its endocrine function, the pancreas may also be considered as an energy gland. The endocrine cells of the pancreas produce two hormones, glucagon and insulin, which regulate blood sugar levels. When blood sugar levels rise, the pancreas releases insulin to help the cells convert the glucose into energy reserves. When blood sugar levels fall, the pancreas releases glucagon and these energy reserves are converted back into glucose.

The gonads refer to both the male and female reproductive organs. The hormones released by these glands (testosterone from the testes, and estrogen and progesterone from the ovaries) promote the production and development of sperm and eggs, secondary sexual characteristics, and influence both male and female behavioral patterns.

Any threat to homeostasis stresses the system. Sources of stress include physical stress, such as illness or injury; emotional stress, such as anxiety or depression; environmental stress, such as temperature extremes and pollution; and metabolic stress, such as improper or inadequate diet. These stressors impact all of the systems of the body and the role of the endocrine system is to respond to them and, through hormonal adjustments, to restore balance to the system.

There are many disorders that derive from the endocrine system. Most of them are linked to abnormal hormone production, either excessive (hyper) or deficient (hypo), and any other system can be damaged as a result of such imbalance.

Conditions of chronic, excessive hormonal production often involve a pathological and tumorous condition. Although an appropriate program of Yoga therapy may be helpful, people with serious hyperfunctioning endocrine conditions are advised to be under the care of a health professional.

Conditions of chronic, deficient hormonal production are more common. A person who is chronically stressed out will eventually become weak, run down, and will not feel well generally. Sooner or later, some of the following common symptoms of hypoendocrine function will begin to manifest: fatigue, depression, low energy, muscular weakness, chills, dry skin, low body temperature, low blood pressure, high cholesterol levels, low blood sugar (hypoglycemia), and weakened immunity. These symptoms may appear in conditions of decreased thyroid and adrenal functioning. When hypothyroid conditions exist, these symptoms are often accompanied by weight gain. When a hypo–adrenal cortex function exists, they are often accompanied by weight loss.

Diabetes mellitus, a serious condition characterized by inappropriately high levels of blood sugar (hyperglycemia), may also be considered in this category, which includes two major types.

Type I diabetes is the result of inadequate production of insulin by the pancreas. It is a condition that usually appears in individuals under forty years of age and most frequently in childhood. Individuals who suffer from Type I diabetes are dependent on insulin treatment, although through careful dietary regulation and a well-conceived program of Yoga therapy, it is possible to reduce the amount of insulin that they need.

Type II diabetes most often affects individuals after forty years of age. In this condition, while insulin levels may be normal or even elevated, the insulin itself is not being properly utilized by the cells. Individuals suffering from this type of diabetes may or may not be insulin dependent, and in this group the most significant improvement can usually be seen. Within this category of diabetes, there are two main types of conditions: the obese and the emaciated. In the first case, the obese condition may be causally related to overeating—particularly a high-fat diet—drinking, and excessive consumption of sweets, and is often complicated by a sedentary lifestyle. Also, secondary complications often arise, including poor circulation and, in extreme cases, gangrene and blindness. In the second case, the emaciated condition is often accompanied by low energy, insomnia, and dehydration, resulting in constant thirst. This condition is usually more difficult to treat.

The Yoga theory for working with any condition involving hypo-functioning is to first consider appropriate lifestyle changes, including taking time for relaxation, modifying diet, and reducing stress by giving up stress-producing habits. In addition, we can use the Yoga techniques of breath, movement, sound, and meditation.

As we have seen, the endocrine system is very complex, requiring balance for proper functioning. Accordingly, the goal of any Yoga practice in relation to the endocrine system is that of restoring and maintaining balance. In this sense, our Yoga practice functions as a kind of homeostatic equalizer. Because there are a wide variety of symptoms, stemming from a wide variety of causes, and because they may manifest in individuals with vastly different structural conditions, the general theory of practice is to utilize techniques that stimulate the area of the body where the involved glands are located, thereby increasing circulation and bringing vital nutrition and oxygen to them.

Following this idea, we present two sequences to stimulate different areas of the body. The first is designed to stimulate the area around the thyroid, parathyroid, and thymus glands, with the intention of balancing the function of these glands by stimulating the immune system and by increasing general strength and metabolic rate.

The second sequence is designed to stimulate the area around the adrenal glands and pancreas. And here again, our intention is to stimulate and nourish these glands and to restore balanced functioning. In the case of type II diabetes, we also want to stimulate the peripheral tissues, activating the nourishing and cleansing function of circulation in order to facilitate the utilization of glucose.

Working with the Thyroid

E.B., a thirty-two-year-old woman, first came to our school for group Yoga classes. She worked as a chef at a fancy and popular restaurant. She was only able to come to one evening class a week, on her day off. In our school, we go around the room to check in with each student to see how they are doing at the beginning of each class. Her response was almost always the same, feeling drained and slightly depressed. She said she would like to come to more classes but was never able to get out of bed to make a morning class. I noticed that she never spoke much with the other people in the class, and invariably left alone at the end of class.

One day I decided to go to her restaurant to eat a meal and to visit her in her work environment. She was happy to see me but only had time for a quick smile and hello. The kitchen was large and hot, and people were moving in and out very quickly. When an order was in or a meal was up, a bell would ring, or someone would shout. It appeared to be a high-stress situation.

That I had come to her work place had touched E.B., and the next time she came to class she asked me if she could come see me privately. I told her I was happy that she was interested and that perhaps we could develop a practice that she could do on her own to help build her energy.

E.B. was slightly overweight, had a flexible body, and had chronically low energy. She told me she had been a "night person" since she could remember. She always woke up feeling tired and had to drag herself out of bed to face another day. She was a single woman who avoided socializing. In her free time, she liked to read books or watch videos. I asked about her eating habits. She told me that she usually ate her main meal after work in front of the TV, or with a book, and often feel asleep on the chair with the lights and TV still on.

E.B. told me that she knew that her thyroid function was low. I decided to develop a practice to stimulate that area of her body, including breathing and sound. From the group classes, I knew she particularly liked to do Matsyāsana. I also included twisting postures to stimulate her elimination.

E.B. made a commitment to see me once a week for one month, during which time we developed the following practice. I suggested that she go for a short walk when she got up in the morning and begin her practice after that. I also suggested that she eat her main meal in the early afternoon before she went to work, and to avoid eating in the night before she went to bed. Finally, I encouraged her to be more physically and socially active.

E.B. told me that it was difficult for her at first to shift some of her habits, but over time she has come to love her morning ritual. She said that the walk helps her wake up and feel ready for her Yoga practice. Now that she doesn't eat before bed, she is less tired in the morning. When she comes to her group class on her day off, her face is brighter, and her sharing is more upbeat. And now I am happy to say that she often leaves class in conversation with another student.

A Practice for Hypothyroid Conditions

1.

POSTURE: Cakravākāsana.
EMPHASIS: To stimulate upper chest and throat area.
TECHNIQUE: Get down on hands and knees, with shoulders vertically above wrists and with hips above knees.

On inhale: Lift chest up and away from belly.

On exhale: Gently contract belly, round low back, and bring chest toward thighs.

NUMBER: 6 times (A two times; B two times; C two times).
DETAILS:

A: *On inhale,* lift chin slightly; *on exhale,* with a soft-pitched humming sound, lower chin.

B: *On inhale,* lift chin. Lower chin while holding after inhale.

C: Keep chin down throughout movement.

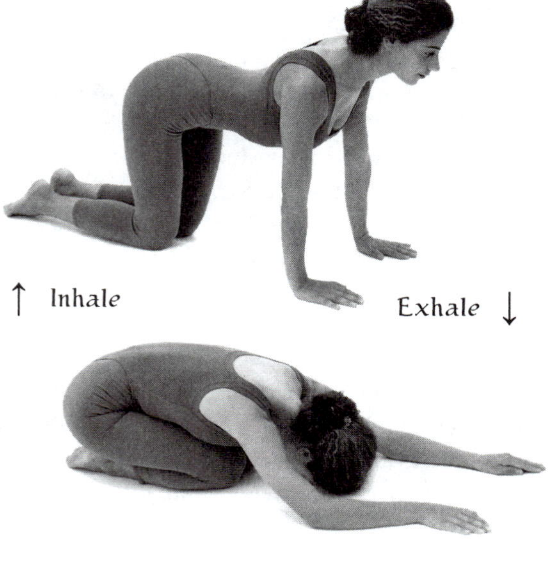

2.

POSTURE: Ardha Uttānāsana.
EMPHASIS: To stimulate upper chest and throat area. To introduce short hold of breath after inhale.
TECHNIQUE: Stand with arms over head.

On exhale: Bend forward, bringing belly and chest toward thighs and hands to feet.

On inhale: Lift chest and arms until parallel to ground. Hold breath 4 seconds.

On exhale: Return to forward bend position.

On inhale: Return to starting position.

NUMBER: 6 times (A two times; B two times; C, two times).
DETAILS:

A: *On inhale,* lift chin slightly; *on exhale,* lower chin.

B: *On inhale,* lift chin. Lower chin while holding after inhale.

C: Keep chin down throughout movement.

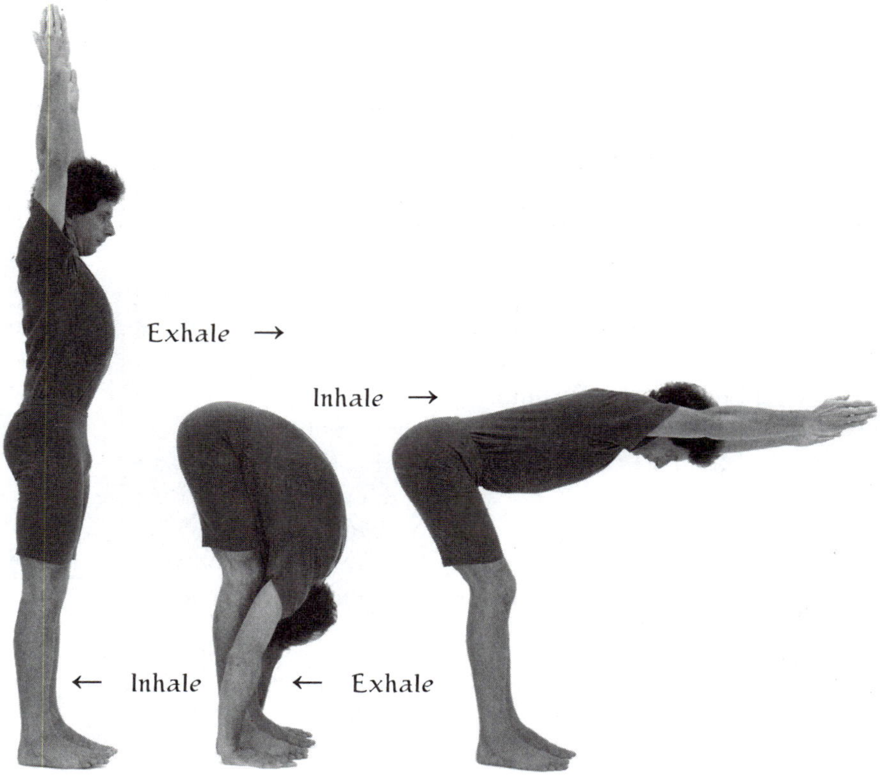

3.

POSTURE: Vajrāsana.
EMPHASIS: To relax back and neck.
TECHNIQUE: Stand on knees with arms over head.

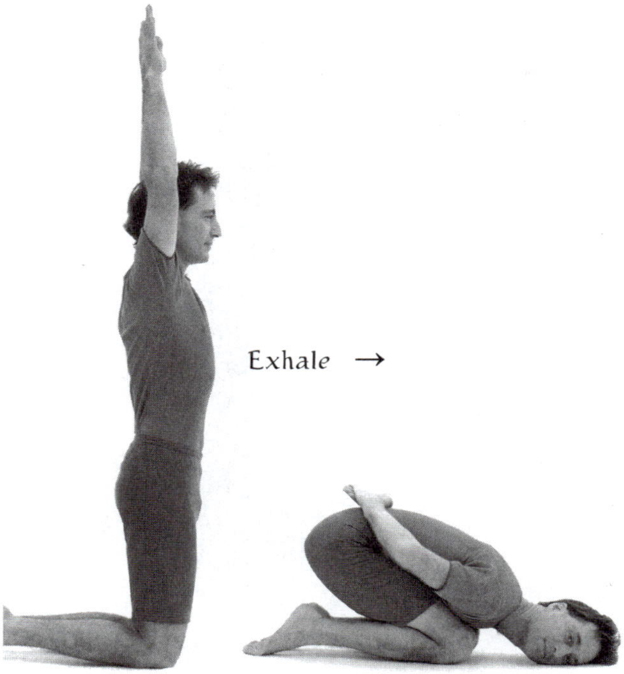

4.

POSTURE: Dvipāda Pīṭham.
EMPHASIS: To stimulate upper chest and throat area.
TECHNIQUE: Lie on back with arms down at sides, knees bent, and feet on floor, slightly apart and comfortably close to buttocks.

On inhale: Pressing down on feet and keeping chin down, raise pelvis up toward ceiling, until neck is gently flattened on floor, while raising arms overhead to floor behind.

On exhale: Return to starting position.

NUMBER: 6 times (A three times; B three times).
DETAILS:

A: *On inhale,* hold chin down; *on exhale,* relax chin.

B: Hold chin down on both *inhale* and *exhale.*

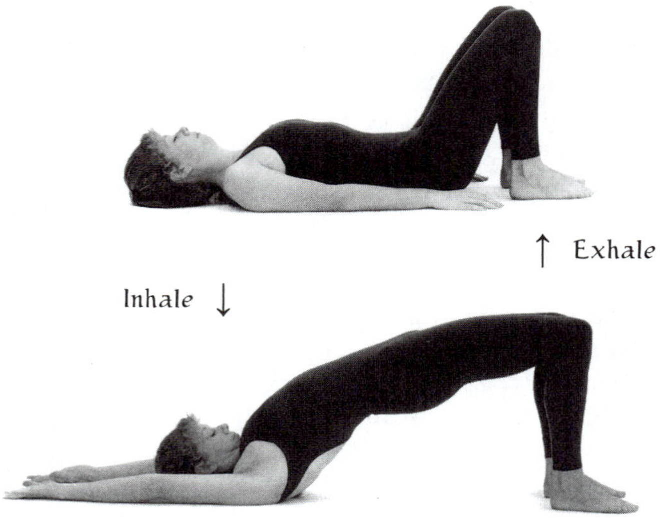

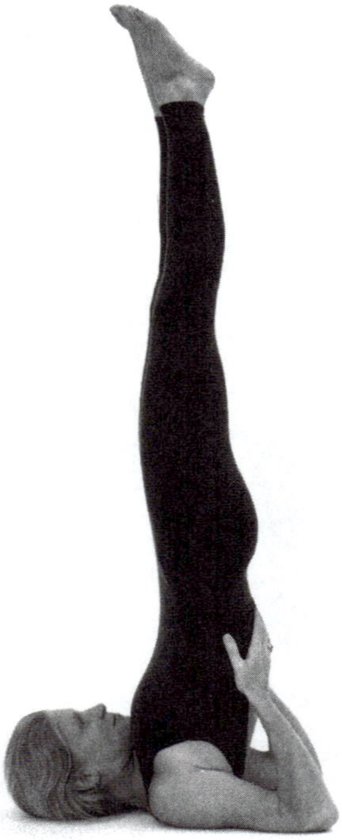

5.

POSTURE: Sarvāṅgāsana.
EMPHASIS: To increase pressure on thyroid/thymus area by inversion and deep breathing.
TECHNIQUE: Lie on back.

On exhale: Raise legs and torso to shoulder stand position, placing palms on middle back for support.

On inhale: Raise legs upward. Stay and breathe deeply.

NUMBER: 18 breaths.
DETAILS: Place hips vertically above elbows, rather than shoulders, and feet slightly beyond head.

6.

POSTURE: Matsyāsana.
EMPHASIS: To stretch and stimulate upper chest and throat area.
TECHNIQUE: Lie flat on back, with hands next to hips. Push down on elbows, lifting shoulders and back off floor, supporting weight on top and center of head. Keep elbows firm and hands firmly on floor for added support. Stay and breathe deeply into thymus/thyroid area.
NUMBER: 8 breaths.
DETAILS: *On inhale:* Arch upper back.

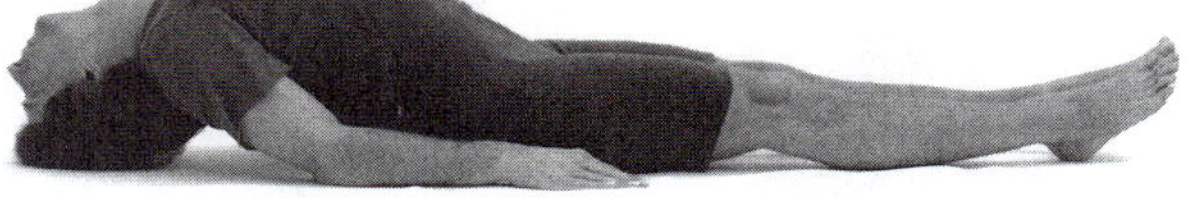

7.

POSTURE: Ūrdhva Prasārita Pādāsana.
EMPHASIS: To extend spine and flatten it onto floor. To stretch legs. To continue stimulating upper chest and throat area.
TECHNIQUE: Lie on back with arms down at sides, legs bent, and knees in toward chest.

On inhale: Raise arms upward all the way to floor behind head and legs upward toward ceiling.

On exhale: return to starting position.

NUMBER: A four times; B four times.
DETAILS: A: *On inhale,* hold chin down; *on exhale,* relax chin.

B: Hold chin down on both *inhale* and *exhale.*

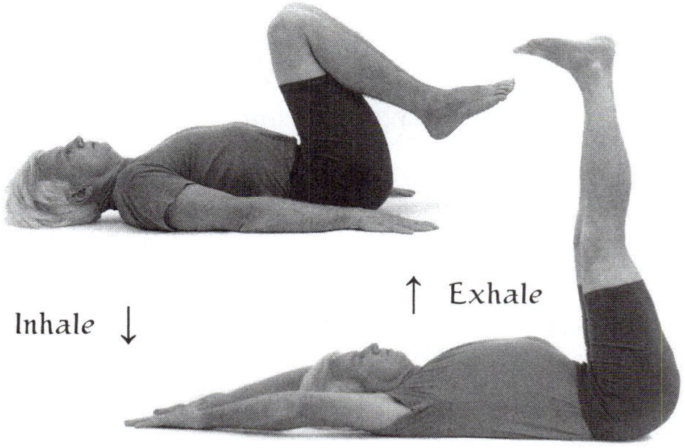

8.

POSTURE: Paśimatānāsana.
EMPHASIS: To compress belly, stretching and strengthening back. To hold after inhale. To continue to stimulate upper chest and throat area.
TECHNIQUE: Sit with legs forward, back straight, and arms raised over head.

On exhale: Bending knees slightly, bend forward, bringing chest to thighs, and palms to balls of feet.

On inhale: Holding feet, lift chest, flattening upper back. Hold 4 seconds after inhale.

On exhale: Return to forward bend position.

On inhale: Return to starting position.

NUMBER: 6 times (A two times; B two times; C two times).
DETAILS:

A: *On inhale,* lift chin slightly; *on exhale,* lower chin.

B: *On inhale,* lift chin. Lower chin while holding after inhale.

C: Keep chin down throughout movement.

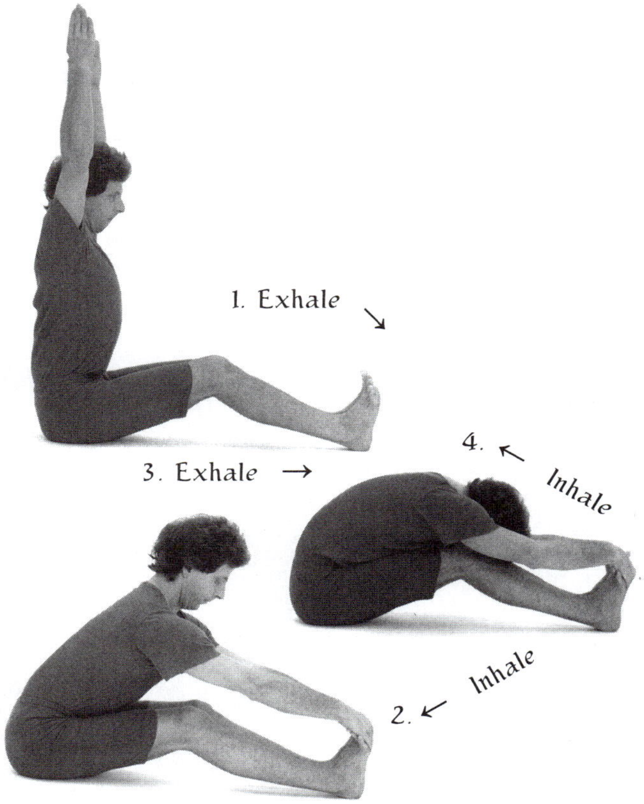

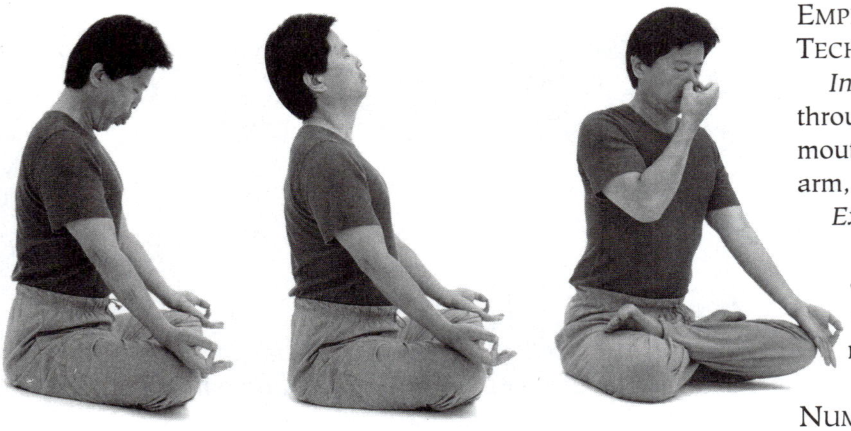

Inhale → Hold after inhale → Exhale in position

9.

POSTURE: Śītalī Prāṇāyāma with alternate nostril exhale.
EMPHASIS: To stimulate upper chest and throat area.
TECHNIQUE: Sit comfortably.

Inhale through an extended curled tongue—like through a straw—while raising chin slightly. Close mouth, curl tongue backward, drop chin, raise right arm, and seal right nostril. Pause.

Exhale through left nostril.

Inhale through curled tongue while raising chin slightly. Close mouth, curl tongue backward, drop chin, raise right arm, and seal left nostril. Pause.

Exhale through right nostril.

NUMBER: 9 times each side, alternately.
DETAILS: Make length of inhale and exhale equal. Make length of holding after inhale one half the length of inhale.

10.

POSTURE: Śavāsana with support.
EMPHASIS: To rest.
TECHNIQUE: Lie flat on back, with arms at sides, palms up, and legs slightly apart. Close eyes. Relax body fully, keeping mind relaxed and alert to sensations in body.
DURATION: Minimum 5 minutes.

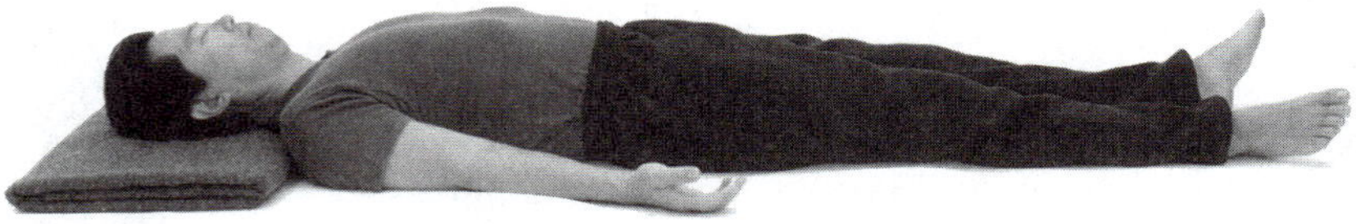

Working with Type II Diabetes

M.K. came to see if a Yoga program could help him with his condition. A fifty-one-year-old professor of archaeology at a midwestern university, he had come to Hawaii with a group of graduate students for a summer research project on native Hawaiian artifacts. He told me that from a routine physical exam for a life insurance policy, he learned that he had elevated blood glucose levels. He had been complaining of blurry vision, which he had attributed to late hours pouring over books, student papers, and his computer terminal. He told me that his doctor linked together the several symptoms he subsequently reported—feelings of fatigue, excessive thirst, and frequent need to urinate—and diagnosed his condition as borderline type II diabetes.

M.K. told me that he had been on a dig in Africa ten years back, had gotten sick, and suffered a lot of physical stress. When he came back, he went right back to the university. He told me that, until his exam, he had eaten a classic low-fiber, high-fat diet. He also said that he had done very little exercise since his own college days. For him, the routine physical exam had been like a wake-up call. Since then he had done his own research, had adopted a more natural and healthy diet, and began to take regular evening walks.

M.K. was not overweight, which is often the case with those suffering from type II diabetes. As we began to work together, I noticed that his belly was flabby and weak. I also noticed that his leg muscles were exceptionally tight.

M.K.'s motivation was high, and he committed himself to the program. He brought his intelligence to his practice, asked a lot of questions about technique, and asked me to keep giving him more work. Over the two months he was with me, I saw him twice a week privately, and he came to group classes on two other days each week.

My plan was to develop a practice that would give him a good overall workout while emphasizing the stimulation of his mid-abdominal region. From his experience with the group classes, he told me that he particularly liked the forward bend variation of the shoulder stand, the deep back bend, and the seated twist. Along with the abdominal lock (Uḍḍīyāna Bandha), these postures formed the core of his practice.

M.K. was back in Hawaii the following summer. He shared with me that coming to our school had been the highlight of his experience in Hawaii. He was able to keep up his practice through the winter, and his blood sugar levels had improved. As a result of his experience, he told me that he wanted to go into a deeper study of Yoga and perhaps become a Yoga teacher himself.

A Practice for Type II Diabetes

1.

POSTURE: Uttānāsana.

EMPHASIS: To stimulate middle of torso. To introduce movement on hold after exhale.

TECHNIQUE:

A: Stand with feet slightly apart, arms over head.

On exhale: Bend forward, bending knees slightly, bringing chest to thighs, and palms to sides of feet.

On inhale: Return to starting position.

B: *Exhale* fully in starting position. Bend forward while holding after exhale.

On inhale: Return to starting position.

Repeat.

NUMBER: 8 times (A four times; B four times).

DETAILS:

B: On *hold after inhale,* feel suction pulling abdomen upward.

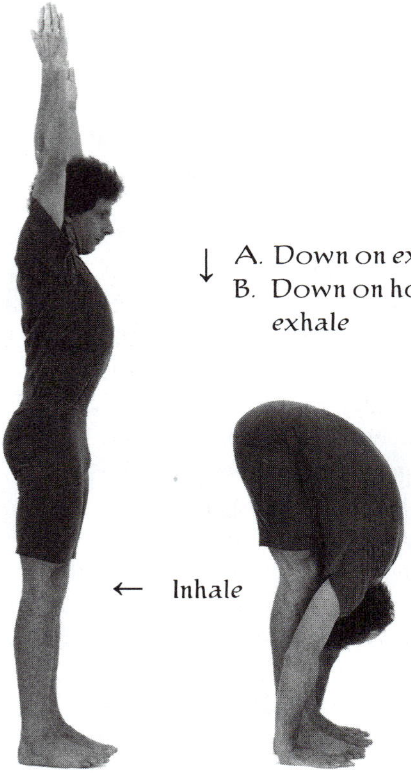
↓ A. Down on exhale
B. Down on hold after exhale
← Inhale

2.

POSTURE: Parivṛtti Trikoṇāsana.

EMPHASIS: To stimulate middle of torso. To continue movement on hold after exhale.

TECHNIQUE:

A: Stand with feet spread wider than shoulders and with arms out to sides and parallel to floor.

On exhale: Bend forward and twist, bringing right hand to floor, pointing left arm upward, and twisting shoulders left. Turn head down toward right hand.

On inhale: Return to starting position.

Repeat on other side.

B: *Exhale* fully in starting position. Bend and twist while holding after exhale.

On inhale: Return to starting position.

Repeat on other side.

C: Stay in twisted position, with right hand down toward left foot.

On inhale: Stay in full twist and extend spine.
On exhale: Stay and deepen twist.
On hold after exhale: Twist slightly further.
Repeat on other side.

NUMBER: A three times each side, alternating; B three times each side, alternating; C, stay six breaths each side.

DETAILS: *On exhale:* Initiate and control torsion through belly contraction. Keep right foot firm while twisting left. Rotate shoulder girdle until left shoulder is vertically above right. *On holding after exhale:* Continue pulling belly gently in and up.

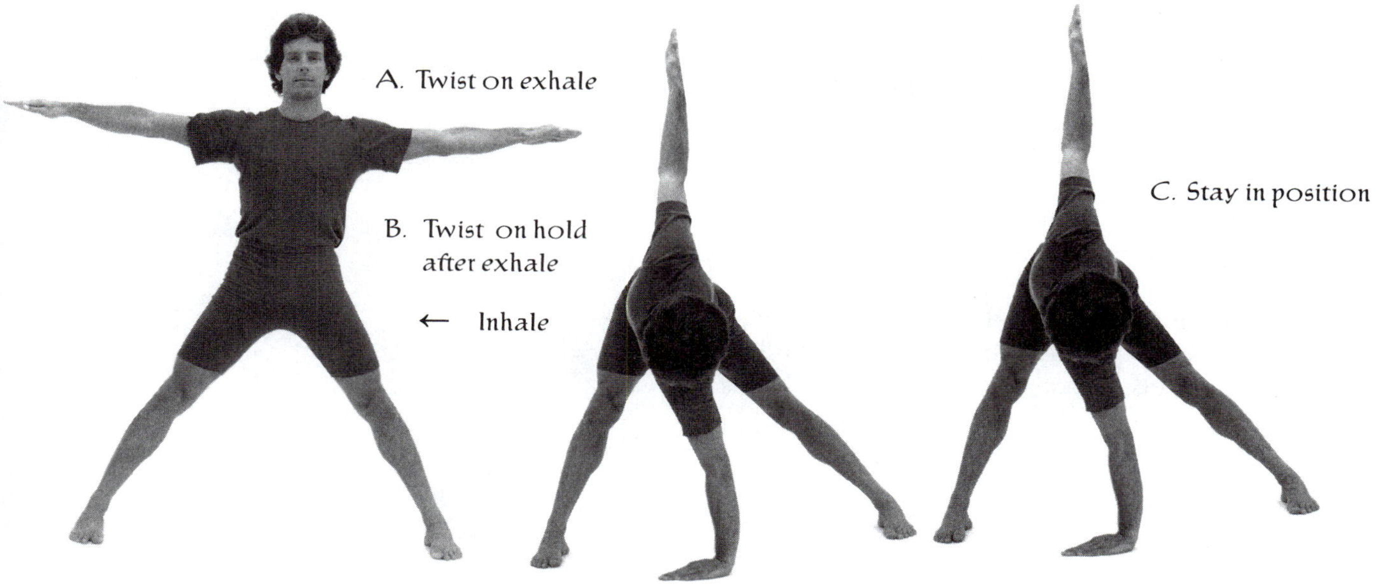
A. Twist on exhale
B. Twist on hold after exhale
← Inhale
C. Stay in position

3.

POSTURE: Adho Mukha Śvānāsana.
EMPHASIS: To stimulate middle of torso. To continue movement while holding breath after exhale.
TECHNIQUE:
A: Get down on hands and knees.
On exhale: Push buttocks upward, lifting knees off ground and pushing chest toward feet.
On inhale: return to starting position.
B: *Exhale* fully in starting position. Push back into posture while holding breath after exhale.
On inhale: Return to starting position.
NUMBER: 8 times (A four times; B four times).
DETAILS: *On exhale:* Keep knees slightly bent, press chest toward feet, flatten upper back, and avoid hyperextension of shoulders. *On hold after exhale:* Feel upward suction of belly while pushing back into posture.

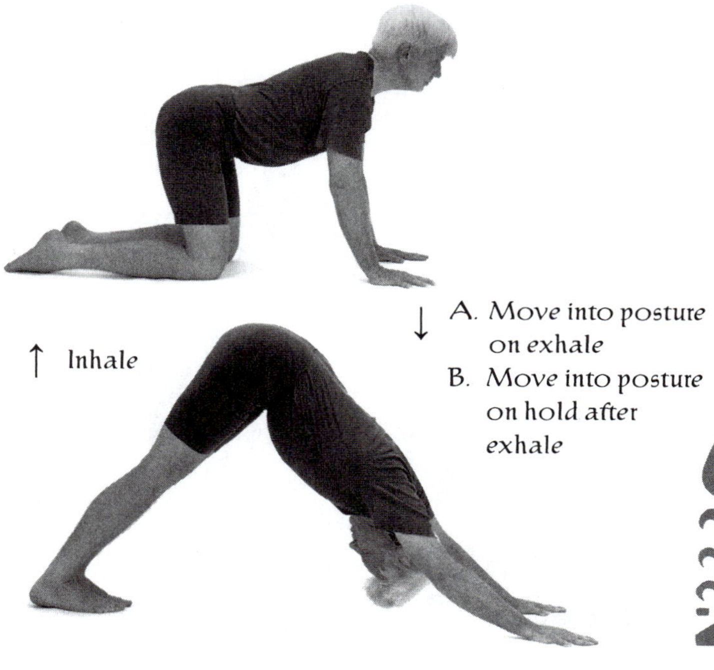
↑ Inhale
↓ A. Move into posture on exhale
B. Move into posture on hold after exhale

4.

POSTURE: Dvipāda Pīṭham.
EMPHASIS: A: To relax upper back. B: To stimulate middle torso.
TECHNIQUE: A: Lie on back with arms down at sides, knees bent, and feet on floor, slightly apart and comfortably close to buttocks.

On inhale: Pressing down on feet and keeping chin down, raise pelvis until neck is gently flattened on floor.

On exhale: Return to starting position.

Repeat.

B: *On inhale:* Pressing down on feet, raise pelvis up toward ceiling while raising arms up over head to floor behind.

On exhale: Remain in position.

On hold after exhale: Bring pelvis back to floor, leaving arms over head.

Repeat.

NUMBER: A four times; B four times.
DETAILS: A: *On inhale,* Lift spine vertebra by vertebra from bottom up.

B: *On hold after exhale,* while lowering pelvis, feel suction pulling abdomen upward.

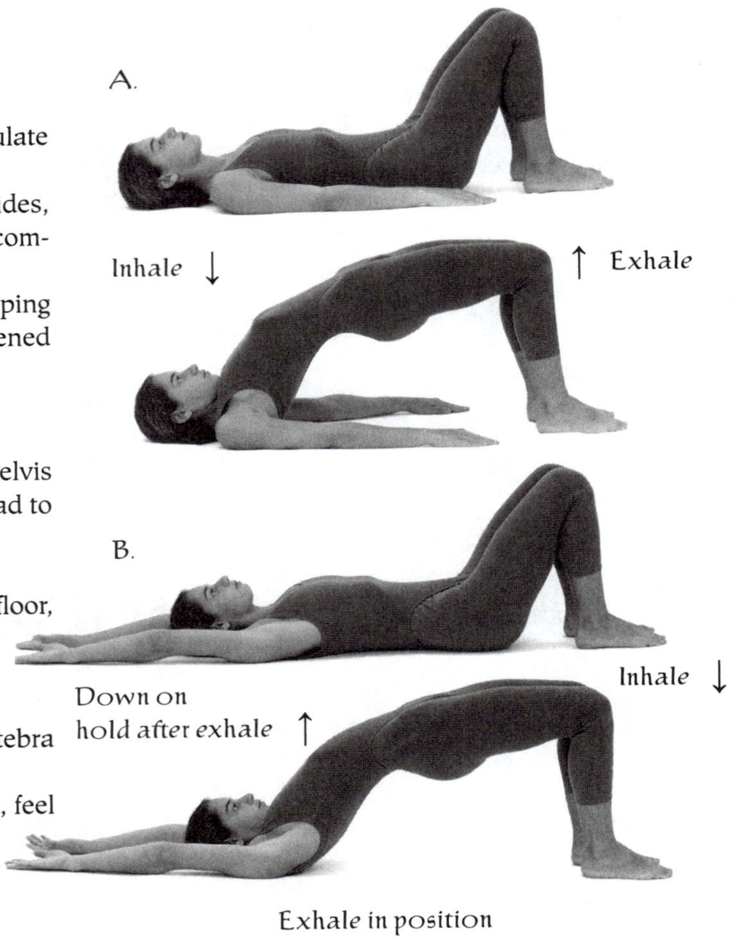
A.
Inhale ↓
↑ Exhale
B.
Inhale ↓
Down on
hold after exhale ↑
Exhale in position

5.

POSTURE: Sarvāṅgāsana and Ākuñcanāsana.
EMPHASIS: To invert. To stimulate middle torso. To progressively lengthen exhale.
TECHNIQUE: Lie on back.

On exhale: Flip legs up over head, lifting buttocks and lower to middle back off floor, placing palms on middle back for support.

On inhale: Raise legs upward.

A: Stay and breathe deeply, progressively lengthening exhale.

B: *On exhale,* bend both knees to shoulders. Remain in position 2 breaths.

On inhale, return to starting position.

NUMBER: A twelve breaths; B three times.

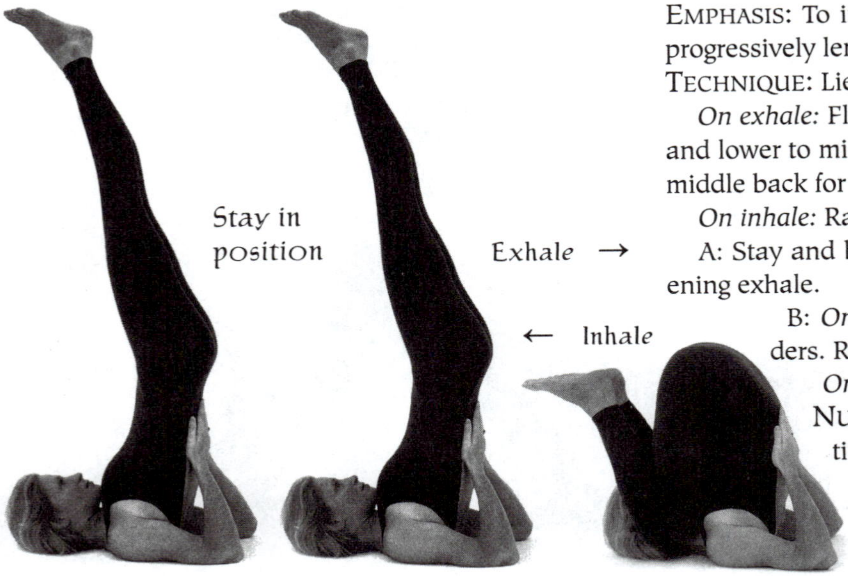
Stay in
position
Exhale →
← Inhale

6.

POSTURE: Bhujaṅgāsana.
EMPHASIS: To gently stretch and expand rib cage, deepening inhalation.
TECHNIQUE: Lie on belly with palms by chest, head turned to one side.

On exhale: Lift chest, turning head to center.

On inhale: Lift chest higher, stretching area of liver and pancreas.

On exhale: Lower chest to floor, turning head to opposite side.

NUMBER: 6 times.
DETAILS: *On inhale:* Use back to lift chest; don't push with arms.

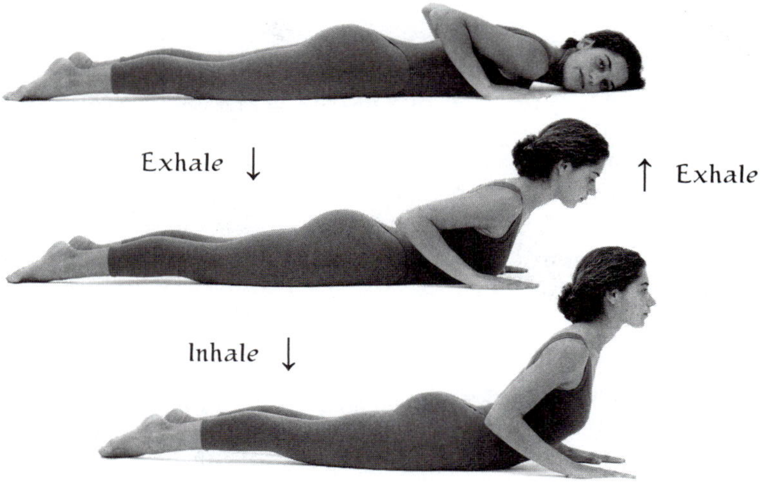

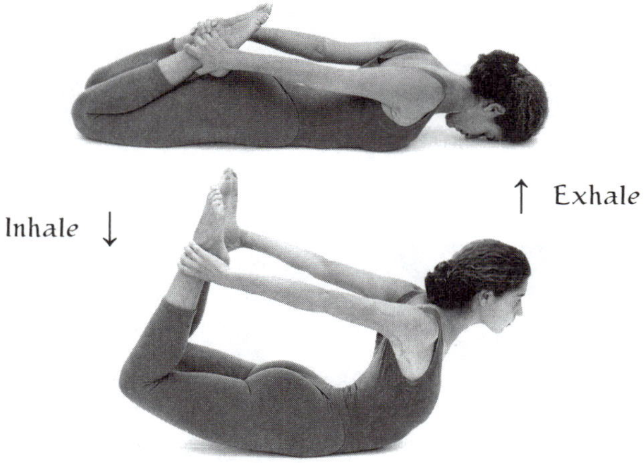

7.

POSTURE: Dhanurāsana.
EMPHASIS: To stretch and stimulate middle of torso.
TECHNIQUE: Lie on stomach, resting on forehead, with knees bent and hands grasping ankles.

A: *On inhale,* simultaneously press feet behind you, pull shoulders back, lift chest, and lift knees off ground.

On exhale, return to starting position.

Repeat.

B: Remain up in position.

NUMBER: A four times; B, stay in position four breaths; two times.
DETAILS: While staying in position, lift chest slightly higher *on inhale.*

8.

POSTURE: Ūrdhva Prasārita Pādāsana.
EMPHASIS: To stimulate middle of torso. To achieve movement while holding after exhale.
TECHNIQUE: Lie on back with arms down at sides, legs bent, and knees in toward chest.

A: *On inhale,* raise arms upward all the way to floor behind head and legs upward toward ceiling.

On exhale, return to starting position.

B: *On hold after exhale,* raise arms upward all the way to floor behind head and legs upward toward ceiling.

On inhale, remain in position.

On exhale, return to starting position.

NUMBER: A four times; B four times.
DETAILS: When raising arms and legs, flex feet as legs are raised upward. Bend knees slightly, keeping angle between legs and torso less than ninety degrees. Push low back and sacrum downward. Bring chin down.

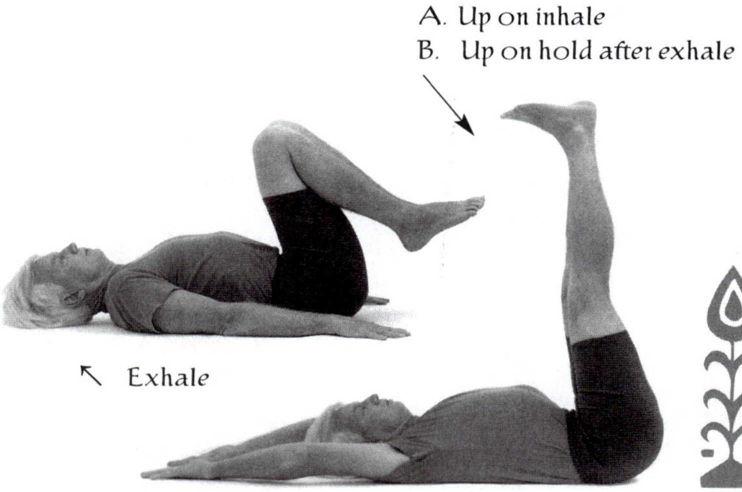

9.

POSTURE: Ardha Matsyendrāsana.
EMPHASIS: To stimulate middle of torso.
TECHNIQUE: Sit with left leg folded on floor, with left foot by right hip, right knee straight up, right foot crossing over on outside of left knee, right arm behind back with palm down on floor by sacrum, and left arm across outside of right thigh with left hand on right foot.

On inhale: Extend spine upward.

On exhale: Twist torso and look over right shoulder.

NUMBER: 8 breaths each side.
DETAILS: *On exhale:* Control torsion from deep in belly, using arm leverage only to augment twist. *On inhale:* Subtly untwist body to facilitate extension of spine.

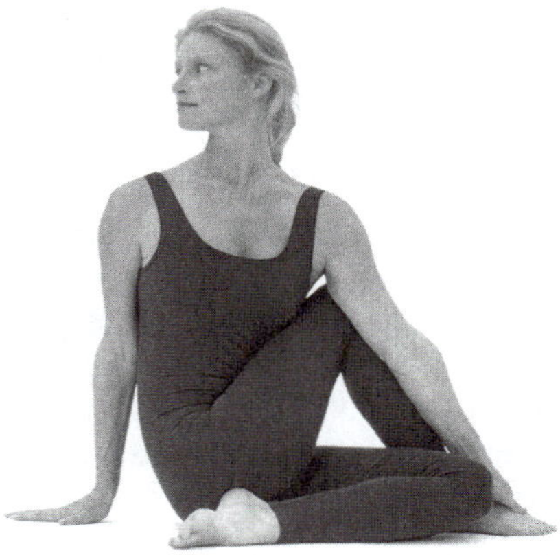

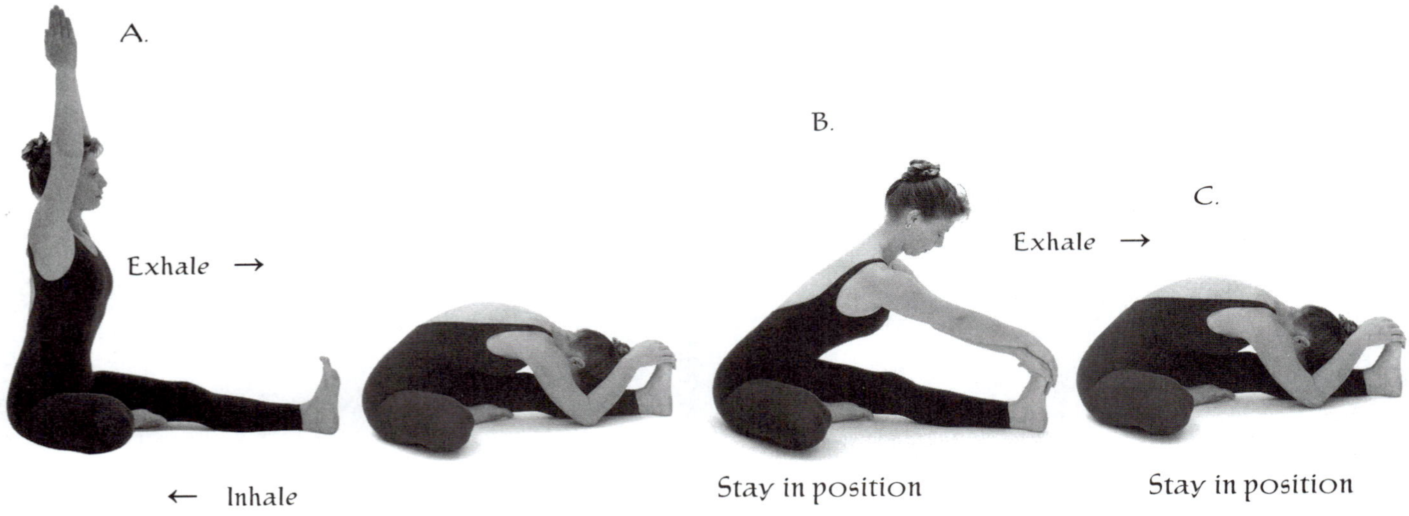
A.
Exhale →
← Inhale
B.
Stay in position
C.
Exhale →
Stay in position

10.

POSTURE: Jānu Śirṣāsana, Mahāmudrā.
EMPHASIS: To stretch back after twist. To introduce abdominal lock (Uḍḍīyāna Bandha).
TECHNIQUE: Sit with right leg folded in, heel to groin, left leg extended forward, and arms overhead.

A: *On exhale:* Bend forward, bringing belly and chest toward left leg and bringing hands to left foot.

On inhale: Return to starting position.

Repeat.

B: *On inhale:* While holding left foot, extend spine upward, expanding chest, flattening upper back, and lengthening in front of torso.

On exhale: Maintain posture while pulling belly firmly in.

On holding after exhale: Continue to pull belly in and up for 4 to 6 seconds.

Release gradually.

Inhale.

Repeat 8 times.

C: *On exhale:* Sink belly and chest to thighs. Rest in position 4 breaths.

Repeat A, B, and C on other side.

DETAILS: Try inhale 8, exhale 12, holding after exhale between 6 and 8 seconds.

11.

POSTURE: Apānāsana.
EMPHASIS: To relax lower back.
TECHNIQUE: Lie on back with both knees bent toward chest and feet off floor. Place each hand on its respective knee.

On exhale: Pull thighs gently but progressively toward chest.

On inhale: Return to starting position.

NUMBER: 12 times.
DETAILS: *On exhale:* Pull gently with arms, keeping shoulders relaxed and on floor. Press low back down into floor and drop chin slightly toward throat.

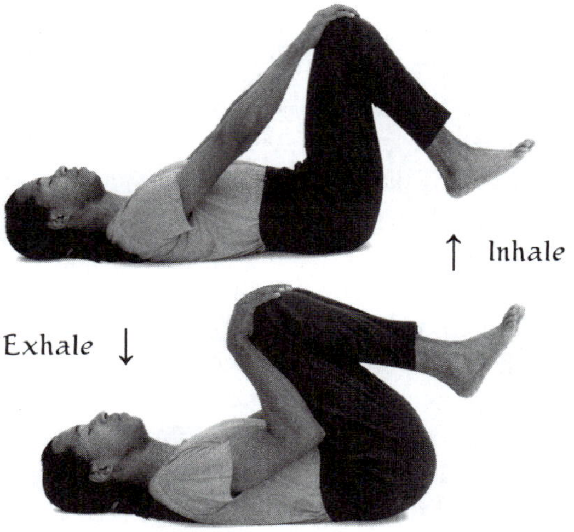

12.

POSTURE: Śavāsana.
EMPHASIS: To rest.
TECHNIQUE: Lie flat on back, with arms at sides, palms up, and legs slightly apart. Close eyes. Relax body fully, keeping mind relaxed and alert to sensations in body.
DURATION: Minimum 5 minutes.

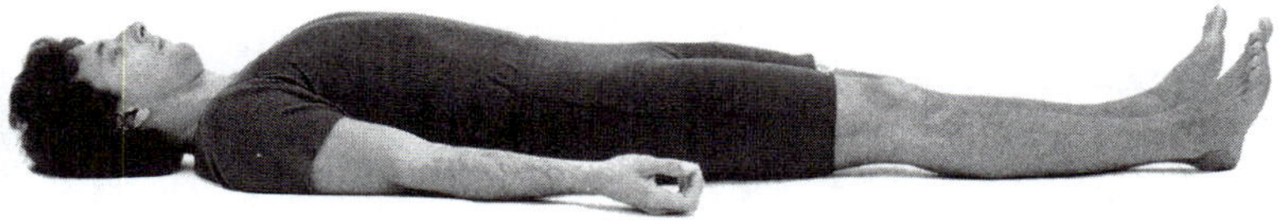

Nervous System

The nervous system coordinates and controls every activity in the body, including organ function, movement, and sensation. It is through the nervous system that we perceive and function in the external world. And it is through the nervous system, in cooperation with the endocrine system, that our internal environment is maintained and continues to function. The components of the nervous system include the brain, spinal cord, various sense organs (such as eyes and ears), and the nerves that interconnect these organs and link the nervous system with the other systems of the body.

In the nervous system, information moves from one location to another through nerve impulses. These impulses travel electrically, but at junctions between nerve cells there are gaps, called synapses, which the signals jump across by converting into chemical form. These chemical messengers include neurotransmitters (e.g. acetylcholine, norepinephrine, and serotonin) and neuromodulators (e.g. endorphines). Neurotransmitters are chemical compounds released at the presynaptic membranes of nerve cells. Neuromodulators are chemicals that determine the postsynaptic cell's response to neurotransmitters. These chemicals can either excite or inhibit nerve function. How much of each transmitter and/or modulator is released, how sensitive the pre- and postsynaptic membranes are to it, its reuptake (reabsorption) or destruction, and its overall effect are influenced by many factors, including stress, diet, emotions, drugs, and toxicity.

Anatomically, the nervous system can be divided into two major subdivisions. The central nervous system (CNS), consisting of the brain and spinal cord, is responsible for integrating, processing, and coordinating all sensory data and motor commands. It is also the seat for the higher functions, such as intelligence, learning, memory, and emotion. The peripheral nervous system (PNS), consisting of all the neural tissue outside the CNS, provides sensory information to the CNS and carries motor commands throughout the body. Its tissues are distributed throughout the body and connect with the CNS at various levels along the spinal cord.

The spinal cord, which is the core of the nervous system, is actually an extension of the brain. Twelve

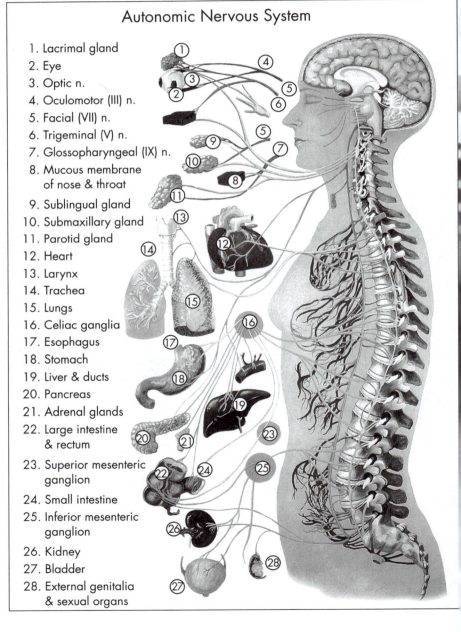

Autonomic Nervous System

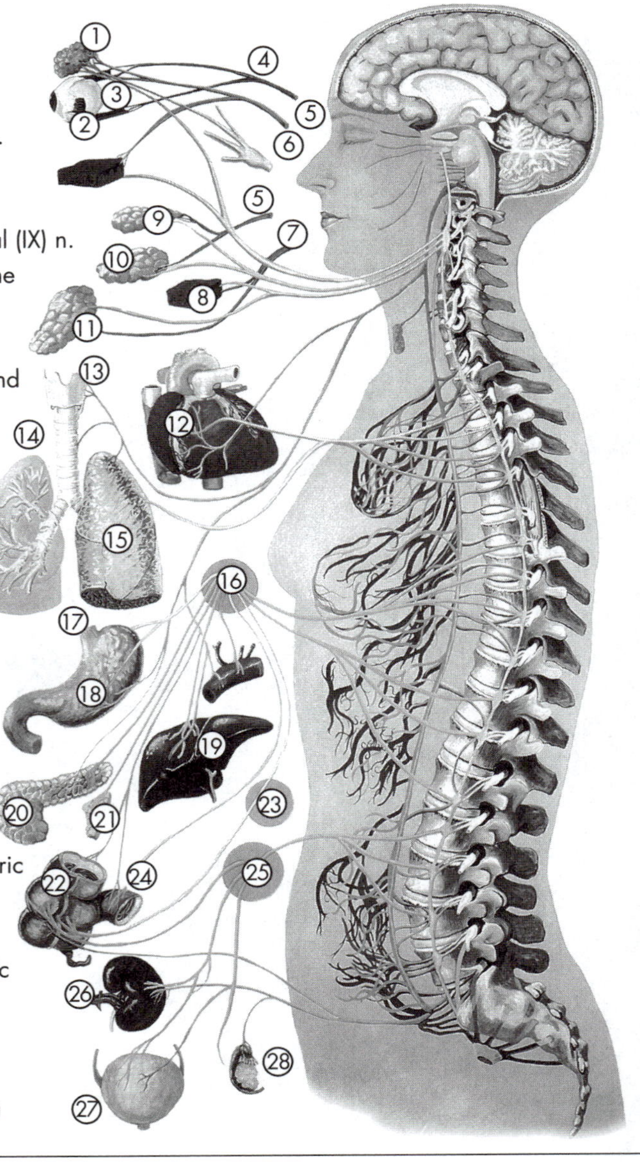

pair of cranial nerves connect the brain to various parts of the head, face, throat, and torso, and thirty-one pair of spinal nerves branch out to either side of the body from the spine, connecting with other nerves and extending to literally every part of the body.

Functionally, the nervous system may be divided into the afferent (carrying toward) and the efferent (carrying away) systems. The afferent system refers to those nerves that carry impulses, originating in the sensory organs, back to the CNS. The sensory organs are the nose, tongue, eyes, skin, and ears. The afferent system thereby supplies information to the brain about the internal and external environment. The efferent system refers to those nerves that carry motor commands from the brain and spinal cord to the rest of the body.

This complex system can be further divided into two basic systems, according to function. These are the autonomic (ANS) and voluntary (VNS) systems.

The autonomic system governs the vegetative and survival responses that keep us alive at an organic level. This includes our cardiovascular, respiratory, digestive, and reproductive functions. The activities of the ANS are primarily involuntary and are controlled without the need for our conscious control. The ANS includes both the sympathetic and parasympathetic systems, and it controls all the basic physiological functions.

When our sympathetic nervous system is activated, we experience increased alertness, a feeling of energy, acceleration of the heart rate, respiratory rhythm, and an elevation in muscle tone. This system, commonly referred to as the flight-or-fight system, excites or arouses activity. The parasympathetic system, on the other hand, functions to increase relaxation, enhance digestion and nutrient absorption, and stimulate elimination. This system, commonly referred to as the "rest-and-repose" system, calms or relaxes activity.

While stimulation of the sympathetic system speeds up circulatory and respiratory functions, it inhibits digestion. Also, the sympathetic nervous system is easily stimulated by strong emotions, which is why responses such as anger, fear, anxiety, and sexual arousal increase heart rate and breathing. It is also why eating in a state of emotional excitement is not recommended, and why chronic tension often leads to the constipation/diarrhea cycle.

When the parasympathetic system takes over, the entire system relaxes. In fact, in cases of acute stress, the parasympathetic system can lower the heart rate to such an extent that the individual loses consciousness. Also, in the case of an asthma attack, excitement of the parasympathetic system creates bronchial constriction.

From these remarks, it can be seen that these two systems act together in a balanced and synergistic way in a healthy individual, and that they both react strongly in stress adaptation mechanisms.

The voluntary nervous system is that part of the nervous system that controls the functions of the skeletal muscles. The activities of the VNS are primarily voluntary, though they usually operate below the level of conscious awareness.

These nerves usually carry motor impulses via the CNS to the muscles, thereby controlling movement. Generally speaking, the spinal nerves of the upper spinal cord innervate the neck and arm muscles, and those of the lower cord innervate the hip and leg muscles. Impulses carried to the muscles along the spinal cord are called motor neurons.

Impulses from motor neurons originate in the motor cortex of the brain. The primary functions of the motor cortex relate to muscle responses. Complicated patterns of movement, involving the coordination of many muscles, are controlled by the pre–motor cortex. When we first learn a movement skill, the motor cortex plays the greatest role and we must pay close attention to each part of the movement. As the skill is learned, the origin of the pattern shifts to the pre–motor cortex, the pathways on which the impulses travel become ingrained, and movements require less conscious attention. Eventually these movement patterns become conditioned reflexes, requiring no thought at all. Such habitual movement patterns often result in cumulative joint stress and eventual degeneration, and the movement aspect of āsana practice, as found in the Viniyoga approach, is designed to replace these dysfunctional patterns with new ones, adapted to the structural and functional needs of our bodies.

Many conditions affect the nervous system. Actually, all conditions resulting from the stresses of daily living are nervous system disorders. These conditions can have an impact on any of the different systems of the body. In fact, most digestive, respiratory, and cardiovascular disorders are linked to the nervous system. Beyond such specific conditions there are also the diverse symptoms that indicate either conditions of excess (hyper) or conditions of deficiency (hypo) in the nervous system.

Hyper Conditions of the Nervous System

Hyper conditions of the nervous system manifest in two different kinds of people: those who are sedentary physically, but hyperactive mentally, such as the high-stressed, overworked professional; and those who are hyperactive mentally and physically, and who obsessively drive themselves in everything they do.

In both cases, hyper people are stressed-out mentally and physically and are often highly reactive emotionally. They may feel tight, tense, wound up, and jittery; they are prone to tension headaches, chronic skin conditions (e.g., eczema), and alternating constipation/diarrhea; and they often have difficulty relaxing and/or sleeping (insomnia). While both types may appear to have lots of energy, they are really running on a hyper energy that actually weakens their systems.

Though both conditions may manifest similar symptoms, they are actually quite different, and, accordingly, their recommended treatment is also different. The strategy for the physically inactive, mentally hyperactive person is relaxation, nourishment, and strengthening, beginning with very simple movements on the back, gradually increasing the intensity until the work is quite strong, and returning to gentle movements with deep breathing. On the other hand, relaxation is the basic need of those hyperactive physically. Because they are so overtrained, the strategy for them is to begin with more intense movements and to gradually simplify, breathing with emphasis on exhalation and ending with deep relaxation.

The following sequence is designed to illustrate an approach to working with the second type of person described above, as the case study that follows will make clear. Of course, it is illustrative of an approach, and further individualization is essential.

Working with Hyper Conditions of the Nervous System

This practice was developed for J.C., a forty-one-year-old entrepreneur. His girlfriend had been taking classes at our school for years. He had been having trouble sleeping, and she recommended he come see me.

J.C. was the type who worked hard and played hard. He told me that he generally worked ten-hour days and on the weekend played aggressive tennis.

J.C. seemed to want to excel in everything he did. He even brought this competitive edge to his Yoga practice, ready to spend whatever amount of energy it took to win.

J.C. didn't have any structural complaints. As we worked together, I saw that his body was strong and tight. He could not make his breath long and smooth and tended to tense his neck and shoulders when he tried.

The strategy I developed for J.C. was to begin with dynamic and stronger standing postures, engaging the bigger muscles of his body, and to gradually bring him to postures that were more relaxing. In order to keep his interest, the sequences had to be challenging. After working with him once a week for a few months, and seeing that in his case there were no contraindications, I decided to teach him the headstand. The effect was significant. He loved both the challenge and the effects. He told me it made him feel mentally and physically centered and relaxed. At the end of the practice, I asked him to rest on his back with his eyes covered for a minimum of ten minutes. He told me that that was the most difficult part of the practice.

The following sequence was developed for J.C. over a period of three months. I asked him to commit to practice at least three days a week, after work and before he ate dinner if possible.

I also suggested that he could try the following simple breathing exercise just before bed: Lying on the back, gradually and progressively lengthen the exhale for several minutes, then relax, then start the same exercise over again. I told him that he could repeat this exercise for a time period up to ten minutes.

J.C. reported to me that he is able to relax more deeply since he began his practice. He feels that the headstand in particular has been of tremendous value to him. He told me that often during the rest period after his practice he completely loses sense of time, and it has lasted up to thirty minutes. He is no longer having problems sleeping the whole night through.

A Practice for Hyperactivity

1.

POSTURE: Uttānāsana/Ardha Utkaṭāsana combination.

EMPHASIS: To activate big muscles of body. To stimulate cardiovascular and respiratory function.

TECHNIQUE: Stand with feet slightly apart, arms over head.

On exhale: Bend forward, bending knees slightly, bringing chest to thighs and palms to sides of feet.

On inhale: Return to starting position.

On exhale: Bend forward, bending knees until thighs are parallel to ground, hips are at knee level, chest to thighs, and palms to sides of feet.

On inhale: Return to starting position.

NUMBER: 8 times.

DETAILS: *On exhale:* Make exhalation progressively longer with each repetition. Bend knees to facilitate stretching in low back. Push heels down firmly, and reach arms forward.

On inhale: Lift chest up and away from thighs, flattening upper back, without exaggerating lumbar curve. Keep knees bent until last part of movement.

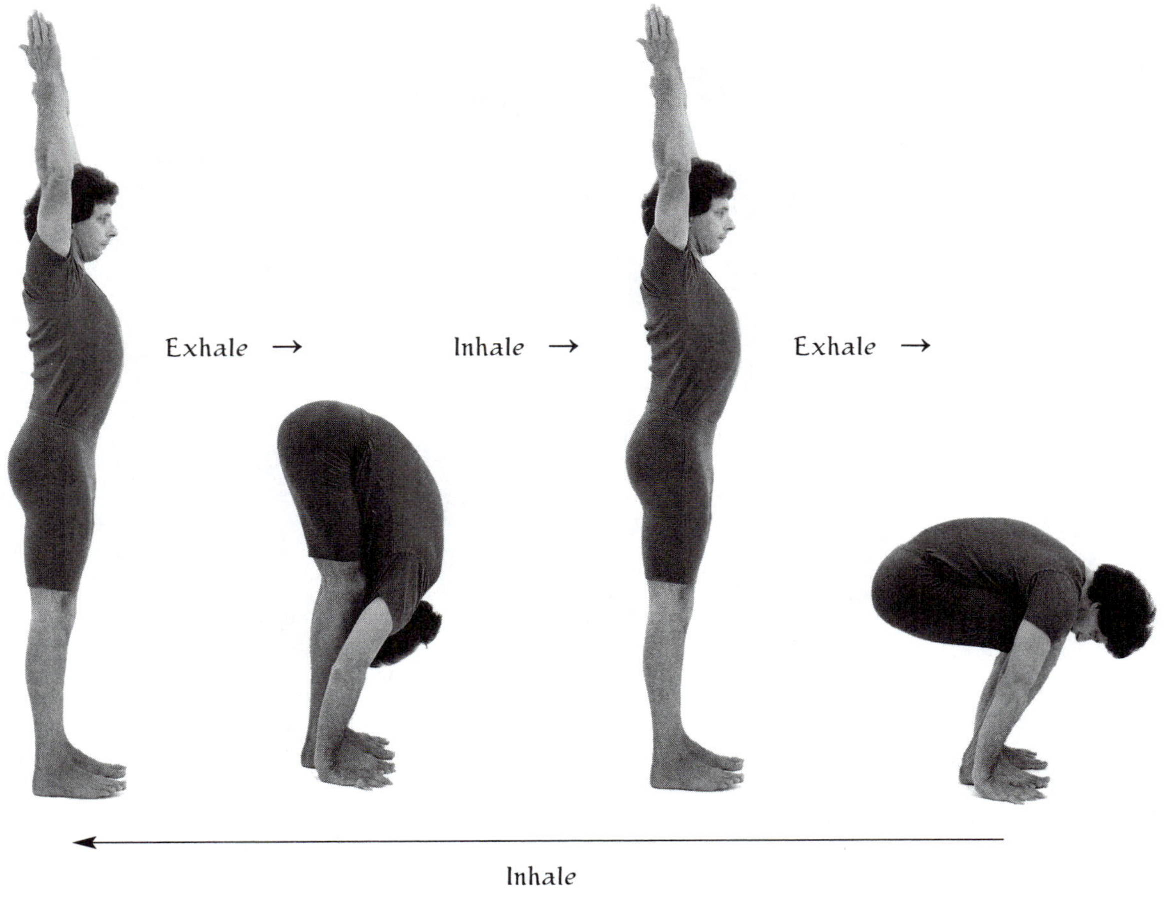

2.

POSTURE: Utthita Trikoṇāsana.
EMPHASIS: To laterally stretch torso and rib cage.
TECHNIQUE:

A: Stand with feet spread wider than shoulders, left foot turned out at a ninety-degree angle to right foot, left arm over head and right arm straight down at waist and slightly rotated externally.

On exhale: Keeping shoulders in same plane as hips, bend laterally, lowering left shoulder and bringing left hand below left knee while turning head down toward left hand.

On inhale: Return to starting position.

Repeat.

B: With left hand down along left leg:

On inhale: bring right arm up and forward while turning head forward toward right hand.

On exhale: return right hand to starting position while turning head down toward left hand.

Repeat.

NUMBER: Repeat A four times, then B four times; then repeat on other side.

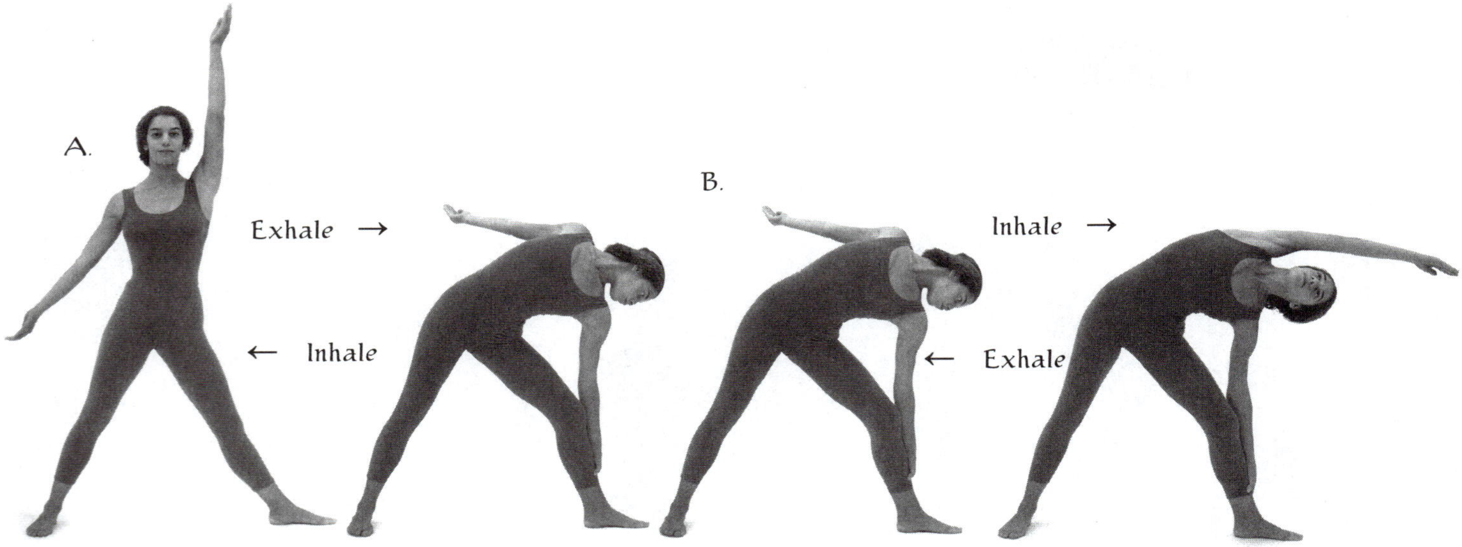

3.

POSTURE: Vajrāsana.
EMPHASIS: To make transition from standing to supine. To stretch low back.
TECHNIQUE: Stand on knees with arms over head.

On exhale: Bend forward, sweeping arms behind back and bringing hands to sacrum with palms up.

On inhale: Return to starting position.

NUMBER: 8 times.
DETAILS: *On exhale:* Bring chest to thighs before buttocks to heels. Rotate arms so palms are up and hands rest on sacrum. *On inhale:* expand chest and lift it up off knees as arms sweep wide.

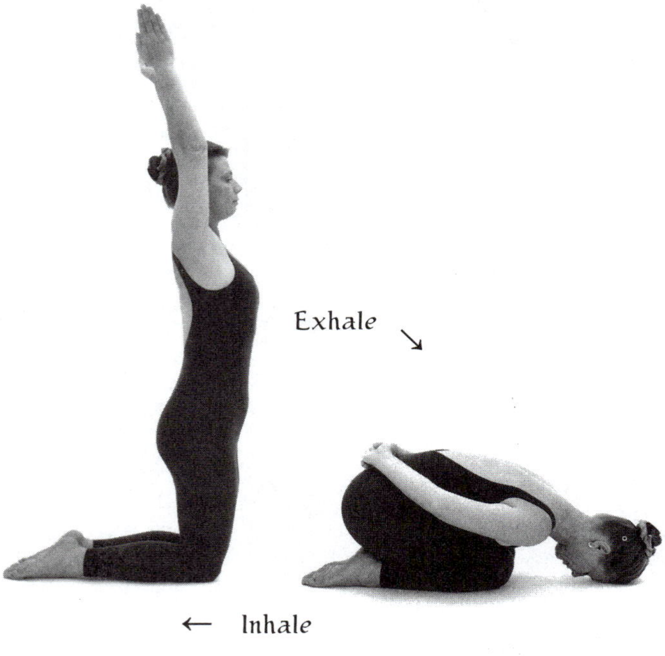

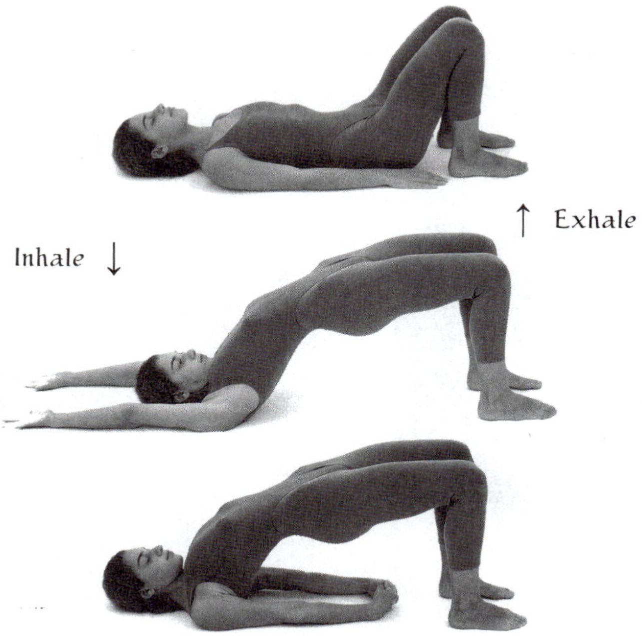

Stay in position

4.

POSTURE: Dvipāda Pīṭham.
EMPHASIS: To stretch upper back and neck.
TECHNIQUE:

A. Lie on back with arms down at sides, knees bent, and feet on floor, slightly apart and comfortably close to buttocks.

On inhale: Pressing down on feet and keeping chin down, raise pelvis while raising arms up overhead to floor behind, until neck is gently flattened on floor.

On exhale: Return to starting position.

B. Stay up in position, fingers interlocked on floor under pelvis, gently pulling shoulders together and stretching upper back and neck.

NUMBER: A four times; B stay four breaths.
DETAILS: *On inhale:* Lift spine, vertebra by vertebra, from bottom up. *On exhale:* Unwind spine, coming down vertebra by vertebra.

5.

POSTURE: Śīrṣāsana.
EMPHASIS: To deepen breathing. To calm and center mind.
TECHNIQUE: From hands and knees, interlock fingers with elbows forearm's length apart. Cupping head in hands, stand on toes, lifting knees off floor. Walk forward with toes until hips are vertically above shoulders. Lift legs to vertical position. Stay.
NUMBER: 12 to 18 breaths.
DETAILS: Position should be comfortable. If there is neck stress, come down. Make inhale and exhale equal, and at a comfortable maximum length.

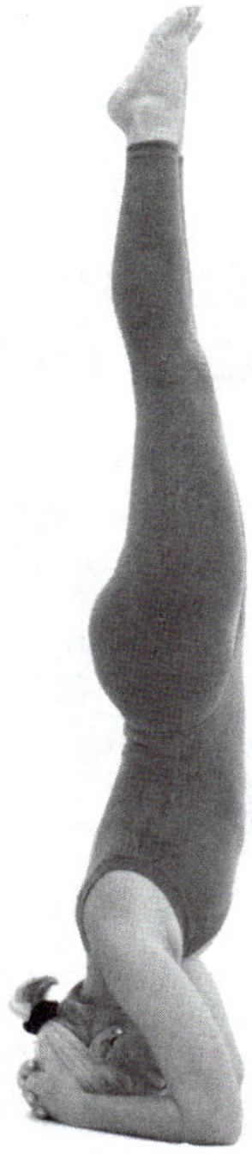

6.

POSTURE: Sarvāṅgāsana.

EMPHASIS: To stretch upper back and neck to counter effects of headstand.

TECHNIQUE: Lie on back.

On exhale: Flip legs up over head, lifting buttocks and lower to middle back off floor, placing palms on middle of back.

On inhale: Raise legs upward. Stay and breathe deeply.

NUMBER: 12 to 18 breaths.

DETAILS: Place hips vertically above elbows, rather than shoulders, and feet slightly beyond head. Make inhale and exhale equal, and at a comfortable maximum length.

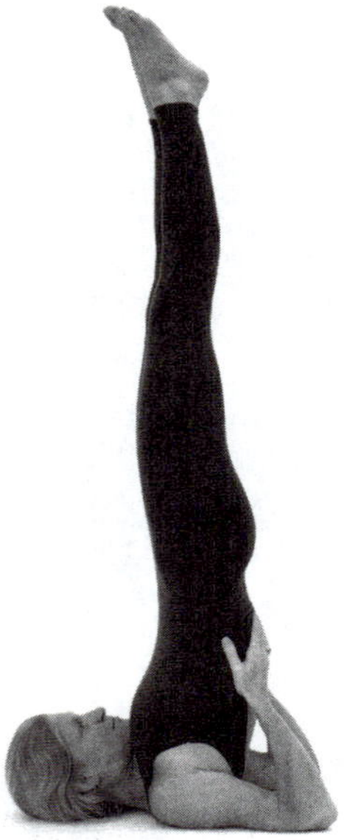

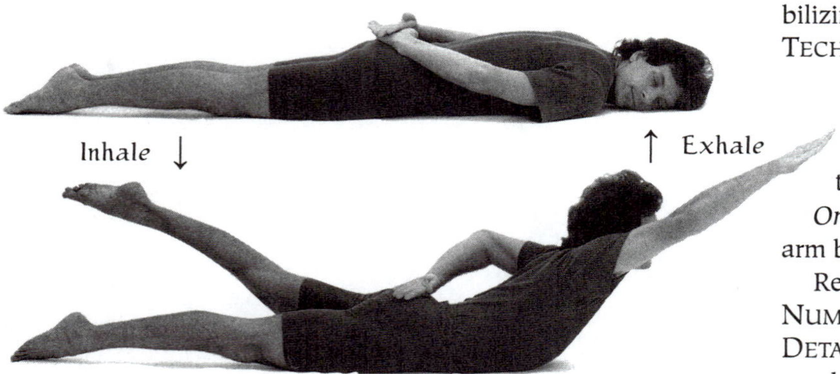

7.

POSTURE: Ardha Śalabhāsana.

EMPHASIS: To arch upper back and neck while mobilizing arms.

TECHNIQUE: Lie on stomach, with head turned to right, hands crossed over sacrum, and palms up.

On inhale: Lift chest, right arm, and left leg, turning head to center.

On exhale: Lower chest and leg, while sweeping arm behind back and turning head to left.

Repeat on other side.

NUMBER: 6 times each side, alternately.

DETAILS: *On inhale:* Lift chest slightly before leg, and emphasize chest height. Keep pelvis level. *On exhale:* Turn head opposite arm being lowered.

8.

POSTURE: Ūrdhva Prasārita Pādāsana.
EMPHASIS: To extend spine and flatten it onto floor. To stretch legs.
TECHNIQUE: Lie on back with arms down at sides, legs bent, and knees in toward chest.

On inhale: Raise arms upward all the way to floor behind head and legs upward toward ceiling.

Stay in stretch 2 full breaths.

On exhale: Return to starting position.

NUMBER: 4 times.

DETAILS: *On inhale,* flex feet as legs are raised upward. Bend knees slightly, keeping angle between legs and torso less than ninety degrees. Push low back and sacrum downward. Bring chin down. While staying in position: *On exhale,* flex knees and elbows slightly; *on inhale,* extend arms and legs straighter.

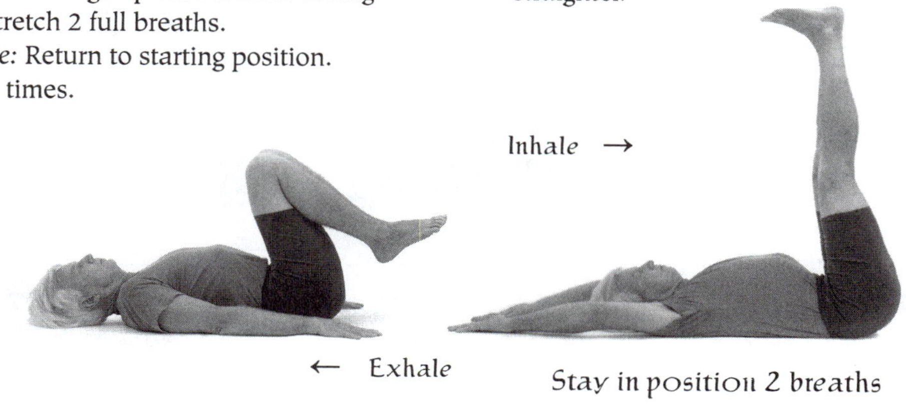
Inhale →
← Exhale
Stay in position 2 breaths

9.

POSTURE: Jaṭhara Parivṛtti.
EMPHASIS: To twist and compress belly. To massage and stretch between shoulders and spine.
TECHNIQUE:

A. Lie flat on back, with arms out to sides, and left knee pulled up toward chest.

On exhale: Twist, bringing left knee toward floor on right side of body while turning head to left.

On inhale: Return to starting position.

Repeat 4 times.

B. Then stay in twist, holding left knee with right hand.

On inhale: With palm up, sweep left arm wide along floor toward ear, turning head to center.

On exhale: Lower arm back to side, turning head to left.

Repeat 6 times.

Repeat on other side.

DETAILS: B: Keep arm that is moving low to floor, palm up *on inhale;* palm down *on exhale.* Hold twisted knee low toward floor.

A.

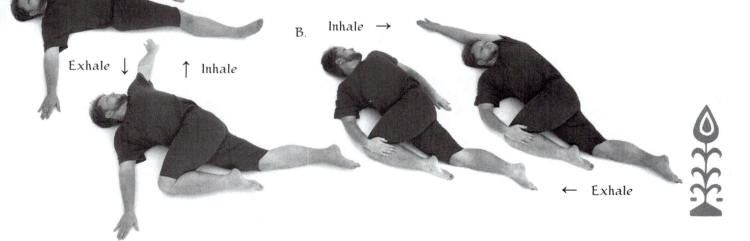

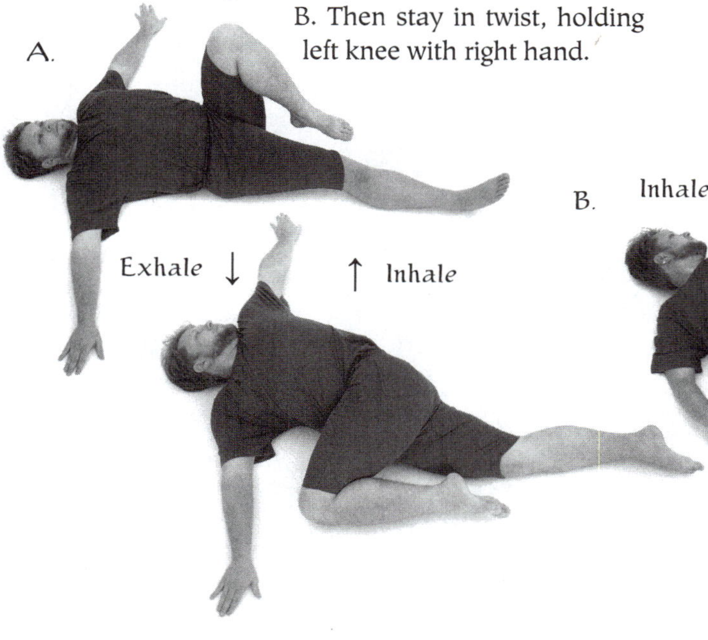
Exhale ↓
↑ Inhale

B.

Inhale →
← Exhale

10.

POSTURE: Paścimatānāsana.
EMPHASIS: To compress belly and stretch and strengthen back. To progressively lengthen exhale. To further calm entire system.
TECHNIQUE: Sit with legs forward, back straight, and arms raised over head.

On exhale: Bending knees slightly, bend forward, bringing chest to thighs and palms to balls of feet.

On inhale: Return to starting position.

Repeat 6 times, progressively lengthening exhale.

Then stay in forward bend 6 breaths, with long *exhale*.

On inhale: Return to starting position.

DETAILS: *On exhale:* Bend knees to facilitate stretching low back and bringing belly and chest to thighs. Move chin down toward throat. *On inhale:* Lift chest up and away from thighs, flattening upper back.

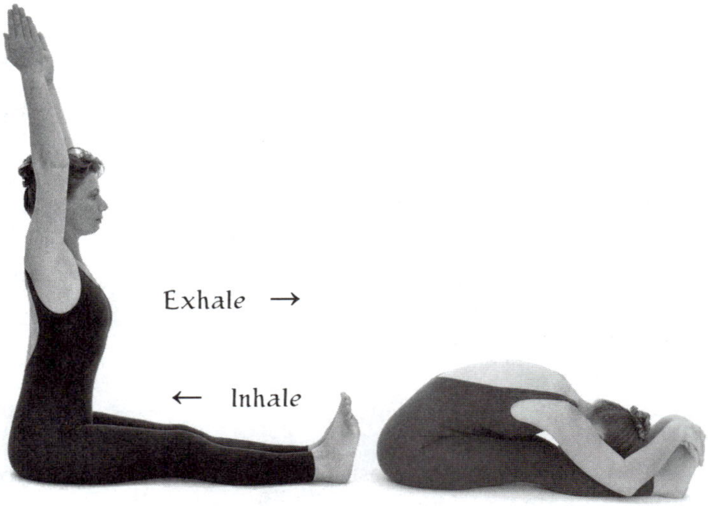

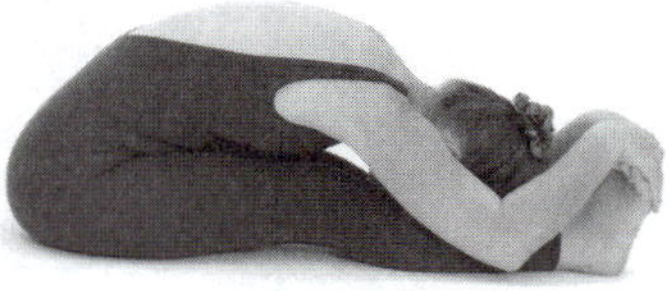

Stay in position

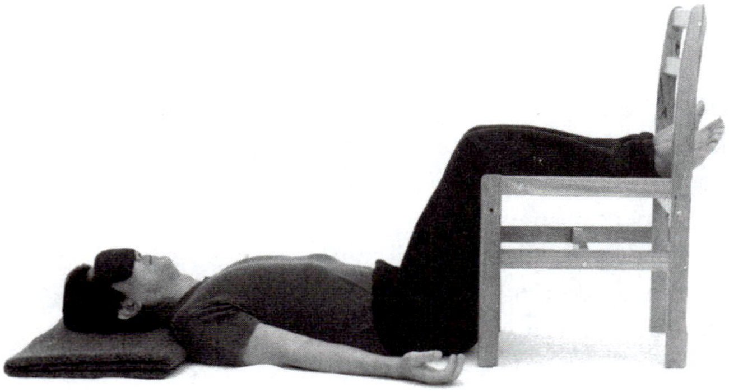

11.

POSTURE: Śavāsana with support.
EMPHASIS: To rest, eyes covered.
TECHNIQUE: Lie flat on back, with arms at sides, palms up, and legs resting comfortably on a chair. Close eyes. Relax body fully, keeping mind relaxed and alert to sensations in body.
DURATION: Minimum 5 to 8 minutes.

12.

POSTURE: Prāṇāyāma—Viloma Krama.
EMPHASIS: To stimulate and compress belly through segmented exhale.
TECHNIQUE:

Inhale deeply and fully.
Exhale 1/2 of breath in 4 to 6 seconds.
Pause in middle of exhale for 4 to 6 seconds.
Exhale remainder of breath in 4 to 6 seconds.
Hold breath out 4 to 6 seconds.
Inhale deeply.
Repeat.

NUMBER: 8 times.
DETAILS: Control first segment of exhale from pubic bone to navel. Control last segment of exhale from navel to solar plexus.

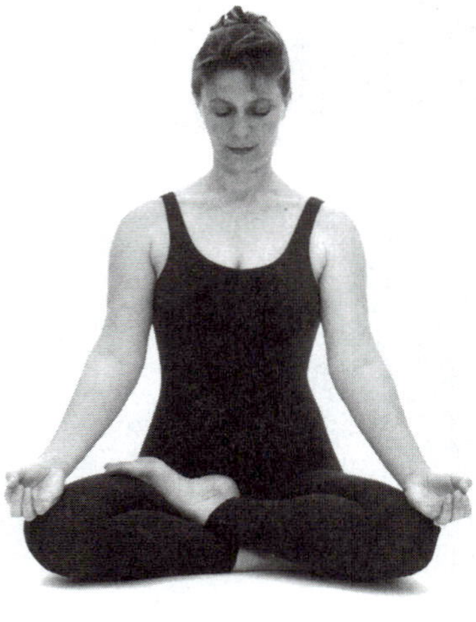

Hypo Conditions of the Nervous System

Symptoms of hypo conditions of the nervous system include sluggishness, dullness, depression, weakness, low blood pressure, constipation, and low energy.

As with hyper conditions, hypo conditions may be of variable origin. People who have been under long-term, low-grade physical or emotional stress often manifest the above symptoms. In addition, there are people suffering from conditions like chronic fatigue (viral) or multiple sclerosis (autoimmune) who manifest similar symptoms.

Although multiple sclerosis (MS) is currently thought to be an autoimmune disease, some of its symptoms parallel those connected with a deficiency in the nervous system. MS is a condition of the spinal cord and spinal nerves that produces weakness, tingling sensations, and loss of control of arms and legs. In later stages, it produces muscular paralysis and possible sensory loss, through the progressive destruction of the nerve tissue (demyelination). MS is thought to be linked to a defect in the immune system that causes it to attack the myelin sheaths surrounding the nerve tissue.

It is tricky to work with this kind of condition. Excessive exercise tends to irritate the person and often makes their symptoms worse. The strategy for working with this condition is to begin very simply, and often on the back with simple movements coordinated with breathing; to move progressively to stronger movements, coordinated with deeper breathing; and often to end sitting in a chair.

The following sequence is designed to demonstrate a methodology for working with a variety of hypo conditions.

Working with Multiple Sclerosis

This practice was developed for M.R., a forty-six-year-old woman suffering with multiple sclerosis. M.R. had been a pediatric nurse but recently had to give up her work because of her condition. She walked into my office with the support of a cane. Her movements were shaky, and she had to sit down immediately for some time to rest.

She told me that in the past two years, she had noticed a slow but progressive decline. M.R. was a mature woman with a solid family life. She told me she felt very discouraged by the deterioration of her health. She said that she was losing her sense of balance and coordination, and that her legs were getting progressively weaker. She also told me that she had very limited endurance and that, if she did too much, it would take her days to recover. She told me that she spent more and more time at home.

Together we developed a strategy of progressively working to strengthen her legs, improve her balance, and deepen her breathing capacity. The sequence that follows developed over about three months, during which she came to see me one time each week. I included in her practice an exercise that she had consistently done on her own, a supine twist, because she felt that it helped her hips.

M.R. and her husband had three children between the ages of eleven and sixteen. One day I asked her if she liked to cook. She said that since she had stopped working, she spent more time in the kitchen. I asked her if she had ever baked bread. She was surprised by my question, and said no. I told her that the exercise of kneading the dough might be very good for her condition. She laughed at my suggestion but said that maybe she would give it a try. I told her to be sure to use her hands and not a machine.

Although M.R.'s multiple sclerosis is uncured, she tells me she is encouraged by small signs of improvement. She is now able to come up on her toes while raising both arms over her head, and doesn't need the wall for balance. Her breathing capacity has deepened, and she feels she can do more without fatigue. She therefore feels much more confident about going out of her home. She comes to see me once every two months now, occasionally bringing me a loaf of bread! The last few times she came, she walked into my office without her cane. She tells me she still has bad days, but that they are fewer and her recovery is quicker.

A Practice for Multiple Sclerosis

1.

Posture: Arm movements in chair.
Emphasis: To gently mobilize rib cage while deepening inhale and exhale.
Technique:

A. Sit on a chair or bench with back straight and hands on knees.

On inhale: Raise one arm forward and up over head.

On exhale: Return to starting position.

Repeat on other side.

B. *On inhale:* sweep both arms out to sides and up over head.

On exhale: Return to starting position.

Number: A four times each side, alternately. Rest. Then B six times.
Details: *On inhale:* Lift chest up and away from belly and lift chin slightly.

A.

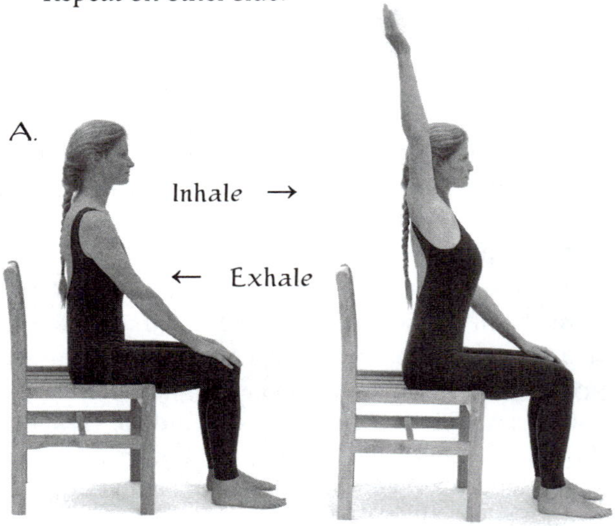

B.

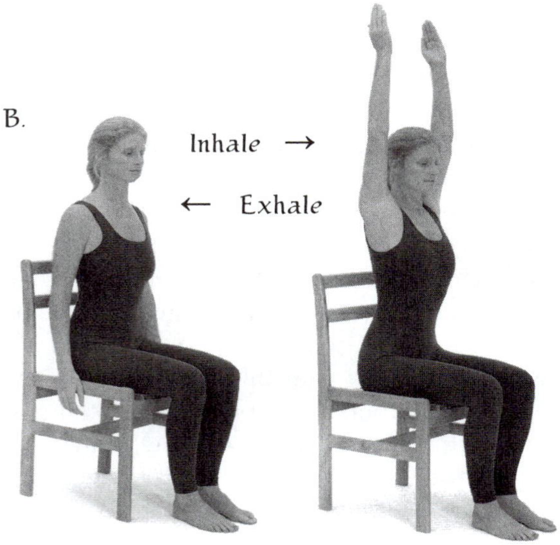

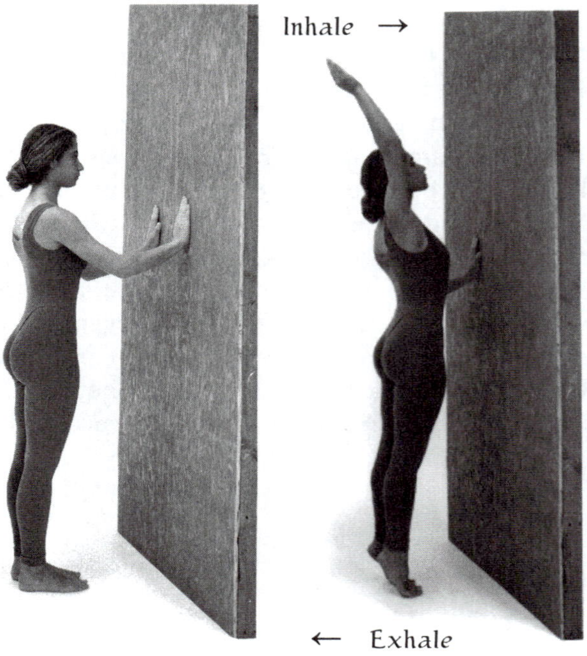

2.

Posture: Tāḍāsana facing a wall.
Emphasis: To encourage balance. To strengthen calves and feet.
Technique: Stand facing a wall, about one foot back, with palms on wall.

On inhale: Raise up on toes while raising right arm up over head.

On exhale: Return to starting point.

Repeat on other side.

Number: 4 times each side, alternately.
Details: *On inhale:* Slightly arch back and lift head. *On exhale:* Slightly round back, chin down.

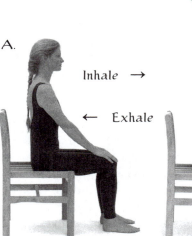

3.

Posture: Forward bending in a chair.
Emphasis: To gently mobilize rib cage while deepening inhale. To stretch back while deepening exhale.
Technique: Sit on a chair or bench with back straight and hands on knees.

On inhale: Raise arms out to sides.

On exhale: Bend forward, bringing hands to feet.

On inhale: Return to previous position.

On exhale: Return to starting position.

Number: 8 times.
Details: *On inhale:* Lift chest up and away from belly, bringing palms to shoulder level with elbows bent and slightly lifted. *On exhale:* Bring hands to knees and slide them down legs towards feet.

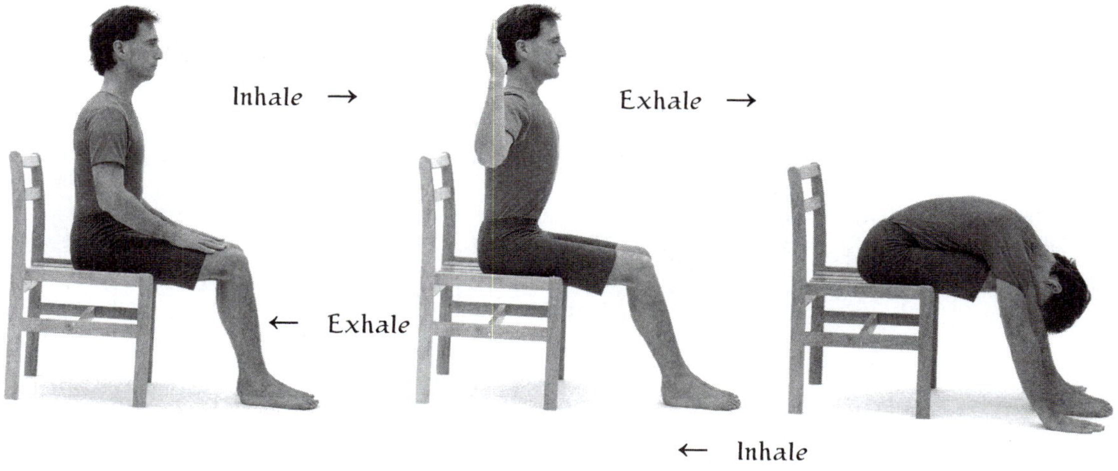

4.

Posture: Vīrabhadrāsana adaptation.
Emphasis: To build energy, strengthen muscles of back, stretch front of torso, and strengthen leg muscles. To increase hold after inhalation.

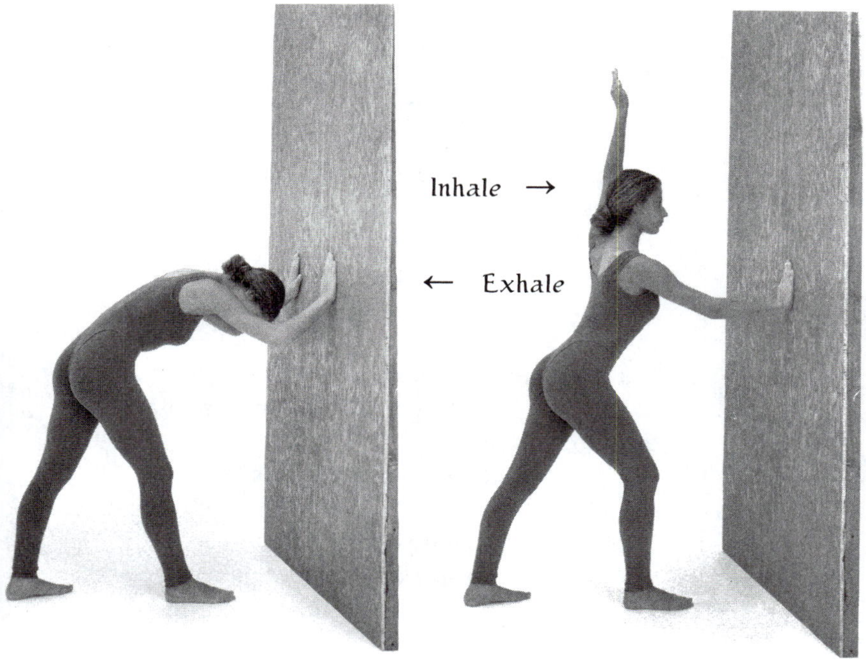

Technique: Stand facing a wall with right foot forward, feet as wide as hips, and palms on wall at shoulder level.

On inhale: Simultaneously bend right knee, displace chest slightly forward and hips slightly backward, lift left arm forward and up and arch back. Hold breath 2, 3, and 4 seconds, 2 times each progressively.

On exhale: Return to starting position.

Number: 6 times each side.
Details: *On inhale:* Slightly press palm on wall down to help arch back. Keep head level. Avoid compressing low back. Keep firm on back heel. *On exhale:* Slightly round back, chin down.

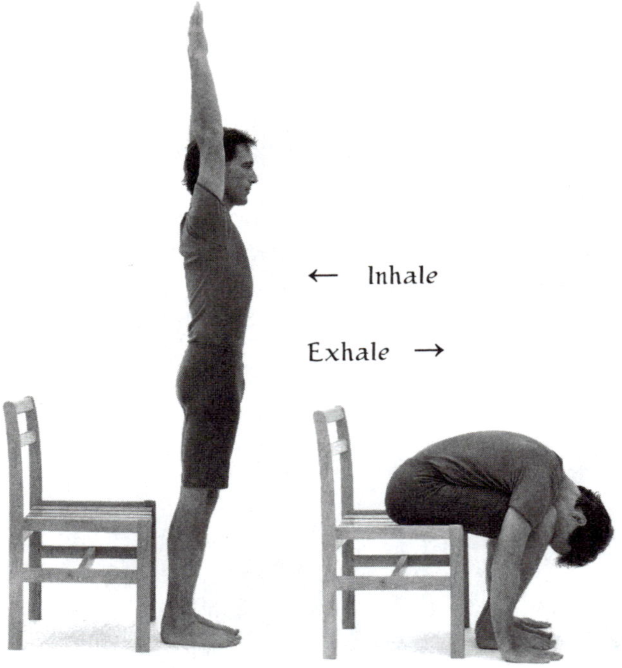

5.

POSTURE: Utkaṭāsana in a chair.
EMPHASIS: To strengthen legs. To increase confidence.
TECHNIQUE: Stand with back to a chair and arms to side.

On inhale: Raise arms forward and up over head.

On exhale: Bend forward, bending knees until sitting on chair, chest to thighs and palms to sides of feet.

On inhale: Return to starting point.

NUMBER: 3 times, then rest on chair, then 3 times again.

6.

POSTURE: Prāṇāyāma-Anuloma Krama—2 stages.
EMPHASIS: To increase capacity to inhale and hold after inhale. To energize system.
TECHNIQUE:

Exhale deeply and fully.

Inhale 1/2 of breath in 4 seconds, feeling expansion in chest.

Pause for 4 seconds.

Inhale other 1/2 of breath in 4 seconds, feeling expansion in belly.

Exhale fully.

Repeat.

NUMBER: 8 times.

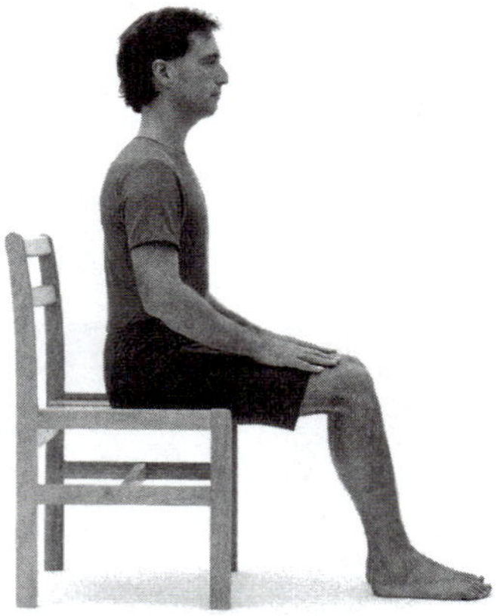

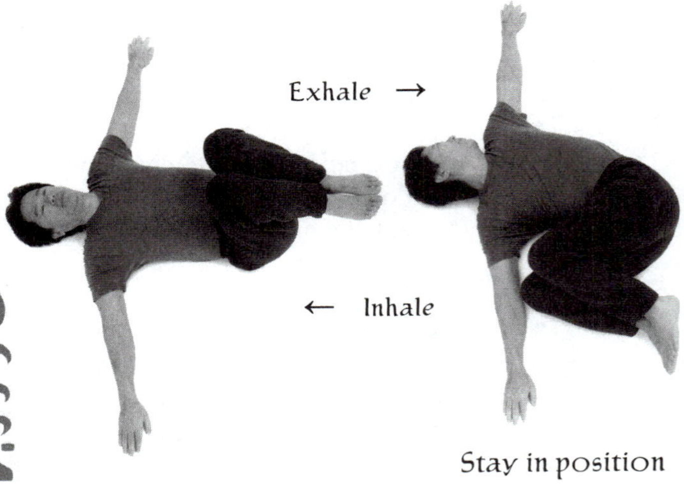

7.

POSTURE: Jaṭhara Parivṛtti variation.
EMPHASIS: To gently twist and compress belly, and stretch hips. To progressively increase number of breaths in posture.
TECHNIQUE: Lie on back with both knees bent, thighs lifted toward chest, and both feet off ground. Arms out to sides, slightly less than right angles to torso.

On exhale: Bring both knees toward floor on right side of body, twisting abdomen and simultaneously turning head left.

On inhale: Return to starting position.

Stay in twist 1, 2, 3, and then 4 full breaths on each side, alternating sides.

DETAILS: *On exhale,* throughout movement, keep knees at an angle to torso that is less than ninety degrees.

8.

POSTURE: Nyāsa technique with sound.
EMPHASIS: To revitalize body through sound and touch.
TECHNIQUE: Sit on a chair or bench with back straight and hands on knees.

On inhale: Raise arms out to sides, open chest, and slightly arch back.

On exhale: Chant **OM** and bring palms to heart. Pause briefly.

Repeat 3 times.

Rest briefly.

On inhale: Raise arms out to sides, open chest, and slightly arch back.

On exhale: Chant **OM** and bring palms to belly. Pause briefly.

Repeat 3 times.

Rest briefly.

DETAILS: Chant: The "**O**" sound should last about 3 seconds, the "**M**" sound about 1 second. *Feel* energy from hands entering heart and belly.

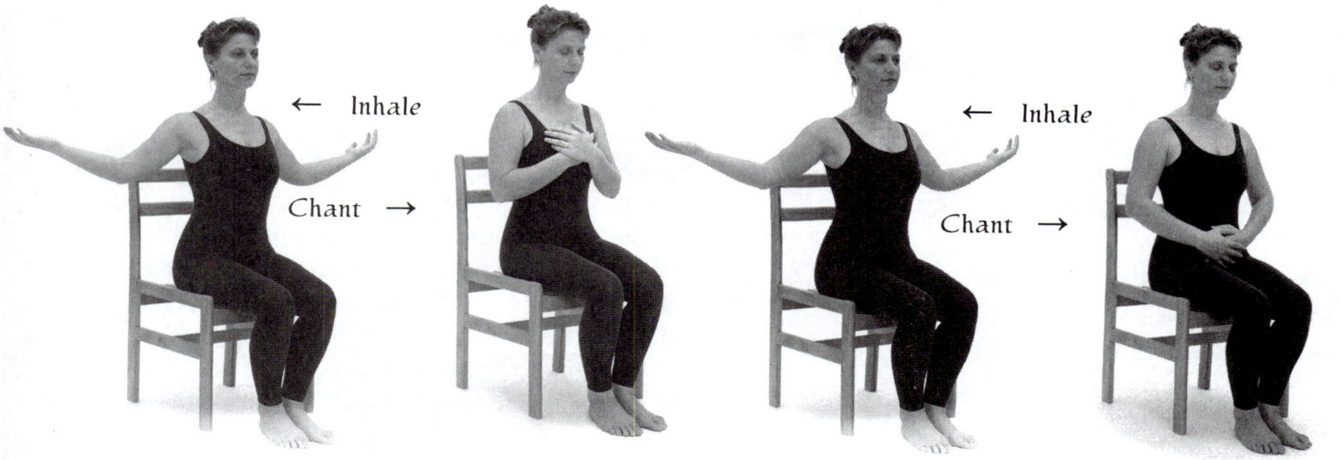

OM on exhale | Touch heart 3 times | OM on exhale | Touch belly 3 times

9.

POSTURE: Sitting on a chair.
EMPHASIS: To relax, feel nourished and alive, while sitting up.
TECHNIQUE: Sit in a comfortable chair, without slumping.
NUMBER: About 5 minutes.

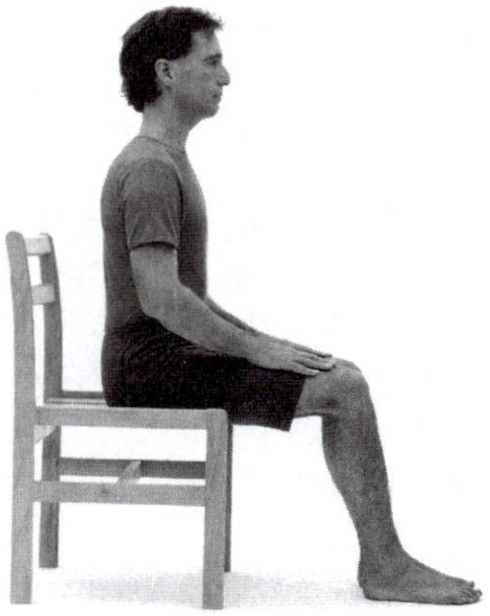

Urinary and Reproductive Systems

Urinary System

The urinary system, along with the digestive and respiratory systems, performs a vital role in eliminating the waste products of our metabolic processes. In addition, this system helps regulate mineral concentrations in our blood, regulates blood volume and blood pressure, and helps the body detoxify poisons.

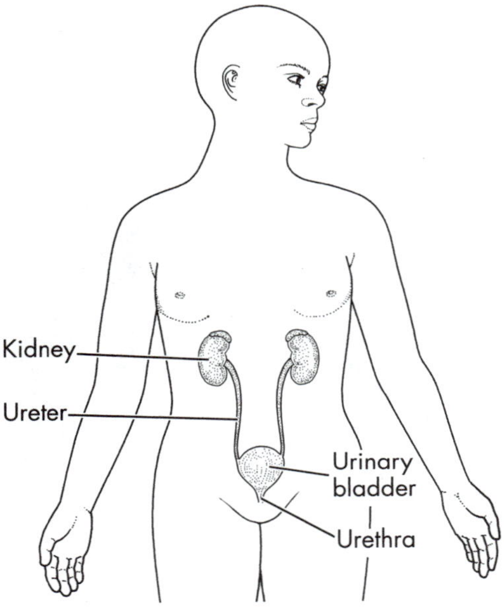

The urinary system consists of the kidneys, ureters, urinary bladder, and the urethra. As blood flows through the kidneys, wastes are filtered out. The kidneys also produce urine, which travels through the ureters to the urinary bladder and is stored in the bladder until it leaves the body, by way of the urethra.

Major problems with the urinary system are serious. If the kidneys are unable to perform their filtration and excretory functions, the entire body is seriously affected. Chronic kidney failure leads to many metabolic disorders, including hypertension and anemia. Acute kidney failure may result in coma and even death.

Less serious are the fairly common inflammations and infections that can effect the urethra (urethritis) or the bladder (cystitis). These conditions usually respond well to some form of medicinal therapy, as well as to dietary modifications. People with these conditions should seek professional care, for if not treated these problems can become chronic and often more serious.

A program of Yoga therapy for the urinary system is oriented toward increased blood flow to the kidneys and toward strengthening the muscles that control the bladder (to help with incontinence). Due to the close relation between the urinary and reproductive organs, practices designed to improve functioning of both systems will be presented together.

Reproductive System

The reproductive system produces, nourishes, stores, and transports reproductive cells and fluids in both male and female bodies. In both cases, the reproductive system includes the reproductive organs (gonads), various glands, ducts, and the external genitals. However, beyond these fundamental similarities, the male and female systems function in very different ways.

The male gonads (testes) produce vast quantities of sperm, which travel through a relatively long duct system and mix with secretions from accessory glands (seminal vesicles, prostate, and bulbourethral glands) to create semen. In the ejaculatory response, this semen is ejected from the body. After ejaculation, it takes some time for the gonads to rebuild their supply of semen, that time period varying from man to man and in relation to stress and age. When the supply is replenished, there is a strong, hormonally based impulse to ejaculate. Unlike the female monthly ovulation cycle, the male semen cycle occurs between three and four times each month. This

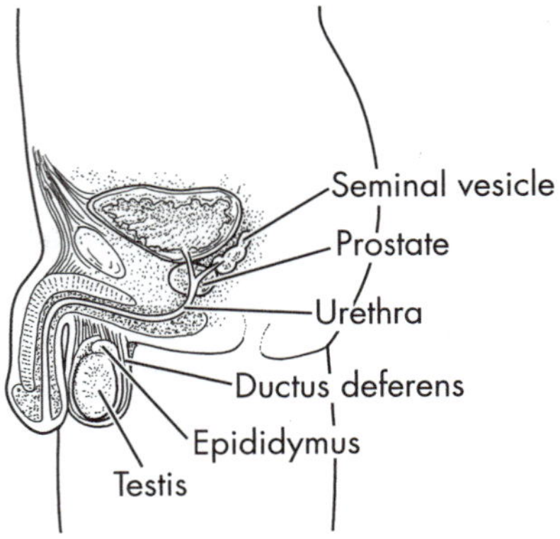

biological fact, not generally considered, has significant psychological implications.

In contrast, the female gonads (ovaries) produce only one egg per month. This egg, after traveling through a relatively short duct system, remains in the uterus until it is either fertilized by a sperm, initiating the development of a new human being, or flushed out of the system during the next menstrual cycle.

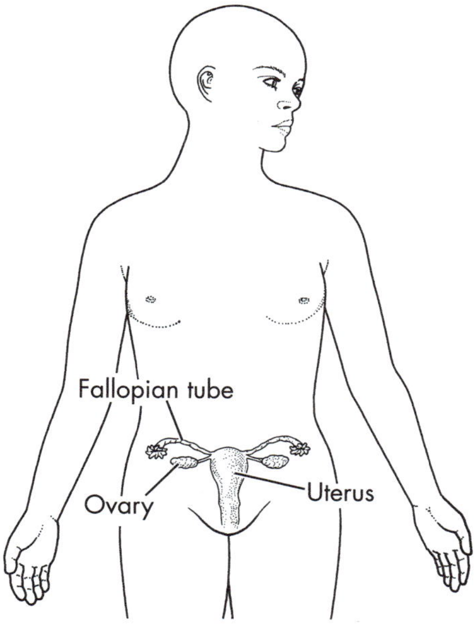

For both male and female, sexual function involves a complex interaction of the conscious mind, emotional states, sensory stimulation, and the coordinated action of the sympathetic and parasympathetic nervous systems. Therefore, there are many factors that can influence proper functioning.

The fulfillment of the biological function of the male and female reproductive systems is pregnancy. There is much of value from the Yoga tradition to help a woman through this passage, which, paradoxically, involves both the most radical transformation of her body and, at the same time, the fulfillment of her biological program. However, we will leave this subject to another publication, keeping the focus of this study on common troubling conditions that can be helped through a well-conceived program of Yoga therapy.

Serious problems of the reproductive system include sexually transmitted diseases, garden variety infections, pelvic inflammatory disease, hormonal problems, sterility or infertility, enlarged prostate, fibroid cysts, and various forms of cancer (e.g., breast and prostate cancers). All of these conditions require some form of professional care, though a good program of Yoga therapy may be a beneficial adjunct to other forms of treatment.

Common, and less serious, problems of the reproductive system for the male usually involve issues of performance, such as difficulty in maintaining an erection or premature ejaculation.

For a female, problems of the reproductive system include PMS, loss of menstruation, or excessive menstrual bleeding. These conditions have a complex of physical and psychological symptoms, including irritability, depression, mood swings, headaches, bloating, and fatigue. In addition to problems associated with menstruation, females may experience pain during intercourse (dyspareunia) or difficulty in achieving orgasm.

Menopause, the completion of the reproductive cycle for a woman, is also an important topic. Symptoms of menopause vary, but generally include hot flashes, night sweats, weight gain, and mood swings. This is a time of significant psychological and hormonal transformation, and there is much of value from the Yoga tradition to help a woman through this passage.

In working with PMS, there are many strategies that can be adopted to help balance the system. Most important, if possible, is to set up external conditions that support what is happening in your body. An example would be to schedule in your calendar, once a month, a day off to take a long walk, or go for a hike or a swim in nature. Often, when women have cramps, they don't want to move, yet movement will significantly improve their condition. We encourage women to walk, starting slowly, gradually increasing the pace, and then, after a little while, reducing the pace. Other adjustments include change of diet, use of appropriate music, oils, and/or massage. The idea is to respect your condition, anticipate it, and be prepared. In addition, a well-conceived program of Yoga therapy can help ease cramps and balance energy and mood swings.

For both the male and female, absence of sexual vitality, lack of sexual desire, or excessive sexual preoccupation are common complaints. These conditions can be caused by overwork, excessive or insufficient exercise, emotional stress, and even poor nutrition.

Sexual drive is as natural to a healthy individual as hunger. Along with survival itself, it is one of the fundamental biological imperatives at the root of our psyches. And yet, the fundamental hormonal differences between male and female, which strongly influence sexual behavior, result in much confusion and misunderstanding between the sexes.

Adding to the confusion, strong religious and social ideals send out mixed messages. From many Western religious traditions comes the message that this deep and natural impulse is somehow bad or even sinful. From the Indian and Oriental Yoga schools comes the teaching about male semen retention, which is often misunderstood and taken out of context. On the one hand we are sinning, and on the other, we are loosing our vital energy. These mixed messages and the ideals that result often lead to psychological complexes, conflict, repression and suppression of our vital energy, the development of imbalances, and even disease.

At the same time, sexual images pervade our society, especially in the advertisement and entertainment industries. A man measures himself against the "macho hunk." His self-image is often linked to his "sexual prowess," and, accordingly, performance anxiety is a common cause of premature ejaculation. A woman is often portrayed as a sexual object, and when, in keeping with such expectations, she measures herself against the young and slim supermodel, the result is often unhappiness, complexes about weight, overtraining, and even more serious conditions such as anorexia and bulimia.

According to the Yoga tradition, it is important to avoid extreme behavior and to understand any set of teachings within its context. For example, the teaching about semen retention must be understood in the context of the tradition in which it developed, and in terms of two distinct practices: those of the celibate monk or yogi; and those of the sexually active tantric. In both cases, retention is not suppression. In fact, a yogi does exercises that both stimulate his sexual vitality and circulate that energy so that it does not accumulate, stagnate, and become a source of disease. On the other hand, that does not mean that there should be excessive loss of this vital energy, for that too can be the source of imbalance and can even weaken immunity. The point of view in this tradition is to avoid either extreme. Don't suppress. Don't indulge. Find a balanced path in relation to your own sexual energy.

Stimulating the Reproductive and Urinary Systems

Some of the conditions described above respond well to practices that strengthen and stimulate the area of the reproductive organs. These practices will include exercises in which the muscles of the perineum are gently contracted and released (Aśvini Mudrā and Mūla Bandha) and are similar to the Kegel exercises taught to women in childbirth classes. In addition, we will use exercises that stretch the muscles of the perineal floor, and which, by alternating contracting and stretching, increase circulation to that area of the body. This approach may be helpful where there is incontinence, lack of sexual vitality, poor sexual functioning, and also in some prostate conditions. The strategy is to balance, stimulate, and rejuvenate the area, through techniques that increase awareness and circulation.

Working with Prostatitis

H.G. was a thirty-nine-year-old Yoga teacher who had been attending seminars and private sessions with me on and off for many years. He was a very strong practitioner, with an ability to do advanced postures.

One day, when I was teaching in New York, he scheduled a private session with me to talk about a problem he had been having. I had not seen him for nearly a year, and when he came I was surprised to see how drained he looked. He told me that for the past six months, he had been suffering from chronic prostatitis and was on yet another round of antibiotics. He wondered if there was any help I could offer.

The good news was that he had fallen in love and was about to move in with his new fiancée. The fact that, in less than one year, he had been suffering from prostatitis for six months *and* had a new fiancée was interesting.

I told him that our strategy would be to develop a cooling langhana course to help him conserve his energy and to reduce the heating effect of the antibiotics. At the same time, we would include techniques to increase the circulation of energy to the perineal area. I also mentioned that, between the antibiotics and the new girlfriend, his kidneys might benefit from some attention. I suggested that he take some time to rebuild his energy and that he explain the situation to his fiancée. He asked me for how long, and I suggested about three months.

Since H.G. was an advanced practitioner, I was comfortable with giving him the following course. For him, it represented a reduction in his normal āsana practice. I included headstand because of its cooling and conserving effects, and because I knew he liked challenging practices. Controlling the exhale from the perineal floor was also new and challenging for him.

As he liked to practice meditation, I asked him to add a visualization of the full moon (*candra*)—which is cooling—to the prāṇāyāma at the end of the practice. On inhale, I asked him to feel like he was drawing moon light from his crown into his perineal floor. On exhale, I asked him to feel like he was spreading that cooling moonlight throughout his entire body.

H.G. reported to me several months later that his condition had cleared. Though he thought that the last round of antibiotics had done the trick, he felt that the practice had helped him regain balance in his system and increase his energy. He told me that he and his girlfriend were happily living together, and he was thankful for having new tools to work with.

A Practice for Prostatitis

1.

POSTURE: Uttānāsana.
EMPHASIS: To warm up back and legs.
TECHNIQUE: Stand with arms over head.
On exhale: Forward bend, bringing belly and chest toward thighs and bringing hands to feet.
On inhale: return to starting position.
NUMBER: 6 times.

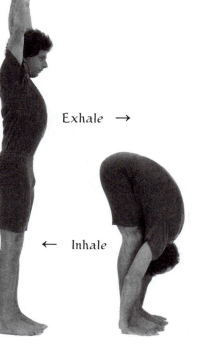

2.

POSTURE: Utthita Trikoṇāsana.

EMPHASIS: To stimulate kidney area by laterally stretching torso. To warm up the neck and shoulders in preparation for headstand.

TECHNIQUE:

A: Stand with feet spread wider than shoulders, left foot turned out at a ninety-degree angle to right foot, left arm over head, and right arm straight down at waist and slightly rotated externally.

On exhale: Keeping shoulders in same plane as hips, bend laterally, lowering left shoulder and bringing left hand below left knee while turning head up toward right hand.

On inhale: Return to starting position.

Repeat.

B: With left hand down along left leg:

On inhale: Bring right arm up and forward while turning head forward toward right hand.

On exhale: Return to starting position while turning head up toward right hand.

NUMBER: Repeat A four times, then B four times; then repeat on other side.

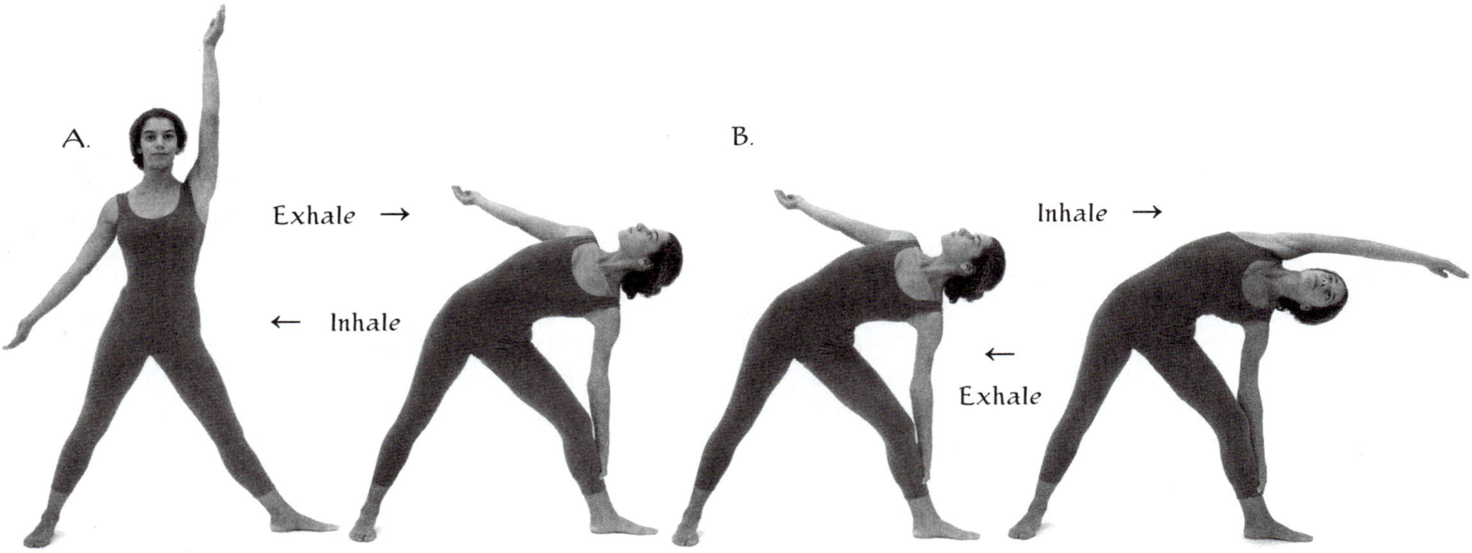

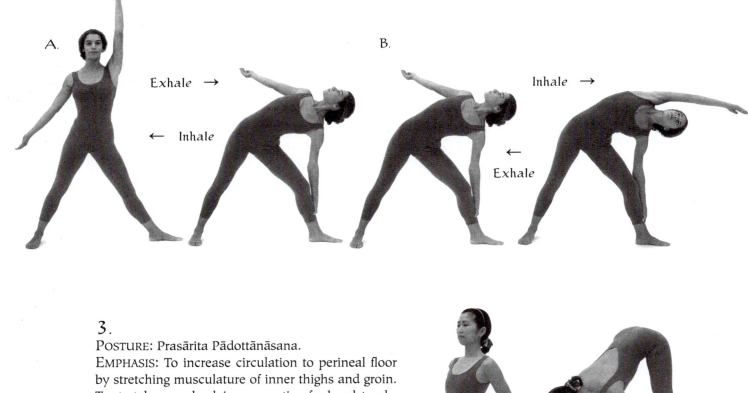

3.

POSTURE: Prasārita Pādottānāsana.

EMPHASIS: To increase circulation to perineal floor by stretching musculature of inner thighs and groin. To stretch upper back in preparation for headstand.

TECHNIQUE: Stand with feet wider than shoulders and hands on buttocks.

On exhale: Bend forward, bringing chest between thighs, sliding hands to ankles.

On inhale: Hold ankles and raise chest, flattening upper back.

On exhale: Return to forward bend position.

Repeat 6 times.

On inhale: return to starting position.

DETAILS: *On exhale:* Bend knees slightly when bending forward, drop chin toward chest. *On inhale:* Lift chin slightly as chest is lifted.

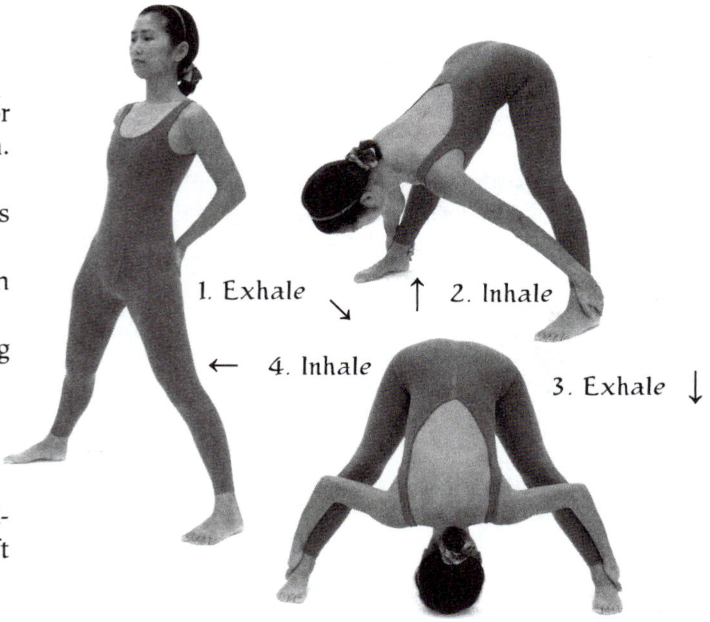

4.

POSTURE: Śīrṣāsana.
EMPHASIS: To deepen calm and cool system.
TECHNIQUE: From hands and knees, interlock fingers with elbows forearm's length apart. Cupping head in hands, stand on toes, lifting knees off floor. Walk forward with toes until hips are vertically above shoulders. Lift legs to vertical position. Stay.

On exhale: Pull upward from perineal floor.

NUMBER: 12 to 18 breaths.
DETAILS: Position should be comfortable. If there is neck stress, come down. Make inhale and exhale equal and at a comfortable maximum length.

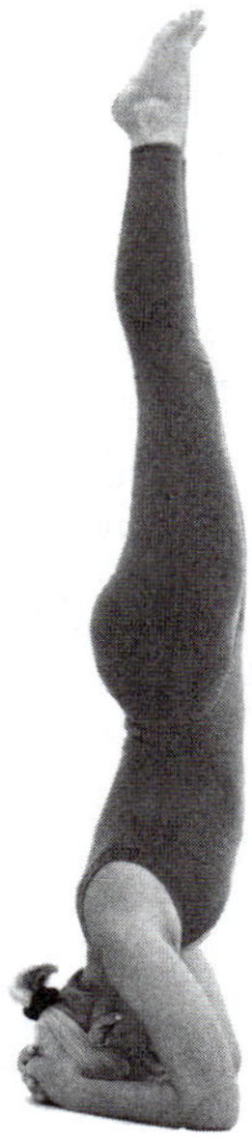

5.

POSTURE: Dvipāda Pīṭham.
EMPHASIS: To balance effects of headstand by stretching upper back and neck.
TECHNIQUE:

A: Lie on back with arms down at sides, knees bent, and feet on floor, slightly apart and comfortably close to buttocks.

On inhale: Pressing down on feet and keeping chin down, raise pelvis until neck is gently flattened on floor, while raising arms up overhead to floor behind head.

On exhale: Return to starting position.

B: Stay up in position, fingers interlocked on floor under pelvis, gently pulling shoulders together and stretching upper back and neck.

NUMBER: A six times; B stay six breaths.
DETAILS: *On inhale:* Lift spine, vertebra by vertebra, from bottom up. *On exhale:* Unwind spine, coming down vertebra by vertebra.

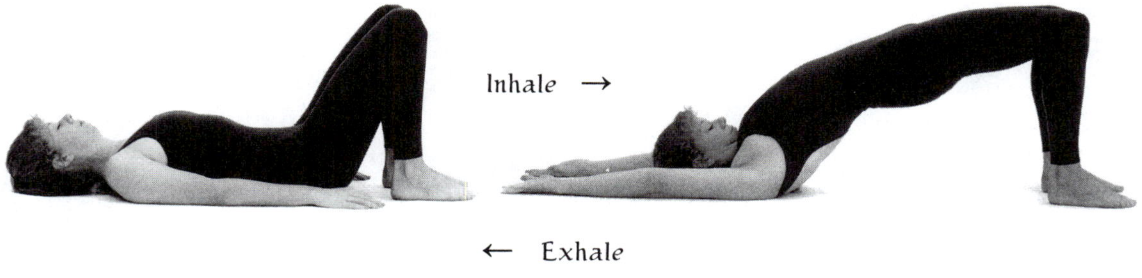

6.

POSTURE: Supta Prasārita Pādāṅguṣṭhāsana.
EMPHASIS: To increase circulation to perineal floor by stretching and contracting musculature of inner thighs and perineal floor.
TECHNIQUE: Lie on back with knees lifted toward chest and with hands placed behind knees.

On inhale: With hands holding legs from behind knees, lift heels upward, straightening legs.

On exhale: Stay in position, placing hands on insides of knees, palms facing outward.

On inhale: Open legs wide, pushing legs apart gently with arms.

On exhale: Close legs, resisting slightly with arms.

Repeat 6 times.

Then stay open 6 breaths.

DETAILS: Keep sacrum, chin, and shoulders down throughout movement. If legs are loose, hold balls of feet while staying in final position.

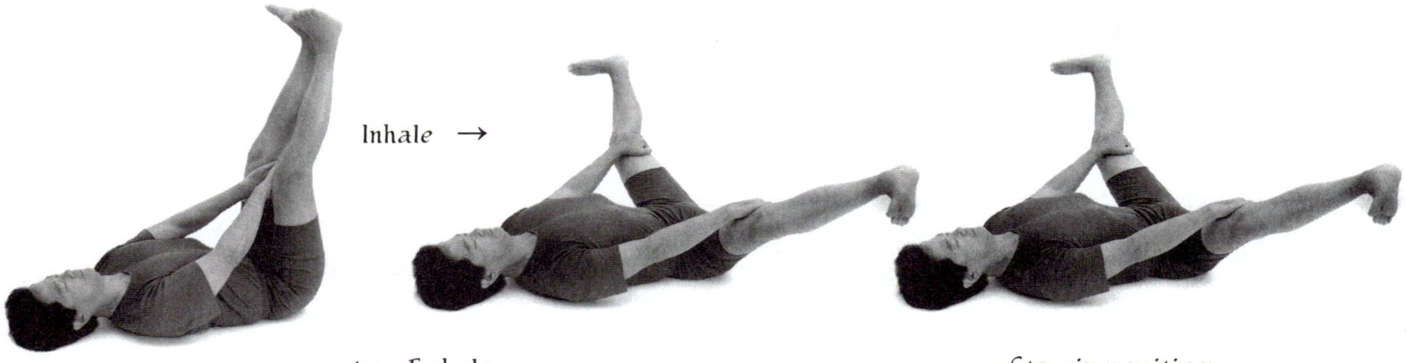

7.

POSTURE: Jaṭhara Parivṛtti.
EMPHASIS: To stimulate kidney area.
TECHNIQUE: Lie flat on back, with arms out to sides and left leg extended upward at an angle of ninety degrees to torso.

On exhale: twist, bringing left foot to floor toward right hand while turning head left.

On inhale: Return to starting position.

Repeat 4 times.

Then stay in twisted position, holding right foot with left hand. Stay 8 breaths.

Repeat on other side.

DETAILS: While staying in position, actively rotate upper back and shoulder opposite leg that is twisting, feeling torsion in kidney area.

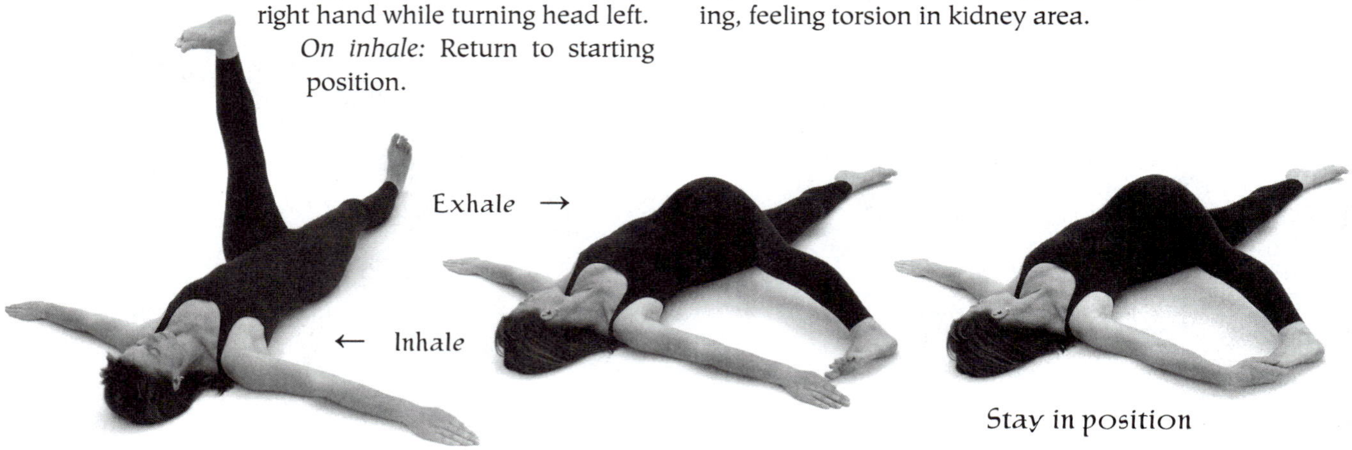

8.

POSTURE: Upaviṣṭha Koṇāsana.
EMPHASIS: To increase circulation to perineal floor by stretching inner thighs and perineal floor.
TECHNIQUE:

A: Sit with legs apart and extended forward, and with arms overhead.

On exhale: Bend forward, bringing hands to feet and chest between thighs.

On inhale: Return to starting position.

B: From forward bend position:

On inhale: Hold feet and lift chest, flattening upper back.

On exhale: Bend forward again.

NUMBER: A four times; B six times.
DETAILS: *On exhale:* Bend knees to avoid collapsing chest over belly. If hips are loose, press sit bones into floor.

A.

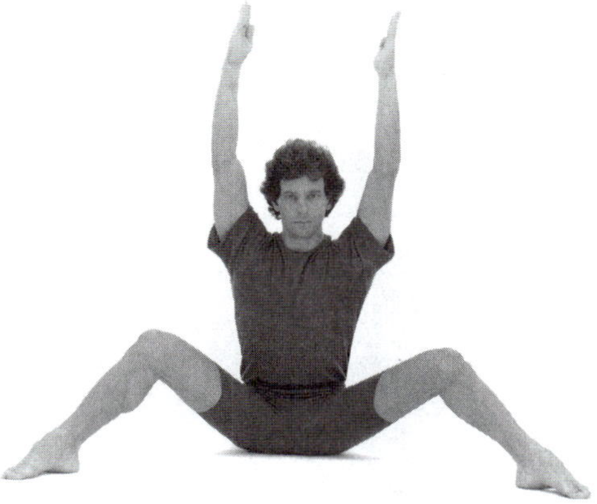

Exhale ↓ ↑ Inhale

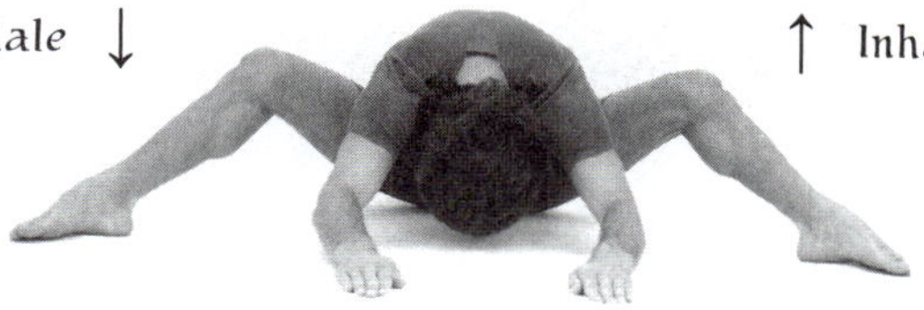

B.

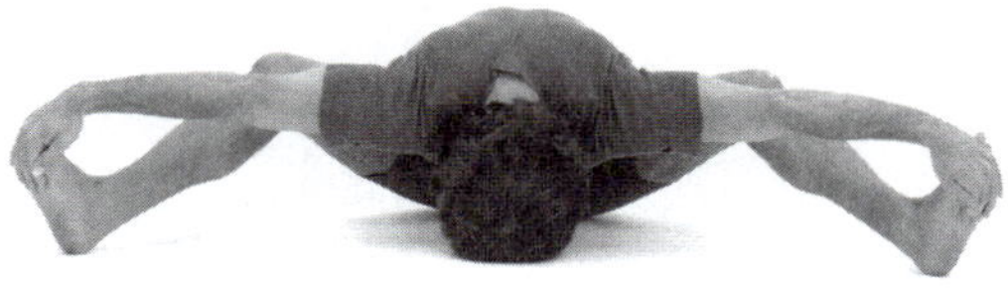

Inhale ↓ ↑ Exhale

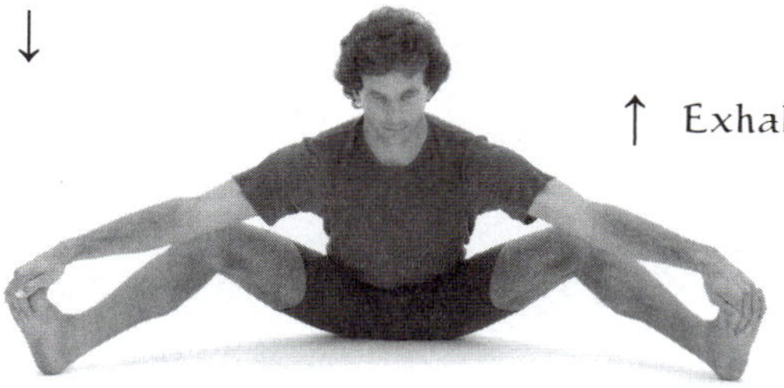

9.

POSTURE: Mahāmudra and Jānu Śirṣāsana.
EMPHASIS: To introduce Mula Bandha. To increase circulation to perineal floor.
TECHNIQUE: Sit with right leg folded in, heel to groin, left leg extended forward, holding left foot with both hands.

On inhale: Extend spine upward, expanding chest, flattening upper back, and lengthening in front of torso.

On exhale: Maintain posture while pulling upward from perineal floor and pulling belly firmly in. Sustain for 4 to 6 seconds.

Repeat 8 times.

Then *on exhale:* Sink belly and chest to thigh.

Rest in position 4 breaths.

Repeat on other side.

DETAILS: *On inhale:* Expand chest, then gradually release first belly and then perineal floor.

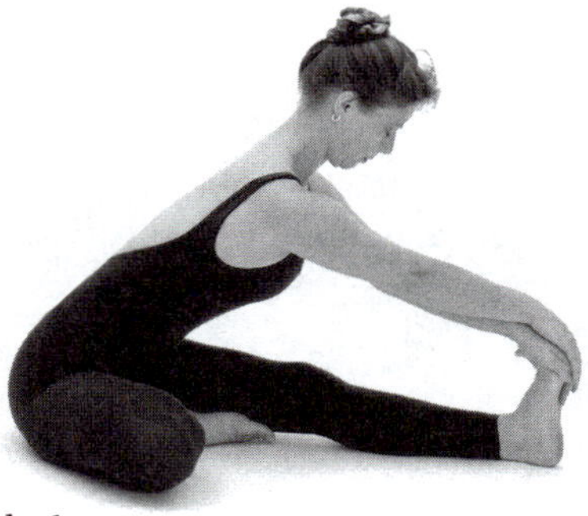

Stay in position

Exhale ↘

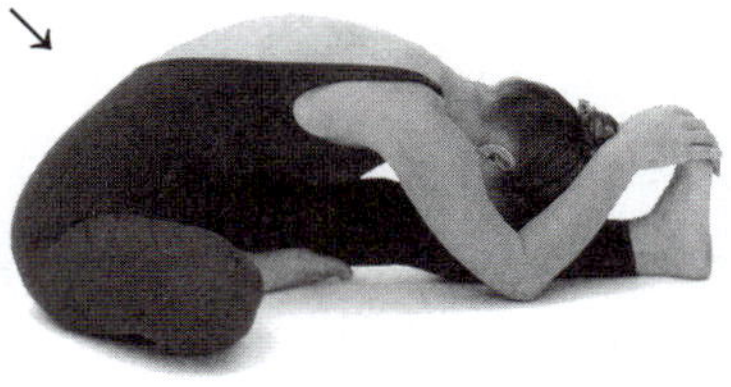

Stay in position

10.

POSTURE: Baddha Koṇāsana.
EMPHASIS: To continue stretching area of inner thighs and groin.
TECHNIQUE: Sit with soles of feet together, heels close to groin.

On inhale: Holding feet with both hands, extend spine upward, flattening upper back.

On exhale: Pull upward from perineal floor, and pull belly firmly in. Sustain 4 to 6 seconds.

Repeat 8 times.

DETAILS: *On inhale:* Expand chest, then gradually release first belly and then perineal floor.

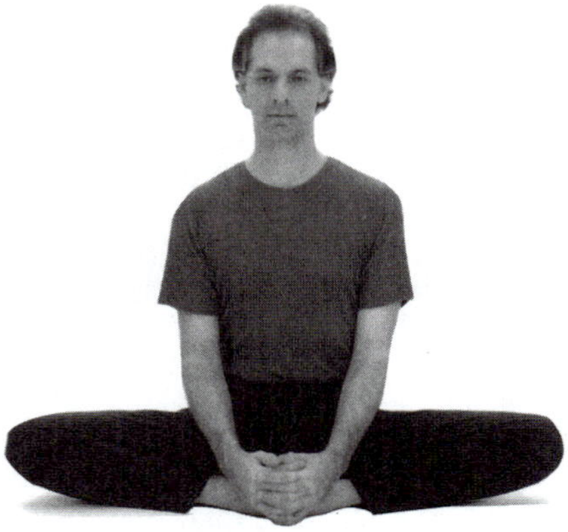

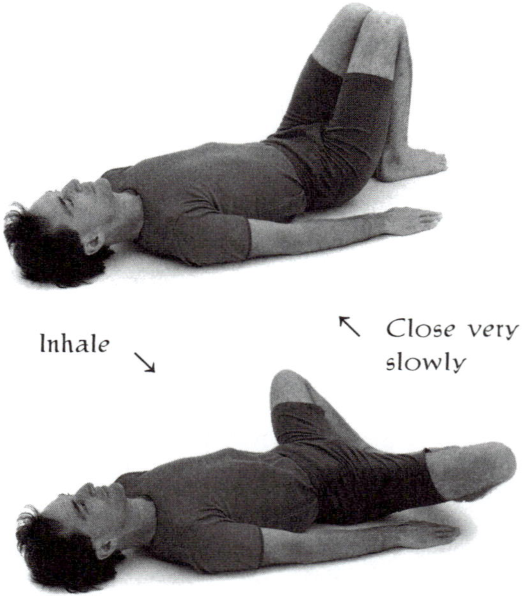

11.

POSTURE: Supta Baddha Koṇāsana.
EMPHASIS: To increase circulation to perineal floor.
TECHNIQUE: Lie on back with knees bent and feet near buttocks. Open legs wide, bringing soles of feet together. Take up to sixty seconds to close knees together. Open legs again naturally.
NUMBER: 6 times.
DETAILS: While closing legs, keep low back flat on floor. Allow any trembling of legs that may occur.

12.

POSTURE: Śavāsana.
EMPHASIS: To rest.
TECHNIQUE: Lie flat on back, arms at sides, palms up, and legs slightly apart. Close eyes. Relax body fully, keeping mind relaxed and alert to sensations in body.
DURATION: Minimum 3 to 5 minutes.

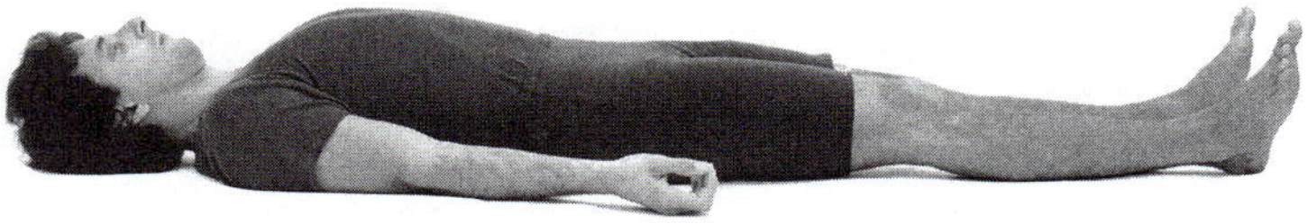

13.

POSTURE: Prāṇāyāma/Viloma Krama, 3-stage exhale with visualization.
EMPHASIS: To strengthen muscles of perineal floor. To introduce visualization to help cool system.
TECHNIQUE:

Inhale deeply and fully.
Exhale 1/3 of breath in 3 seconds.
Pause 3 seconds.
Exhale another 1/3 of breath in 3 seconds.
Pause 3 seconds.
Complete *exhale* in 3 seconds.
Pause 3 seconds.
Inhale deeply and repeat.

NUMBER: 9 times.
DETAILS: *On exhale:* At first stage, contract from perineum to pubic bone. At second stage contract from pubic bone to navel. At third stage contract from navel to solar plexus. *On inhale:* After expanding chest, release progressively from solar plexus to navel to perineum.

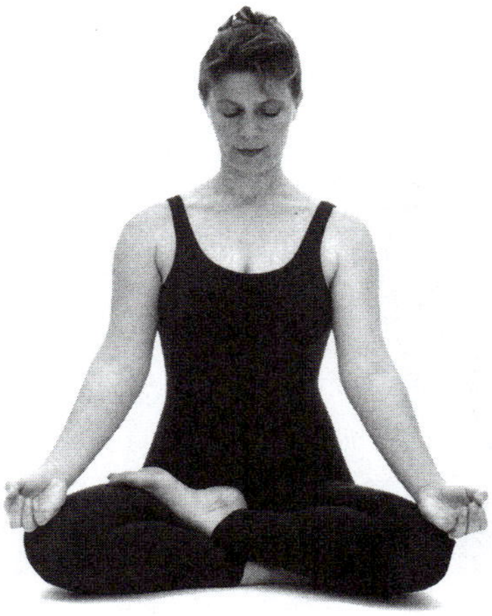

Soothing the Reproductive and Urinary Systems

Other conditions described above respond well to practices that soothe and calm the area of the reproductive organs. Inflammatory, painful, crampy, and tense conditions need relaxation. In working with these conditions, we can use sound techniques, such as chanting a cooling and soothing sound, like *MA* or *SO*, at a low pitch. This can be effective because low-pitched sound increases vibrations lower in the belly, cooling the system when it is overheated, as is the case when cramping occurs, for example. We will also want to emphasize deep breathing, lightly holding after exhale, and gently using the thighs, the belly, and the low back at the same time. When such conditions are present, we will generally **avoid postures that stress the abdominal area**, such as Nāvāsana and deep backbends.

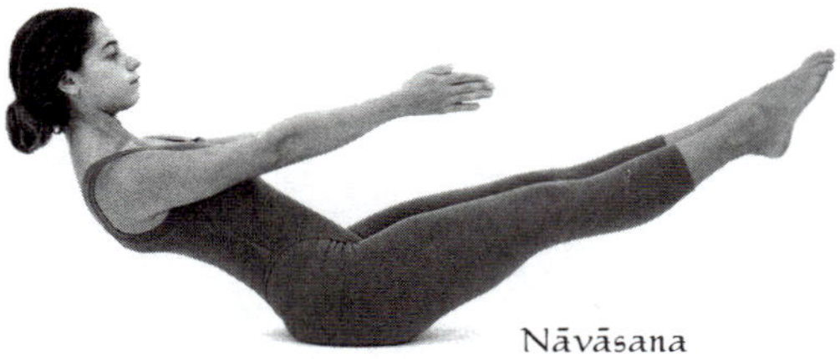

Nāvāsana

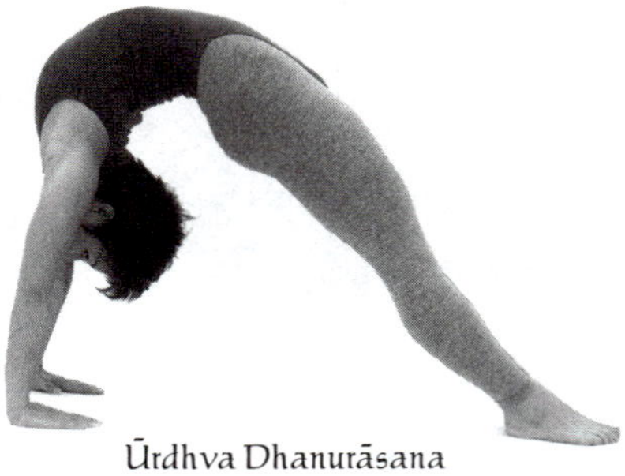

Ūrdhva Dhanurāsana

The following practice may be helpful with menstrual problems, menopause, for women with difficulties experiencing orgasm, and for men and women with problems of excessive sexual preoccupation.

Working with PMS

F.D. was a forty-year-old woman who attended a talk on Yoga therapy I gave in northern Italy. After the talk she approached me to see if I might help her with a recurring condition. We arranged to meet, and she told me that she suffered from terrible premenstrual cramps, accompanied by fatigue and depression. F.D. did not speak English and, at that time, my Italian was very basic.

I told her that I would be in Italy for only two months, and asked if she would commit to seeing me at least four times before I left. She agreed, and we began to work together.

F.D. was married but had no children. She worked as a teller in a bank. In talking to her, I learned that she was a woman of deep faith and went to mass regularly. She seemed to be timid and somewhat fearful.

Knowing that I would only have four sessions with her, I wanted to give her a very simple practice. My strategy was to increase circulation in her lower abdomen, helping it relax, and at the same time, help pick up her energy. As I was working with her, I began to feel that some sound techniques would be helpful, not only for her cramps but also for her mild depression and fear.

Knowing the strong presence of the Holy Mother in Italy, I tactfully asked her if she had faith. When she said yes, I asked her if she would be willing to try some sound techniques that we have found helpful in cases like hers. She agreed. I told her that we would use only two sounds: "OH" and "MA." I told her that "OH MA OH" was an invocation of Mother Mary, calling on her for protection. She liked the image, and we integrated the sounds into the following practice, which we evolved over the four sessions we had together.

The following year, I was in Italy again. I gave another talk in the same town, and F.D. attended. At the end of the talk, she stood up to say that last year she had spent a very brief time with me. She told the audience that the practice I had given her had helped her tremendously. She gratefully reported that she had taught her mother the same practice and that it had even helped her with her chronic stomach problems!

A Practice for PMS

1.

POSTURE: Apānāsana.

EMPHASIS: To gently compress belly while progressively extending exhale.

TECHNIQUE: Lie on back, with knees bent toward chest, feet off floor, and each hand on its respective knee.

On exhale: Pull thighs gently but progressively toward chest, chanting **OH MA OH**.

On inhale: Return to starting position.

NUMBER: 12 times.

DETAILS: *On exhale:* Pull gently with arms, keeping shoulders down on floor and relaxed. Press low back down into floor and drop chin slightly toward throat. Progressively lengthen exhale with each successive repetition.

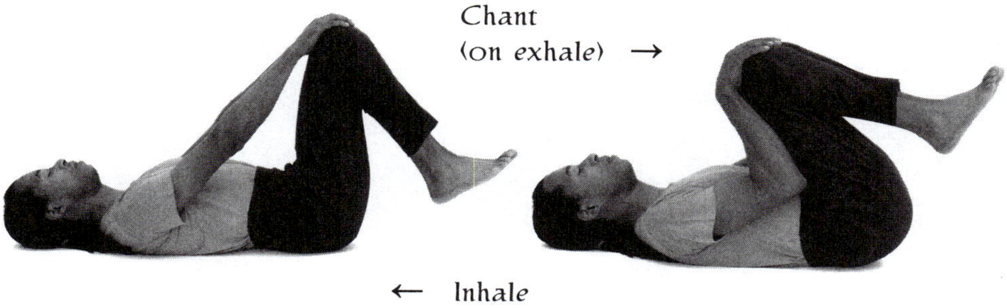

2.

POSTURE: Cakravākāsana.

EMPHASIS: To introduce soothing sound with movement.

TECHNIQUE: Get down on hands and knees, with shoulders vertically above wrists and with hips above knees.

On inhale: Lift chest up and away from belly.

On exhale: While moving hips back down toward heels and lowering chest toward thighs, chant **OH MA OH**.

NUMBER: 8 times.

DETAILS: *On inhale:* Lead with chest, chin slightly down; feel chest expansion. *On exhale:* Bring chest lower toward thighs sooner than hips toward heels; chant **OH MA OH** at a comfortable low pitch, with **MA** slightly lower.

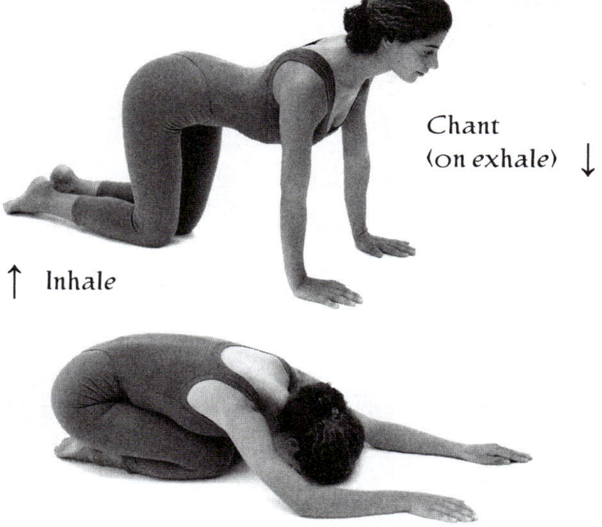

3.

POSTURE: Dvipāda Pīṭham.
EMPHASIS: To increase circulation in pelvic area by relaxing back, gently stretching belly, and lifting hips.
TECHNIQUE: Lie on back with arms down at sides, knees bent, and feet on floor, slightly apart and comfortably close to buttocks.

On inhale: Keep chin down and press down on feet, raising pelvis up toward ceiling, until neck is gently flattened on floor.

On exhale: Return to starting position.

NUMBER: 6 times.
DETAILS: *On inhale:* Lift spine vertebra by vertebra, from bottom up. *On exhale:* Unwind spine, coming down vertebra by vertebra.

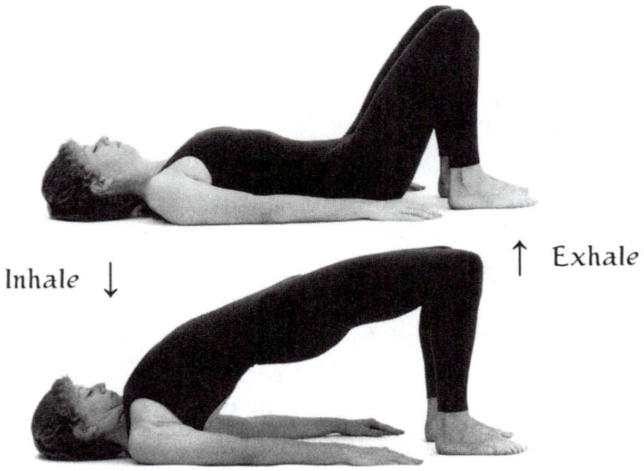

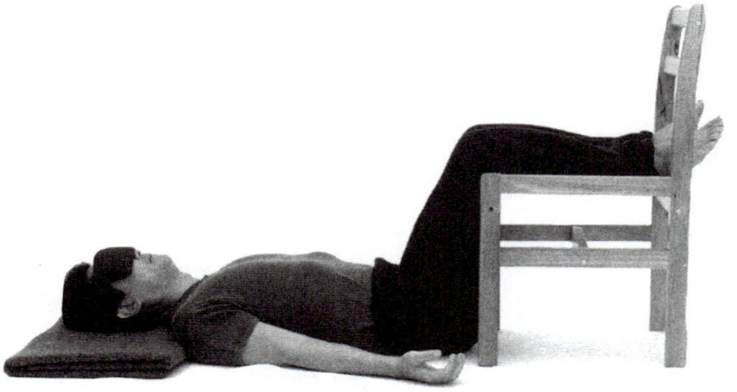

Increase length of exhale

4.

POSTURE: Śavāsana with support.
EMPHASIS: To extend exhale while relaxing on back.
TECHNIQUE: Lie on back with lower legs resting on a chair. Breathe in and out, progressively lengthening exhale.
NUMBER: Stay in position 3 to 5 minutes.
DETAILS: Place a small pillow under head to relax neck, and cover eyes.

5.

POSTURE: Supta Baddha Koṇāsana.
EMPHASIS: To increase circulation to perineal floor.
TECHNIQUE: Lie on back with knees bent and feet near buttocks. Open legs wide, bringing soles of feet together.

On exhale: Close legs 1/3 of way while slowly chanting **OH MA OH**.

On inhale: Stay in position.

On exhale: Close legs another 1/3 of way while chanting **OH MA OH**.

On inhale: Stay in position.

On exhale: Close legs final 1/3 of way while chanting **OH MA OH**.

On inhale: Open legs naturally.

NUMBER: 6 times.
DETAILS: While closing legs, keep low back flat on floor. Allow any trembling of legs that may occur. Chant **OH MA OH** at a comfortable low pitch, with **MA** slightly lower.

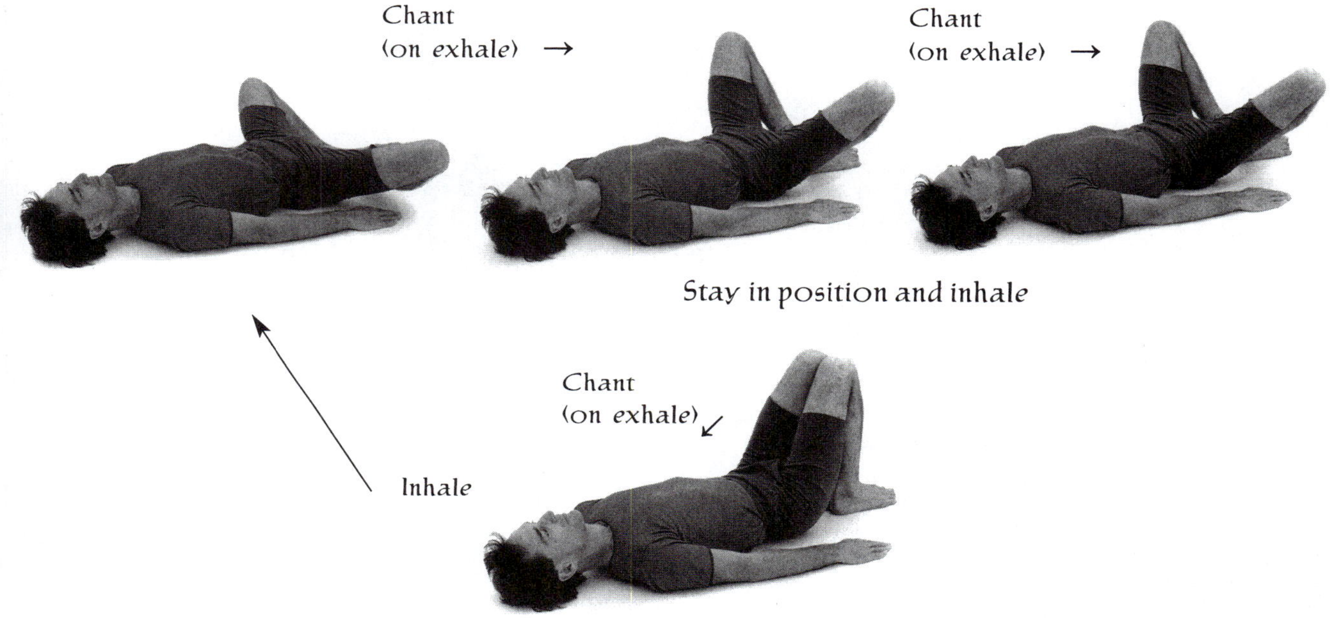

6.

POSTURE: Apānāsana.
EMPHASIS: To gently compress belly while progressively extending exhale.
TECHNIQUE: Lie on back with both knees bent toward chest, feet off floor, and with each hand on its respective knee.

On exhale: Pull thighs gently but progressively toward chest.

On inhale: Return to starting position.

NUMBER: 12 times.
DETAILS: *On exhale:* Pull gently with arms, keeping shoulders down on floor and relaxed. Press low back down into floor and drop chin slightly toward throat. Progressively lengthen exhale with each successive repetition.

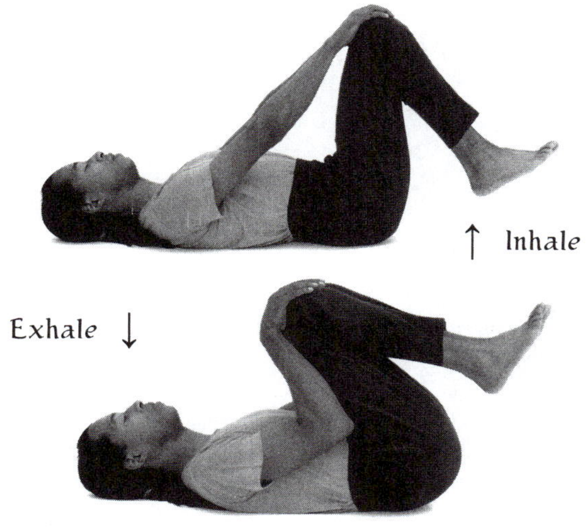

7.

POSTURE: Śītalī Prāṇāyāma with alternate nostril exhale.
EMPHASIS: To cool and soothe system.
TECHNIQUE: Sit comfortably.

Inhale through an extended curled tongue—like through a straw—while raising chin slightly. Close mouth, curl tongue backward, drop chin, raise right arm, and seal right nostril.

Exhale through left nostril.

Inhale through curled tongue.

Then, following same procedure, *exhale* through right nostril.

NUMBER: 9 times each side, alternately.

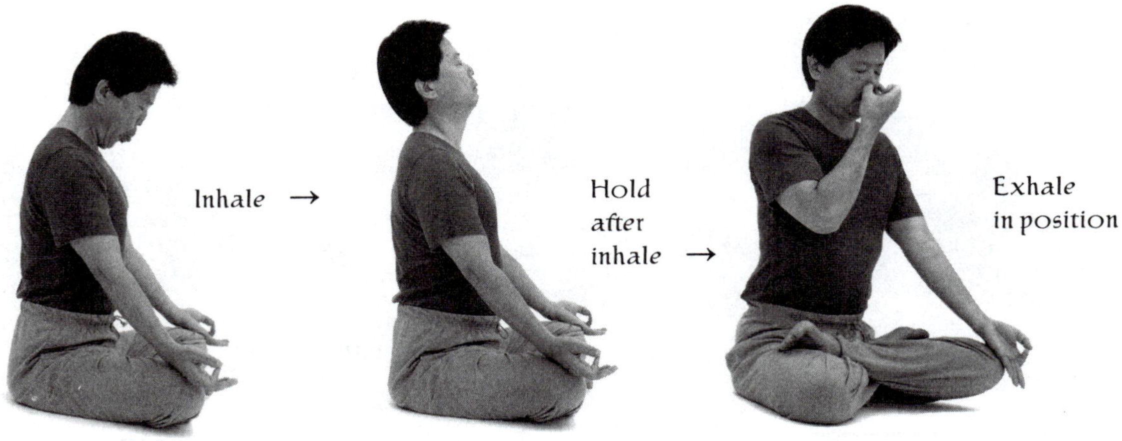

Chapter 5

Emotional Health

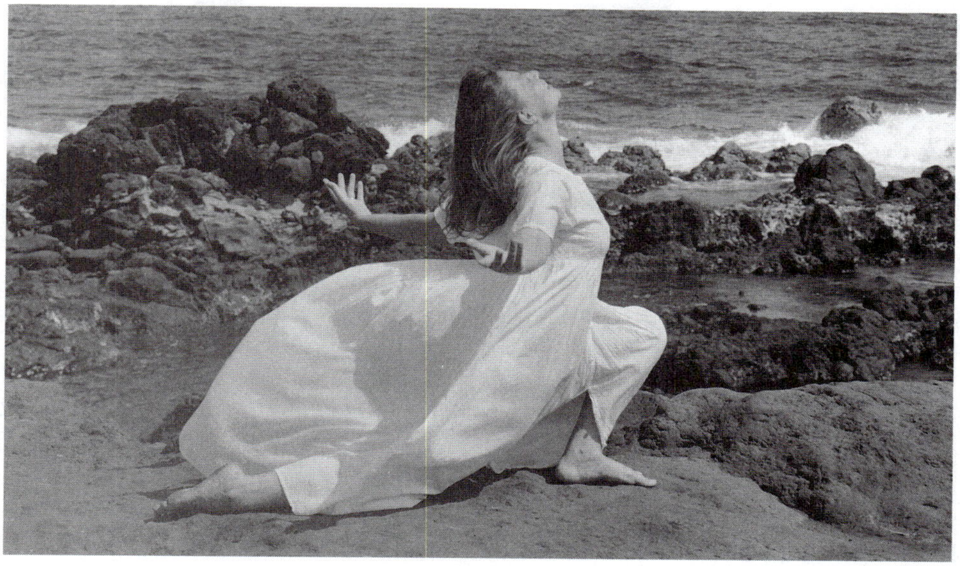

As we have seen, the key to using Yoga practice as therapy lies in our ability to link our conscious minds to the unconscious rhythms of our bodies. This being the case, an understanding of exactly how the body, mind, and emotions interact is essential to the study of Yoga.

From the standpoint of Yoga theory, mind and body always function as one organic whole. Intellectual and emotional processes are regarded in much the same way as physiological and structural ones—as material processes. In fact, according to this view, *all* manifested forms are simply differentiations of a single universal material substance (*prakṛti*). These differentiations extend from the grossest external objects, such as rocks and trees, to the subtlest internal objects, such as our changing emotional states and our self-image.

On the other hand, Yoga theory does makes an important distinction between this perpetually changing substance, which it calls the "seen," and pure, changeless, undifferentiated consciousness (*puruṣa*), which it calls the "seer." In fact, it views identification with the ever-changing differentiations of substance, from the grossest to the subtlest, as the result of misapprehension (*avidyā*), which, in turn, is the cause of suffering. The practice of Yoga involves two goals: the removal of the misapprehension that results in the qualities of mind that perpetuate emotional drama (through the process known as *viyoga*); and the awakening of the discrimination (*viveka*) that results in those qualities of mind that enable us to reach our highest potential (through the process known as *saṃyoga*).

The Spaceship *Voyager*

Many years ago, while watching a program on PBS concerning the process of getting the spaceship *Voyager* out of this solar system, I was struck by the analogy between the goal and challenges of that mission and those of any individual who wishes to overcome suffering and achieve his or her highest potential.

The problem for the rocket scientists was to figure out a way for the spaceship to gain enough momentum to escape the solar system. They realized that they could use the gravity of each planet to pick up sufficient momentum to propel the spaceship outward from the sun and, ultimately, beyond the gravitational pull of the solar system. The challenge was to program the spaceship with the correct velocity and angles of approach to the planets along the way in order to avoid crashing into them or getting stuck in orbit around them. Miscalculating the approach in one way would cause the spaceship to crash and burn in the gravity well of that planet. Miscalculating the approach in another way would cause it go into permanent orbit. However, if the approach were just right, the spaceship would receive a boost from each planet along the way that would enable it to ultimately achieve escape velocity and would propel it beyond the solar system. In much the same way, we can learn to break through the limitations of our own personal solar systems, which include all the particular circumstances of our personal lives. We can learn to avoid crashing into or revolving around our personality and, like the spaceship, use the "gravitational forces" within our own systems to achieve escape velocity and propel ourselves beyond the limitations of our conditioning and onward into new dimensions of our personal evolution.

In his famous commentary on Patañjali's *Yoga Sūtras,* Vyāsa describes five possible levels or states of mind, as follows:

> *Kṣipta:* A seriously disturbed, heavily distracted, and discontinuous state of mind.
>
> *Mūdha:* A seriously depressed mind, covered in darkness and without hope.
>
> *Vikṣipta:* The "normal neurotic" mind, which alternates between distraction and attention.
>
> *Ekāgra:* A mind that is focused and undistracted in one-pointed concentration.
>
> *Nirodha:* The highest potential of mind. It is a state of mind that is freed from conditioned response and, therefore, allows the "seer" to perceive without distortion.

At the first three levels of mental development, we are likely to be so self-absorbed that we either crash into the gravity well of our own personality or go into permanent orbit around ourselves. Another possibility, at these levels of mental development, is that we become magnetically attracted to some other "gravitational center" (such as a lover, community, or guru) and are either absorbed into its mass or locked into orbit around it. In fact, crashing and/or orbiting are inevitable at these three levels of mental development because we have not yet programmed ourselves to use the "gravitationally attractive bodies" within our personal systems to help us reach "escape velocity." At the level of *ekāgra,* we have the capacity to commit to and sustain a personal practice that will enable us to recognize the trap of revolving around the conditioned mind and to continue our journey of personal evolution. And, finally, in the state of *nirodha,* we begin to function at the level of our highest potential as human beings.

The nature of the seer and the process of spiritual development is not the focus here and must wait for a full consideration in our next work. However, some sense of the distinction between seer and seen is important to a correct understanding of the link between our minds (including all of our intellectual and emotional activity) and our bodies (including all of our physiology and anatomy). And the ability to make this distinction is especially important if we are to avoid the mistake of identifying the seer with those subtle functions of the complex brain, which we will now describe, that are part of the seen.

The Limbic Brain

For the sake of simplicity in considering this link between mind and body, we will divide the brain into three main parts:

1. *The brain stem and cerebellum* are involved in the mechanical, and usually unconscious, processes of regulating and processing the sensory, emotional, autonomic, hormonal, and motor functions of the body.

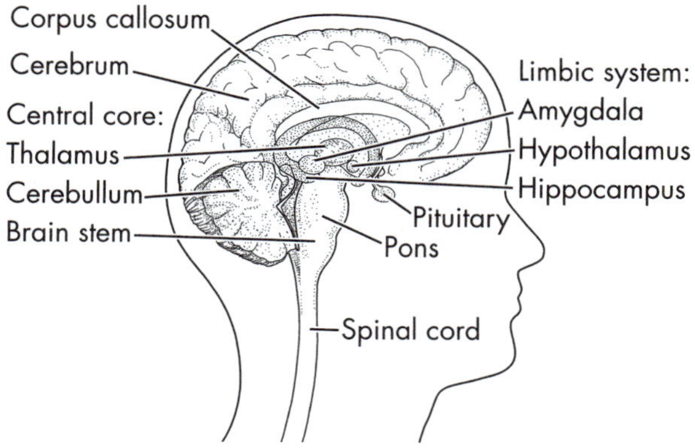

2. *The cerebrum* is involved in conscious processes such as intellectual thought, the processing and comprehension of sensory input, the coordination of voluntary motor commands, and the storing and processing of long-term memory as well as conscious sensory and motor memory.

The cerebrum is divided into two hemispheres, each having four lobes (frontal, parietal, occipital, and temporal). Each hemisphere receives ascending sensory input from and generates descending motor

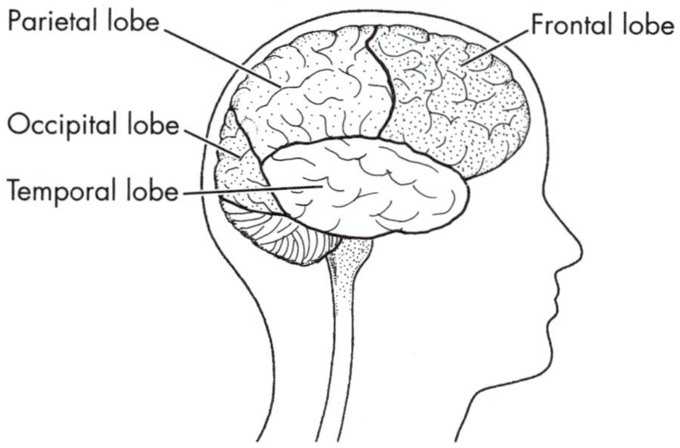

commands to the opposite side of the body, so that the right hemisphere controls the left side of the body and the left hemisphere controls the right. In addition, each lobe contains functional regions associated with the conscious perception of specific sensory information (in the form of touch, sight, sound, smell, and taste) and motor commands (including voluntary control of the skeletal muscles).

The prefrontal lobe of the cerebrum coordinates and analyzes the vast quantity of data received from the senses, and under normal circumstances dictates our responses and contains the perspective we have of ourselves and the external world that surrounds us.

3. *The limbic system* is specifically concerned with learning, memory, and with the emotions and their related behavioral drives. But, of even more importance to our consideration of Yoga therapy, *the limbic system provides the link between the conscious, intellectual functions of the brain and the unconscious, mechanical functions of the body.*

Structurally, the limbic system is located on the border between the seat of conscious functioning (the cerebrum) and the seat of unconscious functioning (the brain stem and cerebellum). One part of the limbic brain (including hippocampus and amygdala) connects directly to the cerebrum; the other part (including thalamus and hypothalamus) connects directly to the brain stem and cerebellum.

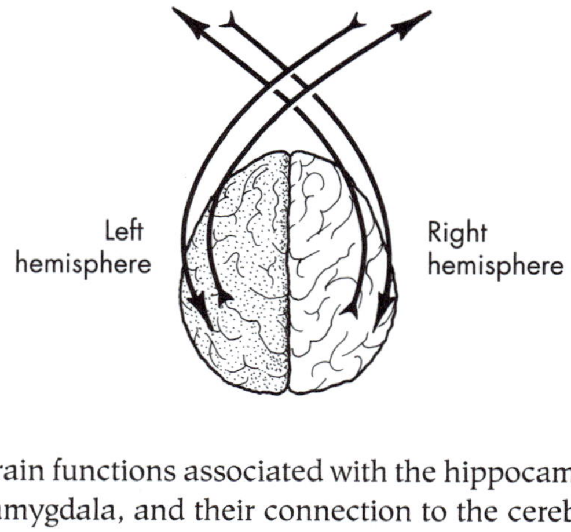

Brain functions associated with the hippocampus, the amygdala, and their connection to the cerebrum appear to be as follows: The hippocampus imprints and subsequently retrieves memory concerned with information. The amygdala imprints and subsequently retrieves memory concerned with emotion, and, in turn, it controls and triggers emotional response. Via the circuit created by the connection between the amygdala and the prefrontal cortex of the cerebrum, thought and emotion are linked. And, via certain direct-circuit links between the amygdala and thalamus, in certain cases, emotional response is directly triggered by sensory input, bypassing the cerebrum and, therefore, avoiding processing by the conscious mind altogether.*

Brain functions associated with the thalamus, the hypothalamus, and their connection with the cerebellum appear to be as follows: The thalamus receives ascending sensory information on its way to processing in the appropriate area of the cerebral cortex. The hypothalamus processes information concerning changing emotional states and related behavioral drives. Through its connection to the brain stem, the hypothalamus directly links the changing emotional states to the nervous and endocrine systems, which, in turn, control and regulate the other organic processes of the body. And, as a result of this connection, imbalances in other systems of the body can also effect hypothalamic activity, producing strong emotion and influencing thought.

Our understanding of the structure and function of the limbic brain continues to grow as neuroscientists become progressively more sophisticated in mapping brain circuitry, and particularly in mapping the pathways of emotional response within the brain. However, we now know for certain that all sensory input (including externally related seeing, hearing, touching, tasting, and smelling, and internally related sensations of the visceral and other internal bodily parts) passes through the limbic brain on its way to the cerebrum for analysis, and back again through the limbic brain, where appropriate responses are regulated via the hypothalamus. It is now clear to neuroscientists that all parts of the brain and nervous system are connected to and converge in the limbic brain.**

*Daniel Goleman, *Emotional Intelligence* (New York: Bantam Books, 1995), pp. 15–32.

**Richard E. Cytowic, *The Man Who Tasted Shapes* (New York: Tarcher/Putnam, 1993), p. 161.

Stress and Disease

The bodily response to stress initiated in the hypothalamus, known as the fight-or-flight response, involves a chain reaction of chemicals released into the bloodstream, as follows: corticotropin-releasing factor (CRF) is released from the hypothalamus; CRF then triggers the release of adrenocorticotropin hormone (ATCH) from the pituitary gland; and, finally, ATCH triggers the release of adrenaline and cortisol from the adrenal glands. The results of this chain reaction are an increase in alertness, muscle tone, heart rate, and blood pressure; a heightening of all sensory reflexes; a deepening of respiration; an increase in the peripheral circulation of blood to the skeletal muscles, as digestion stops and the flow of blood is directed away from the stomach and intestines; a release of red blood cells from the spleen into the bloodstream in order to help supply increased oxygen to the muscles and to aid in the removal of residual carbon dioxide; and a whole range of other complex bodily changes.

Through this mechanism, the body is able to cope with stress and, therefore, to survive. However, if, through chronic physical and/or mental stress, this mechanism is habitually engaged, the result is a depression of the immune response and a weakening of the entire system.* In each of us there exists a unique set of triggering devices, related to how we perceive any given situation. This explains why people respond differently to the same situation because, as Patañjali points out, each of us comes to our experiences with a different set of memories and associations. Depending on those particular memories and associations, any experience can elicit a whole range of emotion—from pleasure to fear. For example, I remember being relaxed and comfortable one night while walking in a dark and quiet but familiar wooded area with a friend from the city, who, unlike myself, was extremely anxious at being in an unfamiliar place and away from the lights and sounds to which he was accustomed. But, whether the source of stress is internal, external, psychological, physical, or some combination of these factors (which is usually the case), it is clear that the link between conscious mind and unconscious body re-

*Deane Juhan, *Job's Body* (Stanton Hill Press, 1987), pp. 309–330.

sponses work in both directions. On the one hand, cerebral activity can directly trigger emotional response, and emotion can stimulate response in the autonomic system. On the other hand, changes in our physiology—due, for example, to hormonal cycles, illness, toxicity, or drugs—can trigger emotional responses that, in turn, influence thought.

Recognition of this fact has led to the development of the relatively new field of psychoneuroimmunology, which studies the links between mind (including thought and emotion), physiology (beginning with the nervous and endocrine systems), and the immune system. The results of the research carried out in this field point to a strong link between state of mind (including habits of thought and emotional response) and physical health; and there is mounting evidence to suggest that people who remain in chronic states of stress and emotional disturbance have a significantly higher incidence of disease, including digestive, respiratory, and cardiovascular.

Ancient Insights for Modern Healing

With the development of new fields such as psychoneuroimmunology, modern science is beginning to confirm what the ancient yogis have recognized for thousands of years: disturbing emotions play a primary role in disease; and, therefore, emotional health is fundamental to the maintenance of health in the physical body. According to Yoga theory, the objects of the senses are like food: the right kind of sensory stimulus is nourishing; the wrong kind is toxic. When the end result of the complex interactions we have been exploring are pleasing sensations, there is a calming and nourishing effect on body, emotion, and thought; when they are unpleasant, there is a sense of disruption. For example, a singing bird or a gently murmuring stream is usually relaxing and restorative, while a violently vibrating jackhammer or excessively loud music often produces anxiety and stress.

The ancient masters developed complete sciences, related to the senses, to help correct imbalances and nourish our systems. For example, the Āyurvedic culinary arts relating to the sense of taste, aromatherapy relating to the sense of smell, color therapy relating to the sense of sight, and traditions of chanting and music relating to the sense of hearing. In addition, the ancient masters recognized the following negative attitudes as particularly overwhelming and tending toward dysfunctional behavior:

Kama: obsessive desire, lust
Krodha: anger, hostility
Lobha: greed, possessiveness
Moha: delusion, self-deception
Matsarya: jealousy, resentment
Mada: arrogance
Bhaya: fear, anxiety

According to the teaching of Krishnamacharya, all these negative emotions stem from the two root attitudes of *ahaṃ* ("I am the doer") and *mama* ("it is for me"); and only when the attitude becomes that of *namama* ("not by or for me") do negative emotions cease to arise. In other words, in terms of our *Voyager* analogy, until we can stop revolving in endless circles of emotional drama and misapprehension around the limiting self-concepts of the conditioned mind, we remain either crashed into or trapped within the narrow confines of the little "me" and, therefore, are fundamentally unable to achieve our own higher potential.

To counteract these attitudes and the limitations they impose, the ancient yogis also taught the importance of *śraddhā* (faith), and where śraddhā was not present, they stressed the value of association with good people (*sat sangha*) and the cultivation of right attitudes, including friendliness toward those who are happy, compassion toward those who are suffering, joy in relation to good actions of others, and equanimity in relation to wrong actions of others.

But most important, on the basis of their understanding of the interconnectedness of all things, they developed the art and science of affecting overall change in our system through the various techniques of Yoga, including āsana, prāṇāyāma, chanting, and meditation. Understanding the direct influence of habits of thought and emotion on biochemistry, and knowing that positive states have a deeply restorative impact on the entire system, they were able to develop certain practices to transform negative qualities of mind and to promote general well-being as a basis for spiritual development.

The effectiveness of the technology they developed has been repeatedly demonstrated by scientific studies. For example, in states of deep meditation, the heart and respiratory rates consistently slow down; the overall metabolic rate drops; as the metabolic rate drops, muscular tension decreases and blood flow increases to the muscles; and the result is a positive influence on biochemistry and an improvement in the overall condition of health—all of which strongly suggests that by changing our state of mind, we can affect an overall qualitative change in our lives.*

Prāṇāyāma

According to theories in neuroscience, the evolutionary origin of the limbic system is linked to the sense of smell and can be traced to that part of the limbic brain known as the olfactory lobe.** It is primarily through the sense of smell that animals identify danger, food, or sexual partners; and it was from the olfactory lobe, in its most primitive form, that reflexive messages were sent to the rest of the nervous system, initiating appropriate behavioral responses. The limbic system still forms the "emotional core" of our own vastly more complex brains and, as we have seen, still has the capacity to powerfully influence and even override the rationality of the cerebral cortex.***

The ancient masters specifically developed the practice of *prāṇāyāma* (regulation of the breath) to balance the emotions, clarify the mental processes, and ultimately to integrate them into one effectively functioning whole. In light of what we now know about the close connections between the various structures of the limbic brain and the prefrontal lobes of the cerebral cortex, it is interesting to speculate about exactly what the ancients actually did understand concerning the power of prāṇāyāma.

*Juhan, *Job's Body,* pp. 309–330.
**Goleman, *Emotional Intelligence,* p. 11.
***Cytowic, *The Man Who Tasted Shapes,* p. 162.

Though a full treatment of the complex and highly evolved science of prāṇāyāma is beyond the scope of this work, it is interesting to note that the practice of prāṇāyāma has a significant impact on the olfactory lobe and, in this way, on the limbic brain. In fact, the ancient masters taught that states of physical and emotional arousal or nonarousal can be regulated via control of the breath at the nostrils. Specifically: inhaling through the right nostril and exhaling through the left (*sūrya bhedana*) is said to activate or stimulate our system; and inhaling through the left nostril and exhaling through the right (*candra bhedana*) is said to calm, soothe, and pacify our system. We can also use both inhalation (brahmaṇa) and exhalation (langhana) techniques to stimulate or soothe our systems respectively; and we use different ratios between the various parts of the breathing cycle—i.e., between inhale, retention after inhale, exhale, and suspension of the breath after exhale—to achieve very specific degrees and types of stimulation and pacification. A detailed exploration of this fascinating and profound science will be the topic of a later work.

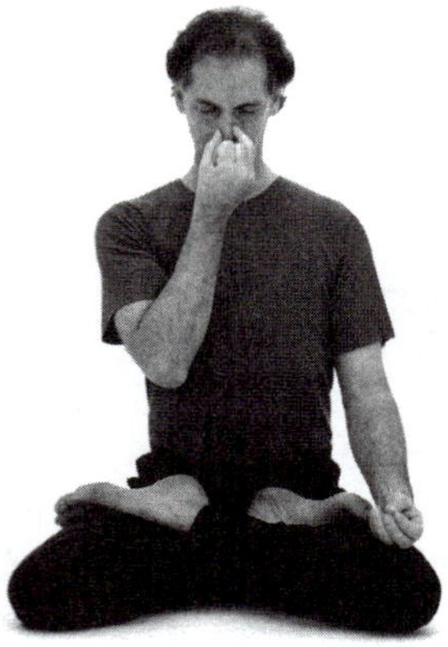

One thing is certain: the ancient masters knew how to use prāṇāyāma techniques to "remove that which covers the light of the mind" (YS, 2:52). In other words, they knew the power of prāṇāyāma to balance and clarify the emotions so that they support rather than obstruct the unfolding of our highest potential.

Yoga Therapy and Mental Illness

Although the whole question of mental illness is very complex and is not our focus here, the following generally recognized conditions of mental aberration are suggestive of the types of problems and range of effects that are often involved:

> *Neuroses:* a wide range of psychological and behavioral responses whose common denominator is anxiety. These vary in seriousness and can impair both work, social adjustment, and health.
>
> *Schizophrenia:* a psychosis marked by progressive withdrawal from reality, grossly inappropriate behavior, aberrations of thought, discrepancies between thought content and mood, delusions or hallucinations, et cetera.
>
> *Depression:* varies from normal reactions to the sorrows of life to serious mood disturbance that can lead even to suicide. Full-blown depression involves weight loss, decreased sexual desire, difficulty sleeping, excessive fatigue, chronic pain or complaints about pain, headaches, a sense of worthlessness, and difficulty concentrating.

Many times conditions of mental and emotional illness have their basis in brain chemistry. When this is the case, the problem is often related to an abnormal concentration of neurotransmitters—the chemicals that trigger and block impulses concerned with the flow and regulation of motor and sensory input to the brain and, therefore, that regulate the nervous system. Other biological causes include the following: certain disorders of the nervous, endocrine, cardiovascular, and respiratory systems; infectious diseases; use of drugs (whether illicit, over-the-counter, or prescription); poor dietary habits; and environmental toxicity and other environmental factors.

A psychiatrist once told me that if a troubling emotional condition is psychologically based, then the appropriate treatment is one of several of a variety of psychotherapeutic technologies; but if that condition is biochemically based, though psychotherapeutic technologies may be helpful, the most appropriate treatment is pharmacological. Our point of view is that the integrative approach of Yoga therapy, working at the level of the body, breath, and mind through the practice of āsana, prāṇāyāma, and meditation, is very effective as an adjunct to any treatment plan. In fact, science has demonstrated the effectiveness of meditation in this regard, and while prāṇāyāma has received little attention from science, we have seen again and again its power with disturbed people to help balance emotion and even to reduce dependence on psychiatric medication.

Although a well-conceived Yoga therapy practice may be helpful in any condition, where there is genetically or disease-based biochemical abnormality, we recommend seeking professional psychiatric or medical care. In this section on emotional health, we are primarily addressing the vast majority of "normally neurotic" people, who have minor to serious emotional imbalance, and for whom Yoga therapy can function as a temporary method of symptom reduction so that they can begin the work of permanently removing the cause of their problems. The ancient teachings on this deeper work have been given to us by Patañjali, in the science of *Kriya Yoga,* which we will explore in detail in our next book.

The Three Primary Energies

According to Yoga theory, our emotional condition fluctuates between states of balance, excess, and deficiency. The ancient yogis explained these states as a result of the predominance of one of the three primary energies (*guṇas*) that are the fundamental constituents of the universal material substance (prakṛti) that makes up the world of the "seen": *sattvic* (balanced), *rajasic* (excessive), and *tamasic* (deficient). And they developed a highly evolved science around these states in relationship to health and disease.

The *sattva guṇa* can be characterized as an energy of balance, harmony, and equilibrium. When it is predominant, and all of the systems of our body and mind are in balance, there is an optimal level of mental clarity, physical health, emotional serenity, and creative inspiration. The sattvic quality of mind can be described as a neutral state of relaxed present awareness; it is described in the Yoga tradition as luminous and clear, and it represents one of the most important goals of Yoga practice.

The attitudes and emotions considered to be sattvic include appreciation, awe, bliss, compassion, contentment, courage, forgiveness, friendliness, goodness, happiness, honesty, joy, kindness, love, patience, peace, serenity, stability, tenderness, tolerance, and wonder. In fact, the emotions of happiness and joy have been scientifically demonstrated to increase the presence of white blood cells and the levels of the antibody immunoglobulin A (IgA), both of which are fundamental to the immune response.*

Anger and Anxiety

The *rajo guna* can be characterized as an energy of activity and creativity. When it predominates, however, it may lead to hyperactive, aggressive behavior, and an inability to control energy in difficult and unpleasant situations. The rajasic quality of mind can be described as a state of agitation. Because unbalanced rajasic energy can lead to violence and other extreme actions that cause suffering both to ourselves and others, it is important to know how to rectify an unbalanced rajasic condition.

Anger can be considered an example of a rajasic emotion. There are many different degrees and kinds of anger, ranging from quiet brooding anger to explosive rage and even violence. The following attitudes and emotions can be included under the general heading of anger: animosity, annoyance, aversion, criticism, cruelty, enmity, hostility, hatred, impatience, indignation, irritation, rage, resentment, violence, and wrath. In any form, strong states of anger trigger the fight-or-flight response, providing the body with a chemical rush that readies it for appropriate or inappropriate response to a given situation.

Anger is impulsive; it leads to a short reaction threshold; and it too often has negative effects on our relationships and on our health. Studies show that heart disease is the direct result of chronic states of anger and hostility; that such states are particularly dangerous for those who already suffer from heart disease; and that anger and hostility represent a particular risk to men. They also show that anger depresses the levels of the antibody immunoglobulin A (IgA), which is fundamental to the immune response.*

Once we recognize that we are in a state of anger, it is possible to defuse it. One way is to use a langhana prāṇāyāma practice to regulate the breathing. For example, by sitting down and focusing on where the breathing starts and where it ends, and by practicing a long exhale and short suspension of the breath after exhale for some time, the tendency to impulsive reaction will be reduced. Because this is a technique to manage, and not suppress emotion, apply the technique and notice what actually happens in your system. Generally, the efftect of this technique will be soothing. Finally, when the anger has subsided, continue using the breathing technique while reflecting on and reevaluating the situation that led to your anger. Because this is a *pratipakṣa* technique (what modern psychology knows as "cognitive reframing") and, therefore, involves reconditioning, once the reaction is over and has been restructured in your mind, your initial anger may even look silly to you.

*Doc Lew Childre, *Freeze Frame* (Boulder Creek, California: Planetary Publications, 1994), pp. 48–53.

*Doc Lew Childre, *Freeze Frame*, pp. 48–53.

Anxiety is another rajasic emotion. There are many different degrees and kinds of anxiety, ranging from chronic, mild worry to obsessive-compulsive disorder to full-blown panic attack. The following attitudes and emotions can be included under the general heading of anxiety: agitation, apprehension, compulsiveness, concern, dread, edginess, fear, horror, insecurity, nervousness, obsessiveness, panic, paranoia, phobia, surprise, terror, uneasiness, wariness, and worry. In any form, strong states of anxiety, like strong states of anger, trigger the fight-or-flight response and can manifest symptoms of sweating, accelerated heart beat, tightness in the belly, muscle tension, shakiness of the limbs, inability to be still or to concentrate, shortness of breath, and insomnia. Increased muscle tension and decreased circulation to the areas of tension are the result of pressure on the capillaries, which together cause an increase in lactic acid.* Lactic acid, in turn, causes muscle fatigue, a tendency toward muscle cramping, and an increase in stress to the liver. Extensive research conclusively links states of anxiety to depressed immune function; to increased susceptibility to gastrointestinal problems, such as IBD and IBS; to infectious disease, such as colds and flus; to respiratory conditions, such as asthma; to the onset of type I and type II diabetes; and even to the metastasis of cancer. Although evidence supports a link between anger and hostility and heart disease in men, in women heart disease is more strongly linked to states of fear and anxiety. There is also evidence suggesting that in many cases anxiety has a genetic component and/or is based in biochemical imbalance.**

In practice, we must make a distinction between normal tension and anxiety and those pathological conditions that reflect a biological disorder rather than a psychological one. For example, where there are serious and persistent conditions of anxiety, obsessive-compulsive disorder, panic attacks, or post-traumatic stress disorder, it is best to seek professional psychiatric help.

One way to reduce anxiety is to use a brahmaṇa/langhana strategy to reduce the hyperarousal in the mind and the subsequent stress in the body. First create a level of physical activity equal to the level of bodily stimulation generated by mental anxiety. Once the muscular and respiratory activity has reached a sufficient level, gradually slow the movement down and introduce deep, slow breathing. We also recommend the use of sound techniques to help shift attention away from anxiety-producing thoughts; and, after that, we recommend either meditation or prayer, depending on one's inclination.

In addition, the support, caring, and touch of loved ones is an invaluable remedy to any condition in which the rajo guṇa is predominant. Finally, in these conditions, we suggest avoiding alcohol, tobacco, and caffeine; we recommend spending time in nature; and, if there is little sunlight, we also recommend sitting in front of a full-spectrum light box for at least twenty minutes each day.

Conditions of anxiety are as variable as the people who suffer from them, and, as we have seen, a Yoga therapy practice is ideally adapted to the uniqueness of each individual. The sequence that follows offers an example of working with conditions of chronic anxiety and, though not prescriptive, is indicative of an approach to these conditions.

*Juhan, *Job's Body*, p. 321.
**Mark S. Gold, *The Good News About Panic, Anxiety, and Phobias* (New York: Bantam Books, 1990), p. 45.

Working with Chronic Anxiety

C.S. was a forty-year-old artist when she first came to our school to study Yoga many years ago. She had been married for a long time, though she had no children. She attended group classes consistently for several years. C.S. was always attentive to the needs of others in the class and had a quality of kindness that was felt and appreciated by all. She was soft spoken and somewhat self-effacing.

I was very surprised, one day, when she told me in private that she could no longer come to class. She had a strange expression on her face and told me in a quiet voice that she couldn't take it anymore. I had no idea what she was talking about. Then it began to come out that she felt that the other members of the class had a bad opinion of her, and that they talked about her behind her back. Fortunately she did not include me in this group. She told me that I must be aware of how the conversation in the room shifted when she arrived, and how the other people looked at each other with little, knowing smiles.

I asked C.S. if she was interested to continue her studies with me in private, and she said yes. She came to see me once a week for nearly a year. Over time, it came out that she had been in a group of artists many years earlier and finally had to leave for the same reasons. I assured her that everybody in this group had a very high opinion of her, and she had their love and respect. Her initial reaction was almost a bit angry, and she couldn't understand why I was hiding the truth from her. So for many months we simply dropped the discussion and focused on her personal practice.

Over the years, she had never complained of discomfort in her body. She did occasionally complain that her breath was shallow and that she had trouble sleeping. Though she didn't experience pain in her body, she was not strong. And she lacked confidence in herself. She told me that she had difficulty being around large groups of people and that she preferred being alone. C.S. confessed that she couldn't go out to the market without anxiety about what other people were thinking and saying to each other about her. She also told me that she had reached an impasse in her work ad had not been able to get beyond it.

My initial strategy included a brahmaṇa āsana practice to strengthen her body and deepen her breathing capacity, and a langhana prāṇāyāma practice to help balance and stabilize her emotional state. I hoped that strengthening her body would also help increase her self-confidence.

C.S. lived in a valley that bordered on state forest. Near her house were paths that led up into the mountains. We developed the following practice, which I asked her to do in the early morning, followed by a brisk hike in the forest before beginning her day.

In my conversations with C.S., I learned that she had a strong and positive memory of her deceased grandmother—who had been a devout Catholic. One day she told me that she had a dream in which she was a little girl and was with her grandmother, who was reading to her. I asked her if she remembered what her grandmother was reading, and she said it was her grandmother's favorite psalm.

I asked C.S. to bring her Bible to her next class, and we read the psalm together. It was the famous Psalm 23, which begins "The Lord is my shepard, I shall not want." In the middle of the psalm is the line "Yea, though I walk through the valley of the shadow of death, I will fear no evil: for thou art with me." We decided to integrate that psalm into her practice. I asked C.S. to read the psalm before each practice and, so she could feel as if she were not alone, to use the words "thou art with me" as a mantra to count certain parts of her breath throughout the practice. She told me how this added element took her practice much deeper, and how much it meant to her.

I left my home in Hawaii to work in the continental United States and in Europe for about four months. While I was away, she practiced the sequence that follows. One evening, after returning home, C.S., whom I had not seen for about five months, arrived for a group class. It was the same class that she used to attend, and many of the friends were very happy to see her. After class, she told me that she had taken a job in an art gallery and, through some connections there, had got a big commission for her own artwork. She told me that she was feeling stronger and more confident, and happy to be back in class.

A Practice for Chronic Anxiety

1.

POSTURE: Dvipāda Piṭham.
EMPHASIS: To warm up the body by engaging thighs and buttocks.
TECHNIQUE: Lie on back with arms down at sides, knees bent, and feet on floor, slightly apart and comfortably close to buttocks.

On inhale: Pressing down on feet and keeping chin down, raise pelvis until neck is gently flattened on floor.

On exhale: Return to starting position.

NUMBER: 6 times.
DETAILS: *On inhale:* Lift spine, vertebra by vertebra, from bottom up. *On exhale:* Unwind spine, coming down vertebra by vertebra.

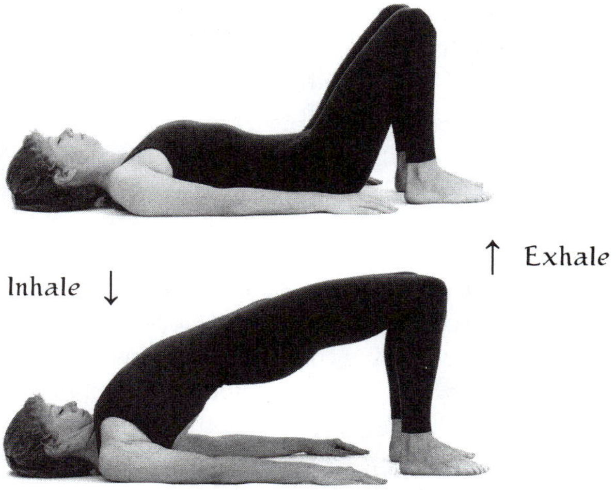

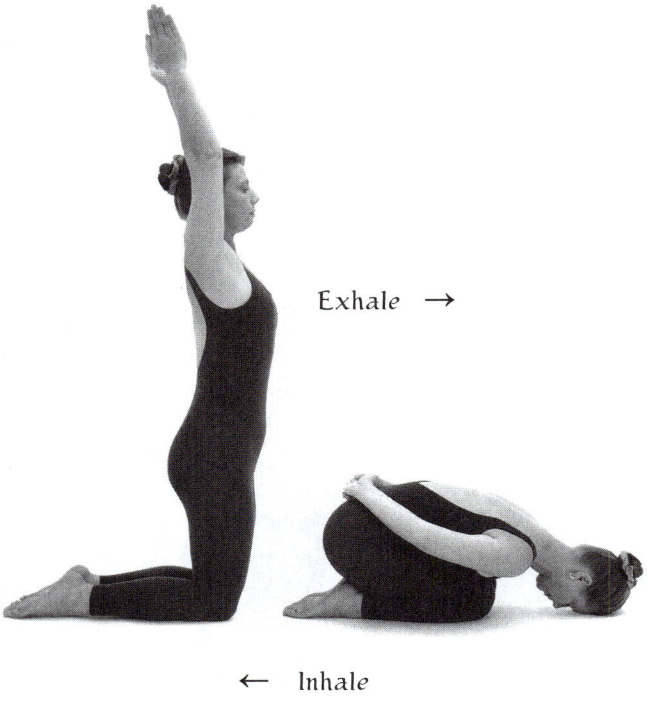

2.

POSTURE: Vajrāsana.
EMPHASIS: To make transition from supine to standing. To stretch low back.
TECHNIQUE: Stand on knees with arms over head.

On exhale: Bend forward, sweeping arms behind back, bringing hands to sacrum with palms up.

On inhale: Return to starting position.

NUMBER: 8 times.
DETAILS: *On exhale:* Bring chest to thighs before buttocks to heels. Rotate arms so palms are up and hands rest on sacrum. *On inhale:* Expand chest and lift it up off knees as arms sweep wide.

3.

Posture: Vīrabhadrāsana.

Emphasis: To build energy, strengthen muscles of back, expand chest and flatten upper back, increase hold after inhalation, and strengthen leg muscles.

Technique: Stand with left foot forward, feet as wide as hips, and arms at sides.

On inhale: Simultaneously, bend left knee, displace chest slightly forward and hips slightly backward, and bring arms out to sides and shoulders back.

On hold after inhale: Mentally recite **thou art with me**.

On exhale: Return to starting position.

Number: 6 times each side.

Details: *On inhale:* Keep hands and elbows in line with shoulders. Feel opening of chest and flattening of upper back, not compression in low back. Keep head forward. Stay firm on back heel. *On hold after inhale:* Recite mantra twice for the first two repetitions, three times for the second two repetitions, and four times for the last two repetitions.

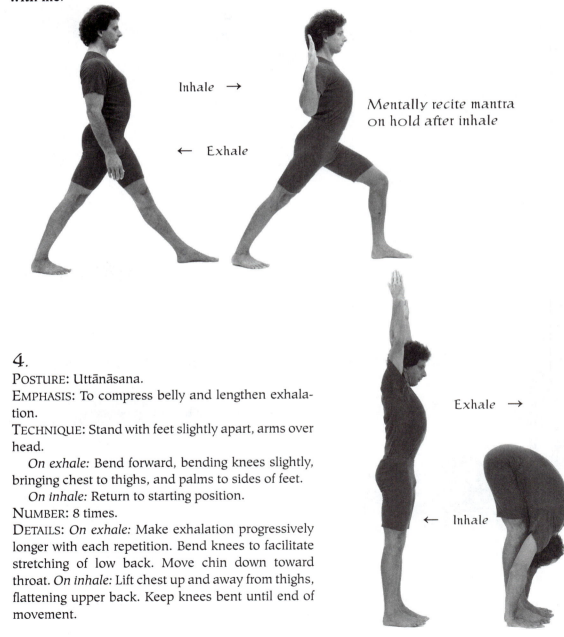

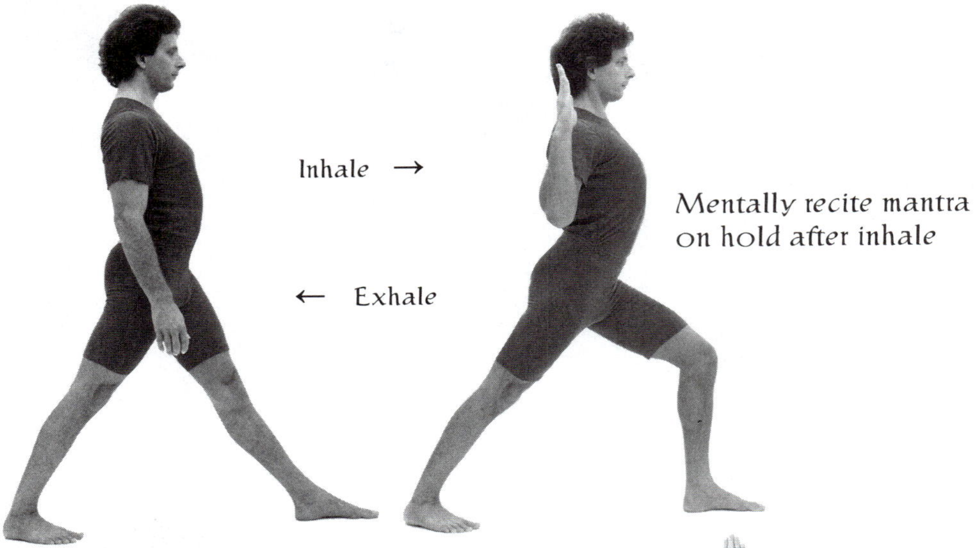

4.

Posture: Uttānāsana.

Emphasis: To compress belly and lengthen exhalation.

Technique: Stand with feet slightly apart, arms over head.

On exhale: Bend forward, bending knees slightly, bringing chest to thighs, and palms to sides of feet.

On inhale: Return to starting position.

Number: 8 times.

Details: *On exhale:* Make exhalation progressively longer with each repetition. Bend knees to facilitate stretching of low back. Move chin down toward throat. *On inhale:* Lift chest up and away from thighs, flattening upper back. Keep knees bent until end of movement.

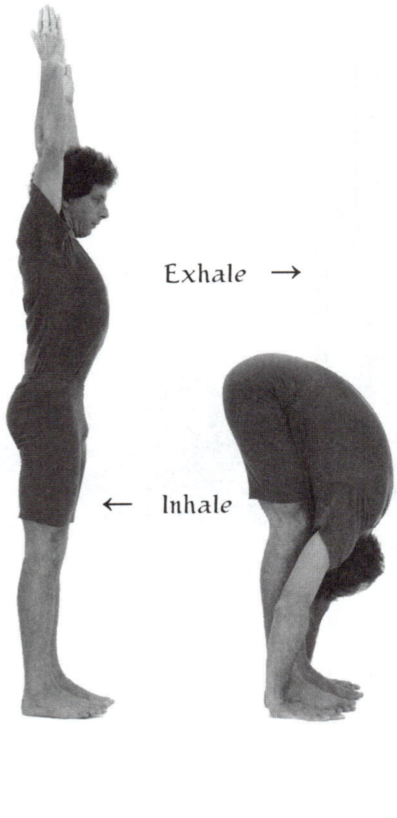

5.

Posture: Vajrāsana/Ūrdhva Mukha Śvānāsana combination.
Emphasis: To energize system by engaging musculature of upper body, expanding chest, and stretching belly.
Technique: From a kneeling forward bend position, place hands on ground in front of body.

On inhale: Stretch body forward and arch back, keeping only hands and from knees to feet on floor.

On hold after inhale: Mentally recite **thou art with me**.

On exhale: Return to starting position.

Number: 6 times.
Details: *On inhale:* Expand chest, stretch belly, and avoid compressing low back. *On hold after inhale:* Mentally recite mantra twice for the first two repetitions, three times for the second two repetitions, and four times for the last two repetitions. End in forward bend position.

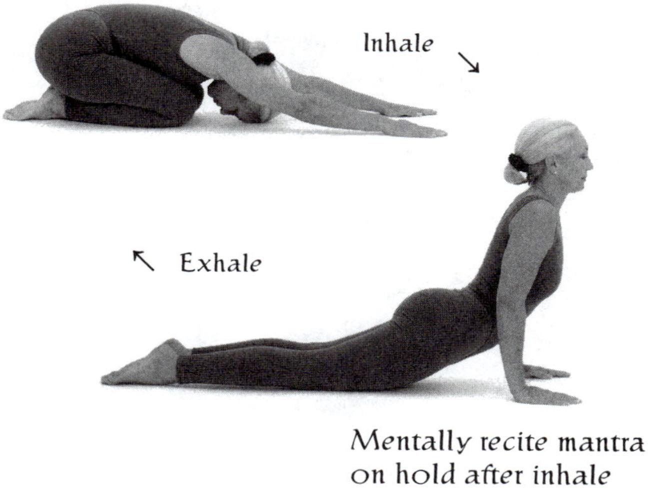

6.

Posture: Bhujaṅgāsana.
Emphasis: To engage big muscles of back, stimulating movement of energy in body.
Technique:

A: Lie on belly, head turned to right, with hands crossed over sacrum and palms up.

On inhale: Lift chest and right arm, turning head to center.

On exhale: Lower chest, sweeping arm behind back and turning head to left.

Repeat on other side.

B: From starting position:

On inhale: Raise both arms up.

On exhale: Bend elbows back towards ribs, and lift chest higher.

On inhale: Straighten arms again.

On exhale: return to starting position.

Number: A four times each side, alternately. B four times.
Details: *On inhale:* Keep knees and feet on floor. B: *On exhale,* Keep palms and elbows level at shoulder height.

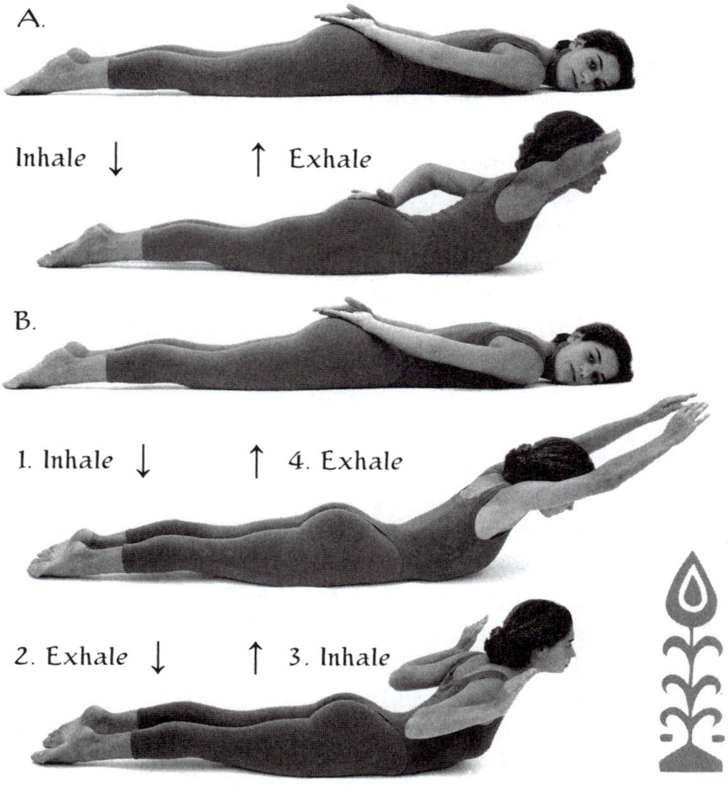

7.

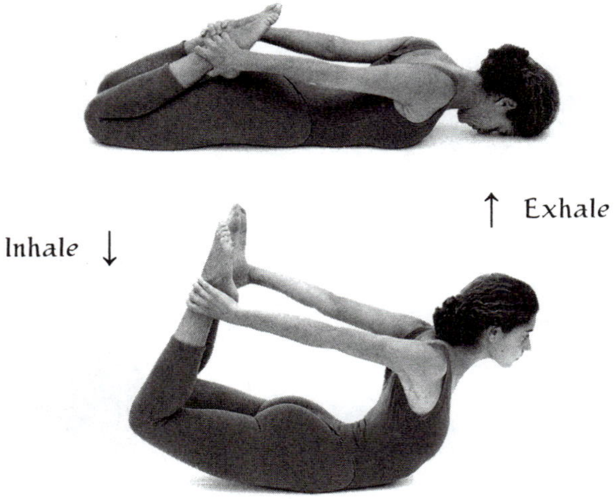

Mentally recite mantra on hold after inhale

POSTURE: Dhanurāsana.
EMPHASIS: To stretch and expand chest, deepen inhale, and strengthen back and legs.
TECHNIQUE: Lie on stomach, resting on forehead, with knees bent and hands grasping ankles.

On inhale: Simultaneously, press feet behind you, pull shoulders back, lift chest, and lift knees off ground.

On hold after inhale: Mentally recite **thou art with me**.

On exhale: Return to starting position.

NUMBER: 6 times.
DETAILS: *On inhale:* Lift head forward, but do not collapse it backward. Keep knees not too wide. *On hold after inhale:* Recite mantra twice for the first two repetitions, three times for the second two repetitions, and four times for the last two repetitions.

8.

POSTURE: Cakravākāsana.
EMPHASIS: To stretch low back. To make transition from prone to sitting position.
TECHNIQUE: Get down on hands and knees, with shoulders vertically above wrists and with hips above knees.

On inhale: Lift chest up and away from belly.

On exhale: Move hips back and down towards heels, lowering chest towards thighs.

NUMBER: 8 times.
DETAILS: *On inhale:* Lead with chest, keeping chin slightly down. Avoid compressing low back; rather, feel chest expanding. *On exhale:* Let chest lower toward thighs sooner than hips toward heels.

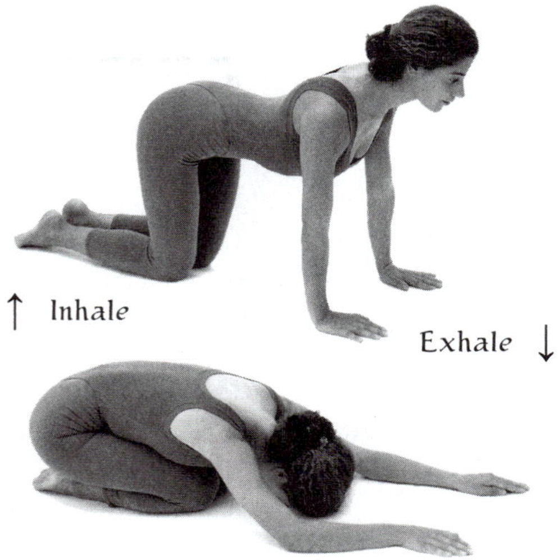

9.

POSTURE: Nāvāsana/Paścimatānāsana combination.
EMPHASIS: To stimulate and strengthen abdomen and low back. To stretch low back and legs.
TECHNIQUE: Sit with legs forward, back straight, and arms raised over head.

On exhale: Lean backward, lifting legs off floor and lowering arms, palms together, until parallel to floor.

On hold after exhale: Mentally recite **thou art with me**.

On inhale: Return to starting position.

On exhale: Bend forward, bending knees slightly, bringing chest to thighs, and palms to balls of feet.

Stay 2 breaths.

On inhale: Return to starting position.

NUMBER: 3 times.

DETAILS: Nāvāsana: Keep low back rounded, eyes and toes at same level, and torso to legs at an angle greater than ninety degrees. *On hold after exhale:* Recite mantra twice for the first two repetitions, three times for the second two repetitions, and four times for the last two repetitions. Paścimatānāsana: Relax low back and belly.

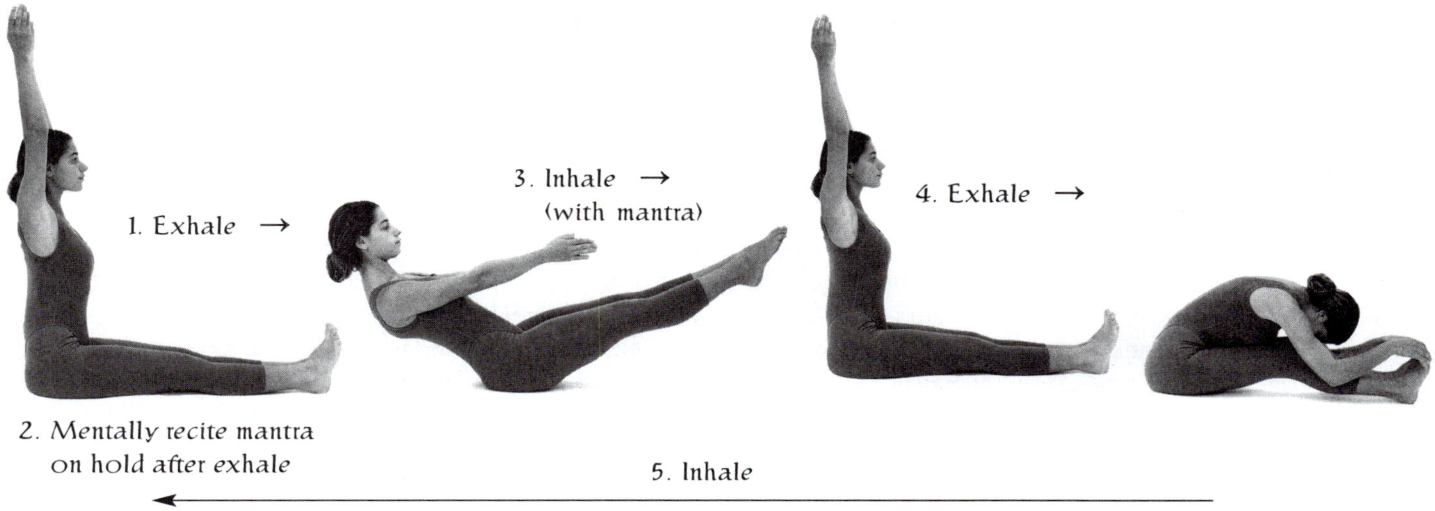
1. Exhale →
3. Inhale →
(with mantra)
4. Exhale →
2. Mentally recite mantra
on hold after exhale
5. Inhale

10.

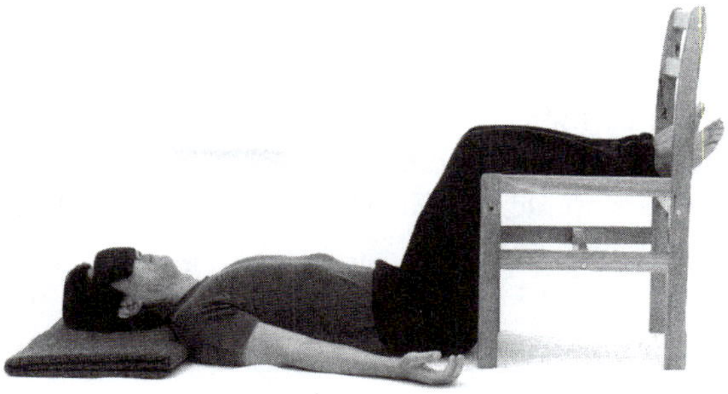

POSTURE: Śavāsana with support.
EMPHASIS: To rest.
TECHNIQUE: Lie flat on back, with arms at sides, palms up, and legs resting comfortably on a chair. Cover eyes. Relax body fully, keeping mind relaxed and alert to sensations in body.
DURATION: Minimum 3 to 5 minutes.
EMPHASIS: To progressively lengthen and then shorten hold after inhale.

11.

POSTURE: Prāṇāyāma, Antaḥ Kumbhaka.
EMPHASIS: To progressively lengthen and then shorten hold after exhale.
To use **thou art with me** on hold after inhale.
TECHNIQUE:
A: Establish deep and equal inhale and exhale, with no breath retention.
B: Initiate and extend length of retention after inhale by mentally reciting two more mantras every two breaths, increasing from two repetitions to six progressively.
C: Reverse the process from six repetitions back to two.
D: Repeat A.

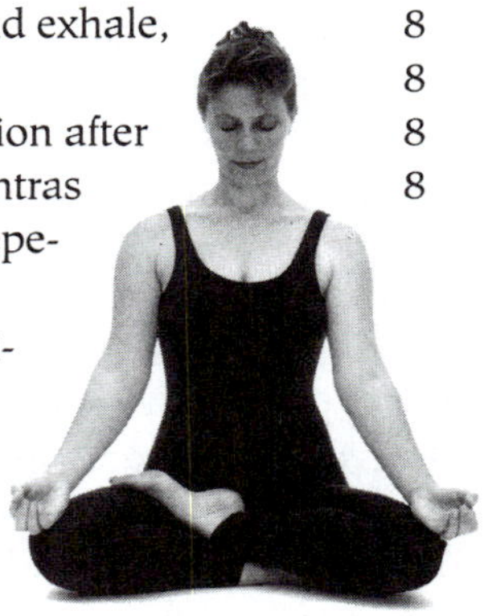

With mantra

DETAILS:

Inhale	*Hold*	*Exhale*	*Hold*	*Number*
8	0	12	0	4
8	2	12	0	4
8	4	12	0	4
8	6	12	0	4
8	4	12	0	4
8	2	12	0	4
8	0	12	0	4

Depression

The *tamo guṇa* can be characterized as a force of stability. When it predominates, however, a great inertia sets in. When this happens, situations that are difficult or unpleasant lead to feelings of helplessness, depression, and, in extreme cases, to drug addiction or even death. The tamasic quality of mind can be described as a state of dullness. Because in this condition there is no movement and no motivation to do anything, what is required is a shift of focus and an awakening of interest that can activate our energy.

Depression can be considered an example of a tamasic emotion. There are many different degrees and kinds of depression, ranging from a lack of direction and purpose in life; to grief due to loss; to chronic sadness, low self-esteem, or helplessness; to an acute clinical depression that can even lead to suicide. The following attitudes and emotions can be included under the general heading of depression: complacency, dejection, despair, disappointment, emptiness, gloom, grief, hopelessness, loneliness, melancholy, sadness, sorrow, self-pity, and shame. Depression differs from anger and anxiety in a fundamental way: while in both anger and anxiety, the body is flooded with the chemicals characteristic of the fight-or-flight response, in depression there is a low level of certain neurotransmitters, such as norepinephrine and serotonin. Genetic research indicates that certain types of depression are inherited; but, whatever the cause, there is mounting evidence that depression significantly inhibits recovery from illness, disease, and surgical procedures. Depression and the other emotions mentioned above are characterized by a loss of energy, appetite, interest, and enthusiasm and are marked by a slowing down of the body's metabolic rate.

A certain amount of depression is a normal reaction to the inevitable losses we suffer in life. However, abnormal or clinical depression is actually a serious illness and often leads to suicide. Thus, when recurring suicidal thoughts are present, it is best to seek professional psychiatric help.

One way to work with depression is to use a brahmaṇa/langhana strategy. First, brahmaṇa postures are used to increase physical activity and energy in the body and to raise the spirit; then langhana prāṇāyāma is used to reduce mental activity, especially the flow of negative thoughts, and to soothe the mind. This is particularly useful when the depression is accompanied by anxiety. Another appropriate method is that of pratipakṣa—a method for assuming another point of view, which corresponds to cognitive reframing and is suggested by Patañjali. For example, a normally self-critical person would begin to recognize and focus on his/her positive qualities.

Other suggestions include getting involved in charitable work, helping others who are less fortunate; playing with or teaching young children, who are generally light and happy; and, if there is faith, getting more involved in prayer and/or a spiritual community. In addition, as with anger and anxiety, the support, caring, and touch of loved ones is an invaluable remedy to any condition in which the tamo guṇa is predominant. Finally, we also recommend that people suffering from depression avoid alcohol and refined sugar, spend time in nature, and, if their environments have a shortage of sunlight, use full-spectrum lights.

As with anxiety, conditions of depression are as variable as the people who suffer from them, and, as we have seen, a Yoga therapy practice is ideally adapted to the uniqueness of each individual. The sequence that follows offers an example of working with conditions of chronic depression and, though not prescriptive, is indicative of an approach to these conditions.

Working with Chronic Depression

S.H. was a forty-five-year-old married woman. She had occasionally attended seminars I taught in Los Angeles. After about five years of seeing me once or twice a year in workshops, she told me that she had decided to come to Hawaii to work with me privately.

I had noticed, over the years, that her body was flexible. She was able to do many postures without much difficulty. I remembered, however, that she was not strong and that her breath was shallow. S.H. complained that she lacked stamina and fatigued easily. She also told me that she often had difficulty sleeping and in concentrating.

As we began to work together, she told me that she had not been able to overcome a deep sense of hopelessness that had been plaguing her for many years. She also told me that she did not have much energy or motivation and had reached a point where she was basically doing nothing.

In the beginning, S.H. told me that she had a good relationship with her husband, who was quite successful in his career, and that they were free of financial worries. They had no children.

As we worked together a little longer however, S.H. told me that her husband was very taken by his work and that they hadn't spent "quality time" together for many years. She told me that they hadn't gone out just to have fun or taken a vacation together in a long time. She said that though he was a good provider, she felt emotionally abandoned.

S.H. told me she had few friends. She said that she had stopped seeing them because she felt guilty about her depressed state.

S.H. told me that she had no enthusiasm for cooking and that she and her husband had gotten into the habit of eating out. They both drank wine, and she expressed to me that perhaps she "drank a bit too much." She said she didn't eat breakfast and usually stayed in bed late into the morning. She said she didn't eat much during the day, except a couple of candy bars!

In my conversations with S.H., I learned that when she was a child, she had spent a lot of time in nature as a Girl Scout. She told me that she remembered that as a happy time. Coming to Hawaii had reminded her of those times, and she realized how much she missed being out in nature and in the company of good friends.

The strategy I developed for S.H. while she was is Hawaii included improved diet, increased physical activity, reconnecting to nature, and developing a personal practice.

We agreed that, at least for the month she was in Hawaii, she would get up early each morning, take a walk on the beach as the sun was coming up, and then do her practice before eating a healthy breakfast. I asked her to focus on the sunrise as she walked, and to keep that in her mind as she did her personal practice. I asked her to feel during her practice as if the sun was rising in her heart and a new day was dawning in her life. I also asked her to spend some time outside in the night looking at the stars before she went to bed and to visualize a happier future.

In addition, I asked her, at least while she was in Hawaii, to give up candy bars and wine. I encouraged her to contact the Sierra Club and go with the groups to hikes in the mountains. One day she came to see me full of excitement. She told me that some people she had met on a hike had invited her to go on a whale watching excursion. She told me that when a whale swam very near the boat she was on, she felt her heart open like she hadn't felt in years. The word she used was "exhilarating." She said that in that moment, she felt a happiness that she hadn't felt in a long time.

We developed the following practice during that month we worked together. My intention was to strengthen her body, deepen her breathing, improve her concentration, increase her energy, help her sleep, and stimulate her interest in life. The use of simple to progressively more complicated series (viṅyāsas) of linked movements were designed to increase her energy. The prāṇāyāma practice was designed to deepen her breath. And the meditation on the sunrise was designed to stimulate her interest in life.

I saw S.H. again the next time I went to Los Angeles, and she came to Hawaii with her husband the following year. She told me that the quality of her life had improved greatly since her last trip to Hawaii. She laughed and told me that she wasn't sure if it was the Yoga practice or the whale! She told me she was spending more time with her husband and was sleeping better. She also told me that she had been inspired by the flowers in Hawaii, and had started getting up early in the morning to go downtown to the flower markets to buy flowers for her new hobby, making flower arrangements. She told me that she has been making gifts of the arrangements to her friends, who love them. Then she thanked me for the "sunrise in the heart" meditation, which, she assured me, she uses every morning.

A Practice for Chronic Depression

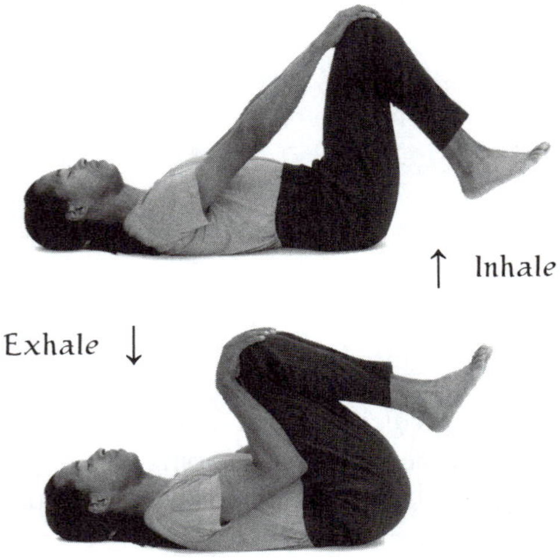

1.

Posture: Apānāsana.
Emphasis: To gently compress belly while stretching low back. To warm up body with gentle movements.
Technique: Lie on back with both knees bent toward chest and feet off floor. Place each hand on its respective knee.

On exhale: Pull thighs gently but progressively toward chest.

On inhale: Return to starting position.

Number: 12 times.
Details: *On exhale:* Pull gently with arms, keeping shoulders relaxed and on floor. Press low back down into floor and drop chin slightly toward throat.

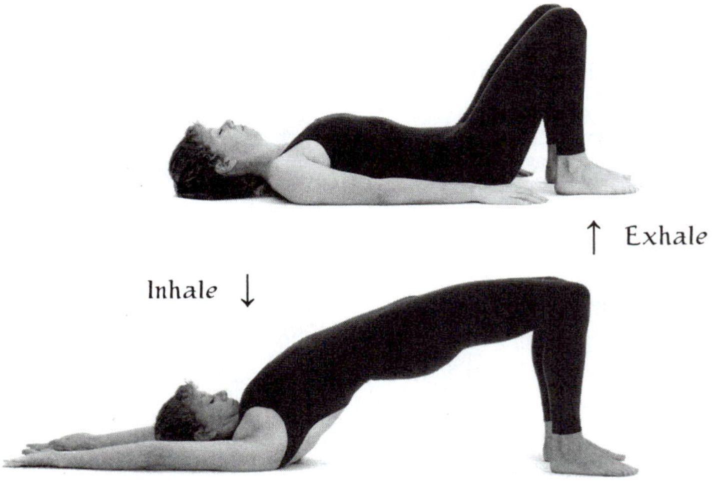

2.

Posture: Dvipāda Pīṭham.
Emphasis: To further warm up body by engaging thighs and buttocks.
Technique: Lie on back with arms down at sides, knees bent, and feet on floor, slightly apart and comfortably close to buttocks.

On inhale: Pressing down on feet and keeping chin down, raise pelvis until neck is gently flattened on floor, while raising arms overhead to floor behind.

On exhale: Return to starting position.

Number: 6 times.
Details: *On inhale:* Lift spine, vertebra by vertebra, from bottom up. *On exhale:* Unwind spine, coming down vertebra by vertebra.

3.

POSTURE: Ūrdhva Prasārita Pādāsana.
EMPHASIS: To extend spine and flatten it onto floor. To stretch legs. To progressively engage the larger muscles.
TECHNIQUE: Lie on back with arms down at sides, legs bent, and knees in toward chest.

On inhale: Raise arms upward all the way to floor behind head and legs upward toward ceiling.

Stay in stretch 2 full breaths.

On exhale: Return to starting position.

NUMBER: 4 times.
DETAILS: *On inhale:* Flex feet as legs are raised upward. Slightly bend knees, keeping angle between legs and torso less than ninety degrees. Push low back and sacrum downward. Bring chin down. While staying in position, *on exhale,* flex knees and elbows slightly; *on inhale,* extend arms and legs straighter.

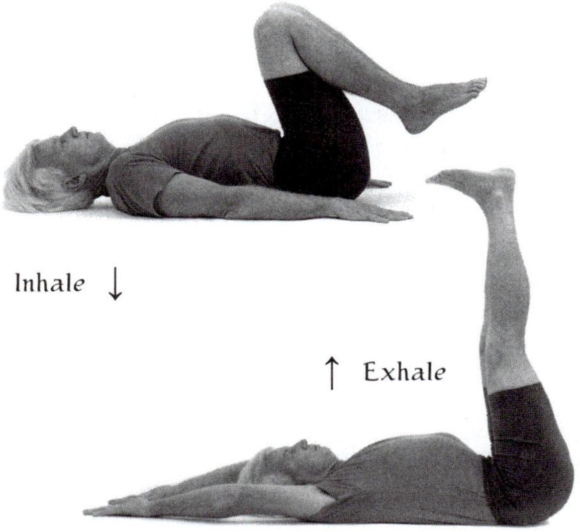
Inhale ↓
↑ Exhale

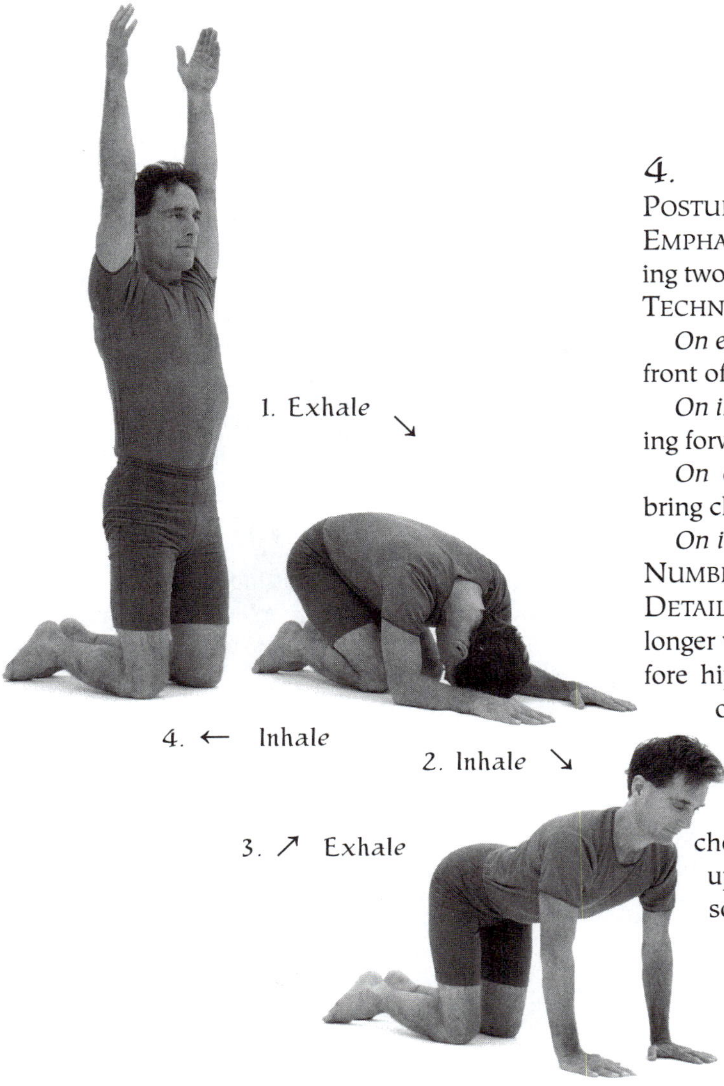
1. Exhale ↘
2. Inhale ↘
3. ↗ Exhale
4. ← Inhale

4.

POSTURE: Vajrāsana/Cakravākāsana Viṅyāsa.
EMPHASIS: To increase activity in body by combining two postures. To introduce lengthening of inhale.
TECHNIQUE: Stand on knees with arms over head.

On exhale: Bend forward, bringing arms to floor in front of you.

On inhale: Lift chest up and away from belly, coming forward onto hands.

On exhale: Tighten belly, round low back, and bring chest toward thighs.

On inhale: Return to starting position.

NUMBER: 8 times.
DETAILS: *On inhale:* Make inhalation progressively longer with each repetition. Bring chest to thighs before hips to heels. Avoid pulling spine with head, overarching neck. Lead with chest, keeping chin slightly down. Avoid overarching low back; rather, feel stretching in belly. *On exhale:* Round low back without collapsing chest over belly. Avoid increasing curvature of upper back. Let chest lower toward thighs sooner than hips toward heels.

5.

POSTURE: Uttānāsana/Ardha Utkaṭāsana combination.
EMPHASIS: To activate big muscles of body, to stimulate cardiovascular and respiratory function.
TECHNIQUE: Stand with feet slightly apart, arms over head.

On exhale: Bend forward, bending knees slightly, bringing chest to thighs, and palms to sides of feet.

On inhale: Return to starting position.

On exhale: Bend forward, bending knees until thighs are parallel to ground, hips are at knee level, chest to thighs, and palms to sides of feet.

On inhale: Return to starting position.

NUMBER: 8 times.
DETAILS: *On exhale:* Make exhalation progressively longer with each repetition. Bend knees to facilitate stretching in low back. Push heels firmly, and reach arms forward. *On inhale:* Lift chest up and away from thighs, flattening upper back without exaggerating lumbar curve. Keep knees bent until last part of movement.

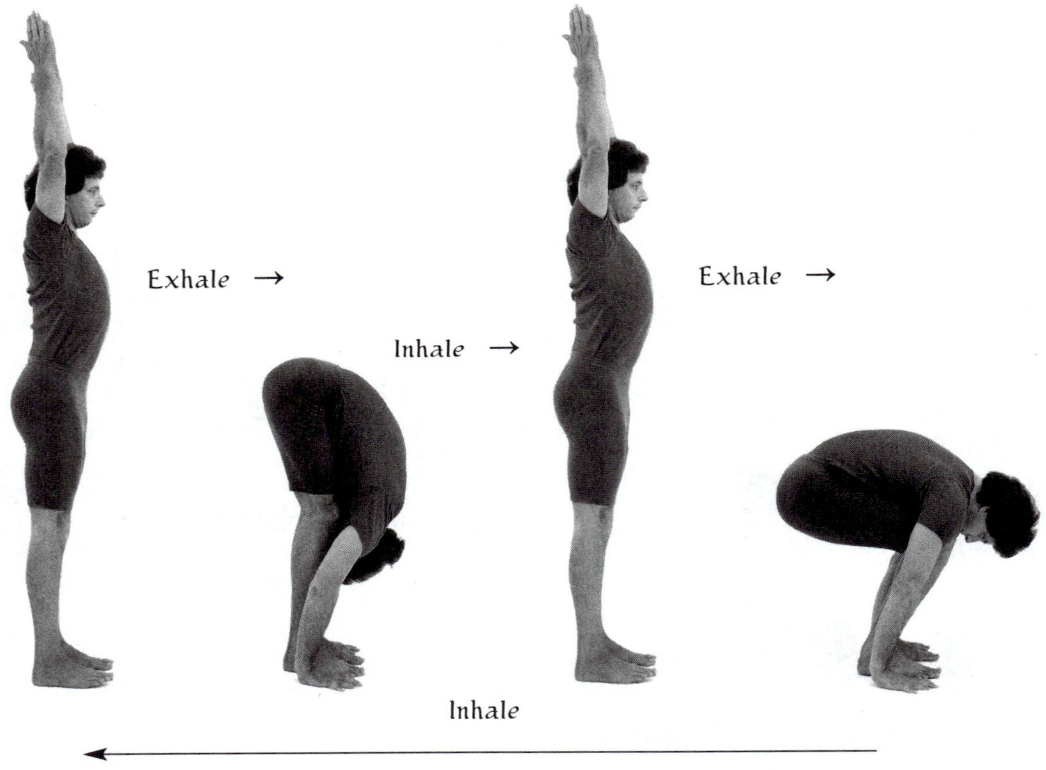

6.

POSTURE: Pārśvottaṇāsana/Vīrabhadrāsana combination.

EMPHASIS: To stretch and strengthen muscles of back and legs.

To expand chest and flatten upper back. To increase hold after inhalation.

To continue to stimulate cardiovascular and respiratory function.

TECHNIQUE: Stand with left foot forward, right foot turned slightly outward, feet as wide as hips, and arms over head.

On exhale: Bend forward, flexing left knee, bringing chest toward left thigh and bringing hands to either side of left foot.

On inhale: Lift torso two-thirds of the way up while bending left knee, arching back, and bringing arms out to sides and shoulders back.

After inhale: Hold breath 4 seconds.

On exhale: Remain in position.

On inhale: Raise arms straight up over head.

On exhale: Return to forward bend position.

On inhale: Return to starting position.

NUMBER: 4 times each side.

DETAILS: Stay stable on back heel and keep shoulders level throughout movement. Vīrabhadrāsana: *On inhale,* keep hands and elbows in line with shoulders. Feel opening of chest and flattening of upper back, not compression in low back. Keep head forward.

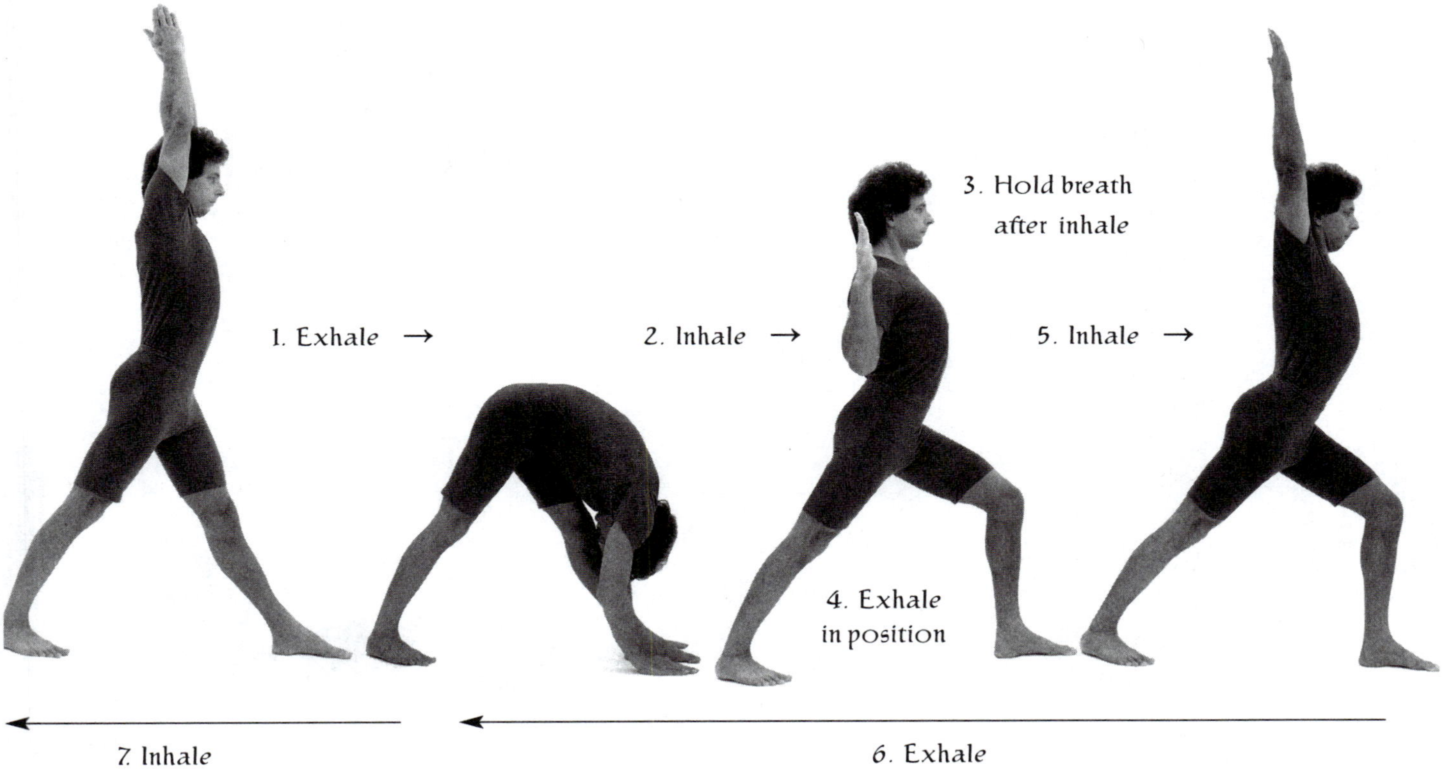

7.

Posture: Vajrāsana/Ūrdhva Mukha Śvānāsana combination.
Emphasis: To further energize system by engaging musculature of upper body, expanding chest, and stretching belly.
Technique: From a kneeling forward bend position, with hands on ground in front of body.

On inhale: Stretch body forward and arch back, keeping only hands and from knees to feet on floor.

Stay 1 breath.

On exhale: Return to starting position.

Number: 6 times.
Details: *On inhale:* Expand chest, stretch belly, and avoid compressing low back. *On exhale:* In arched position, push mid-thoracic forward. End in forward bend position.

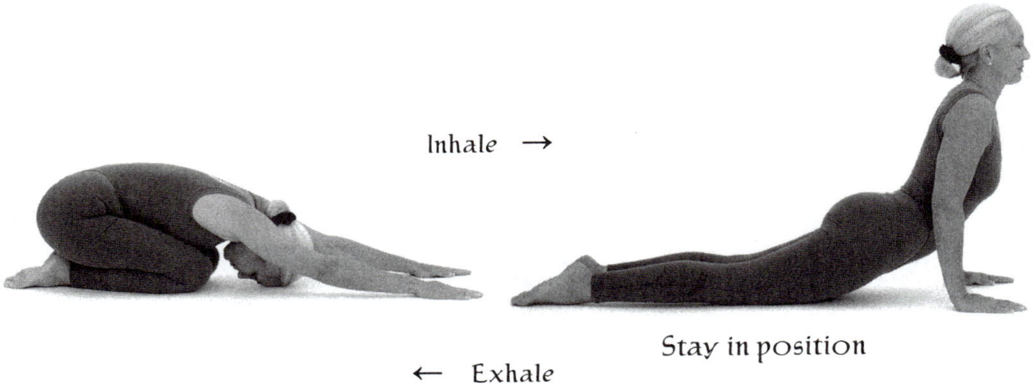

8.

Posture: Dvipāda Piṭham.
Emphasis: To relax upper back, shoulders, and neck.
Technique: Lie on back with arms down at sides, knees bent, and feet on floor, slightly apart and comfortably close to buttocks.

On inhale: Pressing down on feet and keeping chin down, raise pelvis until neck is gently flattened on floor, while raising arms overhead to floor behind.

On exhale: Return to starting position.

Number: 6 times.
Details: *On inhale:* Lift spine, vertebra by vertebra, from bottom up. *On exhale:* Unwind spine, coming down vertebra by vertebra.

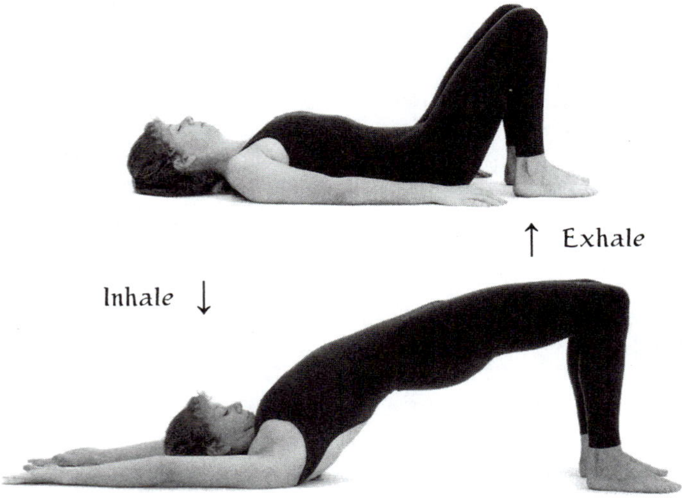

9.

POSTURE: Apānāsana.
EMPHASIS: To relax lower back.
TECHNIQUE: Lie on back with both knees bent toward chest and feet off floor. Place each hand on its respective knee.

On exhale: Pull thighs gently but progressively toward chest.

On inhale: Return to starting position.

NUMBER: 12 times.
DETAILS: *On exhale:* Pull gently with arms, keeping shoulders relaxed and on floor. Press low back down into floor and drop chin slightly toward throat.

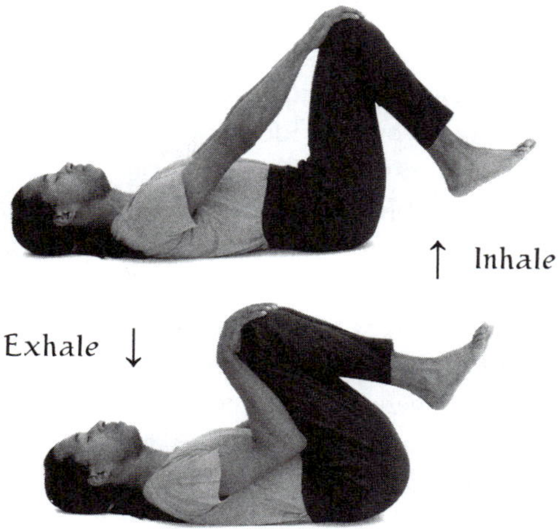

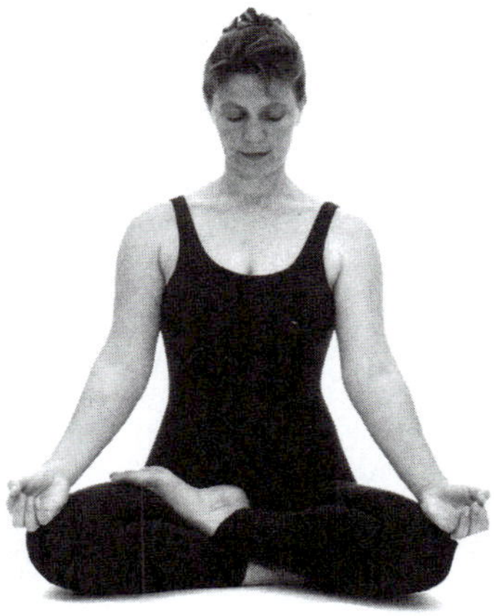

10.

POSTURE: Prāṇāyāma/Anuloma Krama, 2 stages.
EMPHASIS: To expand chest and deepen inhalation capacity. To increase energy and confidence.
TECHNIQUE:

Exhale deeply and fully.
Inhale 1/2 of breath in 4 to 5 seconds.
Pause 4 to 5 seconds.
Inhale remainder of breath in 4 to 5 seconds.
Pause 4 to 5 seconds.
Exhale slowly and fully.
Repeat.

NUMBER: 8 times.
DETAILS: *On inhale:* Expand chest from pit of throat to sternum. Then expand abdomen from solar plexus to pubic bone.

11.

POSTURE: Seated Rest.
EMPHASIS: To rest without lying down.
TECHNIQUE: Sit comfortably with eyes closed. With a relaxed mind, notice the sense of well-being stimulated by the practice.
DURATION: Approximately 5 minutes.

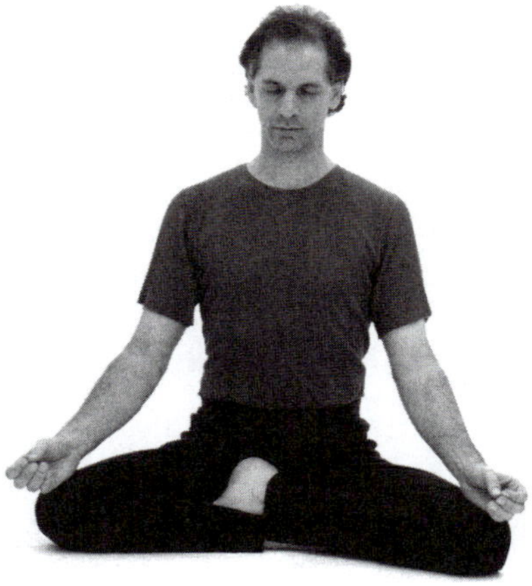

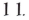

Beyond Therapy

In summary, the therapeutic methods of the Yoga tradition are based on the ideas of *viyoga* (removing something undesirable) and *saṃyoga* (linking to something desirable). From the point of view of emotions, viyoga refers to the reduction of rajasic states of agitation (e.g., emotional states categorized under the general headings of anger and anxiety) and tamasic states of dullness (e.g., emotional states categorized under the general heading of depression); and saṃyoga refers to the sustained effort to develop in ourselves the sattvic state of clarity and contentment. Yoga therapy is used to help people stabilize their emotional lives so they can begin to use Yoga as a process of spiritual transformation; and, for those with rather serious problems, it can function as a "life raft" in the process of getting out of troubled waters. But Yoga therapy is only a preparation for the true intention of Yoga, which is to function as a "launch pad" to new possibilities of personal evolution. While this book has focused on the developmental and therapeutic aspects of Yoga, our next book will focus on Yoga as a spiritual practice.

Pronunciation Guide

I. - (Hyphen) denotes a pause during recitation.

II. There are three accents (svaras) or levels of pitch that fall on the vowels. They are called:

1. Svarita	indicated by the absence of any markings. This is the prime or reference note.
2. Udātta	indicated by a vertical line over the syllable. This has a pitch that is above the reference note.
3. Anudātta	indicated by a horizontal underline. This has a pitch that is below the reference note.

III. Pronunciation guide for the transliteration

GUTTURAL (pronounced from throat)

vowels	a	as in but
	ā	as in father
plain	k	as in kin
	g	as in good
aspirate	kh	as in sinkhole
	gh	as in leghorn
	h	as in hand
nasal	ṅ	as in encore

PALATAL (pronounced from palate)

vowels	i	as in tin
	ī	as in teeth
plain	c	as in church
	j	as in judge
aspirate	ch	as in coachhorse
	jh	as in hedgehog
semi-vowel	y	as in you
sibilant	ś	as in sure

RETROFLEX (pronounced with tip of tongue curled up)

vowels	ṛ	as in sabre
	ṝ	as in chagrin
plain	ṭ	as in cart
	ḍ	as in ardent
aspirate	ṭh	as in carthorse
	ḍh	as in Fordham
nasal	ṇ	as in friend
semi-vowel	r	as in rib
sibilant	ṣ	as in hush

DENTAL (pronounced with tip of tongue against upper teeth)

vowels	ḷ	as in able
	ḹ	(is rare)
plain	t	as in theater
	d	as in they
aspirate	th	as in withheld
	dh	Buddha
nasal	n	as in boon
semi-vowel	l	as in lip
sibilant	s	as in sun

LABIAL (pronounced with lips)

vowel	u	as in bull
	ū	as in rule
plain	p	as in pat
	b	as in bee
aspirate	ph	as in uphill
	bh	as in abhor
nasal	m	as in man

GUTTURAL AND PALATAL

vowel	e	as in prey
	ai	as in aisle

GUTTURAL AND LABIAL

vowel	o	as in go
	au	as in cow

DENTAL AND LABIAL

semi-vowel	v	as in van

NASAL

ṁ or ṅ makes preceding vowel nasal

ASPIRATE

ḥ makes preceding vowel aspirate

Asana Index

Note: Page numbers in ***boldface*** refer to posture sequences.

Halāsana (hala = plough): *plough posture, 101*
Halāsana Parivṛtti (parivṛtti = with twist), *103*
Jānu Śirṣāsana (jānu = knee; śirṣa = head): *head to knee posture, 15, 18, 42, 75, 96, 174, 229, 251, 270, 293*
Jānu Śirṣāsana Parivṛtti (parivṛtti = with twist), *65, 82, 182*
Jaṭhara Parivṛtti (jaṭhara = abdomen; parivṛtti = twist): *abdominal twist, 15, 63, 69, 75, 80, 95, 154, 182, 195, 200, 206, 208, 209, 213, 242, 250, 256, 279, 284, 292*
Karṇapīḍāsana (karṇapīḍa = blocked ears): *blocked ears posture, 101*
Kaundinyāsana (Kaundinya = name of a Vedic sage)
Dvipāda Kaundinyāsana (dvipāda = two-footed), *118*
Ekapāda Kaundinyāsana (ekapāda = one-footed), *118*
Krauñcāsana (krauñca = heron): *heron posture, 27, 28, 36, 42*
Kukkuṭāsana (kukkuṭa = cock): *cock posture, 118*
Ūrdhva Kukkuṭāsana (ūrdhva = up, upward), *118*
Kūrmāsana (kūrma = turtle): *turtle posture, 36, 43,* ***45–48***
Lolāsana (lola = swing): *swing posture, 118*
Mahāmudrā (mahāmudrā = great seal): *great seal posture, 89,* ***93–97****, 229, 251, 270, 293*
Marīcyāsana (Marīci = name of a Vedic sage), *25, 42, 112, 155*
Marīcyāsana Parivṛtti (parivṛtti = with twist), *65*
Matsyāsana (matsya = fish): *fish posture, 54, 263*
Matsyendrāsana (Matsyendra = name of a yogi)
Ardha Matsyendrāsana (ardha = half), *25, 65, 113, 223, 243, 270*
Pūrṇa Matsyendrāsana (purna = full), *65*
Mayūrāsana (mayūra = peacock): *peacock posture*
Uttāna Mayūrāsana (uttāna = upright, stretched out), *102*
Ekapāda Uttāna Mayūrāsana (ekapāda = one-footed)
Prasārita Pāda Uttāna Mayurāsana (prasārita = spread; pāda = foot), *102*
Naṭarājāsana (Naṭarāja = name of a god), *117*
Nāvāsana (nāva = boat): *boat posture, 44, 314–15*
Nyāsa, *285*
Pādahastāsana (pādahasta = feet & hands): *hands to feet posture, 41*
Pādāṅguṣṭhāsana (pādāṅguṣṭha = big toe): *hold toe posture, 41*
Supta Pādāṅguṣṭhāsana (supta = supine), *59, 88, 94, 194*
Supta Eka Pādāṅguṣṭhāsana (ekapāda = one-footed), *174*
Supta Pārśva Pādāṅguṣṭhāsana (pārśva = side), *76, 194*
Supta Prasārita Pādāṅguṣṭhāsana (prasārita = spread), *47, 88, 89, 194, 292*
Ubhaya Pādāṅguṣṭhāsana (ubhaya = two), *41*
Utthita Eka Pādāṅguṣṭhāsana (utthita = standing; ekapāda = one-footed), *116*
Utthita Pārśva Pādāṅguṣṭhāsana (utthita = standing; pārśva = side), *116*
Pādāsana
Uttana Pādāsana (uttāna = upright, stretched out; pāda = foot), *54, 55*
Ūrdhva Prasārita Pādāsana (ūrdhva = up, upward; prasārita = spread), *22, 70, 81, 88, 112, 166, 181, 213, 229, 242, 250, 263, 269, 279, 319*
Padmāsana (padma = lotus): *lotus posture, 14, 90*
Parighāsana (parigha = door bar): *door bar posture, 72, 74,* ***78–84***
Pārśvakoṇāsana Parivṛtti (pārśva = side; koṇa = angle; parivṛtti = with twist): *side angle twisting posture, 63*
Utthita Pārśva Koṇāsana (utthita = standing): *standing side angle posture, 74*
Pārśvottānāsana (pārśva = side; uttāna = upright, stretched out): *side stretch posture, 15, 18, 23, 25, 42, 321*
Ardha Pārśvottānāsana (ardha = half), *42, 78, 93, 121*
Paryaṅkāsana (paryaṅka = bed): *bed posture, 55*
Paścimatānāsana (paścimatāna = stretching the west—back), *13, 17, 23, 25, 29, 41, 47, 60, 71, 81, 113, 167, 183, 214, 223, 243, 251, 263, 280, 314–315*
Ardha Baddha Padma Paścimatānāsana (ardha = half; baddha = bound; padma = lotus), *42*
Ardha Baddha Padma Paścimatānāsana Parivṛtti (parivṛtti = with twist), *65*
Ardha Padma Paścimatānāsana (ardha = half; padma = lotus), *42*
Paścimatānāsana Parivṛtti (parivṛtti = with twist), *75*
Tiryaṅgmukha Ekapāda Paścimatānāsana (tiryaṅgmukha = facing behind; ekapāda = one-foot), *42, 75*
Ūrdhva Mukha Paścimatānāsana (Ūrdhva = up, upward; mukha = face), *101*
Utthita Pāda Paścimatānāsana (utthita = standing; pada = foot), *117*
Piñchamayūrāsana (piñcha = feather; mayūra = peacock): *peacock feather posture, 119*
Pūrvatānāsana (pūrvatāna = stretching the east—front), *54*
Rājakapotāsana (rāja = king; kapota = pigeon): *pigeon-king posture, 52*
Ekapāda Rājakapotāsana (ekapada = one-footed), *53, 69*
Śalabhāsana (śalabha = locust): *locust posture, 25, 52, 189, 193*
Ardha Śalabhāsana (ardha = half), *52, 57, 94, 111, 120, 153, 173, 181, 199, 241, 249, 278*
Samasthiti (sama = equal; sthiti = stable): *equal stability posture, 82*

Sarvāṅgāsana (sarvāṅga = all parts), commonly: *shoulder stand, 98, 99, 100, 102, 103, 104, 105, 110–11, 180, 241, 262, 268, 278*
Ekapāda Sarvāṅgāsana (ekapāda = one-footed), *100, 110–11, 180*
Ekapāda Sarvāṅgāsana Parivṛtti (parivṛtti = with twist), *103*
Niralāmba Sarvāṅgāsana (niralāmba = without support), *105*
Sarvāṅgāsana Parivṛtti (parivṛtti = with twist), *103*
Pārśva Pāda Sarvāṅgāsana (pārśva pāda = foot to side), *104*
Śavāsana (śava = corpse): *corpse posture, 48, 60, 71, 84, 87, 97, 125, 155, 157, 158, 167, 175, 183, 190, 196, 201, 215, 224, 230, 237, 244, 252, 264, 271, 280, 295, 298, 315*
Setu Bhandāsana (setubandha = arch, bridge): *bridge posture, 54*
Siddhāsana (siddha = accomplishment), *14, 85, 90*
Śīrṣāsana (śīrṣa = head): *headstand, 98, 100, 102, 104, 105, 110, 113, 277, 291*
Ekapāda Śīrṣāsana (ekapāda = one-footed)
Niralāmba Śīrṣāsana (niralāmba = without support), *105*
Śīrṣāsana Parivṛtti (parivṛtti = with twist), *102*
Sukhāsana (sukha = at ease): *easy (seated) posture, 14, 90*
Supta Koṇāsana (supta = supine; koṇa = angle): *supine angle posture, 100*
Śvānāsana
Adho Mukha Śvānāsana (adhomukha = face down; śvāna = dog): *downward dog posture, 22, 52, 58, 88, 89, 91, 92, 93, 267*
Ūrdhva Mukha Śvānāsana (ūrdhvamukha = face up; śvāna = dog: *upward dog posture, 22, 58, 313, 322*
Svastikāsana (svastika = auspicious): *auspicious posture, 90*
Tāḍākamudrā (appearance of a tank), *87*
Taḍāsana (tāda = straight tree): *straight tree posture, 87, 115, 282*
Trikoṇāsana (trikoṇa = triangle): *triangle posture*
Parivṛtti Trikoṇāsana (parivṛtti = with twist): *twisting triangle posture, 14, 46, 63, 68, 108, 123, 152, 212, 266–67*
Utthita Trikoṇāsana (utthita = standing): *standing triangle posture, 16, 17, 74, 79, 179, 222, 248, 276, 290*
Upaviṣṭha Koṇāsana (upaviṣṭha = to sit): *seated triangle posture, 18, 20, 43, 75, 196*
Ūrdhva Koṇāsana (ūrdhva = up, upward): *upward triangle posture, 104*
Ūrdhva Koṇāsana Parivṛtti (parivṛtti = with twist), *103*
Uṣṭrāsana (uṣṭra = camel): *camel posture, 54, 55*
Ekapāda Uṣṭrāsana (ekapāda = one-footed), *17, 19, 53, 57, 192*
Utkaṭāsana (utkaṭa = squat): *squat posture, 43, 284*
Ardha Utkaṭāsana (ardha = half), *43, 228, 275, 320*
Ekapāda Utkaṭāsana (ekapāda = one-footed)
Uttānāsana (uttāna = upright, stretched out): *upright stretch posture, 17, 21, 24, 25, 41, 45, 67, 122, 151, 211, 221, 235, 266, 275, 289, 312, 319*
Ardha Baddha Padma Uttānāsana (ardha = half; baddha = bound; padma = lotus), *117*
Ardha Padma Uttānāsana (ardha = half; padma = lotus), *117*
Ardha Uttānāsana (ardha = half), *16, 19, 41, 108, 261*
Ekapāda Uttānāsana (ekapāda = one-footed), *116, 117*
Prasārita Pādottānāsana (prasārita = spread; pāda = foot), *43, 290*
Tiryaṅgmukha Ekapāda Uttānāsana (tiryaṅgmukha = facing behind; ekapāda = one-foot), *116*
Vajrāsana (vajra = diamond, kneel, spine): *kneeling posture, 16, 22, 25, 43, 45, 56, 58, 78, 80, 84, 90, 120, 123, 151, 153, 157, 163, 171, 177, 208, 211, 221, 227, 240, 247, 261, 276, 311, 313, 319, 322*
Vasiṣṭhāsana (Vasiṣṭha = name of a Vedic sage), *75*
Ekapāda Vaśiṣṭhāsana (ekapāda = one-footed), *77*
Vimanāsana (vimana = chariot of the gods): *airplane posture, 18, 52, 189, 193*
Viparīta Daṇḍāsana (viparīta = inversion; daṇḍa = stick): *inverted stick posture, 101*
Ekapāda Viparīta Daṇḍāsana (ekapāda = one-footed), *101*
Prasārita Pāda Viparīta Daṇḍāsana (prasārita = spread; pāda = foot), *101*
Viparīta Karaṇī: *doing inversion, 99*
Dvipāda Viparīta Karaṇī (dvipada = two-footed), *100*
Dvipāda Viparīta Karaṇī Parivṛtti (parivṛtti = with twist), *102*
Ekapāda Viparīta Karaṇī (ekapāda = one-footed), *100*, ***108–13***
Ekapāda Viparīta Karaṇī Parivṛtti (parivṛtti = with twist), *102*
Pārśva Pāda Viparīta Karaṇī (pārśva = side; pāda = foot)
Viparīta Koṇāsana (viparīta = inversion; koṇa = angle): *inverted angle posture, 110*
Viparīta Koṇāsana Parivṛtti (parivṛtti = with twist), *102*
Vīrabhadrāsana (vīrabhadra = a hero): *warrior posture, 13, 23, 53, 56, 117,* ***120–25****, 164, 227, 240, 254, 283, 312, 321*
Vīrāsana (vīra = vitality): *vitality posture, 90*
Vṛkṣāsana (vṛska = tree): *tree posture, 119*
Vṛścikāsana (vṛścika = scorpion): *scorpion posture, 119*

Index

Note: Page numbers in ***boldface*** *refer to posture sequences.*

practice sequence for, **93–97**
primary and secondary intentions in, 85–86
release valves for, 91
risks of, 92
technique, 86
types of postures, 87–90

faith, 131
femurs (thighbones), 138, 185
fibroelastic cartilage, 137
fibromyalgia, 246
fibrosis, 143
fight-or-flight response, 205, 258, 273, 304
flexion, 142
form-function problem, 5, 12
forward bends, 33, 35–48
exhalation and, 168
inversion variations, 100
langhana effect of, 131
leg balances with, 116–17
lumbar-pelvic rhythm in, 36–37, 44
positions for, 40
practice sequence of, **45–48**
primary and secondary intentions in, 35–36
release valves for, 36, 38, 39, 44
risks of, 44
technique, 36–40
types of, 41–44
fuel, and energy, 140–41

genitals, 286
glucose, 258
glycosis, 140
gonads, 257, 258, 286–87
growth hormone, 257
gunas, 308

happiness, 308
Hatha Yoga, 3
hay fever, 246
head, mobility of, 143
headaches, 274
headstands, 34, 98–113
contraindications to, 107
langhana effect of, 131
risks of, 106–7
see also inversions
healing, foundation for, 132
healing insights, 305–6
health problems, causes of, 131, 245, 304–5
heart, 139, 231–44, 257
heart disease, 232–33
heart rate, 232, 273, 306
heat *(agni)*, 131
hernias, 142
hipbones (coxa), 137–38
hippocampus, 303
hips, 184–86
case study, 191
practice sequence for, **192–96**
holding vs. repetition, 5–6, 22
homeostasis, 257
hormones, 257–58, 304
humerus, 137
humming, 24, 131

hyperactivity:
case study, 274
practice sequence for, **275–80**
hyperextension, 142
hypertension, 233–37
case study, 233–34
practice sequence for, **234–37**
hypotension, 238–44
case study, 238
practice sequence for, **239–44**
hypothalamus, 303, 304

IgA (immunoglobulin A), 308
iliopsoas, 168
ilium, 137–38
immortality *(kaya kalpa)*, 130
immune system:
case study, 246–47
and endocrine system, 258
practice sequence for, **247–52**
immunity, 217, 245–46, 308
immunodeficiency, 246, 252–56, 281
case study, 253
practice sequence for, **254–56**
immunoglobulin A (IgA), 308
index of postures, 325–27
indigestion, 204
ingestion, 203
inhalation, 8–10, 160
brahmaṇa effect of, 131, 225
case study, 226
practice sequence for, **226–30**
in *prāṇāyāma*, 306
progression of, 10, 12
variations of, 10
insomnia, 274
intention, in *āsana* sequences, 32
intestines, 205, 210
inversion, 98–113, 142
contraindications to, 107
practice sequence of, **108–13**
primary and secondary intentions in, 98
release valves, 106
risks of, 106–7
techniques, 98–99
types of postures, 98–105
ischium, 137–38
isometric muscle work, 140

jaw, tension in, 143
jet lag, 257
joints, 135–36
knees, 138, 184–86
leverage and, 161
problems with, 186, 273
range of motion in, 135–36
weight-bearing, 186

kama, 305
kaya kalpa, science of immortality, 130
kidneys, 257, 286
kneecaps, 138
kneeling postures, 34
knees, 138, 184–86
case study, 197
practice sequence for, **197–201**
krama breathing, 24, 210
Krishnamacharya, 133, 305

krodha, 305
kyphosis, 138–39, 159
case study, 163
practice sequence for, **163–67**

lactation, 257
lactic acid, buildup of, 140–41, 309
langhana (purification), 130, 131, 206
allergies and, 246
depression and, 316
meditation and, 306
lateral bends, 33, 72–84
practice sequence of, **78–84**
primary and secondary intentions in, 72
release valves, 73, 77
risks of, 77
technique, 73
types of, 74–76
learning, conditioned, 273
leg balances, 115–17, 119
legs, 184
leg variations, 17–19
lengthening the core: extension, 85–97
ligaments, 135, 136, 137, 138
limbic brain, 303–4, 306
limbic system, 303, 306
lipids, 138
liver, 257
lobha, 305
lordosis, 138–39, 159–60, 168
lower back, 168–75
case study, 170
pain in, 37, 159, 184
practice sequence for, **170–75**
lumbar-pelvic rhythm, 36–37, 44
lumbar spine, 137, 138, 159, 168, 184
lumbar-thoraco rhythm, 49, 51
lungs, 216–17
lymphatic system, 245–56
autoimmune conditions of, 246-47; practice sequence for, **247–52**
and cardiovascular system, 231
function of, 245–46
and immunodeficiency diseases, 252, 253; practice sequence for, **254–56**
lymph nodes, lymph glands, 245
lymphocytes, 245, 258

mada, 305
mama, 305
mano maya (mental faculties), 130
matsarya, 305
mayas, 130
medicine *(auṣadhi)*, 130
meditation:
brahmaṇa effect of, 131
and hypertension, 233
langhana effect of, 131, 306
preparation for, 26
melatonin, 257
membranes, 135, 136
meniscus, 138
menopause, 287
menstrual cycle, 287
mental illnesses, 307
metabolic processes, 130, 140
metabolic rate, 258, 306
mind, states of, 302

Contact and Product Order Information

For more information on Gary Kraftsow's Viniyoga Teacher and Therapist Training Programs, as well as retreats, workshops, and educational products, please contact:

Gary Kraftsow
American Viniyoga Institute
P.O. Box 88
Makawao, HI 96768
tel: 808-572-1414
e-mail: info@viniyoga.com
website: www.viniyoga.com

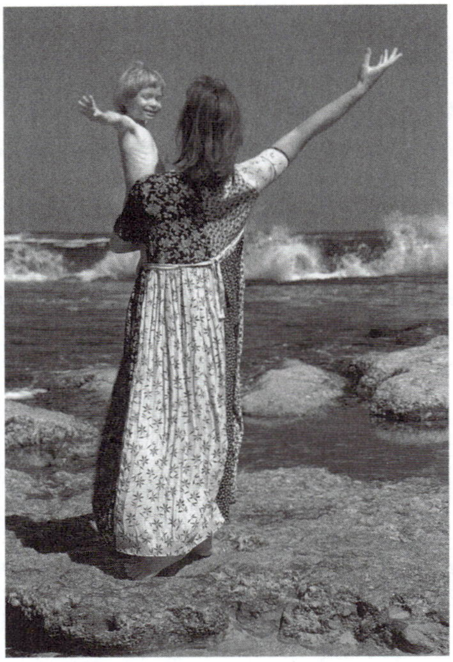

Other Viniyoga training centers:

Antaranga Yoga
Sante Fe, NM
Sonia Nelson
tel: 505-992-0950

The Pierce Yoga Program
Atlanta, GA
Margaret and Martin Pierce
tel: 404-875-7110